CW00690584

1,000,000 Books
are available to read at

Forgotten Books

www.ForgottenBooks.com

Read online
Download PDF
Purchase in print

ISBN 978-1-330-30307-8
PIBN 10019860

This book is a reproduction of an important historical work. Forgotten Books uses state-of-the-art technology to digitally reconstruct the work, preserving the original format whilst repairing imperfections present in the aged copy. In rare cases, an imperfection in the original, such as a blemish or missing page, may be replicated in our edition. We do, however, repair the vast majority of imperfections successfully; any imperfections that remain are intentionally left to preserve the state of such historical works.

Forgotten Books is a registered trademark of FB &c Ltd.
Copyright © 2018 FB &c Ltd.
FB &c Ltd, Dalton House, 60 Windsor Avenue, London, SW19 2RR.
Company number 08720141. Registered in England and Wales.

For support please visit www.forgottenbooks.com

1 MONTH OF
FREE
READING

at

www.ForgottenBooks.com

By purchasing this book you are eligible for one month membership to ForgottenBooks.com, giving you unlimited access to our entire collection of over 1,000,000 titles via our web site and mobile apps.

To claim your free month visit:

www.forgottenbooks.com/free19860

* Offer is valid for 45 days from date of purchase. Terms and conditions apply.

English
Français
Deutsche
Italiano
Español
Português

www.forgottenbooks.com

Mythology Photography **Fiction** Fishing Christianity **Art** Cooking Essays Buddhism Freemasonry Medicine **Biology** Music **Ancient Egypt** Evolution Carpentry Physics Dance Geology **Mathematics** Fitness Shakespeare **Folklore** Yoga Marketing **Confidence** Immortality Biographies Poetry **Psychology** Witchcraft Electronics Chemistry History **Law** Accounting **Philosophy** Anthropology Alchemy Drama Quantum Mechanics Atheism Sexual Health **Ancient History** **Entrepreneurship** Languages Sport Paleontology Needlework Islam **Metaphysics** Investment Archaeology Parenting Statistics Criminology **Motivational**

CANADA

MEDICAL & SURGICAL

JOURNAL.

A Monthly Record of

MEDICAL AND SURGICAL SCIENCE.

EDITED BY

GEORGE ROSS, A.M., M.D.,

Professor of Clinical Medicine, McGill University; Physician to Montreal General Hospital.

AND

W. A. MOLSON, M.D., M.R.C.S., Eng.,

L. M. King's & Queen's College of Physicians, Ireland; Physician to Montreal General Hospital.

VOL. X.

Montreal:

PRINTED & PUBLISHED BY THE GAZETTE PRINTING COMPANY.

1882.

INDEX TO VOL. X.

184872

LIST OF CONTRIBUTORS TO VOL. X.

BAYARD, W., M.D., EDIN.
BELL, JAMES, M.D.
BULLER, F., M.D., M.R.C.S., ENG.
BROWNE, A. A., M.D.
BURLAND, W. H., M.D.
CHIPMAN, C. J. H., M.D.
COLEMAN, F., M.D.
DORLAND, JAMES, M.D.
DUNCAN, W. T., M.D.
FELTON, L. E., M.D.
FENWICK, G. E., M.D.
GARDNER, WM., M.D.
GRAY, HENRY R.
GUERIN, J. J., M.D.
HENDERSON, A., M.D.
HILL, HAMNETT, M.R.C.S., ENG.
HOWARD, R. P., M.D., L.R.C.P., LONDON.
MACCALLUM, D. C., M.D., M.R.C.S., ENG.
MACDONNELL, R, L., M.D., M.R.C.S., ENG.
MAJOR, G. W., M.D.
MCDONALD, J. A., M.D.
MCDONALD, J. M., M.D.
MILLS, T. W., M.D., L.R.C.P., LONDON.
MOLSON, W. A., M.D., M.R.C.S., ENG.
OAKLEY, W. D., M.D.
O'CALLAGHAN, T. A., A.M., M.D.
OSLER, WM., M.D., M.R.C.P., LONDON.
POWELL, R. W., M.D.
REDDY, JOHN, M.D., L.R.C.P.I.
REED, T. D., M.D.
RODDICK, T. G., M.D.
ROSS, GEORGE, A.M., M.D.
SHIRRIFF, F. E., M.D.
SHEPHERD, F. J., M.D., M.R.C.S., ENG.
STEWART, JAMES, M.D.
VINEBERG, H. N., M.D.

CANADA

ICAL & SURGICAL JOURNAL

AUGUST, 1881.

Original Communications.

CT OF A CLINICAL LECTURE BY DR. WIL-N FOX, OF UNIVERSITY COLLEGE HOSPITAL, JUNE 30, 1881.

BY T. W. MILLS, M.A., M.D., L.R.C.P., ENG.

has been long known for his, in some respects, un-ical lectures—which, by the way, are not quite clinical commonly understood,—for this illustrious teacher nfine himself to the points of the case before him, but s it a text for an exhaustive discussion of some sub-icine. The man who follows these lecture for months m told, over the greater part of the entire field of lis lectures, in fact, are rather a combination of what erm didactic lectures, with the clinical lecture as nown to us. I confess I like the combination, and d myself quite see how merely teaching the observ-tom and the attempt at a diagnosis was precisely losophical or useful way to advance students in the f scientific medicine; and that the more so, as no core of cases, it may be, convey an adequate idea e in its various phases to the student's mind, or, in enable him to form that *ideal* for each disease which t of test, measure or standard for comparison; for, ill, *men see commonly only as much as their ideals look for* in any one of Nature's realms. I raise this utset as a centre of suggestion for those who feel interested in education, medical or otherwise. But to return to Dr. Fox.

At the hour of 2 P.M., a tall, rather slightly made man, with a quick, elastic step—though his grey hairs showed that the period of youth and middle age had been passed—stepped from a hansom and proceeded at once to Ward No. 3 of University College Hospital, followed by a small, but most attentive and intelligent-looking band of students, and casting first a glance at the patients, and then taking a keen, observing survey of his class with his large grey eyes, proceeded with a discussion of the case, or, as I should, perhaps, rather say, of the subject—*Phthisis*. The doctor had already discussed some aspects of the subject in one or two previous lectures. The patient was a girl of scrofulous aspect, of about 13 or 15 years of age. The doctor, exposing her neck, pointed to some deep, puckered scars, and then, with only the interruption of two or three brief examinations of the chest (a thorough examination having been made on previous occasions), proceeded to discuss the case in some such fashion as I shall now most imperfectly imitate :—

"These, gentlemen, are the indications of what were and are called 'scrofulous glands.' There has been a great deal of discussion as to the real nature of the changes in the glands so affected ; but at present the changes are generally considered to be of a tuberculous character. In this young girl's lung there is a large cavity ; if you listen behind, or, better still, low in front, on the right side, you will hear large moist sounds and what is commonly called cavernous breathing. In this case it is rather more like large tubular breathing. This is not a case of tuberculous phthisis—that is to say, not primarily so ; there may now be, or may be at a later period, tubercles scattered through the lung ; but the character of the onset, the diathesis of the patient, the extent of the disease, and the immunity of the other lung, all point to 'pneumonic phthisis' as the form of disease here present. Now let us consider the sputa ; it was abundant, purulent, and very fetid. This points either to gangrene, bronchial dilatation, septic processes due to germs, or to a very strong preponderance of the destructive over the formative changes in the body. To the latter we must, in this case, largely attribute the fetor. You observe, too, that this patient has had a strong tendency to sweating, which also points to the same destructive changes I have referred to. The *temperature* in this case is most instructive, and is of the utmost importance in the diagnosis. You will observe from this chart (a large and very fine one it was) that for weeks there has been constant pyrexia—the temperature really may be said never to have been 100°, and generally it has been above that. It shows, it is true, considerable oscillation, but still, be it marked, there is *constant fever*. This indicates that the disease is pursuing an acute course, there is rapid disintegration of tissue, there are constantly preponderating disintegrating changes. Note, also, the delicate aspect of this patient—the thin skin, the light, fine hair, &c. But you who have been following the case will admit there has been very considerable improvement; and this brings me to the very important matter of the *treatment* of this class of cases. The sputa now are no longer fetid. What have we done? We have used inhalations of a disinfecting material (one of the oils) in this, the best thing I know of for the purpose—'Wordsworth's washable respirator,' which, as it can be so easily washed, can be itself kept perfectly clean. But there are other modes of disinfecting the sputa in the air passages. One is to have an atmosphere more or less saturated with carbolic acid; another, to allow iodine to evaporate in the patient's room. But it will not do to check expectoration—such a result would be disastrous, as increasing the very condition we wish to obviate. The next point to be attained is to lessen perspiration, or, rather, to meet the condition which gives rise to it. In getting rid of the fetor of the sputa, we have contributed to this in part already; but as sweating arises when the arteries are dilated, the tension diminished, and, therefore, occurs during sleep, it is obvious we should look for remedies that tend to counteract this. To this class belong belladonna, picrotoxin, &c. Oxide of zinc does good in a large number of cases, though I cannot explain its action. But one of the best remedies is to give the patient alcohol at *the critical time*. If such patients would wake up in the small hours of the night and take a dose of alcohol, they would be saved much discomfort. But here, again, one is met by a theoretical difficulty, for alcohol is considered a dilator of vessels. But in the treatment of cases like this before us, there is nothing so important as to diminish pyrexia; so long as this continues, the patient's course will be retrogressive. In the first place, *absolute rest* in bed must be strictly enforced; the utmost possible tranquillity of mind and body must be enjoined; *all movement*, so far as possible, must be forbidden. This having been done, we are led to ask, What can be accomplished by medicine? And in this matter, gentlemen, we must simply confess our failure and our ignorance. One remedy after another has been vaunted; I have tried them all, and I must say there is no remedy or medicine that will permanently reduce the pyrexia. You may give a large dose of quinine to-day, and find the temperature down to-morrow; but you can never be certain that it will not rise again, you can never know *when* it may rise, and all the while your patient is in other respects subjected, it may be, to much discomfort in consequence of our futile medication; and the same applies to the other so-called antipyretics. You may do something by dieting. Give light, easily digested material. If the pulse is rapid, you may give aconite, or, perhaps better, digitalis, which also, in a certain proportion of cases, diminishes the sweating. The so-called Niemeyer's pill (which dated long antecedent to Niemeyer however) is a very valuable remedy, by the joint action of its ingredients. But among our most useful remedies to lower temperature, induce tranquillity, and prevent tissue waste, &c., is opium: not in doses to induce sleep at night—this is a wretched practice—but in *small* doses. When opium checks expectoration unduly or causes sweating, it, of course, must not be given. But, gentlemen, when you commence to give opium in cases of this kind, as it may be necessary to continue it for some time, you incur a grave responsibility. Remember, you may forge for your patient a most galling chain; for there is no habit that men even of the strongest wills find it so hard to conquer as the habitual use of opium. Take care that you always be sure that at any stage your patient can *leave it off*. But in cases of phthisis, there is another remedy you will find mentioned in your pharmacopœias, viz., Vinum—wine. It is as much a medicine as opium or quinine. Much that I have said of opium, however, applies to it. It is true we sell opium to the natives of the East, by which traffic we rendered it necessary that laws should be enacted to limit its use to prevent the actual extermination of the inhabitants of some of those countries; we sell this "to the great glory of the British nation." But it is to no such abuse of a valuable drug I am now referring, but of alcohol. The distinguished Dr. Flint of America has abundantly shown the great value of alcohol in certain cases in phthisis. Now it is in just such cases as this it is useful. But be careful, as of opium, that your patient can leave it off at any time, and always prescribe alcohol in definite doses. Do not allow it to be slopped about in tumblers, for people often then give it 'as if they loved you.'

"A great deal has been said of *climate*; but in such cases as this one is, you must not put much dependence upon it. It is possible that there may be isolated cases, in which, with even a temperature of 100°, it may be worth while allowing a patient who has plenty of money, and has set his mind upon a journey, to take it; but for patients with high temperatures, as a rule, any sort of move is extremely hazardous. It is better to risk the patient even in a climate such as ours, than to sanction any sort of journey with its excitements of body and mind. To talk to the poor of the advantages of climate is simply to be guilty of cruelty."

I do not know whether I have conveyed to the reader adequately Dr. Fox's meaning or not, but he seemed to lay the greatest stress on the value of absolute rest, opium and alcohol in the treatment of that sort of phthisis of which his case was an example. The entire lecture was most systematic, and so classical the language, that every word might have been reported *verbatim* with the best effect. His auditors were reverently attentive, and must have been deeply impressed by what is not too frequently found in medical lectures in any high degree—the *moral force* of the teacher. Students taught by such a man must go forth to this matter-of-fact world well equipped with the best of all safeguards against degeneracy—a *high ideal.* Such a lecturer must have a double gratification, having taught science well, and in having assisted his students to become men as well as doctors.

TWO CASES OF OPIUM POISONING.

By T. A. O'CALLACHAN, A.M., M.D., Worcester, Mass.

On June 2nd, 1881, I was summoned in haste to a man (J. B., æt. 35) who had, half-an-hour before I arrived, taken six drachms of laudanum. He had been drinking for several days, and in the depression that followed, had taken the poison with suicidal intentions. I found that the drug had already begun to act. He was growing quite stupid, his speech was hardly intelligible, pupils were greatly contracted, and with much difficulty he was kept awake. Mustard water had been given without effect. While waiting for a stomach pump, I administered free doses of sulphate of zinc, and soon had the satisfaction of seeing most of the opium vomited. On the arrival of the pump, I washed the stomach freely till the water returned clear and devoid of the opium smell. I then ordered Tincture of Belladonna in 30 minim doses hourly, gave strict injunctions that the patient should not be allowed to sleep, and left. At 11 p.m., three hours after, I again visited my patient, and found that all the symptoms, with the exception of sleepiness, had disappeared. The pupils were normal in size, and responded readily to light. The belladonna was continued at longer intervals, and the patient kept awake till about 4 o'clock the following morning. No results followed, except a feeling of weakness, which gradually disappeared.

On July 12th, a young lady, aged 18, "tired of life," took four drachms of laudanum. I saw her in about half an hour. She was so cool and unconcerned that I gave her statement little credit. I noticed that her pupils were contracted and enlarged alternately, that one cheek was much flushed, the other pale, and that peppermint, which she afterwards told me she had taken to destroy the taste of the laudanum, was the only odor to be detected on her breath. Seeing no immediate danger, I left an emetic—which was soon thrown away—and departed, with the understanding that I was to be immediately sent for if bad symptoms set in. That evening, just 10½ hours after the dose had been taken, I was hastily summoned, and found that my patient had greatly changed. She was perfectly conscious, but had lost control over her lower limbs, and was unable to stand. On attempting to rise, she was seized with dizziness and a strong desire to vomit. The eyes were surrounded with dark circles, and looked heavy and dull; the pupils were reduced to pin-holes; the pulse, 60, was strong, full and regular. Since taking the poison she had felt no inclination to sleep; on the contrary, she was very wakeful. She now begged piteously for aid, and was willing to do anything to save her life. I administered sulphate of zinc, which soon produced copious vomiting of a dark blue liquid, on which floated mucous-like curds. She swallowed and immediately rejected large draughts of water, thus cleansing the stomach as thoroughly as the pump would have done. When the vomiting had stopped, strong coffee was given her, but not retained. Tincture of Belladonna was prescribed, to be given every hour in 30 minim doses. The patient remained awake till 4 o'clock the following morning, after which she enjoyed several hours natural sleep. The following afternoon she visited my office, and appeared none the worse for her experience, but felt as if she had been sick for a long time. She is now entirely well, and not at all so anxious to leave the world.

TINCTURA FERRI PERCHLOR.

By T. D. REED, M.D., Prof. Mat. Med. Mont. Coll. Phar.

Notwithstanding the numerous preparations of iron which are from time to time being brought forward by the manufacturing chemists, the old tincture keeps its place, and is by many practitioners preferred to all other forms. The prescriber, however, generally feels constrained to combine it with glycerine, or something of the kind, to lessen its unpleasantness in the mouth.

There is a simple method of dealing with this tincture in prescription which is not, perhaps, as widely known as it deserves to be, and I therefore venture to bring the plan before the readers of the CANADA MEDICAL AND SURGICAL JOURNAL.

It is simply the addition of a little alkaline citrate. For every drachm of the tincture, add half a drachm of potas. citras. The result is a liquid of a beautiful green colour, quite free from the peculiar roughness of the iron. For a tablespoonful dose, containing 10 minims, the prescription can be written thus:

℞	Tinct. Ferri Mur., . .	ʒij
	Potas. Citrat., ...	ʒi
	Syrup Limonis, . . .	℥iss
	Aquæ ad	℥vi

This elegant combination ought to suit fastidious patients. If it should be found that "children cry for it," I would not be surprised. Another advantage of this mixture is, that astringent tinctures, as bark, gentian, &c., may be added, without decomposition.

By adopting the combination here described, the prescriber can have the advantage of, while being independent of, the fancy elixirs of iron which at the present time are being pressed on the attention of the profession by enterprising pharmacists.

Hospital Reports.

MEDICAL AND SURGICAL CASES OCCURRING IN THE PRACTICE OF THE MONTREAL GENERAL HOSPITAL.

MEDICAL CASE UNDER THE CARE OF DR. MOLSON.

Case of Obstruction of Rectum by a Cancerous mass—Perforation—Death from Peritonitis. (Reported by Dr. A. HENDERSON.)

S. D., æt. 45, a large, well-nourished man, third officer of S.S. B—. Good family history and of previous good health, with the exception of being subject to attacks of constipation during last three or four years. Has been a hard drinker; history of gonorrhœa, but no distinct history of syphilis. Admitted June 27th, 1881, with following history: Ten days previous to admission, was seized with dull, heavy pain in lower abdominal region, which has continued with more or less severity ever since.

Bowels in the meantime acted regularly up to two days before admission, but motions were never free, in spite of purgatives, which were freely given—castor oil and croton oil (the latter, in two or three drop doses, being given on two or three occasions) and large enemata, consisting of soap suds with olive oil. Two days before admission the stomach began to reject everything that was taken, and at times large amounts of bilious matter were thrown up.

On admission—Patient presented a perfectly healthy appearance, and not in any way cachectic. Temperature normal. Organs generally in an apparently healthy condition. Abdomen a little full. No evidence of abdominal tumour, with exception of slight dulness in region of ascending colon, with some resistance felt on deep palpation. Complains of pain in lower abdominal zone, but no special seat of tenderness can be made out. Appetite poor; tongue moist and furred; urine normal.

June 30*th*.—Castor oil and enemata of soap and water freely used; but without producing more than a slight evacuation of mucus, with a small amount of semi-solid fæcal matter; patient takes only a small quantity of beef-tea and milk, but vomits it shortly after, stomach not being able to retain anything longer than about an hour.

July 6*th*.—Constipated condition still remains unaltered, and vomiting continues; complains intensely of pain, which he locates chiefly in region of umbilicus; enemata of soap-suds, alternating with injections of 4 ozs. linseed oil and 1 oz. turpentine, are being made use of twice daily, and, internally, patient is taking pills containing aloes, nux vomica, and belladonna, but stomach is still irritable, and pills are seldom retained.

July 11*th*.—Patient became suddenly worse, symptoms of general peritonitis setting in during the afternoon, the inflammation spreading rapidly, terminating in death on the night of the 12th.

Autopsy twelve hours after death.—Abdomen excessively distended. Intestines, liver and general contents of abdomen covered with flaky lymph, and cemented together by recent adhesions. Vessels of omentum engorged; about a pint of turbid serum removed from dependent parts. Large intestine distended and coiled up in front of the other organs fully six inches in diameter throughout its whole length, as far as upper part of sigmoid flexure. The bowel was removed with difficulty owing to its extreme friability. On removing intestines, nothing special noted in small bowel, except containing a considerable amount of fæcal matter. The large intestine contained an enormous amount of semi-solid fæces, scybalous masses, milk-curds, and undigested fruits. Just above the brim of pelvis, on left side, and outside the psoas muscle, was a hard mass the size of an orange, bound down posteriorly by adhesions, and containing pus and fæcal matter in its cavity, which was about the size of a hen's egg. The mass was in the interior of the bowel, 8 or 10 inches from the anus, and occupying the whole circumference of the gut, 1½ to 2 inches across, and almost completely obliterating its lumen; moderately firm in consistence, nodular, and in many places ulcerated. Just above the margin of the mass was a small perforation in the bowel, opening posteriorly, through which some fæcal matter had escaped into the abdominal cavity. Other organs healthy.

UNIVERSITY LYING-IN HOSPITAL.

Case of Protracted Labour from Occlusion of the Os Uteri—Incision—Forceps. (Reported by Mr. DUNCAN.)

The patient, E— D—, 37 years of age, a strong, robust, and healthy-looking woman, was admitted into the University Lying-in Hospital on the 6th of April, 1881, expecting her labour about the 20th of the same month. The patient said she had always been exceedingly strong and healthy. She began to menstruate at eleven years of age, and was always regular both as to time and quantity, and never experienced any unusual feelings of pain either before or during the flow. She was married at the age of seventeen, and has always lived with her husband, but never became pregnant before the present time. After marriage the menses were regular and general health good. The menses last appeared on the 17th of July, 1880. After impregnation she suffered from irritation of the bladder, with difficult micturition. She was treated for this by local applications, and the symptoms gradually passed away. During her stay in the hospital she again had difficult and sometimes painful micturition, the urethra presenting a sacculated condition, rendering it exceedingly difficult to introduce a catheter. Patient had considerable morning vomiting, and during the latter months had uneasy feelings in the lower part of the abdomen, but previous to this never had inflammation of the cervix or any uterine disease whatever. On the 12th of April (six days after her admission to the hospital) she felt pains similar to those of labour, but on making a vaginal examination no dilatation of the os uteri could be felt, and on auscultating the abdomen no pulsation of the fætal heart could be heard. These pains were slight, continuing only a few hours, and after passing away the patient again felt quite well, and went about as usual until four o'clock on the morning of the 23rd, when she again felt labour pains, and on making an examination, at 7 A.M., what appearad to be a nearly fully dilated os uteri was felt very high up, with a bag of membranes protruding, and in the interval of a pain a hard substance could be felt, apparently the child's head. The pains continued all that day, with no progress in labour, and also all the following night, recurring every eight or ten minutes. It appeared at this time as if the os was fully dilated, the head of the presenting child being distinctly felt above a fold of mucous membrane of the anterior vaginal wall, which was mistaken for the anterior lip of the os uteri. After 2 P.M. the pains seemed to increase in severity, and at half-past 3 it was thought best to allow the liquor amnii to escape. The supposed bag of membranes, still high up, was very tense during a pain, but resisted all attempts at being ruptured by the finger; accordingly a puncture was made with a stylet, and a considerable amount of fluid came away. The pains became stronger, and the patient, who, up to this time, had not appeared fatigued, now began to show signs of exhaustion. Dr. MacCallum was now sent for to complete the labour with forceps. He arrived at half past nine that evening, and on making a digital examination, found slight shortening of the conjugate diameter, and determined to give an anæsthetic and make a thorough examination. The woman was then put fully under the influence of chloroform, and Dr. MacCallum introduced his hand into the vagina and found that there was no dilatation of the os whatever, and that the supposed bag of membranes that had been punctured was the thin expanded cervix in front of the head of the child. There was no projection whatever at the site of the os, and it was recognized by the part being slightly depressed, and yielding more to pressure of the finger. The os was then opened with the finger, and the patient, after recovering from the effects of the chloroform, was given hydrate of chloral gr. xv. every half hour till four doses had been taken, and then a few minims of chloroform were given during the pains, which became strong, dilating the os, and the head could be felt presenting in the second or right occipito-cotyloid position. At a quarter-past 3 in the morning, the patient was again put fully under the influence of chloroform and Simpson's long forceps applied at the brim. Traction was made in the usual manner, and at ten minutes to 4 the head was delivered and the forceps removed, the body and extremities followed in five minutes without artificial assistance, causing no laceration of the cervix uteri or perineum. The child was a male, weighing 6 lbs. 4 ozs. There was no pulsation in the cord and the child showed no signs of life ; it, however, appeared fully matured and well nourished, but on the soles of the feet and palms of the hands were seen evidences of intra-uterine maceration. The placenta and all the membranes were expelled in an hour and ten minutes, and weighed 1 lb. The uterus contracted firmly, and after a bandage was applied to the abdomen, the patient felt quite comfortable, and continued well until her third day, with scarcely any rise in temperature. On that day she had a chill, and her temperature rose to 104 3-5° ; during the night she threw off her blankets while the nurse was out of the room, and the result was an attack of bronchitis, with sore throat, a hard dry cough, and complete loss of voice. She was given a large dose of quinine, and immediately put upon Tinct. Ferri Mur. ♏ x, with chlorate of potash gr. v every four hours, and was also ordered brandy in small quantities. Her condition rapidly improved under this treatment, and the patient left the hospital on the eighth day after delivery, feeling perfectly well, and had no bad symptoms afterwards.

Reviews and Notices of Books.

Cyclopædia of the Practice of Medicine.—Edited by H. VON ZIEMSSEN, Professor of Clinical Medicine in Munich, Bavaria. Vol. IX—Diseases of the Liver and Portal Vein, with the chapter relating to Interstitial Pneumonia. New York: Wm. Wood & Co.

The appearance of this volume, so long delayed and so anxiously looked for, completes the series. The publishers, who some years ago boldly entered upon this great undertaking, are to be congratulated upon its successful completion. The ability with which the large staff of translators have done their work is worthy of great praise, and the regularity with which the books have followed each other from the very commencement, together with very superior excellence in the typographical department, have served to satisfy the most exacting amongst the subscribers. To add to the good things already furnished, the publishers now announce by circular that, on the completion of the volume on Skin Diseases in Germany, it is their intention to present a copy of the translation to each subscriber who has then completed his set.

The present volume begins with an introductory chapter on certain important anatomical and physiological points—the exact topography, structure and function of the liver, and on jaundice. Then follow in order the various congestive, inflammatory and degenerative disorders to which this important organ is subject. The chapters on the pathology of the various forms of cancer written by Von Schueppel are particularly good, as also is that by Leichtenstern on the clinical aspects of cancer of the liver. A large portion of the volume is devoted to the affections of the biliary passages and portal vein. Catarrh, gall-stones, phlebitis, &c., are all treated of most minutely. Amongst the rarer affections, a case of aneurism of the hepatic artery, with multiple abscesses, reported in this JOURNAL by Drs. Ross and Osler, is mentioned as having presented unusual features.

The volume is an admirable addition to the Cyclopœdia, fully up to the standard of its predecessors, which have been received with such widespread marks of approbation.

A Treatise on Bright's Disease and Diabetes, with especial reference to Pathology and Therapeutics.—By JAMES TYSON, A.M., M.D., Professor of General Pathology and Morbid Anatomy in the University of Pennsylvania, &c. With illustrations, including a section on Retinitis in Bright's Disease. By WM. F. NORRIS, A.M., M.D., Clinical Professor of Ophthalmology in the University of Pennsylvania. Philadelphia: Lindsay & Blakiston. Montreal: Dawson Brothers.

The above is an excellent monograph on these important urinary disorders. It is carefully prepared, and contains all the latest researches. The hulk of the volume is sufficiently reduced to render it an admirable book for the use of students. The section on retinitis, written by a specialist, increases materially its value, although, perhaps, it is rather more curtailed than we should have expected. Several woodcuts of renal sections, &c., are added, as well as colored plates of the urinary tube-casts, and one frontispiece lithograph of a case of albuminuric retinitis.

Photographic Illustrations of Cutaneous Syphilis.—By GEORGE HENRY FOX, A.M., M.D., Clinical Lecturer on Diseases of the Skin, College of Physicians and Surgeons, New York; Surgeon to New Yerk Dispensary, &c. Nos. VII, VIII, and IX. New York: E. B. Treat.

These numbers which we have received in continuation of the series continue to present illustrations from life of some of the various forms assumed by cutaneous syphilis. The photographs are fully equal to any of those of which we have already expressed such a high opinion: and the cases which furnish the plates have evidently been selected with great care, so as to furnish marked examples of the affection it is desired to exemplify. Those which are illustrated on the present occasion are the following: Syphiloderma tuberculosum, S. serpiginosum, S. ulceratiosum, S. pustulo-crustaceum, S. squamosum, and S. gummatosum.

Books and Pamphlets Received.

SUPPLEMENT TO ZIEMSSEN'S CYCLOPÆDIA OF THE PRACTICE OF MEDICINE.—Edited by George L. Peabody, M.D. New York: Wm. Wood & Co.

A TREATISE ON THE CONTINUED FEVERS.—By James C. Wilson, M.D. With an introduction by J. M. DaCosta, M.D. New York: Wm. Wood & Co.

A MEDICAL FORMULARY, BASED ON THE UNITED STATES AND BRITISH PHARMACOPŒIAS.—By Laurence Johnson, A.M., M.D. New York: Wm. Wood & Co.

A TREATISE ON DISEASES OF THE JOINTS.—By Richard Barwell, F.R.C.S. Second edition. New York: Wm. Wood & Co.

THE MOTHER'S GUIDE IN THE MANAGEMENT AND FEEDING OF INFANTS.—By John M. Keating, M.D. Philadelphia: Henry C. Lea's Son & Co.

Society Proceedings.

MEDICO-CHIRURGICAL SOCIETY OF MONTREAL.

A regular meeting was held June 10th, 1881. The President (Dr. Hingston) in the chair.

Dr. Osler exhibited:

1st. Two specimens of fibroid degeneration of the heart. The *first* was from a middle-aged woman who was admitted to the Hospital under Dr. Reddy, with symptoms of advanced mitral disease, and death ensued in a few days. The mitral valves were found thickened and adherent, the orifice much contracted and the edges covered with small vegetations. The aortic valves were competent and not thickened, and covered with small endocardial outgrowths. The left ventricle was much dilated, and the wall in vicinity of apex unusually thin, measuring only 4–5 mm., which in other parts was 15-20 mm. The endocardium was opaque, particularly at the lower part of septum and at apex. The whole of these regions were involved in a fibroid change; on section, presenting scarcely a trace of muscle fibre, but having the greyish-white aspect of connective tissue. There was a change about the tips of the papillary muscles, but the remainder of the heart was free. *Aorta* free from degeneration; smaller arteries not thickened. *Spleen* a little firm. *Kidneys* a little fibroid, not enlarged; arteries not prominent.

The *second* specimen was from a very stout woman admitted into Dr. Osler's wards on June 1st, having suffered for about fourteen days from a moderate general anasarca. This is now present, together with effusions into the peritoneum and right pleura. Complained of weakness, and was somewhat breathless. A large greyish-yellow slough occupied the outer ankle and dorsum of the foot. No organic disease was determined. Heart-sounds only slightly feeble. Diagnosis—Muscular degeneration of the heart. At autopsy, heart enlarged; aortic valves incompetent; two of the segments had united, and the point of junction was firm, calcified, and projected from the arterial wall, preventing both the full opening and the perfect closure of the segments. Ventricle dilated; apex and lower half of septum thin, endocardium opaque, and on section were found in state of fibroid change; muscle substance only seen in small streaks between the greyish-white connective tissue. Over the front and upper parts the muscle substance was increased in thickness, measuring 18–20 mm. Aorta was stiffened and atheromatous; small vessels in various organs very thick; one branch of the front coronary was almost occluded by arteritis, the primary divisions of the renals were much thickened, and the lumen of one nearly closed. Kidneys of average size and weight; capsules a little thick; surfaces not roughened; cortices not diminished; smaller arteries very prominent.

3rd. Specimen of cancer of cœcum; slight stenosis of bowel, perforation; enormous perityphilitic abscess.

Dr. Wilkins read a paper on "Cerebellar Disease," controverting the views lately advanced by Nothnagel in opposition to those of Ferrier; that lesions of either lateral lobe are accompanied by well-marked disturbances of equilibrium. In the reader's case there was a lesion in the left lateral lobe of the cerebellum, 3 centimetres in length, 1 centimetre in breadth, and 8 millimetres deep, besides extravasations in the anterior portion of the frontal lobes. Dr. W. diagnosed cerebellar lesion, from the invariable loss of equilibrium towards the left when the patient attempted to walk: he then always reeled and staggered towards the left side. There was also psychical disturbance due to the large clot in frontal lobe; no persistent motor disturbance; deafness of left side was present, as was also diplopia and ocular incoördination.

Dr. Henry Howard mentioned the facts given by Otto in three cases. First, that of a soldier, who during life had obeyed orders as an ordinary soldier, but at death a *post-mortem* revealed an entire absence of cerebellum; second, that of an imbecile girl, in whom the cerebellum was scarcely seen, and yet there was perfect coördination; a third similar case was quoted. In the last two cases, immoral tendencies were strongly marked. So Otto concluded that the cerebellum was not the centre of coördination.

Dr. Osler said some of the members may remember an old cerebellar cicatrix exhibited to the Society some time ago. In that case there was great loss of power in the lower limbs. In only one or two cases of coarse tubercle in the cerebellum, seen by Dr. Osler, was there any loss of coördination. Dr. Wilkins' case was interesting, in that he had lateral movements. The point of great interest was the hæmorrhage in the left frontal lobe, with no paralysis of the side.

Dr. Buller said complete deafness on the left side was seen. The semi-circular canals play an important part in coördination.

Dr. Wilkins, in reply, stated that the only incoördination present in his case was in the movement of the eyes; that the symptoms to which he particularly directed attention were the disturbances of equilibrium. This, he thought, could be understood, if we viewed the cerebellum, to some extent at least, as an automatic organ. For instance, in an infant attempting to walk, some of the volitional impulses originating in the psychomotor area of the cerebrum are transmitted to the cerebellum, which co-operates with those going directly to the corpora striata, in order to effect the necessary movements to keep erect. After frequent attempts, the cerebellum acquires the power of regulating these movements, and in this way becomes "automatic."

This *acquired* automatic movement explains why, in Dr. W.'s case, sudden destruction of a part of one lateral lobe of cerebellum should cause disturbances of equilibrium, which did not exist in the cases referred to by Dr. Osler, as in the latter cases the slow growths of the lesions permitted other parts of the cerebellum to assume the functions of the parts destroyed. When loss of power was present in connection with cerebellar growths, it was generally due to pressue on the pons. The deafness he (Dr. W.) thought could be explained without reference to semicircular canals, as the auditory nerve was closely connected with the same side of the cerebellum.

Dr. Armstrong read a paper on "Perityphlitis." The patient, aged 38, of medium height and spare build, had been sick for a fortnight; on examination, well marked symptoms of saturnism were evident. Abdomen slightly tympanitic; temperature 99½°, pulse 92; integument œdematous. Pressure showed localized fullness and pain; percussion dull; no fluctuation; liver and spleen slightly enlarged; heart and lungs healthy. The originating cause of his trouble was a strain of the right side in lifting two weeks before. Then, by medical direction, mustard and poultices were used, but from that time till seen by Dr. Armstrong had received no medical aid. On the 20th March he had a rigor; then for 15 days had severe rigors, having two or three in the 24 hours; high fever, up to 106° on one occasion, followed by profuse perspiration, accompanied by retching and vomiting, also epistaxis. Was seen in consultation by Dr. Fenwiek, and for the diarrhœa present a large dose of olive oil was advised. Afterward seen by Dr. R. P. Howard on the 11th April, who deemed it a case of hepatic abscess. On the 15th, there was fœtid diarrhœa, but no pus; after the diarrhœa there were no rigors till the 27th April, during which time he improved. On the 3rd of May, not so well, and complained of severe pain in the stomach. From then till the 15th, got worse, when death ensued. On the 13th, found dullness on percussion; no bulging nor fluctuation. Next day, Dr. Fenwick being present, passed a hypodermic needle and drew off some serum; an aspirator was then passed and a quantity of serum removed. Dr. Osler had, by *post-mortem* examination, found an abscess at the head of the cœcum. The treatment pursued by Dr. Armstrong was, at first, pot. iod. in 10 grain doses, and morphia; ten days after, symptoms of blood poisoning being evident, put him on bark and ammonia, and for vomiting, bismuth and ox. cerium, &c., but with no benefit. Believed the case to be one of inflammation of the cellular tissue behind the cœcum, followed by abscess which opened into the cœcum. Complete cessation of chills followed the bursting of the abscess.

Dr. R. P. Howard said when called to see this case, understood there was no doubt that there had been local peritonitis, which had disappeared. All that remained was symptoms of septicæmia. The question was, where was the abscess? He inferred that there was suppuration in the liver. Had seen a great many such cases, and they had most frequently resolved. When it begins in the cœcum, such is the end; not so in the peri-cœcum. Once we get local peri-cœcal inflammation, the question arises, shall we make an exploratory puncture or not? Many of these cases, under leeches and poultices, resolve; when, however, we have evidence of pus, parts thick and œdematous, then a puncture can be made. Confusion exists in the books: inflammation of the cœcum is one thing, of the appendix quite another. The first is followed nearly always by recovery; the second nearly always fatal. Sands, in his twenty-six published cases, makes no distinction in these two diseases.

Dr. Osler referred to the fact that no part of the body varied so much as the appendix vermiformis. It coils in various directions, and owing to its changed situations may get inflamed. Indeed the cœcum itself changes, as in a case once seen, where it was just about the gall-bladder.

Dr. Geo. Ross said a great difficulty arises in making a correct diagnosis in these cases. He mentioned a case lately seen, where the violence of the symptoms were most intense, as in severe peritonitis, and he had great fears that it was one of perforation, but by leeches and morphia he recovered. Cases that will recover set in just as intensely as those from genuine perforation. Dr. Ross cited a case where a patient had had perforating cœcal ulcer, and the evidence was that it had taken place some time before death. He died afterwards of general peritonitis.

Dr. Hingston exhibited a patient lately referred to in the Society, upon whom he had done the ordinary operation for talipes equino-varus without satisfactory results. A clean cut was made to the bone across the sole of the foot, put in a splint, and extension made. Dr. Hingston said he was not the originator of this operation, it having been done previously by Dr. A. M. Phelps of Chateauguay, N.Y., and the idea of such an operation was derived from the fact of the mode of treatment of wryneck done by Dr. Post of the Presbyterian Hospital, New York city.

The meeting shortly afterwards adjourned.

A regular meeting was held June 24th, 1881. The President, Dr. Hingston, in the chair.

Dr. Fenwick exhibited a fibroid tumour removed from the back of the throat of a girl aged 20. She has a number of these tumours on all parts of the body, which are excessively painful. The incision was made externally. He has since removed others from the same patient, and they are all found to be situated in the vicinity of nerves.

Dr. Gurd reported the following case:

On afternoon of June 17th, 1881, I was sent for to see M. S., a muscular young French-Canadian of 19 years, whom I found suffering agony from a strangulated indirect inguinal hernia of right side. He had had pain and occasional vomitings since previous evening, but this morning went to his work at Hudon Cotton Factory, where he was employed as clerk—had to leave soon as pain was intolerable. On his way home he saw a French doctor, who told him to go to bed, that he had a hernia. As he continued to grow worse, his friends sent for me. He gave a history of chronic constipation, and did not know the nature of the "lump" in the groin, which he had noticed for about six months being there at night but away in the morning. Occasionally he would lift a bale of cotton, but says he had not done so immediately previous to present illness. Some difficulty was experienced in reducing the hernia, which was about size of an egg, tense, red and very sensitive. Simple taxis failing, I applied a bag of ice and gave a dose of morphia. Taxis again failing, I arranged my fingers in the form of a cushion over the tumor, and with moderate pressure, after some minutes, it gradually receded, without making the usual gurgling sound. A slightly thickened feel was left on upper part of canal. Patient felt easier after the reduction. Some one-quarter grain morphia powders were left to be given if necessary.

18*th*—A.M.—Had a poor night; vomited several times; pain is now all over the belly, which feels hard; temperature 98.5. P.M.—Pain less, but is restless and very thirsty; pulse 126; is taking mixture of bismuth, soda, morphia and hydrocyanic acid.

19*th*.—Face anxious looking; tongue coated, dry at tip; vomited through the night; micturition difficult and very painful; belly hard, slightly swollen and tympanitic; gave hypodermic of morphia.

20*th*.—Vomiting continues and is of bilious-looking fluid; pulse 130; skin felt natural; tympanitis worse, so gave injection of turpentine, castor oil and soap-water, but without bringing away either gas or fæces; two hypodermic injections were given to lessen pain to-day.

21*st*.—Had a better night. Dr. Roddick saw him in consultation to-day at 4 P.M.; pulse was then 122, temperature 99 3-5°; dulness on percussion in region of descending colon; elsewhere over abdomen tympanitis rather worse. Dr. R. thought that possibly it might be a case of fæcal obstruction, and recommended that before operating copious injections be thrown high up the bowel by using an O'Beirn's tube. This I did several times, at first trying soap-water, and after sweet oil, without getting away any fæcal matter. Towards evening mind wandered, would only be conscious for a minute or two after being roused and spoken to. Vomiting now became stercoraceous.

22*nd*.—Patient very weak; had bad night; fæcal vomiting continues. Belly less hard, but more swollen; not very sensitive to pressure. Doses with eyes half closed. I saw and explained condition to Dr. Roddick, who concurred in the advisability of an operation; so, after much coaxing, got his parents to allow his being removed to Montreal General Hospital, where, about midnight, Dr. Roddick operated; Dr. Fenwick was present at the operation. The abdomen was opened by an incision 3 in. long in linea alba, below umbilicus. Feeling towards the right inguinal region, Dr. Roddick at once found a small portion of the ilium nipped in the internal ring, and which he easily released by gentle traction and drew it out of the external wound. It was collapsed and darkly congested. For fear of adhesion in inner walls, gas was made to pass through the part from the bowel above, it was then returned, and the wound closed with silver and carbolized catgut sutures. The whole operation, which did not take long, was done under the spray and with full Listerian precautions. The patient's condition, which was very bad before the operation, improved a little for an hour so after, when he vomited a large quantity of dark, stinking fluid, and from this time, in spite of hypodermic of ether, he gradually sank, dying about five hours after the operation. At the *post-mortem*, the portion of intestine which had been nipped was easily detected, being smaller in calibre and much darker than the rest. Signs of recent peritonitis was visible all over the intestines, but more marked at lower end.

Dr. Roddick said when first seen he could see nothing in the vicinity of the ring to account for his condition. Dullness was seen at the left side, and thought that an overloaded colon existed. A large injection was given without any effect. Patient brought to hospital at 7 on Wednesday, and at 10 an incision of 3½ inches in length from the umbilicus down was made. Hand was passed into the wound and down to the right inguinal region, and a knuckle of intestine was found in the internal ring. This was drawn out, and air passod through to see that it was pervious. Stertoraceous vomiting, which had existed, continued, and the patient died at daylight of the day following.

Dr. Rodger mentioned a case of puerperal convulsions which he had at present under his care. The patient, a primipara, aged 20 years, was first seen on Monday night (June 20th), when she was then suffering from violent headache, dimness of vision and more or less general anasarca. Until about within ten days ago she had enjoyed good health, in fact better than before marriage. Confinement not expected before the end of July or end of the first week in August. Procured some of the urine and had it examined that same night, finding about 75 per cent albumen. Early the following morning (June 21st) I was summoned to attend this case, and found the patient in violent convulsions. The husband informed me that the patient had frequently complained during the night of pain over the top of the head, and on that account had been rather restless. Within a very short space of time three convulsions occurred, whereupon I injected hypodermically one-fourth of a grain of morphia at seven o'clock, and on returning at nine o'clock learned that during that time two convulsive seizures had taken place. No apparent return of consciousness had occurred since the first convulsion, and it is quite impossible to arouse the patient by any means whatever. Passed a catheter into the bladder and drew off about two ounces of very dark-coloured urine, which I found perfectly solid with albumen. Examined the os uteri, but found no evidence of dilatation. Administered an enema of turpentine and castor oil, which moved the bowels freely. At 12 o'clock noon, patient was still quite insensible; pupils slightly dilated; breathing slow and stertorous; pulse 120 and temperature 100°. Between the convulsive seizures, the nurse states that the patient is very restless, which I looked upon as due possibly to the action of the uterus. She has had two convulsions since 10 o'clock, which it is thought were more severe than any of those previous. The clonic spasms appearing to continue for an unusually long period, I commenced the use of chloroform, not only with the view of allaying that condition, but also, if possible, aiding in the dilatation of the os uteri. At one o'clock, found the os softer, and could pass the top of my index finger, the uterine action showing itself well marked. I now determined to encourage the action of the uterus, and commenced digital dilatation at once, the patient being kept under the influence of chloroform. Notwithstanding the use of the chloroform, convulsions occurred at intervals of about forty minutes;

and at 4 o'clock, having the os sufficiently dilated, I decided to apply the forceps and deliver. My friend Dr. Alloway very kindly came to my assistance, and we shortly afterwards delivered the patient of a living child. Forty-five minutes from the time of delivery convulsions again set in, and within an hour three had occurred. Hypodermic injections of chloral hydrat. having been spoken highly of lately in cases of this kind, I injected 10 grains, dissolved in 10 minims of water, every half-hour. Two hours were occupied with the use of the chloral, yet during that time patient had two convulsions. Patient very restless ; tossing arms and legs about violently, yet still quite unconscious. Pulse 120 ; temperature 103°. The condition of the pulse at this time being full and bounding (hammer pulse), I resolved to bleed, and, with the aid of Dr. Alloway, took 20 ounces of blood from the right arm, which seemed to give relief, breathing being somewhat more tranquil. There being but little appreciable result upon the condition of the pulse, I opened a vein on the left arm, and this time withdrew 25 ounces of blood, This seemed to have more effect upon the pulse, it being much softer. Scarcely half-an-hour had elapsed when another convulsion took place, though not severe. At 12 o'clock (midnight) again saw the patient, and learned that she had been exeedingly restless since my last visit; this great restlessness I attributed to the chloral, and on that account determined not to resort to its use again. Again passed a catheter, taking off about three ounces of urine, which, on examination, I found perfectly solid from albumen. It was agreed, in conversation with Dr. Alloway, that in the event of there being no change for the better in the condition of the patient, that is, in a reasonable time from the hour of bleeding, to resort to the use of pilocarpin. Let me mention here that I have had experience with pilocarpin lately in two cases of uræmic convulsions following scarlet fever. One of the cases was attended with rapid œdema of the lungs, and was seen by R. P. Howard, who was in consultation upon the case, and at whose suggestion pilocarpin was used. Both these cases did well under its use, profuse perspiration being produced in each, with speedy recovery following. Accordingly, at half-past one o'clock, I injected one-quarter grain of this drug hypodermically, and in about an hour the skin, which previously had been quite dry, was now perceptibly moist. Still at half-past two the general condition was alarming, conjunctiva deeply injected, breathing rapid, loud and stertorous, mouth filled with mucus, but no evidence of any accumulation in the bronchial tubes, pulse 140, temperature 104 3-5°. To all appearances death from coma seemed inevitable at no distant period. The patient having another convulsion, I tried once more the use of morphia sulph., hypodermically, injecting fully a grain. In a short time the restlessness began to subside. Visiting at half-past six, ascertained from the nurse that shortly after I left patient turned over on her left side and has slept quiet ever since. Perspiration during all this time has been most profuse, perfectly saturating the bed linen. Patient up till this time has not shown any evidence of returning consciousness. Pulse 90, temperature 99°.

June 22nd, 10 A.M.—Consciousness returned about 9 o'clock, having recognized her mother, calling her by name. Dr. Gardner saw the case at this time. For slight restlessness, injected ¼ grain of morphia. From this time the case progressed favorably, and to-night (Friday), on examination of the urine for albumen, find no trace whatever.

Dr. Gardner said it is the opinion of Schroeder, also of Fordyce Barker, that labour should not be induced in these cases. Dr. Gardner would not be at all active in inducing labour. He mentioned one case which he left to nature, and succeeded in controlling the convulsions by giving ℳ xxx. of Bat. Sed. Sol. repeatedly. In regard to pilocarpin, it was objected to on account of the mucous secretions which it occasions in the bronchial tubes, and death from apnœa has followed. Success of the morphia is excellent; chloral is of great value in certain cases, but is used too much to the exclusion of morphia.

Dr. Fenwick said in regard to emptying the uterus in these cases, in some half dozen he witnessed, had associated each convulsion with each pain, and he would empty the uterus as soon as possible. In three cases he had attended, the convulsions ceased immediately after the uterus was emptied.

Dr. F. W. Campbell said he had seven or eight cases of convulsions, and where venesection was used, good was done.

Dr. Trenholme said when the uterine spasm causes convulsion, the emptying the uterus is clear; but if not, a large dose of morphia, say 1½ grs., could be given and convulsions controlled.

Dr. Godfrey said his treatment had been to abstract blood and cause free action of the skin.

Dr. Kennedy said that as he had no experience of the use of pilocarpin in puerperal convulsions, he at first did not think of making any remarks upon the case reported; but as Dr. Rodger, as an afterthought, had just mentioned that he had also bled to a large extent, there was the possibility that the benefit experienced was due as much to the bleeding as to the drug. Dr. K. had seen a great many cases of puerperal convulsion, and considered that bleeding was the most efficient remedy when convulsions set in after delivery. Very early in his practice he had met with a case in which the convulsions had thus continued; bleeding was had recourse to, with the greatest benefit, and this had led him to continue the practice. For some years past had not seen convulsions continue after delivery, as in all these cases he favored the uterine flow, which was apt to be very free on account of the large amount of chloroform administered, this being a well known effect of that anæsthetic, and in this way the full benefit of the bleeding was obtained without the necessity of further venesection. He believed in inducing labour in these cases, as it had been his experience to find the exciting cause of the convulsion to be uterine contraction. About two months ago had a very severe case, the woman being in her eighth month; each pain was followed immediately by the convulsion, and this in spite of the free administration of chloroform. Barnes' dilators were used, and delivery rapidly effected by forceps; there was a very free hæmorrhage, and no further attack of convulsions.

The meeting then adjourned.

Extracts from British and Foreign Journals.

Unless otherwise stated the translations are made specially for this Journal.

Pasteur on Rabies.—When a man has a hobby, there is no knowing how far he will go with it; and this may be applied to M. Pasteur, who sees germs everywhere. This eminent biologist has made some most important contributions to science, and his name will ever be connected with his ingenious researches on fermentation, and other important discoveries; but, like most investigators, he has drifted from the right path, and gone into a more speculative kind of scientific experiments. As an example of this may be mentioned his recent experiments with the saliva from the mouth of a child with rabies, with which he inoculated rabbits and guinea-pigs. All the animals died, and their blood was found to contain myriads of micro-organisms, which he concluded to be the specific germs that produced hydrophobia. He then performed a second series of experiments, by inoculating other rabbits with the blood of those that had succumbed from the first inoculation. These also died, and their blood was found to contain the same micro-organisms. He, however, soon discovered by further experiments, but this time with the saliva of children who died from other diseases, that the results were precisely similar to those observed with the saliva of the child. In pushing his experiments still further, but with the saliva of a healthy adult, he met with the same results, and the same germs, as in the preceding cases. This rather puzzled the persevering experimenter, but he is not so easily beaten; and if he has not yet discovered the real nature of the virus of rabies, he fancies he has laid his hand on the organ that secretes it. According to him, the virus of rabies is not secreted by the salivary glands, but by the brain—or rather, the latter is the seat of the malady; and in support of his thesis, he inoculated a small portion of the bulbous extremity of the medulla oblongata of a rabid animal under the cerebral covering of a healthy animal. The latter became rabid. These results were recently communicated to the Academy of Medicine, in a paper read by the general secretary for the learned experimenter, which called forth some trenchant remarks from M. Béchamp, who positively refused to accept the principle on which M. Pasteur has hitherto founded most of his theories, and added that it is not outside the body that one must look for the germs or elements of destruction; but they are to be found in our own body, in the form of microzymes, which are the only cause of all fermentation, and the lowest element to which our organism can be reduced. M. Pasteur has not yet had the time to send in his rejoinder; but it is to be hoped that, when he shall do so, he will read his communication himself, which is sure to be a most interesting one. Nothing daunted, however, M. Pasteur continues his parasitic warfare with unbroken zeal; and, by further experiments with human saliva, he has made the startling discovery that the saliva of a person fasting is venomous, as it contains the same parasites as those found in the saliva of children above described; but that, on the person breaking his fast, his saliva is deprived of the venomous quality, as the parasites are taken into the stomach with the food. All this is terrible to contemplate; and even M. Pasteur was confounded, as the result of his experiment was as awful as it was unexpected. The learned biologist made no attempt to offer any explanation, but said that he would for the present only point to the fact, which, he added, was in itself very suggestive.—*Brit. Med. Journal.*

Washing out of the Stomach.—M. Bucquoy and M. Constantin Paul have recently published some interesting details on this subject, which are analysed in the *Journal de Médecine Pratique.* M. Bucquoy, who was one of the first promoters in France of this method, borrowed from Kussmaul, relates a new case concerning a man suffering from a considerable dilatation of the stomach, consecutive on a stricture of the pylorus itself, which supervened after the ingestion of nitric acid. He was dying literally from hunger, in consequence of complete gastric intolerance, when he was submitted to washing out of the stomach with Fancher's tube; a considerable improvement was then quickly produced, and the patient increased in weight more than two kilogrammes in a fortnight; however, he was attacked by new troubles, and succumbed to pulmonary phthisis shortly afterwards. M. Bucquoy enlarged greatly on the various indications which might be met by washing out the stomach.

M. Constantin Paul has especially studied this question at great length, and has published some very useful hints on the method of employing the operative proceeding. It must first be noted that, for the operation in question, the sitting position of the patient is most favourable; certain timorous and nervous persons, however, should be put in the reclining position for the first few times. The instrument used is Faucher's tube, with this restriction, however, that it may be useful during the first few days to use the ordinary stiff sound to overcome the œsophageal spasm which sometimes occurs at this moment, but which disappears after a few applications. In order to remedy this inconvenience, M. Debove has had a screw constructed which much facilitates, in this case, the introduction of a flexible India-rubber tube. When, however, the patient himself introduces his sound, which he always does very rapidly, a stiff tube is, on the contrary, a necessary condition, since it enters by a true swallowing movement. M. Audhoui has had constructed a flexible tube with a double stream, which much facilitates the washing out of the stomach, but in which the tube whence the liquids issue is, as a matter of necessity, restricted, which is a serious inconvenience. The method of introduction, as described by M. Bucquoy, is as follows: The tube being slightly moistened with water (M. C. Paul recommends that it should be greased with vaseline during the first few days only), the patient takes the free end of the tube, places it in the pharynx, and pushes it slightly, making a swallowing movement. He repeats this swallowing movement a certain number of times, guiding the tube with the hand; this penetrates into the stomach rather rapidly; and the patient stops when he sees near his lips a mark traced at from 45 to 50 centimètres from the free end then lying along the large curve of the stomach. To charge the siphon, the patient pours alkaline water into the receiver; and, after having filled it, raises it above his head until the liquid has entered almost entirely. At this moment, he lowers the receiver below the level of the stomach, and above the basin. The cylinder becomes filled immediately with the contents of the stomach; and it will be seen that there returns a more considerable quantity of liquid than has been introduced, bringing with it the residue of digestion. The operation is repeated a certain number of times, and as often as necessary, until the water returns in an almost limpid state. Alkaline water is generally employed for these operations. M. Constantin Paul has found that the silicated water of Sail, or an antiseptic solution containing thymol or hyposulphite of soda, is useful. To conclude the operation, he pours into the stomach two or three hundred grammes of milk.

The first liquids injected are tepid, because they cleanse the parts better; the later ones are cold, because they form a better coating for the mucous membrane, and induce contraction more easily. In certain serious cases, the operation is renewed twice daily; in ordinary cases, once only at the beginning, then less frequently afterwards. Whatever may be the nature of the gastric affection thus treated, according to M. Paul, good results are almost immediately obtained; in the first place, cessation of the pain; then the appearance, at the end of some days, of spontaneous action (in the case of dilatation); finally, a reappearance of the appetite, and a much more rapid augmentation of weight than would be believed. At the present time, washing out of the stomach is no longer limited to dilatation, as it was at first. It is applied to various affections. M. Paul quotes cases of gastralgia, of hysterical vomiting, of gastric ulcer, which have been thus completely cured. He has thus been able to greatly relieve the sufferings of a woman who had fæcal vomiting, and who suffered from an umbilical hernia; finally, in cancer of the stomach, the symptoms are very much relieved, and it is possible even to bring on a notable temporary improvement. M. Bucquoy and M. Ferrand have also observed cases of cure of simple ulcer. M. Debove likewise has reported, in the *Progrès Médical*, an extremely remarkable case of cure of a patient suffering from a simple ulcer, probably very old in origin, with absolute intolerance of the stomach, and a state of extreme cachexia. The favourable results obtained were almost immediate; and, at the end of six weeks, the patient, who had increased from 100 to 125 grammes daily, was on the road to complete recovery.

Professor Germain Sée, in his treatise on gastro-intestinal dyspepsia, relates a certain number of cases which well demonstrate the utility of this method in gastric affections of very different kinds. He speaks of the case of a young girl suffering from serious anorexia, with invincible refusal of all nourishment, who had reached the last stage of marasmus, and who was treated for six months with this mechanical treatment. Dr. Sée has also seen obstinate vomiting thus stopped; cancer is greatly relieved, and dyspepsia of the cachectic form, which seemed of the nature of cancer, has been completely cured. In the last case, as well as being a means of treatment, it forms a true method of diagnosis. This brief enumeration shows the great importance of this new mode of treatment, which unites perfect harmlessness to very great faciiity of employment, since, up to the present time, not a single accident has been known to occur from the operation.—*Brit. Med. Journal.*

Action of Coffee and Sugar on the Stomach.—In a paper presented to the Société de Biologie (*Rev. Méd.*, May 14), M. Leven states that coffee, so far, as is often supposed, from accelerating the digestive process of the stomach, rather tends to impede this. When thirty grams of coffee, diluted in 150 of water, is given to a dog, which is killed five hours and a half afterwards, the stomach is found pale, its mucous surface being anæmic, and the vessels of its external membrane contracted. The whole organ exhibits a marked appearance of anæmia. Coffee thus determining anæmia of the mucous membrane, preventing rather than favoring vascular congestion, and opposing rather than facilitating the secretion of gastric juice, how comes it that the sense of comfort is procured for so many people who are accustomed to take coffee after a meal? A repast, in fact, produces, in those whose digestion is torpid, a heaviness of the intellectual faculties and embarrassment of the power of thinking; and these effects, and the disturbance of the head, are promptly dissipated by the stimulant effect which the coffee produces on the nervous centres, as shown by experiments with cafein. Coffee and tea, when taken in excess, are a frequent cause of dyspepsia, for the anæmic condition of the mucous membrane being periodically renewed, a permanent state of congestion is at last produced, which constitutes dyspepsia. Sugar, which with many doctors has a bad reputation, is an excellent aliment, which assists digestion, and should not be proscribed in dyspepsia. By experiment, digestion of meat is found to take place much more completely when sugar is added. Coffee exerts both a local and general action, operating locally by means of its tannin, by diminishing the calibre of the vessels, but acting on the general economy by exciting the nervous centres and the muscular system. It renders digestion slower, and is only of good effect by relieving the feeling of torpor after meals. Its injurious action on digestion may be corrected by adding sugar so as to counterbalance its effects on the mucous membrane. This adding sugar to coffee is not only a pleasant practice, but one contributing to digestion.

A Hint to Chloroformists.—When in Paris I was invited by Dr. Labbé to assist in a case of ovariotomy at a private hospital. The patient was given chloroform. When the anæsthesia was complete, the surgeon made his incision in the linea alba, through the skin and cellular tissue. Suddenly the respiration stopped, and the heart ceased to beat, as clearly shown by the cessation of bleeding and the bloodless appearance of the lips of the wound. The mouth was cleansed from mucus, the tongue drawn forwards, the patient's head thrown well back, and artificial respiration was practised for quite ten minutes, but without result. The case appeared desperate, when Dr. Labbé put a large cloth in boiling water and applied it to the cardiac region. Instantly the heart commenced to beat and the patient to respire. She was saved. The operation was not terminated. The cloth which had been applied was of such a heat that a large blister was raised at the seat of its application. Such simple and ever at hand means, which has succeeded several times with Dr. Labbé, may be unknown to a few of your readers, and possibly useful to all.—*Dr. Adolphi Paggi in London Lancet.*

Cantharides Poisoning.—Mr. Clark treats almost every case of gonorrhœa during its primary symptoms—*e.g.*, scalding, chordee, etc.—with thick discharge, by saline medicines with tepid-water injections. When the discharge becomes thinner and all active inflammation has abated, iron and cantharides are prescribed internally in the form of tincture of the perchloride of iron and tincture of cantharides, of each five minims three times a day, and an injection of sulphate of zinc of the strength of two grains to the ounce. In the first case of poisoning, the patient had been taking the cantharides mixture for five days, at the end of which time he was virtually cured. A week after the discontinuance of the medicine he was attacked with violent pain over the bladder. and this was accompanied upon the following day with strangury. The symptoms which, at first were very severe, passed off at the end of about four days under the use of nitric acid and hyoscyamus internally and hot baths upon the recurrence of the strangury. In the second case the patient after taking two doses only of the cantharides mixture had some of the symptoms of poisoning, viz. frequent desire to pass urine, burning pain during micturition, which was very difficult and was always accompanied towards the end of the process by a few drops of blood. Half the dose was then ordered but the directions were not followed, the full dose being continued, yet the symptoms rapidly abated. In each case every trace of the gonorrhœa was removed, and as soon as the active symptoms produced by the cantharides had passed off the patient felt as well as ever, and had not the slighest discomfort in the urinary organs. The delay of the symptoms in the first case may probably be explained by the supposition that the drug became stored up in the kidneys, and that after a short time its cumulative action gives rise to the symptoms of poisoning.—*London Lancet.*

Skin-Grafting with Grafts taken from the Dead Subject.—In the latter part of June, 1880, while sitting on a door on which there was a steel hinge, the patient was struck by lightning, and became comatose, in which condition he remained for several hours. He was brought to Bellevue Hospital and placed in Ward 12, at that time, under my charge. When his clothes were removed the skin came off his left arm and scapula, leaving a large raw surface. This surface was treated by different means for some weeks, until a healthy granulating surface was obtained all over the affected part. About this time, a healthy young German, who had attempted suicide by cutting his throat, was brought to the hospital, and died within a few hours. Six hours after his death, I went to the dead-house and removed a portion of skin from the inner side of the thigh, where there was least hair, and the skin most delicate. Having cut this piece of skin into a great many small pieces, I applied them and dressed the surface after my own method, which is to apply first, next to the grafted surface, a piece of the green protective used in Lister's dressing; over this I strap the ulcer with ordinary rubber or adhesive plaster, and over the whole throw a roller loosely. The object of the green protective is to prevent the grafts from adhering to the plaster and being torn off when the dressing is removed. The strapping is simply to make pressure, which must be firm and evenly applied. After the dressings had remained on for four days, they were removed, and after some little discharge had been washed off, I had the patient photographed. About one-fourth of the grafts had failed to take, and were washed off when the wound was cleansed. The remainder have attached themselves to the ulcer, and the lower and central portions of the ulcer on the arm are already covered with a thin, delicate skin, as a result of the fusing together of the little islands of skin, each graft serving as a point of departure for the formation of these islands. As in other and similar cases, cicatrization would have doubtless gone on to complete cure in a short time, but for an attack of erysipelatous inflammation, resulting from the low condition of the boy's general health, and his exposure to other cases of that disease, which destroyed a large portion of the newly formed skin, requiring subsequent graftings, but finally resulted in a cure, with much less of contracting cicatricial tissue than is commonly witnessed after recovery from such extensive burns.

Skin and mucous membrane removed from the living in surgical operations have been often used for grafts. But I wish to state here my claim, that the idea of removing skin from the cadaver and grafting it on to the living subject is original with me, and that I was the first to perform this operation, which has since been done many times successfully by other gentlemen. It seems to me that any one who has witnessed, as I have done repeatedly, skin taken from the dead body several hours after death return again to life, adhere to a granulating surface, and with surprising rapidity send out prolongations of delicate skin in all directions, covering the surface with a new skin comparatively free from contraction, must agree with me that skin-grafting is in its infancy, and that when men of ability have given it more attention, and found out the possibilities of the proceeding, we may expect to see frightfully contracting cicatrices which follow burns and nævi removed by excision, and their places filled with a skin almost as perfect as the surrounding, and which has been removed from the dead or living body of another person.—*Dr. J. H. Girdner in N.Y. Med. Record.*

Simple Tests of Water.—The complete analysis of water requires much chemical skill, but the more common impurities may be detected by simple tests and various injurious salts thus recognized. "Among them," says the *Boston Journal of Chemistry*, "are the nitrates, whose presence is chiefly significant, as showing that organic matter has been acted upon, and may be present. The danger is not in the salts themselves, but in their source, which should, if possible, be ascertained. To examine water for nitrates, put a small quantity of it in a test tube, add an equal quantity of pure sulphuric acid, using care that the fluids shall not mix; to this add carefully a few drops of a saturated solution of sulphate of iron. The stratum where the two fluids meet will, if nitric acid be present, show a purple, afterward a brown colour. If the nitric be in minute quantities, a reddish colour will result. The presence of ammonia, if in excess, can be determined by treating the water with a small quantity of potassic hydrate. Ammonia, if present, will be liberated, and may be recognized by its odor, or by the white fumes of chloride of ammonium, when a glass rod wet with muriatic acid is passed over the mouth of the test tube. If chlorine is present in any form in water used for drinking, it is evidence that sewage contamination in some form exists. The presence and amount of chlorine may be ascertained by the following simple method: Take 9 grains of nitrate of silver, chemically pure, and dissolve it in 200 units (say, cubic centimetres) of distilled water. One unit of the solution will represent 1-100th of a grain of chlorine. Take a small measured quantity of water to be examined, and put it into a glass vessel more than large enough to hold it. Add to the water a small quantity of the solution; if chlorine be present, a white precipitate will result. Repeat the addition, after short intervals, until no precipitate results. The units of the solution used will determine the hundredth of a grain of chlorine present. If more than a grain of chlorine in a gallon be present, reject the water, unless it can be clearly determined that the excess does not come from sewage. The water should be slightly acidulated with nitric acid before the test is applied. Heisch's sugar test for the presence of dangerous organic matter is at once simple and trustworthy. Place a quantity of the water to be examined in a clean glass stoppered bottle; add a few grains of pure sugar, and expose to the light in a window of a warm room. If the water becomes turbid even after exposure for a week, reject; if it remains clear it is safe."

Transfusion in Profuse Menorrhagia.—Mr. T. Whiteside Hime has performed this operation with success in a sterile married woman, aged 35. Menorrhagia had existed for five years, commencing from fatigue and severe shock during a catamenial period. The anæmia was very marked; the cervix uteri was conical, the os narrow; it was incised and the uterine cavity painted with a strong solution of perchloride of iron, but with little good effect. Mr. Hime drew six ounces of blood from the patient's husband, and, using a special transfuser, introduced the blood through the patient's medio-cephalic vein. During the process her breathing stopped; a drachm of ether was immediately injected subcutaneously, and artificial respiration employed; she rallied, and the transfusion was completed. This was done in November, 1878; since then menstruation has never been excessive. The transfusion was indirect, the blood being first whipped and defibrinated in a warm vessel, then strained into the apparatus, which is double-chambered, so that the blood may be surrounded by hot water. The blood runs, by gravitation, out of the apparatus, through an elastic tube into the vein. The apparatus is very cheap, and cannot easily get out of order.—*Brit. Med. Journal.*

Nurses.—There has been much discussion recently concerning the stated objection of certain sisterhood nursing associations to send nurses to small-pox cases. Mr. Lewis Wingfield has written strongly to the papers on the subject, and the *Gentleman's Magazine*, in commenting on his published letters, observes that "not the least serious question opened out by Mr. Wingfield's letter is that of the value of our nursing sisterhoods. One and all of these to whom Mr. Wingfield applied declined to send a nurse to serve in a house in which there was small-pox. I do not deny that a woman may well hesitate to face the risk of so serious and loathsome a disease. For those, however, who, in the profession of religion, have formed a sisterhood, to decline such a call is like a soldier refusing to join a forlorn hope. They may be volunteers. That, however, does nothing to free them from responsibility. Fancy our volunteer soldiers refusing, on account of the danger, to front an enemy when he had once landed! I hope this refusal to face danger will open men's eyes to the real value of not a few of the institutions in which women play at being nurses. In our hospitals the presence of lady nurses is not an unmixed blessing. I have spoken to patients who have felt the weariness and suffering of life in hospital augmented by the fact that they dared not ask ladies of gentle birth for the menial service they required. Though less brutal in language, moreover, than the nurse of former times, the lady nurse knows how to make the patient wince when he has the misfortune to get into her black books. We are in a curious transition stage in many matters. When we have settled down to the new order of things we shall find that in nursing, as in other matters, professional service is better than amateur, and shall learn that the sufferer is as often pained as cheered by ministrations that not seldom owe their origin to forms of mysticism, fanaticism or hysteria.—*British Medical Journal.*

Billroth's Patient Dead.—The patient on whom Billroth operated, January 29th, for cancer of the pylorus, died May 23rd, symptoms of a return of the disease having shown themselves three weeks before. The autopsy revealed a recurrent colloid cancer, which in all probability had arisen from the retro-peritoneal lymphatic glands and had spread over the entire abdominal peritoneum. The outer surface of the stomach, the transverse colon, as also the neighbouring parts of the duodenum and jejunum, were covered with colloid cancer, so that it was difficult to isolate the stomach and duodenum. The stomach was of a natural shape, so that no one would have suspected that a piece 5½ inches long had been removed from it. A sort of sac-like dilatation was found in the site of the greater curvature; notwithstanding this, however, the patient had borne and digested her food well up to the time of her death. There was no stenosis at the point of union of the stomach and duodenum, and it was with difficulty that the line of suture could be distinguished.—*Deutsche Medizin. Wochensch.*, June 4th.

The proper way to give Aconite.—In the London *Medical Record*, Dr. Wm. Murrell makes some judicious observations on the correct plan for administering aconite so as to secure its most advantageous action. He observes that aconite does act best in small doses frequently repeated. Many practitioners get no good from aconite, because they do not know now to use it. The dose of the tincture recommended in the *British Pharmacopœia*—from 5 to 15 minims—is absurdly large, and no one with any respect for his patient's safety or his own reputation would ever think of giving it. The best way is to put half a drachm of the tincture in a four-ounce bottle of water, and to tell the patient to take a teaspoonful of this every ten minutes for the first hour, and after this hourly for some hours. Even smaller doses may be given in the case of children. The great indication for the use of aconite is elevation of temperature; the clinical thermometer and aconite bottle should go hand in hand. If properly used, aconite is one of the most valuable and indispensable drugs in the pharmacopœia.

Out-Patient Treatment of Rickety Tibiæ.—Dr. T. F. Chavasse of Birmingham, finding that osteotomy can be safely performed under antiseptic precautions for the relief of rickety curves in long bones, has successfully operated for deformity of the tibia on twelve children, all under five years of age. In these cases the curves were mostly lateral; and in none was it necessary to remove a ridge of bone to bring the leg into a straight position. After cutting down on the concavity of the curve of the tibia, along the inner edge of that bone, the chisel is employed to cut from within outwards until the tibia is so far divided that the fracture may be completed with the hands. The fibula breaks close to the fracture of the tibia. Antiseptic dressing is then applied, and suitable splints secured by a plaster-of-Paris bandage; the patient is then sent home. At the end of six weeks—the plaster bandage being removed about the fifteenth day—the splints are taken of, and the child is able to run about.—*Brit. Med. Journal.*

Small-Pox and the Efficacy of Vaccination.—This question has recently had new facts brought to bear upon it by Dr. Buchanan. During the past year the death-rate per million in London, from small-pox, was ninety among the vaccinated against three thousand three hundred and fifty among the unvaccinated. Similar statistics show that the mortality among children under five years of age was forty and one-half per million among the vaccinated, against five thousand nine hundred and fifty among the unvaccinated. Among adults the mortality rates are one hundred and eleven for vaccinated, to one thousand nine hundred and six for unvaccinated. These figures show very clearly the efficiency of vaccination, and also the need of revaccination.

CANADA

Medical and Surgical Journal.

MONTREAL, AUGUST, 1881.

THE ANNUAL MEETING.

We devote as large a space as possible this month to giving a full Report of the Proceedings at the Annual Meeting of the Canada Medical Association, at Halifax. Although the attendance was not large, still it may be considered to have been successful. The papers read had been carefully prepared, and contained much that was of interest. We are glad to see that the Association is to continue its well-directed efforts towards obtaining legislation tending to establish some systematic supervision of the public health. The important matter of animal vaccine received a good deal of attention, there being a strong feeling that it would be well if a proper supply of reliable lymph could be constantly maintained by the public authorities for use throughout the country.

Socially, everything was done by the profession of Halifax to render the meeting pleasant as well as profitable. On the second day, at noon, a steamer was placed at the disposal of members and friends, and, after a pleasant sail down the harbour, landed them at the Provincial Lunatic Asylum, where a bountiful lunch had been prepared. In the evening, there was an illumination in the public gardens, with music and torchlight procession.

The place of meeting for next year is to be Toronto, and Dr. Geo. E. Fenwick is the President-elect. We congratulate our predecessor of the JOURNAL upon this high mark of confidence and respect from the united profession, one to which his long services in many ways in the service of the public have rendered him fully entitled.

CANADA MEDICAL ASSOCIATION.

The annual meeting of the Canada Medical Association was held in the Legislative Council Chamber, Halifax, on the 3rd and 4th August, 1881.

On the first day, the meeting was called to order at 10 o'clock, by Dr. Canniff, the President of the Association.

Hon. Dr. Parker, as chairman of the Committee of Arrangements, presented a verbal report.

Moved by Dr. Clark, seconded by Dr. Oldright, that Dr. Strong, Superintendent of the Cleveland (Ohio) Lunatic Asylum, be elected a member of the Association "by invitation."—*Carried.*

The military and naval surgeons of Halifax were also elected members by invitation.

Dr. Strong and the ex-presidents present were requested to take seats by the President.

The minutes of last session at Ottawa were read and approved. Dr. McDonald of Londonderry, Drs. Slayter and Lanigan of Halifax, Dr. Townshend of Parrsboro, and Drs. Somers and Fitch of Halifax, were elected permanent members.

An invitation was read from the Sandy Cove Bathing Establishment, asking the members to avail themselves of the privileges of the baths.

Dr. Reid, Halifax, read the report on Medicine. Special attention was drawn to the disease known as General Paralysis of the Insane—a malady of most fatal character and on the increase, and not receiving sufficient attention. The report was received for discussion.

Dr. Stewart, of Brucefield, Ontario, read the report on Therapeutics.

The President of the Association, Dr. Canniff, read a paper on "Vital Statistics and Pnblic Health." The President stated that the committee appointed at the last meeting had waited upon Sir John A. Macdonald, and had been accompanied and assisted by many of the medical men now in Parliament, that the Government are heartily inclined to assist in forwarding the movement to provide for the public health, and that if it had not been for the very indifferent health of the Premier himself, it is probable that legislation on this important matter would, before this, have been introduced into the Dominion Parliament. He believed that the Association was doing a good work in keeping the subject before the country, and hoped they would continue their efforts until brought to a satisfactory issue.

Hon. Dr. Parker considered this a most important matter; hoped that further action of a decided nature would soon be taken. His idea is that our aim should be to have a committee formed of good representative men from each Province to initiate and watch the progress of a bill for this object. This law-making should begin with the separate Provinces, each for itself, and the whole should be consolidated under some Act governing the entire Dominion, and passed by the House of Commons. Sir J. A. Macdonald used formerly to say that all matters connected with statistics belonged to the Provincial Legislatures, but he has seen reason to change this opinion, and would be ready to admit the control of the general government over statistics and such like matters which are necessarily intimately connected with sanitary legislation. They had recently held a meeting of the profession of Nova Scotia at Antigonish, and had been able to lay the foundations for taking their share in the proposed plan of concerted action.

The report of the President was received, and laid on the table for future discussion.

Moved by Dr. Botsford, seconded by Dr. Steeves, that the following compose the Nominating Committee: Drs. Robillard, Ross and Fenwick of Montreal, Dr. Eccles of London, Drs. D. Clark and A. H. Wright of Toronto, Drs. Lawson and K. F. Black of Halifax, Dr. Steeves of St. John, and Dr. Atherton of Fredericton.—*Carried.*

Dr. Hill of Ottawa then read for Dr. Grant of Ottawa a short paper descriptive of a method of using the ordinary enema-syringe for a stomach-pump. This method has already been described by Dr. Grant in the last volume of the CANADA MEDICAL AND SURGICAL JOURNAL, to which we would refer our readers.

Some members objected to the method, that it would be found very difficult to introduce a flexible and soft tube down the esophagus, but Dr. Hill said that he had been assured by Dr. Grant that in trying the instrument he had not experienced this difficulty.

The Association adjourned at 1 p.m.

AFTERNOON SESSION.

The President took the chair at 2.30 p.m., and proceeded to read his address on "Medical Ethics." He stated that it was with some difficulty he had selected a subject for an address which might be of practical interest to the Association, and he finally determined to review the present code of ethics by which we are guided, and make some remarks upon certain of the clauses. He entered fully into the duties of the members of the profession towards the public, towards each other, and towards themselves. Towards the public, in leaving nothing undone tending to the restoration to health of those entrusted to their care; towards each other, in the most delicately honorable bearing; towards themselves, in not neglecting those much-needed recreations and moments of rest which the generally overworked practitioner so much requires. He strongly deprecated any assumption of superiority, pointing out that the proper line of conduct for a physician was that of the unobtrusive gentleman; advised free, untrammelled consultations in all cases when difficulty or doubt presented themselves; and endeavored, throughout his address, to show that a code of medical ethics could not be otherwise than in harmony with a Christian code of ethics. But charlatanism, in or out of the profession, received a severe castigation. The address was of a very practical character, and cannot fail of having a beneficial tendency in recalling attention to many of those points upon the strict observance of which depends the existence of harmony amongst our *confrères*.

In accordance with a previous resolution, a discussion on Dr. Reid's paper followed, in which Dr. Clarke, of Toronto, Dr. Jennings, of Halifax, Dr. Botsford, of St. John, Dr. Hill, of Ottawa, Dr. Morse, of Amherst, and Dr. Oldright, of Toronto, took part.

The report on Therapeutics, read by Dr. Stewart, was next discussed. Several members gave their views on the comparative safety of chloroform and ether, the former being the favorite.

Dr. Atherton said that in his opinion the bad results in Great Britain from chloroform were chiefly to be attributed to two causes. 1st, the complicated apparatus frequently made use of, and 2nd, the dread which they appear to have of it. In Edinburgh it is given freely and he thinks carelessly. In judging of the comparative merits of various anæsthetics we should be guided more by the opinions arrived at by those who are in the habit of daily administering it, and not so much from the results obtained by experiments. He gave some particulars concerning a case (published in the *Canada Lancet*) where he had performed Tracheotomy for the purpose of resuscitation from chloroform poisoning.

Dr. Hingston asked why, in this case, a tube might not have been passed *per vias naturales*, avoiding the operation. The answer was that, opening the trachea was the idea which first presented itself in the urgency of the moment, and it was fortunately successful.

Dr. Fitch spoke strongly in favor of ether which he uses exclusively. He thinks that drawing the tongue forcibly forward should always answer every purpose for admission of air into the trachea.

Dr. Stewart said that many were in the habit of entirely neglecting the pulse, regarding the respiration only. He thought that this was a mistake, that the pulse should be carefully observed. Kepler has shown by sphygmographic tracings that, in all dangerous cases, there is great fall in the blood-pressure. He knew of three deaths in three years in Edinburgh alone. French experimenters have shown that the application of very hot water to the cardiac region is of great service in stimulating the heart's action.

Dr. Oldright referred to the anæmia observed in chloroform administration as indicative of syncopal tendency, and to the frequency of accidents in dentists' chairs, the latter being due perhaps to two causes, the semi-erect position, and the known danger of interference with the fifth nerve. He had made one trial with Bromide of Ethyl, using f. ʒ i. He entirely failed to anæsthetize the patient and has never used it again.

Dr. Oldright then exhibited his method of treating empyema. After the chest is punctured with a trocar, and the pus drawn off, he attaches a tubing, passing through a vessel containing an antiseptic solution, and held some distance above the patient, the pleural cavity is then washed out and fluid is passed through until it returns quite clear, and this is repeated every few days. Dr. O. gave several cases treated in this way, in which the results had been very satisfactory. In one the expansion of the lung had been such that subsequently no difference could be detected between the two sides.

Dr. Jennings preferred a counter opening, but also advocated washing by syphon.

Dr. Fenwick thought the plan had no advantage over simple incision. This plan was now used by him in the Montreal General Hospital and was very satisfactory. He employed Lister's dressings. Never advises aspiration, for the pus always re-collects. Does not think recovery is ever complete, but that there always remains some shrinking of the affected side.

Dr. Atherton formerly treated it by washings but had abandoned the plan, finding it inconvenient and reaching as good results by incision and dressings of carbolized oil. He agreed with Dr. Fenwick as far as concerned operations on adults or aged persons, but believed that in the young, perfect expansion of a lung could be obtained. He alluded to the fact that sudden death had occurred from injecting the pleura.

Dr. Farrell advocated draining by a tube with the extremity beneath an antiseptic solution, as being cleanly and effectual. Always used an oval and not a round tube, as fitting better between the ribs.

Dr. Geo. Ross said that the procedure of Dr. Oldright contained nothing novel. It was better than syringing, as giving a less forcible stream. The principle of very copious washings was that taught by Fraentzel and the Germans.

He alluded to the plan by valvular drainage advocated by Dr. Phelps, of Chateauguay, N. Y., but could not admit that any other proceedure ever gave better results than a large incision and Lister's dressings, without any injections.

EVENING SESSION.

The President took the chair at 7.30 p.m.

Dr. Bessey, of Montreal, read a very interesting paper on "Vaccination from animal vaccine." In the paper he refered to the prominence which vaccination with lymph direct from the animal had already attained. He called attention to the bad results which had followed vaccination in the past especially in former years in the city of Montreal, when done with long humanised lymph which had in spite of every care used in its collection, conveyed various materies morbi associated with the vaccinal disease.

He took it for granted that certain propositions were now accepted by the profession from which other prepositions naturally followed. 1st, That vaccination was our best prophylactic against small-pox. 2nd, That not to be disappointing it must be well and thoroughly done with lymph capable of reproducing a perfect vaccine vesicle. 3rd, That to avoid "accidents" the lymph must be pure. That to fulfil the obligation resting upon the practitioner it was necessary to avoid the use of either degenerated lymph from too long human transmission, or lymph containing blood impurities, which it could hardly fail to do if taken promiscuously from human subjects. He showed by drawings of the disease when in full bloom and the resulting scars, 15 varieties of typical vaccinal cicatrices here given, that bovine lymph or heifer transmitted lymph induces a development of vaccinia in a greater state of perfection, and of more protective efficacy, in consequence, than humanised lymph. That the calf lymph was benigner in its action and gave all the results of true Jennerian vaccination. He would not deny that humanised lymph might by carefulness in selection, in the hands of careful men, be used for even 30 or 40 years with apparently satisfactory results as regards accidents, but it was now established beyond cavil that each remove a greater distance from the animal preceptibly shortened the period of duration of the disease and diminished its effect on the constitution, thus lessening the amount of protection afforded by the operation. That vaccine being indigenous to the heifer, does not degenerate: the painting of the arm shown is from a child vaccinated from lymph taken from the 240th heifer, from the original spontaneous cases which occurred at Longue Pointe, near Montreal, in Nov. 1877, during which year an epidemic of animal pox prevailed among cows and horses. He traced the progress of animal vaccination, and mentioned the various new stocks of animal lymph that have been introduced to the profession since the time of Jenner, 1798, which were, Woodville in 1800, Passey of France in 1836, Galbeata's retro-vaccination in Italy 1810 followed later by Prof. Negri. The introduction of animal vaccination into France by Janvix, discovery of the Beaugency stock in 1868 by Prof. Depaul, the Longue Pointe stock by himself in 1877, and the progress of animal vaccination under Dr. Warlomont in Brussels, and last of all its introduction into England by Act of Parliament in 1881. That he had vaccinated three children of a family with lymph from a case of horse pox, and two of the same family with the cow pox, as an experiment upon the same day, the result was in both cases the development of typical vaccinal vesicle, the horse pox producing rather more local disturbance but running its course and terminating satisfactorily. That accidents follow vaccination and lack of prophylactic effect, are directly traceable to an imperfect vaccination with imperfectly developed or impure lymph. That a perfect vaccination consisted in the reproduction of a perfect vaccine vesicle with its attendant constitutional fever, and nothing else; that he feared, and believed in the possibility of conveying syphilis, skin affections, scrofulous taints, &c., with humanised lymph. He described a number of spurious vaccinations which might result from the operation, none of them protective, and suggested revaccination at an early date in all doubtful cases, which is not like past vaccinal inoculation—illegal. He concluded by instancing the following advantages to be derived from the use of heifer lymph: 1st, It guarantees against the possibility of transmitting any other blood contamination. 2nd, The advantages of constant supplies of reliable lymph. 3rd, It gives the greatest possible guarantee of protection by emulating perfectly spontaneous vaccination, as observed by Jenner on the hands of milkers, and which has always been found to give absolute security against future contagion. 4th, It enables the practitioner to be independent of his patients as to his stock of lymph. It had been objected to it that it was hard to take, this objection would be entirely removed with due care in its propagation and use, which he very fully explained, showing that both producer and user must use considerable judgment in the matter to secure success. He concluded a most interesting paper with the hope that the Association would press upon the attention of the Government the duty of establishing a National Vaccine Institution for the benefit of the whole country.

Dr. Slayter does not believe that syphilis can be communicated by vaccination. He has always used lymph supplied by the Royal Institution, and has never been dissatisfied with the results. He thinks with Dr. Bessey that there should be some means by which the public could be supplied with pure vaccine lymph.

Dr. Robillard said that in 1874, during an epidemic of smallpox, he vaccinated two children with lymph procured in Liverpool from the Royal Institution. In both of these, eruptions showed themselves, one of which he felt satisfied was of a syphilitic nature, and which disappeared under mercurial treatment. He had never felt safe with that lymph since.

Dr. McDonald (Londonderry) procured his vaccine from Boston. He found that animal lymph was more insoluble than humanized lymph, and ignorance of this fact probably led to some of the failures when the former was used. He would also urge on the Government the importance of their taking charge of this matter.

Dr. Cowie said that formerly the lymph used in Halifax was perfectly satisfactory. In 1860 he had, in one day, vaccinated 120 persons; only six or seven failed, and in none were there any troublesome symptoms. During the past two or three years it had not been so satisfactory. There were now many more failures, and he had recently seen a man, vaccinated a month before, with large unhealed ulcers and enlarged glands.

Dr. Geo. Ross said that he would like to bear testimony from his own observation to the excellent results which had followed the introduction of animal vaccine in Montreal. Previous to this, with the ordinary crusts and lymph which were passed along from one to another, not only were failures comparatively frequent, but unpleasant consequences were often met with. He had seen long-standing ulcers, axillary abscesses, erysipelas and cellulitis, and even, in rare cases, pyæmia with multiple abscesses. These unfortunate occurrences had led to the widespread opposition to vaccination which had prevailed in Montreal. Now, however, we had a supply of pure animal lymph, which we used with perfect confidence, and could say that such accidents as the above never occurred. He was satisfied that animal lymph should always be used when procurable, and that to that end it was highly desirable that the Government should arrange some plan for perpetuating and disseminating a generous supply of the pure article.

Dr. Bessey, in reply to certain enquiries by members, said that he was in the habit of personally selecting perfectly healthy young animals exposed for sale for the purpose of inoculation. He keeps always two in the stable—one in the later stages and the other partly vaccinated. He once used a lean, poor heifer, but found that the lymph was bad, and caused weak, unhealthy sores. He was obliged to recall all the results of that inoculation. He found from experience that for human vaccination it was better to charge points on the sixth day and not wait till the vesicles were at their heighth on the eighth day; but that for inoculating another heifer, he would wait till the eighth day or later. The reason for this is, that in the first case, for complete absorption, you require a thinner lymph than in the latter case. Full maturity also implies a larger size of the lymph vesicles which renders them unsuitable for use on the human subject, but has no effect when used for bovine inoculation.

On motion of Dr. Black, seconded by Dr. McDonald, it was resolved that, as the time was limited, no discussion on any paper should exceed ten minutes.

Dr. Worthington (Clinton, Ont.) then read a paper on "The Treatment of Scarlatina Maligna by Cold Water and Ice." He selected a number of instances where, during the epidemic prevalence of this disease in his locality, he had adopted this treatment in apparently very desperate cases, accompanied by high temperatures and the usual concomitants of delirium or coma, and had saved many cases thereby. In these frightful attacks, such is his confidence in these antipyretic measures, that if he cannot gain the consent of the friends to their employment, he prefers to retire from the responsibility of their treatment. He urged very strongly the more general adoption of these very valuable measures of combating this formidable complaint.

Dr. Jennings spoke highly of the plan of inunction for reducing fever, and

Dr. Fitch said that he had latterly employed glycerine for the same purpose, and found it answer well.

Dr. Coleman advocated the repeated cold-water bathing in this as well as in typhoid fever.

Dr. Eccles remarked that the same principle as advocated in the paper applied to all febrile diseases when violent symptoms seemed purely due to fever-heat.

Dr. Fenwick then read a paper on "Antiseptics in Ovariotomy and other Surgical Operations." (This article, which contains a number of Dr. F.'s hospital and private cases, will appear later in this JOURNAL.)

No discussion owing to the lateness of the hour.

The next paper was by Dr. Hingston, "On certain features in Ovariotomy." The reader of the paper dealt hurriedly with the history of the operation in Canada, giving credit to the late Dr. Robert Nelson of having performed the first ovariotomy here. He went into some of the reasons why ovariotomy had not, until recently, been as successful in Canada as in Great

Britain, one chief reason being that the operation had been performed too much like other operations, with a view rather to speed than thoroughness. He disposed of the claims from time to time put forward to cure ovarian cysts by other than surgical means. He admitted that spontaneous cure sometimes occurred, and mentioned two instances under his own observation. He discouraged too early operation, while yet no discomfort is felt, and while yet the tumor is insignificantly small and when the parietes of the abdomen had not undergone that process of thinning which fits it for the operation. He deprecated that eager hunting for cases which led to unnecessary operations on the one hand, and, on the other, that avoidance of an operation which seemed more than usually hazardous lest the fair average in statistics should be disturbed. He spoke of the circumstance noticed by operators generally that good cases run in succession and bad ones in like manner, and thought it due to atmospheric conditions which we could not at the moment recognize, but which we soon learned to respect. Dr. Hingston then gave the particulars of his last fifteen operations, dismissing his successful ones with a few words, but dwelling at length on the cause of death in the unsuccessful ones. All the operations were completed, though the adhesions in two cases were of a nature to almost demand discontinuance. He had learned to regard adhesions to the parietes as of small moment; more formidable were those to liver, spleen or intestines, but what he most dreaded was intimate connection with the omentum, from the difficulty of separating them and proneness of that viscus to hæmorrhage, and the great difficulty of controlling it without extensive ligaturing. He considered the length of time occupied in the operation of small moment, and he did not think the length of the incision (under certain limits) of great moment, yet he thought an incision greater than necessary was unpardonable, and an instant more time in the performance of an operation equally unjustifiable. He thought limiting the number of spectators of the first moment, and that the direction of the wind in blowing in at, instead of out, should not be overlooked, especially in hospitals. He was averse to the use of the clamp; he had seldom used it, and had regretted its use. He had found the thermo-cautery unreliable as a hæmostatic, except with very small vessels, and in these compression forceps usually sufficed. The anæsthetics used were always the same—chloroform till complete anæsthesia, and ether during the continuance of the operation.

In reply to Dr. Slayter, Dr. Hingston said, with reference to antiseptics, that in most of the cases Listerism had been carried out thoroughly; in a few, not. He could not, so far, recognize any difference in the two methods.

Dr. Slayter was surprised to find Dr. Hingston not in favor of Listerism. Compare any old statistics of this operation with those of the present day, such as those of Spencer Wells and Knowesly Thornton. It is Listerism which has been the means of enabling these operators to shew their marvellous successes The term absolute cleanliness is very vague. He had seen what was called Listerism in many of London Hospitals, and he called it a perfect parody, and therefore they did not believe in it. The truth is that the lukewarm men never did the system justice and thus failed to look on it with favor. Let us give it a *fair* trial, that is all its advocates want. Why, operators did things now they would not have dreamt of doing before the introduction of Lister's dressings.

Dr. Black supported the same views.

The Association adjourned at 11.10 P.M.

MORNING SESSION, AUG. 4.

The Association met at 9 A.M.

The Treasurer's report was submitted, and Drs. Hill and Atherton were appointed auditors to examine and report upon it.

The Secretary, by direction of the President, exhibited some spruce shaving splints sent by Dr. Grant, of Ottawa.

Dr. Slayter exhibited an ingeniously-contrived self-retaining speculum, which enables the surgeon in certain cases to dispense with the service of an assistant.

Dr. J. W. Macdonald, of Londonderry, read a paper on

"Water Analysis," and at the same time exhibited a case containing chemicals and apparatus for the examination of water. He answered questions put him by Drs· Coleman and Hill.

Dr. Stewart of Brucefield, read a paper on "Treatment of Exophthalmic Goitre by ergot," and, at its conclusion, replied to questions by Drs. Steeves and Coleman.

Dr. Coleman read a paper on "The use of the Ophthalmoscope in the diagnosis of brain disease." He cited several cases and their mode of treatment, and his success in such treatment.

Dr. Jennings read a report of some cases in practice, shewing the effect on the temperature of a patient on a water bed by using hot or cold water; also some cases shewing the effect of constant irrigation with carbolized water as compared with the ordinary Listerian spray and gauze. At the same time he exhibited an instrument used in the process of irrigation, which was worked on the syphon principle.

The accounts of the acting General Secretary, Dr. A. H. Wright, for $11.39, and of the Local Secretary, for $21.40, were ordered to be paid.

Dr. Slayter gave notice of the following resolution:

"WHEREAS,—The system of specialism and specialists, which at present obtains to a certain extent in the Dominion, and which has developed to a very large proportion in the neighboring Republic, is for the most part the outgrowth of superficial professional education and want of success as practitioners of medicine and surgery;

"THEREFORE RESOLVED,—That it is the opinion of this society that specialism should be discountenanced by the members of this society, and that specialists should be treated and looked upon as irregular practitioners, except in rare cases, where long experience, extended study, and peculiar aptitude have placed a medical man in a special positon towards his brethren;

"BE IT THEREFORE RESOLVED,—That the members of this society pledge themselves to do all in their power to check the growth of this species of evil."

In supporting his resolution, Dr. Slayter said the evil complained of was ruining their profession in America, and must be stopped if they ever expected to come up to the European standard.

Dr. Farrell spoke of the difficulty of the doctors getting together in these annual meetings, as now held, and thought the smaller societies in the Maritime Provinces should be consolidated into a branch of the Dominion Association. He moved that a committee be appointed to consider the matter and confer with the various provincial medical societies for the purpose of bringing about a plan of organization of the medical societies in the Dominion in connection with the Canada Medical Association. Drs. Clark, Canniff, Hill, Fenwick, Hingston, Steeves, Atherton, J. F. Black, Farrell and the Secretary were appointed such committee.

Dr. Fenwick of Montreal, for Dr. Howard, brought up a notice of motion made at last session to amend chap. 7, sec. 2, of the by-laws, so as to impose a fee of $2, to be paid by each member only at every annual meeting attended.

The motion passed.

Dr. Page made a short speech on sanitary legislation, and moved that Drs. Canniff, Oldright, Grant, Hill, Bruce, of Ontario; the President-elect (Dr. Fenwick), Drs. Osler, Larocque, of Quebec; Botsford and Atherton, New Brunswick; and Hon. Dr. Parker and J. W. Macdonald, of Nova Scotia, be a committee to seek from the Dominion Government improved legislation in respect to sanitation and vital statistics, and to insist upon the organization of the profession as a condition of political support at the next election.—The motion passed.

On motion of Dr. J. F. Black, seconded by Dr. Slayter, the Committee on Public Health was instructed to hold a conference with the committee on the same subject of the Nova Scotia Medical Society.

It was decided to defray the travelling expenses of the Secretary and Treasurer from the funds of the Associaton.

The President of the Association having announced that Dr. A. H. David had withdrawn from the office of General Secretary of the Association, a resolution was passed expressive of the Association's deep regret that any cause should prevent him from continuing his services, and more especially that this cause should depend upon personal indisposition The success of the Association had heretofore largely arisen from the steady and persevering efforts of Dr. David, and the Association trusted that he might for many years witness the continued success of an institution to which he had been so devoted.

The auditors, Drs. Hill and Atherton, reported having carefully examined the Treasurer's accounts, which they find to be intelligently and well kept and quite correct. They show $188.35 received since last September and $133.66 expended, leaving a balance on hand of $4.69.

Dr. Oldright gave notice that at next meeting he would move that clause 18 of by-laws should be amended by substituting the words "Public health, vital statistics and climatology," for the words, "Climatology and epidemic diseases."

On motion of Dr. Slayter a vote of thanks was passed to the railway companies for reduced fares.

On motion of Dr. Atherton a vote of thanks was passed to the Sandy Cove Bathing Company and the Local Government, the former for the use of baths, and the latter for the use of the Provincial building.

On motion of Dr. Hill a vote of thanks was passed to the medical profession of Halifax for their kindness to visiting members.

The following is the report of the nominating committee which was read by the chairman, Dr. Robillard:

President—Dr. Fenwick, of Montreal.

General Secretary—Dr. W. Osler, of Montreal.

Treasurer—Dr. E. Robillard, Montreal.

Vice-President of Ontario—Dr. D. Clark, of Toronto.

Local Secretary of Ontario—Dr. A. H. Wright, Toronto.

Vice-President of Quebec—Dr. F. W. Campbell, Montreal.

Local Secretary of Quebec—Dr. Belleau of Quebec.

Vice-President of Nova Scotia—Dr. R. S. Black, Halifax.

Local Secretary of Nova Scotia—Dr. C. D. Rigby, Halifax.

Vice-President of New Brunswick—Dr. P. R. Inches, St. John.

Local Secretary of New Brunswick—Dr. C. Holden, St. John.

Committee on Arrangements—Dr. D. Clark, Oldright, Temple, A. A. McDonald, of Toronto, with power to add to their number.

Committee on Necrology—Drs. Fulton, Toronto; Atherton, Fredericton; Lachapelle, Montreal.

Committee on Education—Drs. Eccles, London; Holmes, Chatham, and Bessey, Montreal.

Committee on Climatology and Public Health—Drs. Botsford, St. John; Worthington, Clinton, Ont.; Larocque, Montreal; McDonald, Londonderry, and Coleman, St. John.

Committee on Ethics—Drs. Canniff, Toronto; Malloch, Hamilton; Gardner, Montreal; Marsden, Quebec; Bayard, St. John; Parker and W. J. Almon, Halifax; Steeves, St. John; Beaudry, Montreal, and Chas. Moore, Sr., London.

Committee on Publication—Drs. Ross, Montreal; Cameron and Fulton, Toronto; the general Secretary and Treasurer.

Committee on Practice and Medicine—Drs Lawson, Halifax; Graham, of Toronto; Duncan, of Bathurst.

Committee on Surgery—Drs. Shepherd, of Montreal; J. F. Black, Halifax; and McFarlane, Toronto.

Committee on Obstetrics—Drs. Temple, of Toronto; Trudel, Montreal, and McKarren, St. John.

Committee on Therapeutics—Drs. Tye, Thamesville; Wilkins, Montreal, and Somers, Halifax.

The Committee recommended that the next meeting be held in Toronto, the time to be decided by the Association.

The report was adopted *en bloc*.

On motion of Dr. Hingston a vote of thanks was passed to the retiring President for his able conduct in the chair and his admirable address, containing many useful and practical hints. This was acknowledged by Dr. Canniff amidst applause.

The association then adjourned to meet in Toronto on the first Wednesday of September, 1882.

DR. ANDREW CLARK.

The *Whitehall Review* has an article on Dr. Andrew Clark. As this eminent physician is well known in Canada owing to his having accompanied H.R.H. the Princess Louise, and from the fact that he is at present in attendance upon Sir John A. Macdonald, the following may be found of interest:—

"Generally speaking, we may say of medical men that we have a new school and an old one. The old school were wonderful conversationalists. The patients looked forward to a brief, chatty, brilliant talk as the best part of the interview. The new school is much more business-like. At once you come to the point. The examination is a piece of work to be got through, and in as workmanlike a way as possible. The patient is simply 'a case.' The patient of this celebrated physician will be unfortunate if he do not carry away some wise suggestion or interesting remark from Dr. Clark. He will certainly be struck by what is said to himself. A full, clear interpretation will be put on the facts that have seemed so baffling to him. There will be no reticence or obscurity in the opinion formed. A prescription, of course, will be written, for it seems to be *de rigueur;* a doctor seems always writing a prescription. But the patient sees that the doctor is watching, following, and assisting nature. He understands that the treatment is philosophical and physiological. He is to put himself under regimen. His cure will depend much on his own resolution and self-government. As, in most cases, the illness has been superinduced by chronic causes, so it must be met by chronic treatment. Such I take to be the ordinary line adopted by the patients whose ailments still permit them to make personal calls. Of course the whole field of therapeutics in which modern science has made such rapid advance is open to our doctor, but the basis of all solid treatment is the obvious, common-sense, natural procedure, of which the patient is himself able to judge, and by which he is most impressed. Dr. Clark is a younger and more athletic-looking man than you would expect from the long period during which he has been before the public. He bears the traces of labour and care, and no one has better reasons to appreciate the advantages of a holiday, especially if it be in one of Sir Donald Currie's steamers. He has a Scottish name and descent, and is a very Scotchman of the Scotch. There is something that is almost suggestive of the Hebrew in the cast of his face and features, but they wear an expression of kindness and sympathy which in itself has a soothing efficacy. He has been long and intimately connected with the London Hospital, of which he is physician. Twice a week, at an immense personal sacrifice, he is there to lecture, and he is a man who is never five minutes after his time. In his waiting-room you will not fail to notice a large and elaborate ornament presented to him in recognition of priceless services rendered in the awful cholera time. The London Hospital, the poorest in point of endowment, is largest in the number of its beds and the range of its usefulness, and Dr. Clark may claim his full share in its development. I once heard it casually stated as a curious fact that the Radical section of the Cabinet are patients of Dr. Clark. Well, I suppose they appreciate radical treatment in their own individual cases. City men come in crowds to him. A good dietetic treatment was probably the very thing they wanted, and would receive. Those who dine not wisely but too well will find the stern, undeviating regimen, which would most likely be imposed, decidedly salutary. A large proportion of our most successful physicians come from the city westwards. I could cite many names both of the present and the last generation. Dr. Clark, without losing his old friends, has acquired troops of others, from Royalty downwards. He is probably one of those physicians whose lot it is to be baroneted. Why not make some great physician or surgeon a peer at once? The French had their Barons Larrey and Nélaton; why should we not follow such worthy precedents?

"For a man on whom the public has no mercy, and who is supposed to be sometimes obliged to work his eighteen hours a day, Dr. Clark has a remarkable breadth of intellectual interests. The two subjects to which his attention seems specially directed are metaphysics and theology. No doubt these have a direct relation to the higher problems of life and mind. 'In natural science,' as George Eliot truly says, 'there is nothing petty to the mind that has a large vision of relations, and to which every single object suggests a vast sum of conditions.' I believe that very often a serious and complicated case may have much light thrown upon it by material derived from a region that seems altogether remote from pathology. The higher problems of mind will frequently cast a light on obscure conditions of body. Dr. Andrew Clark is extensively read in patristic literature. He was a Greek prizeman in his day, and has a natural affinity for the Greek Fathers. And not only is he ecclesiastical, but ecclesiological. His line of life necessarily takes him all over the country, and I believe I am correct in saying that his first thought in any brief season of leisure is to visit the church of the locality. Then, as for the general conversation, there are, indeed, very few items of talk which you can carry away. You are impressed, not so much by what our doctor says as by what he does *not* say. As Mezzofanti knew how to hold his tongue in thirty languages, so a physician is silent about three thousand cases. His conversation is literary and scientific; perhaps I ought to call it philosophical. When names are used, it is simply the names that are indicative of systems. He puts his mind fairly to yours; he brings matters to a direct issue. I will put down a few remarks of Dr. Clark on the subjects arising in conversation, or addressed to his students in lecture. 'Every Monday and Thursday I go to the London Hospital. It is work I love and glory in beyond everything. I consider that nothing is little, nothing is unimportant. What seem slight directions must be scrupulously carried out. I have been an hour and a half in the London Hospital investigating a case. I was two hours over a case yesterday. In the mystery of the human will, in the play of human thought which connects the visible with the unseen, in the emotions which agitate the human breast, there is an element of disturbance, which, in the phenomena of disease, is almost always in action, and which, in the calculation of causality, can never be precisely estimated.' (This illustrates the intercommunication of body and mind.)

"Dr. Clark is not opposed to the infliction of suffering on animals, though I will not say that he goes the length of vivisection. 'What is all the suffering,' he asks his students in one of his lectures, 'inflicted by all the vivisectionists of all the world in comparison with the hecatomb of suffering which political experimenters have inflicted upon mankind in their attempts to settle the question of the balance of power in Europe? Are the sufferings of men of less account than the sufferings of brutes? Are the countless woes of human hearts to be reckoned but as dust in the balance against the wounds of guinea-pigs and frogs? Doctors are not like publicans—those ardent promoters of health, morality and happiness—a numerous and powerful body that can turn the tide of political party. We are still political nobodies. When we are sufficiently represented in Parliament and upon the Privy Council, and when we have a Minister of Health, who shall be also a member of the Cabinet, we shall probably take our just place.'

"I asked him whether he believed there was a general concert of scientific opinion in favour of the doctrine of Evolution. No; his own opinions were certainly not that way. Unbelief is spreading rapidly. There is no absolute scientific argument for a resurrection; he accepted the doctrine, but accepted it as a matter of faith. 'I am particularly fond of St. Chrysostom. From what one reads of him, and especially when one is able from other sources to read between the lines, I am persuaded that modern Ritualism is to be found in the early Greek Church, say at the beginning of the fifth century. The Anglican clergy only accept the first four General Councils, while the Greek Church take the six. The clauses of the first four Councils do not occupy much space, but most Anglicans are not acquainted with their contents or know to how much they are pledged.'

"This seems a favourite aphorism. 'Pathological changes grow out of long-continued mental disturbances;' which illustrates the medical epigram, 'All acute illnesses are chronic.' Finally, I may quote his own high standard set forth to his students and characteristic of his own career. He defines it as 'that spirit of sacrifice, sincerity, and faith which should rule your ways and works in life, and will place you in filial relations to the Eternal Mind.'"

—The *Popular Science Monthly* for August contains the following:—The Herring, by Professor T. H. Huxley, F.R.S.; Physical Education—Recreation, by F. L. Oswald, M.D.; The Blood and its Circulation (illustrated), by Herman L. Fairchild; The Teachings of Modern Spectroscopy (illustrated), by Dr. A. Schuster, F.R.S.; Origin and History of Life Insurance, by

Theodore Wehle; The Insufficient Use of Milk, by Dyce Duckworth, M.D.; Intelligence of Ants, by George J. Romanes; Lunar Lore and Portraiture, by F. E. Fryatt; The Visions of Sane Persons, by F. Galton, F.R.S.; School-room Ventilation, by Dr. P. J. Higgins; Origin and Uses of Asphalt (illustrated), by Leon Malo, C.E.; The Unit in Plant-Life, by Byron D. Halstead, Sc.D.; The Electric Storage of Energy; Sketch of Robert Wilhelm Bunsen (with portrait); Correspondence, Editor's Table, Literary Notices, Popular Miscellany, and Notes.

Medical Items.

PERSONAL.—Mr. Rankine Dawson, student in medicine of McGill, passed his primary examination in anatomy and physiology for the degree of M.R.C.S., at the meeting held in London on the 4th July.

RIDEAU AND BATHURST MEDICAL ASSOCIATION.—The following are the officers elect for the ensuing year: *President*, Dr. Cranston; *1st Vice-President*, Dr. Lafferty; *2nd Vice-President*, Dr. Baird; *Secretary*, Dr. Bentley; *Treasurer*, Dr. Hill.

—The following appointments have been made in the Toronto School of Medicine: *Adjunct Lecturer on Midwifery*, Dr. W. W. Ogden; *Adjunct Lecturer on Surgery*, Dr. M. H. Aikins; *Adjunct Lecturer on Medical Jurisprudence*, Dr. W. Oldright; *Adjunct Lecturer on Anatomy*, Dr. L. McFarlane; *Adjunct Lecturer on Materia Medica and Therapeutics*, Dr. George Wright; *Assistant Demonstrator of Anatomy*, Dr. John Ferguson; *Assistant Secretary*, Dr. A. H. Wright.

THE TRANSPLANTATION OF BONE.—The greatest discovery in surgery, thus far in the year 1881, is that of Dr. William MacEwen. He has successfully transplanted bone—fragments of wedges of bone taken from patients for curved tibiæ—into the arm of a child whose limb was useless by reason of extensive necrosis: two-thirds of the humerus had been destroyed and no repair of bone had taken place. A good new humerus was the result, less than an inch shorter than its fellow.

STATISTICS OF NEPHRECTOMY.—Dr. Barker, *Lancet*, April, 1881 : Number of cases on record, 54 ; recoveries, 26 ; deaths, 28. In eleven of the cases a wrong diagnosis was made. The lumbar operations show rather better results than those in the linea alba.

—A prominent physician of Cincinnati who was taking a mixture of cascara sagrada and strychnia for constipatation, discovered that the alkaloid was acting as an aphrodisiac ; not being in need of such a remedy, he wrote a note to a neighboring druggist, in which he stated the case, and requested that the prescription be refilled, minus the strychnia. His messenger returned with the medicine and the following laconic reply: "Here's your cascara ; for G—d's sake send me the strychnia !"

—A sick boy : "Oh, Doctor, I'm so glad you've come. I don't know what's the matter with Charley, at all. He complains of the febrile rise in his peritoneum, and he says his hypochondrion is all twisted out of shape. Oh, he's an awful sick boy, Doctor." "I should say. Must have been reading the Presidential bulletins." The doctor leaves a seidlitz powder and departs.—*New Haven Register*.

—In Old England, marsh poison in ancient times swept down the haughtiest heads of the nobility and of royalty. Henry of Agincourt, Wolsey, Devereux, Lord Deputy of Ireland, and a host of distinguished persons died of dysentery or some cognate disease. Mary of England, Pole, James I, Cromwell and Charles II. died of marsh fever. It is a fact, albeit a quaint one, that the Reformation was, validly, the first step in the march of sanitary reform in England. It led to the filling up of the moats and stews, fish-ponds and lakes, which furnished diet for fast-days, and which maintained a constant supply of paludal poison at the very door-step of every country house in England, just as the tank or water-pit does to-day beside each hovel in Bengal.—*Chevers on the Physician's Leisure*.

—Anent doctor's signs, the *N. Y. Record* says : The brazen sign is large ; it covers the whole door-post, it stretches from window to window ; its lettering is brilliant, and it is set off with scroll-work in the corners; the passer-by sees it, and cannot but read it; small boys shout out the name as they go by, and adults mutter it over till they reach another block. It is judiciously placed so that the street-lamp illumines it at night. It affects the more public ways, and it indicates the astute and enterprising physician. He is one who maintains a dignified equipoise between the Code which says, "Thou shalt not advertise," and the Bible which says, "Let thy light so shine." In these days, when æstheticism is in the ascendant, when every man of thorough culture lunches at least once a week on the sight of a lily, it would be strange if a love of the beautiful did not affect the style of that corner slab of modern civilization—the subject of this discourse. The Æsthetic Sign, in its supremest development, consists of a black marble slab, in which the physician's name is carved and gilded. When especially "intense," the letters are old Roman, with golden punctuation marks, which delicately suggest to the looker-on that he come to a full stop. Some superficial critics have already classified these evidences of the union of the beautiful with the pilular, as "mortuary signs"—a name which is uncanny and which stamps its user as a Philistine.

—If the President's recovery is much longer retarded, there will be but little further use for Medical Journals, as the newspapers are giving daily essays on the subject of his wound, treatment, etc. Some of them combine science and poesy in a manner wonderful to read. For instance: "There are sleeping organisms in the blood which fever wakes at 102° Fah. Then death summons its drowsy cohorts in tiny legions for their ghastly work. But they have slept there since babyhood, waiting for the signal. We begin to die when we begin to live. In all parts of the body are colonies of animalculæ as independent of us as we are of the stars, but no more so. As complete is their organization as ours, and with as good a reason for existence, as clear an office, and possibly as bright a future. In the crystal chambers of that masterpiece of Nature, the eye, they revel or rest, living out like us their day. And more wonderful still, even they have parasites as dependent and as independent. All this we say we know, but we know it in that misty, hazy way we know the stars go round, because somebody said so, and nobody contradicted him." The author of the above is an Indiana man, and the only way it can be explained is, that he was taking his usual daily anti-ague medicine—whiskey and quinine.—*Peoria Monthly.*

FELLOWS' HYPOPHOSPHITES.—The attention of our readers is called to the advertisement of Fellows' Compound Syrup of the Hypophosphites, which appears for the first time in our pages. Having used this preparation for some years, we have no hesitation in recommending it in cases of overwork and where a good, reliable and pleasant tonic is required.

WYETH'S PEPTONIC PILLS.—This pill will give immediate relief in many forms of dyspepsia and indigestion, and will prove of permanent benefit in all cases of enfeebled digestion produced from want of proper secretion of the gastric juice. By supplementing the action of the stomach, and rendering the food capable of assimilation, they enable the organ to recover its healthy tone and thus permanent relief is afforded. One great advantage of the mode of preparation of these pills is the absence of sugar, which is present in all the ordinary pepsin and pancreatin compounds; in this form the dose is much smaller, more pleasant to take, and is less apt to offend the already weak and irritable stomach. The results of their use have been so abundantly satisfactory, that we are confident that further trials will secure for them the cordial approval of the medical profession.

MALTOPEPSYN —The following letter from a Toronto physician speaks for itself:—

TORONTO, 26th July, 1881.

HAZEN MORSE, ESQ.

DEAR SIR,—In reply to your letter of the 12th inst., asking our experience of the use of Maltopepsyn in the Infants' Home, I beg to say, on my own account and for Doctors McDonald and Pyne, whom I have spoken to on the subject, that much benefit has been derived from the employment of your preparation wherever the use of agents required to promote digestion was indicated.

It has been found beneficial, also, in vomiting accompanying diarrhœa among the infants of the Home, and is advantageously administered in certain forms of diarrhœa.

Yours truly,

J. H. BURNS, M.D.,

Consulting Physician at Infants' Home.

CANADA

MEDICAL & SURGICAL JOURNAL

SEPTEMBER, 1881.

Original Communications.

ON WATER ANALYSIS.

By J. M. MACDONALD, M.D., L.R.C.S.E.
Medical Officer, Steel Company of Canada, Londonderry, N.S.

(Read before the Canada Medical Association, at Halifax, 3rd August, 1881.)

I am frequently asked, by both medical men and laymen, to give some ready method by which the fitness or unfitness of water for domestic purposes can be ascertained. For answering the question several difficulties present themselves. The cost of apparatus for a complete examination of water is a serious matter; few persons have the time or inclination to carry out detailed chemical analysis, and, lastly, a conclusion as to the purity or impurity of water must be based upon a collection of all the evidence that can be obtained, rather than from the results of one or two tests. The vital importance of the subject and the lively interest which is being awakened in regard to it, have led me to attempt the description of water analysis, which will be sufficient for ordinary purposes, and at the same time fall within the means and the opportunities of every medical practitioner. Two years ago I imported from Savory and Moore of London, one of the Parks' cabinets for water analysis. It cost me, inclusive of duty about $150.00, and nearly one half of the contents were destroyed by breakage. As few would care to go to that expense, I have endeavoured to meet the difficulty by preparing a small, cheap, and at the same time efficient case of chemicals and apparatus, which should not cost more than $12.00 or $14.00. The case is 18 inches long, 5 inches wide, and 9 inches high. Inside it contains the following chemicals in three ounce bottles :

Standard solution of Nitrate of Silver.
Sol. of yellow Chromate of Potash.
Solution of Soap.
Solution of Nitrate of Barium.
Two shaking bottles for soap test.
Nessler's solution.
Dilute Sulphuric Acid.
Sol. of Iodide of Potassium and Starch.
Standard Solution of Ammonium Chloride.
" " Permanganate of Potassium.
Oxalate of Ammonium.

The apparatus consists of :

1 Flask with ring for boiling.
2 India rubber caps with two necks.
1 retort stand.
1 Burette with clamp.
India rubber tubing.
Spirit lamp.
5 Test tubes
Glass rod.
" measure 50 C. C.

In the examination of water, the coarser physical characters such as colour, smell, taste and transparency should first be noted. The *colour* is best observed by pouring the water into a tall glass vessel and looking down upon it. A perfectly pure water has a bluish tint, and the bottom of the vessel is clearly seen through several feet of water, while some waters are so turbid as to obscure the bottom when only a few inches are looked through. A green colour as a rule indicates vegetable impurity, a yellow or brown colour (excepting in peat water), animal impurity. *Smell* is best observed by warming, boiling, or distilling the water, when characteristic odors are frequently given off. The evidence derived from an examination of the physical characters is very unreliable, we must therefore proceed to an examination of the dissolved solids, which gives us the most valuable evidence. The examination is divided into the qualitative and quantitative.

I. *Qualitative.*—The most useful tests are the following:

SUBSTANCES SOUGHT FOR.	REAGENTS TO BE USED AND EFFECTS.
Reaction	Litmus and turmeric papers—Usual red and brown reactions.
Lime	Oxalate of Ammonium—white precipitate.
Chlorine	Nitrate of Silver and dilute Nitric Acid—White precipitate becoming lead colour.
Nitrous Acid	Iodide of Potassium and Starch in solution and dilute Sulphuric Acid—A blue colour.
Ammonia	Nessler's Solution—A yellow color or yellow-brown precipitate.
Nitric Acid.............	Sol. of Sulphate of iron and pure Sulphuric Acid —Olive colored zone.
Oxidisable matter including organic matter ...	Permanganate of Potassium—Red colour disappears.

II. *Quantitative.*—1st, Determination of chlorine: Prepare a solution of Nitrate of Silver by dissolving 17 grammes in one litre of water. Take 100 C. C. of the water to be examined, place it in a white porcelain dish. Add enough solution of yellow chromate of potash to make it just yellow. Then add the nitrate of silver solution from a burette and stir. A red colour is produced which disappears as long as any chlorine is present. Stop when the least red tint is permanent, then read off the number of C. C. of nitrate of silver used, each of these represents 3.55 milligrammes of chlorine. Multiply by 10 to give the amount per litre, and this again by .07 for grains per gallon. Chlorine in water is very suspicious of the presence of the liquid excreta of men or animals. If in addition we find nitric and nitrous acid, ammonia and phosphoric acid the evidence is very strong. Chlorine however may be due to strata containing chloride of sodium or calcium. In this case the water is alkaline from sodium carbonate. In some cases the chlorine is due to impregnation from sea water. It is then large in quantity, there is also magnesia, and little evidence of organic matter.

2nd, *Hardness.*—This is estimated by Clarke's soap test and by it we determine—

1st, *Total hardness*, representing the aggregete earthy salts and free carbonic acid.

2nd, The *removable hardness* or that which disappears on boiling.

3rd, The *permanent hardness* which is unaffected by boiling.

By the soap test can also be determined the amount of certain constituents such as lime, magnesia, sulphuric acid and free carbonic acid.

Apparatus required for the soap test.—Measure of 50 or 100 C. C. Burette divided into tenths of a cubic centimetre, two or more stoppered bottles to hold about 4 ounces. We also require the following solutions :

1 *Standard solution of Barium Nitrate.*—Dissolve 26 grammes of pure barium nitrate in 1 litre of water, or 18.2 grains to 1 gallon. A concentrated solution of ten times this strength may be made and diluted with nine parts of water when used.

1 *Solution of soap.*—Dissolve a piece of soft potash soap of the British Pharmacopœia in equal parts of water and alcohol ; filter and then graduate as follows :

Put 50 C. C. of the standard solution of barium nitrate into the shaking bottle and add to it slowly the soap solution from the finely graduated burette. After each addition shake vigorously and place the bottle on its side. Continue this until you have a thin beady lather over the whole surface permanent for five minutes. Read off the amonnt of soap solution used ; if exactly 2.2 C. C. have been taken the solution is correct. If less the soap solution must be diluted with spirit and water. The amount of dilution can be ascertained by a simple rule. Suppose 1.8 C. C. bave been used and the whole of the unused soap solution measures 200 C. C. then

$$\text{As } 1.8 : 2.2 :: 200 : x.$$
$$x = 244.4 \text{ C.C.}$$

The 200 C.C. must then be diluted with equal parts of spirit and water to 244.4 C.C.

With these solutions, and having all glasses, burette, etc., perfectly clean, for the least quantity of acid would destroy the accuracy of the process, we can proceed as follows :—

1. *To determine the total hardness of the water.*—Take 50 C.C.

of the water in a stoppered bottle, and add the soap solution from the burette, shaking strongly after each addition until a lather permanent for five minutes spreads over the whole surface without any break; then read off the number of tenths of soap solution used; from this number subtract 2, as that quantity is necessary to give a lather with 50 C.C. of the purest water. The soap solution which has been used indicates the hardness due to all the ingredients which can act upon it; as a rule, they are lime, magnesian salts, iron, and free carbonic acid. It is usual to express this hardness by degrees of Clarke's scale. Though dependent upon various causes, it is considered as so much calcium carbonate per gallon, one grain of calcium carbonate per gallon being one degree of Clark's scale.

The calculation is as follows: Each tenth of the soap solution corresponds to .25 milligrammes of calcium carbonate; multiply this co-efficient by the number of tenths of soap solution used, and the result is the hardness of 50 C.C. Multiply by 20 for the amount per litre, and by .07 for grains per gallon or degrees of Clark's scale.

To obtain the permanent hardness.—Boil a known quantity briskly for half-an-hour, replacing the loss with distilled water from time to time; cork the vessel and allow it to cool. Then determine the hardness in 50 C.C. as before.

Removable hardness.—This is very easily calculated, for we have only to take the difference between the total hardness and the permanent hardness and express the result as removable hardness. The permanent hardness is the most important, for it represents the most objectionable earthy salts, viz., calcium, sulphate and chloride, and the magnesian salts. The permanent hardness of good water should not exceed 3 or 4° of Clark's scale.

The next step in our investigation is the

Determination of free or saline Ammonia, and of Nitrogenous Organic matter.—Ammonia in water is chiefly derived from organic substances, either vegetable or animal. In the detection and estimation of ammonia, the very delicate test known as Nessler's solution is of the greatest value. Nessler's solution is thus prepared: Dissolve 50 grammes of iodide of potassium in 250 C.C. of distilled water; reserve a small quantity; warm the larger portion, and add a strong aqueous solution of corrosive sublimate until the precipitate ceases to disappear, then add the reserved solution of iodide so as to just dissolve the red precipitate; filter, and add to the filtrate 200 grammes of solid potash dissolved in boiled water. Dilute to 1 litre, and add 5 C.C. of a saturated aqueous solution of mercury bichloride. Allow to subside, decant the clear liquid, and keep in a dark place. In addition to this solution, we require *Standard Solution of Ammonium Chloride*, which is of the strength of .0315 grammes to 1 litre of water; each C.C. represents .01 milligrammes of ammonia. The mode of procedure is as follows: Place in a flask 250 C.C. of the water to be examined; distill off about 120 C.C.; measure this distillate carefully, test a little with Nessler's solution in a test-tube, and observe the colour; if not too dark, take 100 C.C. of the distillate and put it into a cylindrical glass vessel, and place it upon a piece of white paper. Add to it 1½ C.C. of Nessler. Put into another similar cylinder as many C.C. of ammonium chloride as may be thought neessary, and fill up to 100 C.C. of pure distilled water which has previously been proved to be free from ammonia; drop in 1½ of Nessler. If the colours correspond, the process is finished, and the amount of ammonium chloride used is read off. If the colours are not the same, add a little more ammonium chloride, so long as no haze shows itself; if it does, then a fresh glass must be taken and another test made. When the colours correspond, read off the C.C. of ammonium chloride used; allow for the portion of distillate not used; multiply by .01 and we have the number of milligrammes of free ammonia in the 250 C.C. acted upon; multiply this amount by 4, and we have the number of milligramme per litre.

Example.—From 250 C.C. of water 123 were distilled; 100 C.C. were taken for the experiment; 4.5 C.C. of ammonium chloride were required to give the proper colour; then $4.5 \times \frac{123}{100} \times .01 \times 4 = 0.2214$ milligrammes of free ammonia per litre.

The free ammonia or saline ammonia is the ammonia combined with carbonic, nitric, or other acids, and also what may be derived from any easily decomposable substance such as urea. The quantity should not exceed .02 milligrammes per litre in good water. Having calculated the free ammonia, the residue of the water in the retort is used to determine the nitrogenous organic matter as measured by albuminoid ammonia. The nitrogen is converted into ammonia by means of potassium permanganate, in presence of an alkali; the ammonia is then distilled off and estimated as above.

Dissolve 8 grammes of permanganate of potassium and 200 grammes of solid caustic potash in one litre of water; boil thoroughly to drive off any ammonia and destroy any nitrogenous matter. This is known as Wankhyn's solution. Add to the residue in the retort 25 C.C. of this solution; distil over 110 to 120. Calculate the ammonia as before, and state the results in this case as *albuminoid ammonia*. The standard limit of albuminoid ammonia in good water is stated by Wankhyn to be .05 milligrammes per litre; some other authorities place it at .08. Much albuminoid ammonia, little free ammonia, and almost entire absence of chlorides, is, according to Wankhyn, indicative of vegetable contamination.

Oxidisable Matter.—The chief sources of oxidisable matter in water are oxidisable organic matter and nitrous acid as nitrites. The estimation of these affords valuable evidence of the character of water and are conveniently determined by means of permanganate of potassium. We calculate first, *total oxidisable matter* in terms of oxygen required for its oxidation. Make a solution of permanganate by dissolving 395 grammes of the crystallized salt in 1 litre of water. Each C. C. of this solution yields 0.1 milligramme of oxygen in presence of an acid. Test its accuracy by a solution of crystallized oxalic acid, of the strength of .7875 grammes to the litre of water. This solution, acidulated with diluted sulphuric acid, should exactly decolorise an equal quantity of the solution of permanganate. The process as recommended by Woods is as follows:

"Take a convenient quantity of the water to be examined, say 250 C.C.; add 5 C.C. of dilute sulphuric acid (1 to 10); drop in the permanganate solution from a burette until a pink colour is established; warm the water up to a 140° F., dropping in more permanganate if the colour disappears; when the temperature reaches 140 remove the lamp, continue to drop in the permanganate till the color is permanent for about ten minutes. Then read off the number of C. C. and multiply by 0.1 to get the milligrammes of oxygen and by 4 to get the amount per litre." The amount of oxygen obtained by this process includes that from organic matter and nitrous acid. To separate these we must drive off the nitrous acid by boiling with sulphuric acid as follows: Take 250 C. C. of the water under examination; add 5 C. C. of dilute sulphuric acid as before; boil briskly for 20 minutes, then allow it to cool down to 140° F. add the permanganate solution until a pink colour remains for ten minutes; then calculate as before. The result in this case must be stated as milligrammes per litre of oxidisable organic matter or *organic oxygen.*

Nitrous acid is now easily determined for it is represented by the difference between the two preceeding processes. Each milligramme of oxygen is equivalent to 2.875 milligrammes of nitrous acid, the difference must therefore be multiplied by this factor and the result is nitrous acid in milligrammes per litre. From the foregoing tests we can gain sufficient evidence to form an opinion of the character of a given sample of water. The inferences from this evidence can be drawn as follows: A large quantity of nitric and nitrous acids, much oxidisable and nitrogenous organic matter, with much chlorine indicates recent sewage impregnation. With little oxidisable organic matter and nitric acid in large amount, we assume that more or less complete conversion of organic matter has taken place. Albuminoid ammonia and nitric acid in abundance, and free ammonia and chlorine in small amount is indicative of vegetable contamination. Little chlorine with much albuminoid and free ammonia, nitrous and nitric acids show contamination from gaseous emanations.

To those who have not the inclination or the opportunity to carry out an analysis such as I have described, a few ready tests may be useful. Any druggist can prepare from the formulæ already given the following solutions: Nitrate of silver, Nessler's solution, solution of permanganate of potassium and solution of Iodide of Potassium and starch. Provided with these they can proceed as follows:

1. Observe the colour.
2. Observe the smell, particularly when the water is boiling.
3. The taste.
4. Add to a small quantity of the water, in a test tube or wine-glass, a little of the solution of nitrate of silver. If it gives a white colour it contains chlorides. This is a very suspicious sign.

To another portion of the water add a small quantity of Nessler's solution. A yellow colour or yellow-brown precipitate shows the presence of ammonia.

6. Add a few drops of the solution of permanganate of potassium. The pink colour remains if the water is pure; it disappears if the water contains organic matter.

These simple tests would in most cases settle the question of the purity or impurity of a suspected water. The amount of disease and suffering caused by the use of impure water is in this country assuming terrible proportions. Epidemics of typhoid and other zymotics are constantly occurring which could be easily prevented by a little care in examining the water and discontinuing the use of impure wells. This is one of the evils arising from the want of public health legislation. Surely the day is near at hand when our Legislature will protect the lives of our people from this as it does from other forms of poisoning, and furnish us with the means whereby we can control the causes of preventible disease. Then shall we gain a happy victory over those dread enemies which are desolating the homes and destroying the lives of so many of the brave sons and daughters of this prosperous Dominion.

A QUARTERLY RETROSPECT OF SURGERY.

Prepared by FRANCIS J. SHEPHERD, M.D., C.M., M.R.C.S., Eng.
Demonstrator of Anatomy and Lecturer on Operative and Minor Surgery, McGill University; Surgeon to the Out-Door Department of the Montreal General Hospital.

Resection of the Stomach and Intestines.—Prof. Nussbaum of Munich says that it is not so very long since a suggestion, made by the surgeon, Carl Theodor Merren, to remove cancer of the stomach, was looked upon as a "beautiful dream of youth." However, Prof. Czerny demonstrated practically five years ago that a person can continue to live after the whole stomach has been removed; he cut out the entire stomach and stitched the œsophagus to the intestine, the digestive functions were carried on very well, and the patient had good health. Three cases of resection of the intestine have lately been recorded by Czerny. In two, a coil of intestine, which had become gangrenous as a strangulated hernia, was removed; and in the third, a malignant tumour of the colon was excised. In one of the first two instances the patient recovered without fever or reaction of any sort; in the second, the patient died during the operation in a fit of vomiting. In the third case, a woman, aged 47, had a large tumour of the transverse colon, which was attached to a coil of the sigmoid flexure. Part of the sigmoid was first resected and the ends brought together with thirty-three sutures, and then a wedge-shaped piece of the meso-colon was removed and ligatured. A drainage-tube was inserted, and the wound in the abdomen closed by deep and superficial sutures. The patient recovered, and was living half a year after the operation. Antiseptic dressings were used.—(*Berlin Klin. Woch.* and *Dublin Journal of Medical Science*, July, 1881.)

A still more remarkable case of resection of the intestine, which was seccessful, has been reported by Koeberlé of Strasburg (*Gazette Hebdom.*, 1881), and in this case the operation was not done antiseptically. A young lady, aged 22, had suffered frequently from colic, and in October, 1880, symptoms of intestinal strangulation occurred twice in fifteen days. Since then she had suffered from persistent colic, which could hardly be subdued by hypodermic injections of morphia. Gastrotomy was performed on November 27th. Four strictures were found involving six and a-half feet of small intestine, the slighest having a diameter of one-sixth of an inch. He removed *six and a-half feet* of intestine, and tied twelve vessels. Tne ligatures from the two free ends of the intestine were tied together and attached to the fibrous tissue of the linea alba through a suture, which retained them in contact with the peritoneum at the inferior angle of the abdominal incision. The ligatures of the mesentery were brought out at the inferior angle also, and were retained, together with the sutures of the intestine, in a fixed position. The superior part of the wound was partially closed. Enterotomy was performed on the third day; the ligatures and sloughs separated on from the 12th to the 13th day; the first alvine discharge took place on the 20th day. On the 25th day, communication with the intestine was almost closed, and six weeks after the operation the external wound was also closed and healed. According to latest accounts the patient feels quite well, and suffers no gastric disturbance

The series of successful operations for *Resection of the Stomach* by Prof. Billroth and his assistant is perhaps the most remarkable advance which has of late been made in operative surgery, not even excepting the successful cases of excision of the kidney which are now not infrequently reported in the various medical journals. The fourth patient on whom Prof. Billroth performed the operation of resection of the stomach lived for several months, sufficiently long to establish the occasional advisability of undertaking this operation. An additional interest attaches itself to this patient from the fact that an autopsy was obtained (*Wiener Medizinische Wochenschrift*, No. 22.) Dr. Zemann, who directed the post-mortem, found that death had resulted from metastatic deposits of cancer throughout the entire peritoneum, duodenum and jejunum. The stomach remained quite natural in form, and no one would have guessed that fourteen centimetres had been removed from it. The woman had not suffered from any digestive troubles, but had taken and retained her food. At the point of junction of the duodenum with the lesser curvature of the stomach there was no stenosis, the thumb being easily passed through the orifice. The union was perfect in all respects, so that hardly a scar could be perceived along the line of suture.

Removal of the Spleen.—This old operation, which was formerly recommended for the cure of melancholy, has, from time to time, been performed, and quite lately a prominent surgeon of Detroit has incurred a great deal of obloquy by removing this organ for hypertrophy. Of course the operation was unsuccessful. It seems to be much more dangerous to remove it in human beings than in animals; in dogs it has been frequently removed without bad results. The *Gaz. Med. Lombardia* describes a recent operation as follows: "Dr. Chiarleoni performed, at the Casa di Salute, Milan, March 26th, splenectomy on a female patient suffering from paludal cachexia, in the presence of a large number of distinguished colleagues. The operation, executed with great method and freedom, was very laborious, owing to the extensive and strong adhesions of the spleen to the left edge of the liver and the diaphragm. It was impossible to tie all these adhesions before removing them, and a very considerable hæmorrhage from the surface ensued; and this, conjoined with a certain amount of nervous exhaustion, caused the woman's death a few hours after the termination of the operation. As far as we are aware, so bold an operation has not been executed in Italy except on one occasion by Drs. Zaccharelli and Fioravanti, at Naples, in 1549." (*Med. Times and Gazette.*) The propriety of such heroic operations is, to say the least, questionable, notwithstanding the "great method and freedom" with which they are "executed." Whilst on the subject of "heroic operations," I shall quote the following: "*Surprising Surgery.*—Those who are interested in the advance of operative surgery will not fail to be struck by some of the recommendations of German surgeons. During the proceedings of a congress held in April last, Dr. Zeller of Berlin suggested that, as a prophylactic measure in operations about the mouth and throat, the trachea should be divided about the 3rd and 4th rings. The lower end should be fastened at one corner of the transverse incision in the skin, the upper end at the other corner, so that the discharges from the operation wound may be prevented from obtaining access to the lungs. After the operation, the two ends of the divided trachea may be brought together again. That this operation would be attended with danger to the patient probably few persons would be prepared to deny—perhaps with a danger as great, or greater, than that it is intended to guard against,—and we must congratulate Dr. Zeller's dogs on having so well recovered from it. But in ingenuity of suggestion and in boldness of performance, this operation of Dr. Zeller's cannot compare with that of Dr. Gluck (Berlin), for this gentleman hopes that, sooner or later, the complete removal of the bladder and prostate—which he has carried out successfully in dogs—may be introduced into surgery. It may, says Dr. Gluck, be performed on men without opening the peritoneum, and the ureters should be fastened to the abdominal wall; for in dogs, the sewing of them into the rectum has not well been borne, and the attachment of them to the cut urethra can scarcely be recommended. We shall watch with interest for Dr. Gluck's account of the first operation of this kind performed upon the human subject. We fear that not many even of our most brilliant surgeons will care much to perform it, and not many patients will care to submit to it when the most favourable result which can be hoped for has been explained to them."—*Beilage Zum Centralblatt für Chirurgie*; quoted in *Practitioner*, July, 1881.

Transplantation of Bone.—Dr. MacEwen, well known for the great success he has had with his osteotomies, presented a paper to the Royal Society on a case in which he had successfully transplanted bone (*Lancet*, May 28). The patient was a child 4 years of age, who had lost two-thirds of the shaft of the humerus by necrosis fifteen months previously, and in whom no osseous repair had occurred. The limb was of course useless. Dr. MacEwen proceeded first to make a groove in the soft tissues in the position of the bone, relying for this on his anatomical knowledge, and then placed in this groove small fragments of wedges of bone removed from other patients for curved tibiæ. The result has been that a good new bone has been formed, the new portion has united firmly to the upper epiphysis and lower part of original shaft, and the bone is only half-an-inch shorter than its fellow. The operations were performed with strict antiseptic precautions. This is the first time this operation has been performed in a scientific manner. The necessity for the operation is fortunately rare, as nature generally is so skilful in the repair of bone that the interference of the surgeon is seldom needed. It is strange that before Dr. MacEwen had made his case public, Mr. McNamara, of the Westminster Hospital, intimated to his class his intention of transplanting bone to supply a deficiency in the tibia of a child. This he has since done, using part of an amputated metatarsus in the transplantation.

This operation resembles greatly that which is said to have been in vogue amongst the Bulgarian peasants for years, viz., when a man has had a compound fracture of the humerus, tibia or other long bone, with considerable loss of substance, they cut out a piece of bone from a living sheep or cow and transplant it into the human subject. Travellers say the results are marvellous, and that the patient almost invariably recovers without any shortening. The transplantation of teeth is now an established operatien in dentistry.

Treatment of Hydrocele.—Many new methods for the treatment and radical cure of hydrocele are being continually brought before the profession. According to most authorities, only a very small percentage of the cases treated by the injection of iodine fail to be cured, and after all, the treatment by this method on the whole gives the best results. In obstinate cases, or where the risk of injection of iodine is too great, other means must be resorted to. Dr. Ogilvie Wills, in the *Edinburgh Med. Journal* for July, relates a case of hydrocele of the cord, where, from the age and infirmity of the patient, he was unwilling to risk the iodine treatment, cure was effected by the introduction of catgut drainage, under full Listerian precautions; in another case of vaginal hydrocele, this method completely failed. His favourite treatment, when not contraindicated, is the injection of iodine according to Mr. Syme's plan, and he has rarely seen it fail. When considerable inflammatory reaction ensues, Dr. Wills has found much relief to accrue from the application of a tobacco poultice, made by boiling an ounce of cut tobacco with a sufficiency of water to make a cataplasm, and then adding linseed until a proper consistency is reached.

Mr. Lister has lately had some successful cases treated by Volkmann's "Schnitt" method—transfixing the skin and sac with two needles and cutting into the sac between them, then stitching the cut edge of sac to cut edge of skin, and applying salicylic jute dressings under the spray. This, without the Listerian precautions, is a modification of an old method, as is also the insertion of setons and drainage-tubes, and it is hardly fair for gentlemen who merely add the Listerian method, to claim these methods as something quite new. The favourite method in Bellevue Hospital, New York, of treating hydrocele in children is by scarifying the inside of the sac. In my hands this has not been at all successful. Mr. S. Osborn lately read before the Medical Society of London the notes of two cases of hydrocele treated successfully by a single tapping, with the subsequent use of the galvano-suspension bandage. The first case was a hydrocele of the tunica vaginalis, which had been present for seven or eight years; and the second was a case of double encysted hydrocele, present for six years—ages 70 and 63 respectively. The galvanism was believed not only to cause contraction of the muscular fibres of the scrotum, but to impart a healthy action to the serous sac, aiding absorption. Mr. Osborn recommended a trial of this bandage in other diseases of the testicle, such as varicocele and neuralgia of the testis.

Subcutaneous Ligature of Varix and Varicocele.—Mr. John Duncan of Edinburgh, in a lecture published in the *British Medical Journal*, July 9th, advocates the subcutaneous catgut ligature for the above affections. He holds that it is singularly easy of application, free from risk and very certain in its results. This is certainly high praise and if these assertions can be substantiated, surgeons will be inclined to perform the operation for radical cure of varix or varicocele much more frequently than heretofore. Most surgeons in the treatment of varicocele have felt it unnecessary and inadvisable to resort to severe measures and have contented themselves with palliative ones, such as suspension, truss, cold douche, etc. Sir James Paget says, "the cases in which varicocele is more than a trivial affair are very few, and in these few it is not such as the sexual hypochondriacs imagine," again, "varicocele is troublesome because of the sense of weight and aching which sometimes, though not always attends it, and in some cases the veins are apt to become inflamed or very sensitive. But this, I believe, is the widest limit of the harm that varicocele ever does." Even after a successful operation the depressed mental condition often continues. To return to Mr. Duncan's operation, from which I fear I have rather strayed. His mode of procedure is as follows: "The veins are carefully separated by the fingers from the artery and vas deferens, and a needle armed with catgut is thrust through at the point of separation; it is again introduced at the orifice of emergence, made to pass between the veins and the skin and finally brought out at the original entrance. The two ends are then firmly knotted, with as much force as strong catgut will bear, and cut short. By traction on the loose skin of the scrotum, the knot is made entirely to disappear, and the punctures are covered with salicylic wool saturated with collodion. The same manœuvre is repeated at the distance of an inch or a little more. The effect is the formation of a hard lump of coagulum between the ligatures, at first slightly tender, but which soon becomes perfectly callous. Mr. Duncan has performed this operation six times with complete success.

He treats varix of the leg in the same way, but does not advise an early operation. He first tries the elastic stocking, even in advanced cases, but when solid œdema and eczema and ulceration cannot thus be kept in check, or perpetually recur, he advises the subcutaneous ligature as being the safest and surest operation. He has had eight successful cases.

So-called Rupture of the Internal Lateral Ligament of Knee Joint.—In a thesis submitted for graduation at the College of Physicians and Surgeons, New York, and published in the *New York Medical Journal* for June, 1881, Dr. Charles A. Jersey questions the existence of the condition known under the above name, and expresses his opinion, on the strength of clinical observations and experiments on the cadaver (the latter having been performed in the prosectors room at the College under the direction of Dr. Wm. T. Bull), that the injury in question really consists in a fracture of the tuberosity, into which the ligament is inserted. His conclusions are as follows: 1. Many cases of so-called rupture of the internal lateral ligament of the knee joint are, in reality, cases of fracture of the internal tuberosity of the condyle. 2. Many of the more severe sprains are fractures of the tuberosity. 3. The absence of bony crepitus is no certain sign of non-existence of fracture at this part. 4. The diagnosis rests on the extreme lateral motion, the severity of the pain on manipulation, the localized pain always found at a certain point, and the length of time required for complete recovery.

Tracheotomy.—Dr. Foulis of Glasgow, well known for his successful case of extirpation of the larynx, says that the tubes generally made for children are too large, and that, as a rule, when used in very young children, completely fill the trachea, and if left in for any length of time, might cause erosion. Dr. Foulis employs five tubes; they are as follows: below 18 months, diameter, 4 mm.; 18 months to 2½ years, 6 mm.; 2½ to 10 years, 8 mm.; 10 to 20 years, 10 mm.; largest size, 12 mm. As to the point for opening the windpipe, he, contrary to the rules generally given, recommends that the incision should be made through the isthmus of the thyroid, in the middle line, where it is, he says, as destitute of blood-vessels as the middle line of the tongue or perineum. He says the high operation requires, especially in children, the dislodgement of the isthmus or division of the cricoid. If a tube is to be worn, it is better not to have the cricoid cut, for its elastic spring keeps up a continual pressure on the tube, leading slowly to irritation and, it may be, perichondritis. In the after treatment, he disapproves of the use of steam.—(*Glasgow Medical Journal*, Feb., 1881.)

Mr. Golding Bird (*Lancet*, March 12th, 1881,) holds that it is improper to introduce the tracheotomy tube immediately after the trachea has been opened. He says no tube should be introduced until the trachea has been cleansed, as far as possible, from all foreign bodies, as membrane, blood-clots, &c., but that other means should be adopted to keep the tracheal wound open. He has acted on this rule in his last eight cases, employing a German nose speculum, the blades of the instrument being inserted into the tracheal wound and then screwed open. He has improved upon this, and now uses his instrument instead of tracheotomy tubes. Mr. Golding Bird remarks that under the old method the greatest anxiety is felt lest the tube should become blocked, and constant cleansing with feathers, &c., has to be carried out at frequent intervals; that the foreign matters can scarcely be expelled *via* the glottis, while the chances of their finding their way out through a rigid bent tube, the end of which hangs freely in the trachea, are very remote. He therefore advises the use of some such method as he has made use of, as being safer, surer, and more rational.

Tubeless Tracheotomy.—Dr. Alfred C. Post of New York, in the *Annals of Anatomy and Surgery* for April, in a short paper, gives his experience of tracheotomy without tubes, according to the method suggested by Dr. H. A. Martin of Boston. He has had two cases; in each, the operation was performed as a preliminary measure to facilitate the continued administration of anæsthetics, and to guard against the entrance of blood into the bronchial tubes in protracted and bloody operations involving the nasal and buccal cavities. In each case the practical result was in the highest degree satisfactory. The opening into the trachea was larger and more direct than in the usual operation, not liable to be clogged with mucus, and unattended by the irritation which is often occasioned by the presence of the tube. He is fully persuaded that the use of the tracheal tube is a source of irritation, and that it is very desirable to dispense with it if possible.

There are objections to both these latter methods. In Dr. Golding Bird's, the constant presence of an instrument pressing against the sides of the trachea would be a continual source of irritation, and might possibly give rise to erosion. What Dr. Bird says with regard to the too early insertion of the tube is sound, and worth making a note of. Dr. Martin's tubeless tracheotomy may be useful as a prophylactic measure in operations about the throat and mouth, but where a permanent opening is needed, there would be great difficulty in keeping it free from exuberant granulations and preventing too early closure. Dr. Zeller of Berlin has, at the congress of German surgeons lately, strongly advocated this operation as a prophylactic measure, as I have noticed above under the heading of "Surprising Surgery."

Thermo-Cautery in Tracheotomy.—Dr. Jules Bœkel, who

advocates this method, gives an epitome of twenty-four cases, in which he thus operated in two years. Previously he had published seven cases. In these cases he employed the thermo-cautery to divide all the tissues down to the trachea, generally using it at a white heat, but the trachea he opened with a bistoury for fear of subsequent contraction, a fear which he has since learnt to be hypothetical. He summarises thus: To-day that I have acquired in the manipulation of this instrument a greater experience, I can affirm its superiority . . . The fear of consecutive narrowing of the trachea after the use of the thermo-cautery, enters into the domain of hypothesis." There is rarely, he says, fear of primary hemorrhage and he has never experienced any trouble from secondary hemorrhage. In twenty-four cases there was complete absence of hemorrhage. (*Gaz. Méd. de Strasbourg*, 1880, in *Dublin Med. Journal*, Aug., 1881).

The use of Antiseptics in Surgery to be made compulsory by legal enactment.—Prof. Nussbaum has of late been strenuously advocating that a law should be passed, making the employment of antiseptics in surgery compulsory or rather that the neglect of their employment should be accounted a criminal act. He states that to his personal knowledge fatal cases are constantly occurring, which could be prevented by the use of even the simplest forms of antiseptics. Now this is strong language and Prof. Nussbaum must look through very green spectacles, in an atmosphere rendered dim by carbolized spray. His experience surely has been a very sad one and surgery in Germany must be at a very low ebb indeed. He out-Lister's Lister and must believe we have at last reached perfection in the treatment of wounds. Such legislation would effectually put a stop to any further improvements in the treatment of wounds and an effective bar would be placed on all advance in surgery. It would be a return to the despotism and stagnation of the Middle Ages. This would be only the thin edge of the wedge, soon the State would make it compulsory to treat fevers by cold baths, to cut off limbs by the galvanic wire (under the spray of course), to employ internal urethrotomy in every case of gleet and many other methods might be enforced, which will readily suggest themselves to my readers. Prof. Nussbaum has been considerably abused for his extreme views and German surgeons hold that the State has no right to enforce the use of any particular method, but, that as long as the surgeon has to bear the responsibility, he must be left free to choose which form of treatment he shall use. It is a pity that the antiseptic system, which has done so much for modern surgery should be thrown into disrepute by the over zeal of its advocates. Prof. Nussbaum after all his tirade would commence his legislation in a very mild manner. There is nothing very objectionable in the following more than the principle involved. "Any person summoned to treat an accidental case or wound, must no longer close it up with charpie and adhesive plaster, nor examine or disturb it with a finger which has not been disinfected; but, after the surgeon has washed his hands and also the wound with some disinfectant (for which purpose a five per cent. solution of carbolic acid seems to be the most convenient), the wound must be thoroughly protected, with an antiseptic dressing. Such dressing may consist of carbolic jute or wadding, chloride of zinc wadding, or some other well known antiseptic material," Such a law he is convinced, would save in his own city alone, the lives of dozens of wounded people and deliver hundreds from a tedious and dangerous suppurative process. Prof. Volkmann, at the recent International Medical Congress in London, delivered a most eloquent address on the advantages of antiseptic surgery or rather Listerism, which has done so much for modern German Surgery. Previous to its introduction the German Hospitals were regarded as *pest houses*, and Listerism has certainly contended successfully against the horrible results of dirt and wound contagion, which were so common a few years ago in Continental hospitals. This great change affords the key to Prof. Nussbaum's vigorous advocacy of compulsory antisepticism. The *Lancet* (Aug. 13, 1881) remarks, that "our admiration for the change effected is only equalled by our horror at the previous condition."

Early Diagnosis of Hip Joint Disease.—Mr. John H. Morgan, in Vol. X. St. George's Hospital Reports, says that among a very large number of patients that are brought to the Hospital for Sick Children on account of lameness, the proportion in which it is due to morbus coxæ, is very considerable. The lameness of morbus coxæ is peculiar. The action of the joint itself is very limited, so that in progression there is a tendency for the pelvis of that side to move, and for the sacro-iliac articulation to take on the part of the more or less fixed hip-joint. Often in hip-joint disease the lameness is hardly perceptible after rest, and only becomes evident when the joint is over-worked and possibly inflamed, and thus the lameness varies in the same patient under different conditions. In congenital dislocation of the hip it is otherwise; the lameness is constant, and the head of the bone in its new position freely movable. (In rheumatism, the lameness is more at first, and wears off after exercise.) The best method of examination is by laying the child naked on a couch, and first grasping the sound limb a little below the knee, and flexing the leg upon the thigh, bend the femur on the pelvis until the thigh touches the abdomen; extension should then be made to the full, and the head of the bone rotated in the acetabulum and made to perform all the movements the joint is capable of. This gives confidence to the patient and affords a standard of comparison to the surgeon. If the same course be pursued with the affected limb, it will be found that a point is reached at which further movement in some direction is impossible, and it is checked by firm muscular action; and any attempt at further movement causes the joint to be fixed and the pelvis to be carried in the direction in which the force is applied. This locking of the joint is a certain evidence of disease, one that is never absent and rarely to be mistaken. Verneuil has stated that he has never come across any case of this disease in which abduction of the thigh was not painful; and Mr. Morgan has found no exception to this rule, though he has carefully sought for it. Extreme extension is next to abduction, the movement in which this fixity of the joint is most frequently found. Fixity of the joint due to rheumatism is sometimes seen in children; but this affection is rare in young children, and in them there is no shortening or wasting of the limb, or flattening of the buttock; all the movements of the joint, except flexion, can usually be performed without pain, and there is no pain on pressure over the trochanter. Chronic rheumatic arthritis occurs only in the elderly, so may be dismissed without further remark. Mr. Morgan states that there is one most important disease which, in an early stage, gives rise to all the appearances which have been above described, namely, disease of the lumbar vertebræ, which, by implicating the psoas, causes it to remain in permanent contraction; and thus to render the femur flexed and somewhat adducted on the pelvis. This contraction may be overcome by manipulation under an anæsthetic (though it is by no means advisable to do so); as soon as the influence of the anæsthetic has passed away, the former condition will be regained. Wasting of the muscles of the limb and gluteal region is a feature which is constantly present at very early periods in hip-joint disease. This wasting is, as Sir James Paget has pointed out, far in excess of that which would result from disease of the muscles alone, and to this wasting he aptly gives the name of "reflex atrophy," and he says "it depends on disordered nervous influence, and seems proportionate to the coincident pain, as if it were due to the disturbance of some nerve centre irritated by the painful state of the sensitive nerve fibres."

This wasting of the muscles forms a valuable aid towards the detection of disease in its early stage; and when it is not due to any central cause, as the condition of the cord which exists in infantile paralysis, is not likely to be symptomatic of any other disease.

In long standing cases of hip joint disease there is observed a shortening of the limb, which is not due to any displacement of the head of the bone or actual shortening of the limb, but to the result of an altered position of the pelvis, which on the affected side is raised to a higher level than that of the opposite side. This Mr. Morgan believes is due to the constant contraction of the iliac portion of the erector spinæ and quadratus lumborum muscles, in obedience to reflex nerve irritation.

BI-MONTHLY RETROSPECT OF OBSTETRICS AND GYNÆCOLOGY.

PREPARED BY WM. GARDNER, M.D.,

Prof. Medical Jurisprudence and Hygiene, McGill University; Attending Physician to the University Dispensary for Diseases of Women; Physician to the Out-Patient Department, Montreal General Hospital.

The Treatment of Rupture of the Uterus by Drainage.—This method of treatment continues to excite much attention in Germany, and cases are occasionally reported. One of the latest of these is by Dr. J. Mann, of the University Obstetrical Clinic of Buda-Pest. The report appears in the *Centralblatt fur Gynakologie* for August 6th, 1881. The patient was aged 24, unmarried. She had already been attended at the clinic, premature labour having been induced on account of generally contracted, flat pelvis, of rachitic origin. She made a good recovery. She again became pregnant, and at what appeared to be the end of the thirty-second week, labour was induced by introduction of a bougie to the uterus. Labour pains began an hour afterwards; 30 hours subsequently the membranes ruptured. There was, however, little dilatation, and the head was still high in the pelvis. An hour and a quarter later bi-polarversion was resorted to. During the operation rupture took place. On vaginal examination after extraction, it was found to be in a transverse direction on the anterior uterine wall. The hæmatoma about the site of rupture, which is believed by some observers to be pathognomonic, was present in this case. After thorough antiseptic vaginal irrigation, a large drainage-tube was introduced through the rent. The vagina was then plugged with carbolized cotton wool. A "T" bandage, with protective over the end of the tube, was applied to the vulva, and an ice-bag placed over the fundus uteri. The irrigation of the laceration with carbolized water was performed through the drainage-tube twice a day. On the fifth day the tube was expelled. The patient made a tedious, but satisfactory recovery, and was discharged on the thirtieth day.

On Hemorrhage and excessive Sickness during Pregnancy; and on Abortion in connection with Inflammation of the Uterus and its Cervix.—By J. Henry Bennet, M.D. *Brit. Med. Journal*, July 9th, 1881.

Messrs Boys de Loury and Costilles at the St. Lazare Hospital, Paris, first brought to light the frequent existence of inflammation of the neck of the uterus, and pointed out that it is frequently a cause of hemorrhage and abortion. Dr. Bennet published the first edition of his work on inflammation of the uterus in 1845 and therein brought forward facts new to the profession, confirmatory of those adduced by French observers already mentioned. A long professional career has confirmed Dr. Bennet in the views then enunciated, and these views have proved to him the key to many obscure phenomena and to their successful treatment.

Briefly stated, the great clinical fact, believed in and taught by Dr. Bennet, is that many women become pregnant while suffering from inflammatory and ulcerative disease of the cervix uteri, or from chronic inflammatory disease of the body of the uterus. A train of erratic and morbid phenomena result and modify the usual course of pregnancy, of parturition, and of the puerperium.

During pregnancy, uterine inflammation causes a variety of pains, aches and sympathetic reactions; intractable sickness, profuse leucorrhœa; erratic, periodical or constant hemorrhage; the formation of moles or blighted ova; abortion, and its concomitants and sequelæ. If the patient have had previous healthy pregnancies, she at once recognizes that she "feels differently." Dr. Bennet believes this to be an important element in forming the diagnosis. He believes intractable vomiting in pregnancy to be caused most frequently by inflammation of the body and cervix of the womb, and contends that if such vomiting does not speedily yield to medicinal treatment, the woman must be examined with the speculum and subjected to local treatment if necessary. The so-called menstruation of pregnancy, Dr. Bennet believes to be nearly always due to inflammation of the cervix.

During parturition, Dr. Bennet believes that many of the accidents of parturition, are due to the co-existence of uterine inflammation. Such are hemorrhage, rigidity of the os, laceration of the cervix, retained placenta and post partum hemorrhage. During the puerperal state, the author believes that uterine inflammation strongly predisposes to most of the accidents of the puerperal period, such as hemorrhage, metritis, puerperal fever, phlebitis, prolonged red or purulent lochial discharge, prolonged inability to stand or walk.

If, on examination, inflammatory disease be found, it ought, Dr. Bennet says, to be treated exactly as in the non-pregnant state, by emollient and astringent injections and if necessary by vitally modifying caustics, such as nitrate of silver, nitric acid, or acid nitrate of mercury, applied to the vaginal cervix and to its cavity if need be. These applications may be made repeatedly if necessary, at 5-days interval for the silver-nitrate and 7 days for the others. Leeches may, and have often been applied by Dr. Bennet to the os with good results and without disturbing the course of pregnancy.

Remembering the frequency of abortion in chronic womb disease, it is well to avail of a hint offered by Dr. Bennet as to the management of such cases. The pregnant woman ought to be told that the fœtus may be actually dead or die soon after the examination. Such being the case, it may be cast off with or without bleeding, and that these results must not be attributed to the treatment.

While we cannot accept *in toto* Dr. Bennet's opinions, we yet believe that uterine inflammatory disease often operates in the manner he has indicated. In any case the presence of the subjective symptoms will at least warrant an examination. One important out-come, if no other will result from such an examination. The practitioner will be prepared for accidents. He will know that he has a bad case to deal with ; "that rigidity of the os ; slow painful labour ; laceration of the cervix ; hæmorrhage, during or after parturition ; adherent placenta ; metritis ; ovaritis ; hemorrhage, purulent, long-continued lochial discharges—in a word, a bad labour and a bad getting up may be expected, in the natural course of things."

An Improved Method of Treating Uterine Displacements.—Dr. Robert Bell of Glasgow, in the *Edinburgh Medical Journal* for July, 1881, gives the result of his experience in the treatment of uterine displacements by vaginal tampons of cotton-wool soaked in a solution of alum and carbolic acid in glycerine. The principle is not new, for Emmet and Bozeman of New York, and others, have advocated similar methods. Emmet, however, prefers oakum to cotton. Dr. Bell's solution is the following: Glycerine, 80 oz.; alum, 10 oz; carbolic acid, 1½ oz. This solution, it will be observed, theoretically—and Dr. Bell claims to have found, practically—fulfils most desirable indications. The glycerine depletes, and so lessens congestion by its affinity for water; the alum constringes, and so braces up the vaginal walls; and the carbolic acid, by its antiseptic properties, renders it possible for the cotton to be retained for a convenient length of time. Dr. Bell at first used the glycerine of tannin of the Pharmacopœia, but although it answered the purpose well, it is expensive, and stains the patient's underclothing. The author of the paper has, during the last two years, treated 200 cases by his method, and for eighteen months has not used a pessary at all. He usually employs only one large tampon, but in some cases of flexion, uses two—a small one pushed well up in front or behind the uterus, and a larger one beneath it. In the case of prolapsus, if there be laceration of the perineum, this must first be rectified. The uterus is elevated as nearly as possible to its normal position, and there retained by a suitable-sized tampon of cotton soaked in the solution. This can be retained for three or four days without becoming offensive, on account of the antiseptic ingredient. The watery depleting discharge excited by the glycerine is believed by Dr. Bell to be much increased by the astringent. He claims to have seen patients thus completely cured of procidentia, which had existed from three to eight years, by perseverance in the treatment for from two to seven months.

Amongst other gratifying results, the author especially mentions the speedy disappearance of bladder symptoms in anteflexions and versions. To sum up, the advantages are: freedom from the dangers of hard pessaries, such as erosions of vaginal mucous membrane, peri-uterine inflammation, &c.; the depleting effect of the glycerine and alum in diminishing congestion and hyperplasia; the rare necessity for the use of the (always more or less dangerous) probe or elevator in flexions; and, lastly, the fact that the physician, with only an ordinary amount of experience and intelligence, can, under proper directions, manage an ordinary case of displacement requiring treatment.

The disadvantages are, to the busy physician, the tedious, prolonged nature of the treatment; and to the patient, the annoyance of such frequent repetitions of unpleasant applications, with the watery discharge consequent upon them. In a certain proportion of cases, we believe that these objections will not weigh as against the good effects to be obtained. On the other hand, the practitioner who has the necessary mechanical ingenuity, and has acquired some experience in the use of pessaries, will not readily give up a means of treatment which, combined with the anti-congestive hot water vaginal injections of Emmet, yields such frequent satisfactory results to his patients, with comparatively little trouble to himself.

The Treatment of Uterine Myoma.—Mr. Lawson Tait of Birmingham discusses this subject in a paper in the number of the *Brooklyn Annals of Anatomy and Surgery* for June of the present year. At the outset, Mr. Tait lays down a proposition with which every practitioner who has seen many cases of uterine fibroid will agree. It is, that the larger number of cases need no surgical interference. The experience of the autopsy room shows how often such tumours exist without symptoms and unsuspected. They either do not grow to such size as to endanger the life or disturb the comfort of the patient, or they do not press upon neighbouring organs so as to cause distress and danger; or they are not accompanied by the most formidable of all their symptoms—hemorrhage. The explanation of this is various. They either grow slowly and imperceptibly. The growth is often absolutely arrested at the menopause, or (very rarely) they completely disappear or undergo chalky degeneration; or their relation to the uterine structure is such that they do not cause bleeding.

Myomata requiring surgical treatment for mere size are rare.

Mr. Tait has met with but two cases. In both he removed the tumour by abdominal section ; successfully in one case, unsuccessfully in the other. Distress from pressure on neighbouring organs (bladder and rectum) are more numerous. Mr. Tait has treated many such, but has succeeded in relieving most of them by pessaries placed so as to ease the weight of the tumour, so that in one case only has operation been resorted to by him. Here enucleation was the method resorted to, and the result was successful.

As regards the hæmorrhage, by far the most frequent condition requiring interference, Mr. Tait gives his experience. It does not support two impressions rather widely entertained about these tumours. He has not found ergot, however administered, alone or combined, to have a decided influence in restraining such bleeding. The intra-uterine injection of astringents has yielded occasional successes, but these have rarely been permanent, and in two cases death was produced directly from the method. In the second place, he has not found (as is generally supposed) the hemorrhage to cease at the ordinary climacteric period. The tumour generally causes prolongation of the menstrual activity for some time, occasionally ten years, after the ordinary period has been reached.

In discussing the results of surgical treatment of such cases, Mr. Tait states his belief that it is not generally recognized how often, what he believes to be, a special risk after uterine operatione in spanæmic patients obtains, namely, that from the formation of fatal heart-clot. If this be true, its bearing upon the question as to the time when operation shall be undertaken is obvious and important. Here a sound judgment by the light of experience will be needed to enable the surgeon to steer between two difficulties—unnecessary operations and operations too long delayed.

As regards enucleation, Tait's experience has been so unfavourable that he has resolved never to undertake it again. He has not always been successful in securing the expulsion of the tumour, and when this was attained, the subsequent recoveries were slow and unsatisfactory. As regards removal by abdominal section, it is to be remarked at the outset that a large number cannot thus be removed, as from their formation and relations they afford no pedicle. In two cases Mr. Tait attempted enucleation by the abdomen, but was obliged to desist, and both patients died. In six pediculated cases he has operated with two successes; using the clamp or ligature. The recoveries were in cases treated by his own clamp. All the cases treated by the ligature died from continuous oozing from the stump. Mr. Tait states that the idea occurred to him in 1871 that removal of the ovaries might be an effectual means of controlling the hæmorrhage, which is, as every one knows, almost exclusively menstrual. He put the idea into practice on August 1st, 1871, in the case of a tumour with menorrhagia. This patient recovered. The case is, however, very vaguely stated. The author operated on two other cases, one in 1873, the other in 1874; both died. Mr. Tait has, since then, operated by ovariotomy ten times for menorrhagia due to uterine myoma, with only one death, and with success in arresting the bleeding. The death was due to heart-clot, in a very much weakened patient. He makes the smallest possible incision, often barely two inches in length, and searches with his left and middle fore-finger for one ovary after the other. He does not remove one until he is satisfied that he can remove both. He transfixes the mesovarium with a hooked needle, and brings a loop of silk through. This he ties by a special knot devised by himself, and called the Staffordshire knot. He has never found it to slip or fail, but does not describe it. The ovaries are then removed by scissors or knife, as may be most convenient.

The treatment of Nerve-pain and other Nervous Symptoms in the Diseases of Women.—It is now some years since Dr. Weir Mitchell of Philadelphia, the eminent specialist in diseases of the nervous system, announced to the profession the splendid results which he had obtained by a new method of treatment, for the hitherto obstinately rebellious condition of neurasthenia, with its multifarious symptoms and associated conditions. These results were announced in a little book entitled "Fat and Blood, How to make them." During the last few months the author has published another and larger book, "Lectures on the

Diseases of the Nervous System, especially in Women," in which he confirms all that he has previously asserted.

Two years ago, Dr. Goodell of Philadelphia, in his presidential address, before the American Gynecological Association, announced the great success he had experienced from the method in the neurasthenia of womb disease. Since then the treatment has become very popular in the United States, and from time to time very gratifying results have been recorded.

Dr. Horatio R. Bigelow of Washington, has recently published the results in two cases, (*American Journal of Obstetrics*, July 1881), representing the extremes of bodily habit, the one being thin, sallow, wan and extremely nervous, the other being stout, phlegmatic and well nourished.

In the first case in addition to the features already mentioned, there was scanty irregular menses, backache, headache, inability to walk, extreme nervous depression, rectal and vesical tenesmus, pain in the region of the right ovary and down the right leg. On examination a short vagina, retroflected uterus, doughy swollen cervix, and tenderness at the neck of the bladder. Mechanical treatment by replacement, Sims' position, proper adjustment of clothing and pessaries did no good, on the contrary seemed to aggravate the symptoms. A variety of other local and general tonic and sedative treatment was tried without avail, as the patient grew worse. She was now placed on the "rest" treatment, with speedy gratifying results. Sleep became natural and refreshing, the circulation of hands and feet became natural, the pains disappeared, the complexion which had been subicteroid, became clear, the digestion perfect, the muscles became developed and the weight of body increased.

The results in the second case were equally gratifying.

If there be one lesson more important than another for the practitioner in the diseases of women to learn, it is this, that the most intelligent local treatment without concurrent appropriate general treatment will often utterly fail to remove the symptoms. The pains complained of often persist after the local difficulties have been remedied. "The rapid strides gynecology bas made, within a few years, the advancement which it must continue to make, and the laudable enthusiasm of its desciples, while productive of great general good, have not been without a measure of harm. There is a tendency to meddlesome interference in many cases, that would be better if left alone, and a proneness to attribute all of her suffering to a uterine cause, in the woman who may have some trouble with her sexual organs. "It is a practice as common as it is unscientific and cruel, to attribute all of these manifestations to the womb, and to suppose that they will subside with the alleviation of the local disturbance." Experience shows the association of uterine disease, chiefly versions and nerve-pain to be most frequent in delicate, sensitive natures, who have known grief or abused themselves in fashionable dissipation. A wifely anxiety for the conduct of a husband, domestic worries, and literary ambition, also frequently conduce to the bringing on of the condition. In some cases the nerve pain is the cry of the whole cerebro-spinal nervous system, rebelling against the extra tax put upon it and demanding rest and nutriment. It indicates the condition of neurasthenia and is associated with dyspepsia, inability to concentrate the mind on a given subject, defective eyesight, gloominess, constipation and insomnia. The primary condition and these its aecessaries, often exist independently of any womb complications. On the other hand, thousands of women with dislocated wombs go through life, with a certain measure of comfort, without any nervous irritability.

The so-called "rest treatment" consists in absolute rest in bed of body and mind, full feeding with nutritious easily digested food; massage and champooing, swedish movements and electricity. In addition to these, various tonic and analeptic drugs may be administered if there be a clear necessity. A careful, experienced, firm nurse is selected; the patient is put to bed in a large darkened room. She is not allowed to assist herself or move in any way. She is not allowed to see her husband or friends or to receive letters from them. She is not allowed to read, sew, or converse on any subject requiring mental effort. Her diet at first is milk only; skimmed milk at first, then eggs, poultry etc. Then massage, which when appropriately practised has a wonderfully soothing effect on the nervous system. At the same time electricity, in the form of both currents may be used, the galvanic for its sedative effect on the nervous system and stimulant effects on general nutrition, the faradic to develop the muscles. This is continued in most cases about six weeks. It may be supposed that the restraint will prove irksome to the patient. Experience shows that it is not so, or at all events only for the first few days.

It will be at once apparent from the above description of the method, that the expense of such a course of treatment must prove a serious draw back to its general employment.

Dr. W. S. Playfair, the eminent London obstetrician, is the first to report the results of the treatment in Britain. This he does in a paper in the *London Lancet* for May 28 and June 11 ult., in which he gives an account of four cases of neurasthenia, neuralgia, hysteria, chloral and morphia-habit connected with uterine disease. All were cured. Dr. Playfair concludes by saying:—"My own conviction is that Dr. Weir-Mitchell has made a most important contribution to practical medicine by the introduction of the method I have been describing"

Reviews and Notices of Books.

The Principles of Myo-Dynamics.—By J. S. Wight, M.D., Professor of Surgery and Lecturer on Physical Science at the Long Island College Hospital. 8 vo. New York: Bermingham & Co.

This little volume treats of the application of mechanics to the muscles and joints of the body. Prof. Wight defines myo-dynamics as treating of the forces of muscles and their effects. He says there are two kinds of myodynamics, viz., *myostatics*, which treats of muscular forces when they are in equilibrium with some other force or forces, acting on a bony lever, as when the hand holds a weight; *myokinetics*, which treats of muscular forces, when they are moving some other force or forces, acting on a bony lever, as when the hand moves a weight. He then proceeds to describe the different kinds of levers very fully, illustrating, by diagrams, formulæ, and giving examples of each kind of lever in the human frame, and laying down certain statements which may be regarded as axioms, *e.g.*, the longer the fibres of a muscle the more extensive is the motion it can make and the greater its power; the energy of a contracting muscle is proportioned to the energy of the volition, &c The whole book is divided into sections, numbering 144; these are again divided into subsections, which in many instances are illustrated by examples. In the main section an assertion is made, and in the subsection this assertion is illustrated or explained. The whole book is stuffed with facts, and in that, according to M. Taine, is truly Anglo-Saxon. We fear that it will be perused by few, except enthusiastic mathematicians, and that for general purposes it will not be much made use of by the surgeon, but will be very valuable as a book of reference. Each articulation is described in the manner I have above related, and tho action of each muscle and group of muscle is explained, but the terse, axiomatic manner in which it is done makes it rather difficult reading for an ordinary mortal without a marked taste for dynamics. The last dozen pages are taken up with a description of the myometer. The work is profusely illustrated with diagrams, which will be much appreciated by teachers of anatomy who use the blackboard.

In conclusion, we must congratulate Prof. Wight in publishing such a scientific volume, the first of the kind that we know of.

A Treatise on the Diseases of the Nervous System.—By WM. A. HAMMOND, M.D., Professor of Diseases of the Mind and Nervous System in the Medical Department of the University of the City of New York, &c. With 112 illustrations. Seventh edition, rewritten, enlarged and improved. New York: D. Appleton & Co. Montreal: Dawson Bros.

This new edition of a deservedly popular work on nervous affections will no doubt be well received. The book itself is so well known that we need do nothing further than point out a few of the more important additions which have been made. These are: considerable amplification of the chapter on cerebral congestion, and chapters on Myxœdema, on Syphilis of the Brain, the Spinal Cord and the Nerves, and on the Symptomatology of Cerebral and Cerebellar Lesions, and a new section on Diseases of the Sympathetic Nervous System. Besides these entirely new parts, we find, on comparing this with the last edition, a great number of minor additions in several chapters, including many changes necessitated by the investigations of late years in this branch of medical science.

In its present form, with the above considerable amount of new matter, Dr. Hammond's treatise is rendered complete, and will continue to be accepted as one of the foremost text-books on Neurology, one not containing a repetition of the ideas of others, but in many parts showing distinct indications of the strong, if occasionally peculiar, views held by the author.

Therapeutic and Operative Measures for Chronic Catarrhal Inflammation of the Nose, Throat and Ears. Part II.—By THOS. F. RUMBOLD, M.D. Forty illustrations. St. Louis: Geo. O. Rumbold & Co.

This volume composes the latter part of a work which we noticed a short time ago, entitled "The Hygiene and Treatment of Catarrh," by the same author. It contains full directions concerning the instruments which are requisite and the procedures to be adopted, in all the various disorders of a catarrhal nature involving the nares, fauces and aural apparatus. It is the work of a practical man who has had extensive experience in these affections, and will no doubt be useful to general practitioners. A number of cases are appended, illustrative of the treatment recommended in some of the more unusual diseases described.

Traité de l'Acide Phenique.—Par le Docteur DECLAT. Paris: Chez Lemerre, Libraire-Editien.

The enormous extent to which the employment of this favourite antiseptic has grown is shown by the appearance of this work of no less than 1070 pages devoted to a discussion of the value of carbolic acid and the various complaints in which it has been successfully employed. The author devotes, in the introductory chapters, considerable space to finding out when this agent was first introduced, and to furthering his claims to be considered in some sense the originator. Then external parasites, both animal and vegetable, are considered, and the carbolic acid shown to be the most reliable destructive agent. Various febrile affections are reviewed in connection with their origin from minute parasitic origin. Charbon and several other diseases of the lower animals, communicable to man, also naturally claim a large share of attention. In all of these, and a great many others, the remedial powers of the phenic acid are highly extolled. This work is of considerable interest to every one concerned with the study of the extensive influence and power for good of carbolic acid as a remedial agent in the numerous diseases which are the result of the presence of parasitic organisms or germs.

Extracts from British and Foreign Journals.

Unless otherwise stated the translations are made specially for this Journal.

Discussion on Listerism.—At the International Medical Congress, London, Aug. 6th, Mr. Spencer Wells read a paper. He took strong Listerian ground, and said that now he had given up drainage altogether, so great was his faith in antiseptic surgery. Several others, Volkman especially, followed in a similar strain. Then Marion Sims arose, and while he declared for Listerism he advocated drainage, and reminded Mr. Wells of a case (ovariotomy), in which he assisted him in a bad operation,—bad on account of adhesions,—and the patient *almost* died, but at last nature opened the abdominal wound and discharged a large amount of fetid fluid, and immediately she recovered. Finally came Mr. Keith to close the discussion. Never in the history of surgery did a few modest words make such a recoil in the "currents of expectant thought" as his.

It has been said, and was repeated by Volkman and Kuget, in this discussion, that intra-peritoneal surgery was the "touchstone of Listerism." Professor Keith has been quoted the world over, again and again, as not only a warm disciple of Lister, but as illustrating in his remarkable success in ovariotomy, *more than any other surgeon*, the value of antiseptic, or rather, the Listerian method. No one can deny this.

So slow were his few words uttered that I can almost repeat overy one *verbatim*.

You can imagine the effect much better than I can describe it when he said that for several months past he had " abandoned the antiseptic treatment altogether." " True," he said, " I had eighty successful recoveries under Lister's medhod, and *stopping there* it would be a wonderful showing. *But out of the next twenty-five I lost seven.* One died of acute septicæmia, in spite of the most thorough antiseptic precautions : three of " nnquestionable carbolic acid poisoning; one of renal hemorrhage." He went on to say that out of the eighty consecutive cases (or rather he said it first) many came too near dying; that a large number got a high temperature—105°, 106°, 107° Fahrenheit —the evening following the operation, but, he said, " they happened to pull through." He then said that since he had for four months back abandoned the antiseptic method, and relied upon perfect cleanliness, care in controlling hæmorrhage, and thorough drainage, his cases were giving him much less trouble, and he was getting more satisfactory results.

He now stopped for a few moments, hesitating, as he must have realized the importance of his words, knowing that the whole world—surgical—was lending a " listening ear " to his utterances. The silence was " audible." Then he raised his head, and looking his audience square in the face, he said, " Gentlemen, I have felt it my duty to make these statements, for *they are true*," and took his seat. I shall not attempt to describe the applause, nor the effect of his statements. Professor Keith, by the way, told me privately that he almost died himself from using the carbolic acid so much. He got renal hæmorrhage and debility to an alarming degree. He said, moreover, that he never had great faith in it, and should not have continued its use so long—I mean the " Lister method " —but for the fact that so many eminent men were carried away with it; and if, after his remarkable series of cases, he had changed, and lost seven out of the twenty-five, as he did, without Listerism, all the world—he himself—would have attributed the result to the change.

One thing is certain: Mr. Keith's statements, in connection with those of others *and his own experience*, put Mr. Lister in a very unpleasant position; for he was put down on the programme to close the discussion on the treatment of wounds to secure union by first intention, which took place on Monday, 8th inst. Although four days had elapsed, he had no answer. To show how deeply he was impressed by all that had been said, he began his remarks, which were extemporaneous instead of written, as was expected, by saying that he never had admitted that abdominal surgery was the "touchstone of Listerism," and to the surprise and dismay of his followers went on to argue that, with the rapidity with which wounds of the peritonæum heal and the remarkable absorbing power of that membrane, and therefore its ability to take care of its exudates, he "doubted very much" whether, in the hands of a skillful, careful operator, it was not better to dispense with the antiseptic plan. I realize how important are the statements I am making, and lest some of your readers may think that they are open to criticism as to accuracy, I will say that I sat near enough to hear every syllable uttered, and I pledge my honor as a man and a surgeon for the absolute accuracy of every statement, though I took few notes.

Then, seeming to realize the danger of admitting such wonderful absorbent qualities to the peritonæum, he went on to say that he had recently made some experiments that surprised him very much, which proved that serum or bloody serum was "a very poor soil for the development of germs from contact with air-dust, and that blood clots were still more sterile. Indeed, it was very difficult to make them grow or develop at all, unless diluted with water." By the way, he declared that he had witnessed free cell development in a blood clot.

And these remarkable facts, said he, "at once call into question the necessity of the spray."

He then went on to say that he was not yet ready to give up the spray, but if simple irrigation or lavation should prove as good, he would say, "*Fort mit dem spray;*" and he further said, "I am not certain but I shall give it up. I am not at all sure but that before the next meeting, two years hence, I shall have abandoned the spray altogether." (His recent house surgeon says that he has lost all confidence in its utility.)

As to carbolic acid, he said, "I am forced to admit its unfortunate character." That was all; not a word about oil of eucalyptus or any other substitute. He kept referring again and again to abdominal surgery, but his manner showed to everybody that he was upset.

He gave no statistics, no large comparisons, as was expected by his disciples. He referred to the excellent results in two cases of recent operation, saying that "I could hardly believe I should have got such results without the antiseptic plan; I did not before I used it."

And this is the fault that the best surgeons here find with him. They are all ready and glad to give him or any other man credit for all he has really done, and they all admit that Mr. Lister has done much to improve surgery. I need not explain. But they very properly say, "With his unprecedented opportunities, both in his own practice and in that of his host of followers, why don't he give us large and complete statistics? Instead, he only gives either isolated cases or a small group of successful ones, such as may be found under almost any plan." I quote one of London's most eminent and fair-minded men.

It was curious to watch the effect of the thing. I have alluded to the impression produced by Keith's remarks. As Lister was speaking, one of his ardent admirers—I mean an admirer of his mode of dressing; I am not discussing the man, who is an earnest hardworking, accomplished gentleman—turned to me, and said, "My God, I would never have believed Professor Lister would have admitted that." Another said, "Well, if Lister abandons the spray and carbolic acid, giving us no substitute, where is 'Listerism?' We had drainage, we had animal ligatures, we had air-proof dressings, before." And so on. Every little group of surgeons was discussing the matter; those who had never accepted the Listerian method being quite as much surprised as its warmest adherents.

"Mein Gott!" said a German whom I did not know, "Lishterism ist todt." "Fort dem Spray? Fort dem Acid Carbolique? Was giebts zu bleiben?"

And so the pendulum swings.—*Cor. Boston Med. and Surg. Journal.*

How to render Septic Wounds Aseptic. —The proper measures to render foul wounds aseptic are well illustrated in a recent lecture of Prof. von Nussbaum of Munich, translated in the *Edinburgh Medical Journal.* They are so instructive that we quote them fully:—

In July last a student received a sabre-cut of the head in a duel, which ran parallel to the sagittal suture, to the left of it, and was 11 centimetres long. The bone was denuded and laid bare, so that it seemed like a fissure. One of his friends, a military surgeon, had cut away some of the hair, washed off the blood, and dressed the wound with olive oil and Brun's wadding. For five days it went on very well. The patient then wished to get up, and asked for more to eat. The surgeon, however, noticed a considerable swelling of the edges of the wound, and refused both requests. The next day, at 1 a.m., the patient had a severe rigor, and when the surgeon came he found some erysipelas and the wound dry and smelling badly. The temperature, which had hitherto never been above 38°C., had now risen to 40.7°C., and the patient spoke in such an excited manner that one immediately suspected the onset of delirium. The patient's relatives, who had now arrived, insisted that he should be brought to my clinic. This required a few hours' time to carry out, and and when the patient came under my care, at 4 p.m., he was very delirious, had a temperature of 40.9°C., a small pulse of 130 per minute, and the erysipelas had spread over the whole scalp. There was here a probability of getting that unfortunate termination which was formerly so much dreaded in all cases of severe head-injury. Evidently there had been foul-smelling pus pent up in the wound, and this had led to erysipelas. The septic condition of the secretions had affected the small blood-clots which lay in the deep crevices of the wound, and there could be little doubt that secondary meningitis was imminent. I confess that, having regard to the severity of the septic symptoms, I had very little hope of being able to bring about a favourable state of affairs; however, careful disinfection is always useful and can never do any harm, so I had the patient put under chloroform, then I cut away more of the hair from round about the wound, washed the surrounding parts, which were soiled with blood and discharge, with a five per cent. solution of carbolic acid, slit up the overlapping edges of the wound with the scissors to such an extent that the whole floor of the wound was laid bare. By this means I could evacuate some foul pus and blood-clots, the retention of which had doubtless been the cause of the erysipelas and the serious symptoms. I dipped a pad of Brun's wadding in an eight per cent. solution of chloride of zinc, and disinfected with this the whole floor of the wound, carefully washing and syringing the exposed bare bone. I then put two drainage-tubes in the wound, sewed up the other parts with catgut sutures, injected some five per cent. carbolic lotion through the drainage-tubes, washed the surface of the skin with the same, and then put on a Lister's dressing, but without "protective," so that the gauze, which was soaked in two-and-a-half per cent. carbolic lotion, might come into direct contact with the secretions from the wound. I ordered the patient an acid drink and some light soup. He passed a quiet night, after getting a hypodermic injection of two cg. acetate of morphia. The next morning I was as much astonished as pleased when the patient, perfectly conscious, held out his hand and quietly wished me "Good morning." The delirium was quite gone, the temperature 38°C., and the pulse 98 per minute. Everything had changed so much for the better that we hoped the meningitis had been warded off. As the dressings had shifted a little, I changed them under the steam-spray, and found then that the wound in a satisfactory condition. The erysipelas was quite gone, and there was no retention of the discharge. The temperature soon fell still further, and in sixteen days after his admission to my clinic the happy patient left for his home, having only a strip of plaster about the breadth of a finger upon the cicatrix on his scalp.

As a second illustration, I may relate a case which was recently under my care. A servant-girl was pushed from her chair in jest, and fell so heavily that she fractured her radius and ulna, and the ends of the bones protruded through the skin. A practitioner who lived near put adhesive plaster upon the wound and bound up the arm in splints in the ordinary way; as it bled rather freely during the night, he sprinkled some styptic powder over the plaster. On the third day the arm was so much swollen, and there were so many blue and green blebs upon it, that the practitioner was afraid to go on treating the case, and called in another medical man, as the patient was strongly opposed to going into hospital. The surgeon who was called in requested to have a consultation with me, and spoke of the possibility of amputation being necessary. The mention of amputation caused great con sternation in the house, for the foolish joke had been perpetrated by the son of the girl's master. When I saw the patient the arm was greatly swollen and tense, the wound had a grayish surface, and was covered with foul-smelling pus; round about it there were also numerous blebs of different sizes. The small ones—about as large as a pin's head—were like transparent yellow glassy beads, and were very numerous, and lying close together; the larger ones were black and blue in colour, and filled with blood-tinged serum. There was high fever. The patient's countenance was of a yellowish-brown colour, and the morning temperature was as high as 40.3°C. Under these circumstances I could not say positively that the arm might be saved; but, on account of the patient's youth and good constitution, I said that with the utmost care a good result might probably be obtained. Both the patient and her medical attendant gave me full permission to do what I thought proper. I first put the patient under the influence of an anæsthetic. I then shaved the whole arm, washed it with a five per cent. carbolic lotion, and let two steam sprays play upon the wound. I made a semi-circular incision, which extended about half round the arm, avoiding nerves, etc., and by this means exposed the fragments of the broken bones lying at the bottom of the wound. The arm could then be bent in the middle, so that it was possible to have the floor of the wound thoroughly washed and purified with 5 per cent. carbolic lotion. (In cases where there is no bleeding, but only foul pus, I prefer to use the 8 per cent. solution of chloride of zinc.) I next ligatured some bleeding vessels, cut off the sharp ends of the broken bones, syringed and washed everything clean, put short drainage-tubes in each corner of the wound, and bandaged the arm on a splint, leaving the widely-gaping wound uncovered; over this wound—which was about half the size of an amputation wound—I put some absorptive gauze, and arrange that a three per cent. carbolic lotion should drop upon this day and night, the drops following each other so rapidly that they formed really a fine continuous stream. In 24 hours about 28 litres of this lotion passed over the arm. After two days, however, the wound became free from odor, and the temperature fell to 37.7°C. to 38.2°C., so I diminished the irrigation considerably, and allowed from 16 to 18 litres of carbolic lotion to flow over the wound in the 24 hours. In a few days the wound looked so well that an ordinary Lister's dressing was applied, and the wound soon healed up like a fresh injury.—*Med. & Surg. Reporter*.

Pyæmia from an Unusual Source Simulating Enteric Fever.—Enteric fever is so frequently under our observation that its easy recognition would be thought to follow from constant attention to its special features. Nevertheless, those amongst us who are occasionally called upon to give an opinion upon the more complicated cases of this disorder are obliged to confess that, in spite of clinical and pathological knowledge, our diagnostic acumen may be every now and then hampered, if not entirely baffled. To rightly interpret anomalous phases of the disease in question we are often compelled to pass in review other complaints which produce symptoms akin to those that are perplexing us. There are several such, too well known to need enumerating. I recite the following cases because, in our researches to explain its somewhat obscure symptoms, we detect an unexpected source of evil, which we believe to have been the means of enabling us to arrive at a precise diagnosis of our patient's illness. Moreover, in my opinion its peculiar features recall forcibly to one's mind the notable observations on the absorption of septic products, published as a leading article in the August number of *The Lancet*, under the title of "Blood Disease and the Germ Theory."

I was requested to see in consultation a young man, in good circumstances, reported to be suffering from typhoid fever. I am indebted to a medical friend for the following notes:—

F. B—— was first visited on December 6th 1880, suffering from diarrhœa without abdominal tenderness, temperature 103°; pulse frequent, 120; white tremulous tongue, not red on the tip or edges. Complained of having, for about a fortnight, what he termed a severe cold, aching limbs, and general depression. He had taken medicine from a chemist. He gradually became worse. The pulse became more frequent, with a peculiar thrill, very compressible, and for two days before death, which occurred on December 14th, it rose to 140 and 150. The temperature rose and fell rapidly without any corresponding alternative in the general symptoms. He passed on several occasions copious stools, much resembling the discharges from the bowels in enteric fever. Throughout the illness there were "no spots." During the last week pleuropneumonia supervened, affecting the lower half of the right lung. In the night of December 10th he had a prolonged rigor, and for the last four or five days profuse cold sweats. No enlargement of the spleen could be detected. His urine was high colored and slightly albuminous. He became very deaf, but his mind was clear till four days before his decease; he was without headache or obscurity of thought. The last forty-eight hours he was delirious, talking and shouting. About ten months previous to this last illness he contracted a chancre, which was followed by an unusually severe attack of eczema.

In running through the various symptoms presented by this patient, notwithstanding that many of them resembled to a certain extent those of enteric fever, yet two were wanting, and these two so frequently found in the fully developed form of this disorder that my attention was at once arrested by their absence.

(1) The tongue was not covered with a thin or thick white fur, nor were its margins red; (2) there was no eruption, rose-colored or otherwise. There was no special sanitary defect about the house or premises; during the last few years no case of enteric fever in the village had come under observation; and I may here add that in the five months which have elapsed since the decease no case of fever has occurred in the young man's family. There were no signs of any affection of the joints, or evidence of subperiosteal abscess. We drew back a long prepuce, and exposed the glans penis; this was covered with an abundant creamy pus, and half its surface was occupied by a soft chancre in a sloughing state. We determined that there had been absorption into the system of this pent-up matter, and that our patient was suffering from pyæmia. As the symptoms were acute—that form of pyæmia, in fact, from which patients rarely recover—we gave a most unfavorable opinion to the parents, without detailing our discovery.

It will, of course, be asked how it came to pass that an examination of the penis should have been made. In this way. Some months previously I saw this patient, who was then covered from head to foot with a most copious eruption of acute eczema. He confessed to having had a chancre, was treated with mercury, and gradually recovered. Fortunately, in the above difficulty our researches were thus aided, and our perplexity, as we believe, solved, by a previous acquaintance with our patient's proclivities. No post-mortem examination could be obtained.—*E. F. Russell, M.B., M.R.C.P., in London Lancet.*

The Local Treatment of Phthisis by Carbolic Acid.—By Robert Hamilton, F.R.C.S., Senior Surgeon, Southern Hospital, Liverpool.—A paper which Dr. W. Williams lately read before the North Wales Branch of the British Medical association, draws attention to a mode of treatment of phthisis, which, I believe, will prove extremely valuable, and, I am sanguine enough to think, will be more successful than any other in many allied diseases of the lungs. The inhalation of carbolic acid vapor, in the continuous mode suggested by my colleague, meets a difficulty which, I have always felt, has stood in the way of all previous methods of conveying drugs to the lungs. He utilizes the carbolic gauze of Lister, and merely saturates it occasionally with an aqueous solution of the acid. The old form of inhalers, as well as the modern spray-producers, necessitate a quantity of aqueous vapour being introduced into the bronchial tubes and into the air-cells, much in excess of what is ever naturally taken in. There is a positive evil in this, such vapor condensing, and being then deposited on the delicate epithelial lining of the air-tubes and cells, interferes with the osmic movements which respiration induces. That respiration is practically impeded is shown by the coughing and the suffocating sensation produced, so that a very few minutes' use, at one time, of inhalers and vaporizers is all that is possible. The suspension put to natural processes is apt to be overlooked in our eagerness to get the drug brought into actual contact with diseased lung-tissue; and the evil produced by the water is far more than commensurate with the good that the drug can do. The mode of conveyance of the minute particles of carbolic acid by Dr. Williams' respirator is not open to the above objection; and as the drug itself has been tested in surgical practice, and found to be of invaluable service in the treatment of all suppurating surfaces which are accessible, it is fair to infer that, if it can be applied *per se* to the lungs, it may be equally efficacious in checking the growth and development of morbific germs in them, and thus allow tissue to be reconstructed.

I have treated several cases of phthisis in the way suggested by Dr. Williams, with good results. The almost constant wearing of the respirator whilst under treatment may be an obstacle to the rapid adoption of the method; bnt it is, as he says, astonishing how soon the patients become accustomed to the wearing of them. They are only one degree more unsightly than the respirators which many people wear out of doors without hesitation. Further improvement in their shape and appearance is sure to follow, if their value be established. I have desired to draw attention to this mode of treatment of phthisis, because it is following in the lines of thought in which surgical procedure has run for some time, with marked success. It approves itself to the views of those who uphold the germ theory of disease; and as an undoubted germicide, and nothing more when used in moderation, it carries out another great desideratum—non-interference with natural processes of nutrition and repair of material.—*Brit. Med. Journal.*

Treatment of Diarrhœa in Phthisis.—Mr. Williams states that the diarrhœa arising in cases of phthisis from the ulceration of the alimentary tract requires very careful treatment. The great point to be kept in view is the healing of the ulcers, and this can only be attained by shielding them from all irritable substances and by promoting a healthy granulating action. The treatment in fact resolves itself into three sets of measures, (1) Rest in bed and the administration of only such food as can be quickly and easily assimilated without causing much distension of the intestine or accumulation of flatus. (2) Warm applications to the abdomen in the form of linseed poultices, &c., to reduce the pain and promote a certain degree of derivation to the skin. If the pain be severe a small blister over the area of tenderness to the touch is advisable. (3) Internal medicines. Where there is reason to suppose that the ulceration is slight and is confined to the small intestines, the diarrhœa may be treated by bismuth and opium, or by some astringents. The liquor bismuthi et ammon. cit. (B.P.) is a convenient form, but not always so effective as the powered carbonate or nitrate of bismuth in ten to twenty grain doses. Dover's powder combined with it in ten grain doses is often effective. The most powerful astringent is sulphate of copper in a quarter to half grain doses, combined with half a grain to a grain of solid opium. Of the various vegetable astringents tannic acid in four grain doses answers best; but it should, in every case, be combined with a certain amount of opium to reduce the irritability of the ulcers. Indian bael, especially a preparation of the fresh fruit, is often efficacious in checking the diarrhœa, if the ulceration be limited. If, however, the ulceration attack the large intestine as well as the small, recourse must be had to injections and suppositories. The enema opii (B. P.) administered twice a day, is sometimes sufficient, and may be strengthened by the addition of acetate of lead (four grains to an injection) or of tannic acid, five grains. When the ulceration is very extensive and involves the greater part of the large intestine, an attempt should be made to apply the remedies more thoroughly to the mucous membrane, and for this purpose injections of larger amount—from a pint to a pint and a-half—may be used, consisting of gruel or of starch, or best of all, of linseed tea, and all containing a certain quantity of opium (thirty to forty minims of the tincture). The linseed tea appears to exercise the same beneficial effect on the ulcers of the large intestines as it does on follicular ulceration of the throat. In cases where the stools are very fœtid, glycerine of carbolic acid may be added with advantage to the injection. In many cases where it is desirable not to distend the large intestines, suppositories of morphia (from half a grain to a grain) or of compound lead one, or of those of tannic acid are indicated. When the lardaceous degeneration has so far advanced as to reach the intestine, Dr. Williams thinks that the case is beyond any effectual general treatment; he is therefore content to restrain the diarrhœa by astringents, the more powerful the better. Tannic acid in from two to four grain doses, with dilute sulphuric acid, sulphate of copper, or sulphate of zinc, are the most useful, and injections of these substances do some good.—(*The Lancet*, June 11 & 18, 1881.)

Statistics of Medical Literature.—At the International Medical Conference, in London, Dr. J. S. Billings, of Washington, D.C., read a paper upon medical literature, with especial reference to its character and distribution. The paper opens with the following statistics:—

It is usual to estimate that about one thirtieth of the world's literature belongs to medicine and allied sciences. The number of volumes is computed to be about 120,000, and about twice that number of pamphlets, and this amount is increasing at the rate of about 1500 volumes and 2500 pamphlets annually. Out of the 180,000 medical men in the civilized world about 11,600 are producers of or contributors to this literature. These are divided among the different countries as follows:

	Number of physicians.	Number of medical writers.
United States	65,000	2,800
France and colonies	26,000	2,600
German Empire	32,000	2,300
Great Britain and colonies	35,000	2,000
Italy	10,000	600
Spain	5,000	300
All others	17,000	1,000

The number of physicians who are writers is proportionally greatest in France and least in the United States. In 1879 the total number of Medical books and pamphlets published was 1643, according to the *Index Medicus*. Of these France published more than any other country, the contributions of the United States ranking third. The special characteristics of the medical literature of the present day are largely due to journals and transactions of societies. These form about one half of the current medical literature, and are by far the most widely read and studied. They amounted in 1879 to 655 volumes, containing about 20,000 original articles which were judged worthy of notice in the *Index Medicus*. Classifying the literary product of 1879 by subjects, we find the scientific or biological side of medicine represented by 167 books and 1543 articles. In this branch Germany leads, while the United States is very low in the list. The practical side of medicine was represented by 1200 books and 18,000 articles. Here France showed the greatest production, the United States next and then Germany. In scientific medicine we go to Germany to school, as that country at present leads the world. It was not long ago that the scientific student of medicine found his career anything but a profitable one. This condition is, however, rapidly changing, with the increasing specialization of his profession, and with the general tendency of science toward achieving practical results. So vast is the present range of medical science that we must now look, for original discoveries, mainly to specialists.—*Phil. Med. and Surg. Reporter.*

The Cotton Pellet as an Artificial Drum Head.—After giving a short historical review of the artificial drum head, Knapp reports four cases in which its application rendered decided services to the patient. In Case I, a lady of 41, who had copious and offensive discharge following scarlet fever, and who at the age of 12 was so deaf as to necessitate people to speak loud directly into her ears, was treated by Dr. F. A. Caldwell, who put cotton pellets into her ears. He attended her himself until the discharge had almost disappeared. "Since then (29 years) she has worn the cotton pellets, and by their aid has always enjoyed good hearing, and has been free from pain and inflammation." At present, without the pellets, she understands conversation at the distance of a few feet—with them at twenty. In Cases II, III and IV, the results obtained were also excellent. The points which Dr. K. desires to make in regard to the use of the cotton pellets are summarized in the following statements quoted from his article:—

1. "Cotton pellets moistened with glycerine and water (1.4), and worn as artificial drum heads, are a great aid to hearing in many cases of partial or total defect of the natural drum-head, with or without otorrhœa."

2. "Their therapeutical action in arresting profuse discharge on the one hand, and preventing the mucous membrane of the drum cavity from drying up, on the other, is most valuable."

3. "They protect, like natural drum-heads, the deeper parts of the ear against injurious influences of the atmosphere."

4. "In some cases they are quite indispensable, and may be worn for a lifetime with permanent comfort and benefit."

5. "In other cases they are needed only periodically, according to the copiousness of the discharge, or the exsiccation of the mucous membrane requires their action, in the one or other direction."

6. "The period during which a pellet may be left in the ear varies with the condition of the parts. They should be changed frequently—*i.e.*, every day, or every few days, so long as the discharge is considerable. They should not be worn at all when the discharge is abundant and offensive. When there is no dis-

charge, they may be left in as long as they are comfortable and the hearing is good. So far as my experience goes, they are apt to become unclean in a week or two. They then ought to be removed, the ear cleansed, either with dry cotton or cotton steeped in warm soap-suds, and new pellets introduced."

7. "The management of the ear disease should remain in the hands of the physician until a stationary condition, either of slight or no discharge, has been reached. During the time the patient is under treatment, he can be taught how to cleanse his ear and remove and replace the pellets."—*H. Knapp, M.D., in Archives of Otology.*

The Latest Scope.—Ophthalmoscopes, laryngoscopes, *et id omne genus* of explorative agencies have very recently been called upon to welcome an addition to their number at the hands of M. Trouvé at the Paris Observatory. This novel instrument is called the Polyscope, and well deserves its name, if we can realize the numerous uses to which it may be applied. It was exhibited as introduced in the interior of a live fish, the little animal having, in the most accommodating manner, swallowed it, probably for the benefit of science. Through wires held in the band of the operator, the whole interior of the fish became illuminated, so that its vertebræ could be clearly seen and counted. Already have its applications to the uses of the physiologist and the surgeon been practically tested. According to *La Nature*, it has been employed to demonstrate the texture of the rectum and bladder, to assist in the localization and extraction of a projectile in the posterior nasal region, and to examine the interior of the stomach of a bull suffering from gastric fistula. In this wonderful age of progress, what novel sights may we not hope to see through such polyscopic media ; what light we not expect to be thrown upon obscure points of diagnostic value, to guide us through therapeutic intricacies ! We hear much said, in these days of moral perversity, about the "true inwardness" of things, but what can equal in personal interest the interior of the human body when brilliantly lighted up under the dazzling rays emitted from a polyscope ! We are not yet informed whether, like the fish, we shall be compelled to swallow this new instrument of diagnosis, in order to detect the quality or amount of our back bone; but we stand ready to go to the full extent of human endurance to be enabled to pass in review all our internal viscera, in which for so many years we have had a direct and vital interest. —*College & Clinical Record.*

May Iodide of Potassium excite Bright's Disease?—In view of the very large doses which have been advised and are frequently administered in the treatment of syphilis, the question whether iodide of potassium may excite Bright's disease becomes one of considerable importance. In the *American Journal of the Medical Sciences* for July, 1881, Prof. I. Edmondson Atkinson, of the University of Maryland, calls attention to the large proportion of cases treated for advanced syphilis that present, after death, evidences of marked kidney disease; and, in this connection, to the fact that syphilitic renal disorder in its characteristic lesion, the gumma, is comparatively rare, while the forms the most frequently encountered are not in themselves syphilitic. In searching for a cause that might produce these changes quite independently of the syphilitic poison, Dr. Atkinson concludes that since iodide of potassium has decided diuretic action, and, as is known to clinical observers, may cause both albumen and casts to appear in the urine, the continuance of this remedy in some cases might lead to the changes observed. He therefore made a series of observations upon seventy cases of late syphilis, of which nineteen presented evidences of renal alterations more or less grave. The relation existing between the administration of iodide in these cases, and the appearance of mucous or hyaline casts and albuminuria, was quite evident; as in a number, the abnormal elements gradually disappeared after the cessation of the remedy. The condition appeared to be catarrhal in character, and the casts were the results of renal irritation. In no case, however, was extensive parenchymatous inflammation of the kidneys excited; but an obvious syphilitic disorder of the kidney in one case disappeared under the full and systematic use of the iodide. The author's conclusion is that while the evil effects of the iodide of potassium are small and for the most part transitory, the occurrence of more severe alterations is not impossible, nay is probable. To these evil effects some individuals are more susceptible than others.

The Value of Belladonna in Intestinal Occlusion.—Dr. C. J. Edlefsen relates, in *Norsk Magazin for Lægevidenskaben*, the ease of a ship carpenter, 48 years of age, who had always enjoyed previous good health, but during seven days had had no evacuation of the bowels, and during the past two days had vomited fæcal matter. The abdomen was distended and very tender to the touch, the extremities cold, pulse frequent, but feeble; no excrements in the rectum. Various laxatives and injections had been tried in vain. Patient was now ordered 3-5ths of a grain of extract of belladonna every hour. After five doses (three grains) had been taken, the vomiting ceased, and after five more doses, the patient was relieved of about one gallon of thin, gruel-like excrements, after which he improved rapidly. There were no symptoms of belladonna poisoning, although six grains of the extract were given.—*Med. & Surg. Reporter.*

A Study of Primary, Immediate, or DIRECT HEMORRHAGE INTO THE VENTRICLES OF THE BRAIN.—Dr. E. Sanders of New York, in an instructive paper upon this subject in the *American Journal of the Medical Sciences* for July, 1881, says: "Strange as it may seem, though important as the subject undoubtedly is, primary intra-ventricular hemorrhage is either passed by unnoticed, or if noticed, receives a passing mention only, being characterized as very rare, unimportant, and not to be diagnosed (Northnagel, Hughlings-Jackson, Brichetau, and others)." On the contrary, Dr. Sanders considers primary hemorrhage into the ventricles as their most common disease, and says: "Like many other diseases that were formerly classed as very uncommon, but have by later research and observation been found more frequently present by merely being looked for, primary hemorrhage into the ventricles of the brain when sought for in the post-mortem room will, I am sure, share a like fate." Dr. Sanders has collected and studied 94 cases of this form of apoplexy, which, as compared with ordinary cerebral hemorrhage, is remarkably frequent at the two extremes of life. As regards the diagnosis, Dr. Sanders says, "given a patient with sudden complete coma, partial or complete paralysis, or even without any paralysis at all, contracture and convulsion, with rapidly following death,—in fact, that collection of symptoms which we have come to recognize under the term '*apoplexie foudroyante*,'—the probabilities are that we are dealing with a primary intra-ventricular extravasation." The effusion most frequently occurs in the lateral ventricles. The prognosis is almost always fatal. This important contribution to cerebral pathology contains the clinical histories of 28 cases, with the notes of the autopsies, and several comparative tables, which greatly enhance its value for reference.

Rare Result in an attempt to Deliver with the Forceps.—I was summoned on the night of December 8th, 1880, to attend A. S. in labour, in consultation with Dr. A. B. I arrived at the bedside at midnight and obtained the following history: A. S., aged 20, short, thick and muscular, was taken with labour pains at 10 a.m., December 8th. The family physician was summoned at 2 p.m., and at 3 p.m. membranes ruptured, vertex presentation, contractions vigorous. The position was not detected, as the sequel of the case will abundantly demonstrate. The second stage progressed slowly, notwithstanding the pains were frequent and powerful. At 8 p.m. the forceps was applied in the pelvic position. The forceps used was that known as the "Reamy forceps." From this time until a short time before my arrival (midnight) every effort was made to deliver, aided by chloroform and the most powerful contractions, but without success. When I arrived I found the woman greatly exhausted; the pains still strong and frequent. Examination revealed an occipito-posterior position; the head at the inferior strait and thoroughly impacted, with the male-blade of the forceps resting beneath the pubic arch, and buried in the vagina to the shank and embracing the head firmly in the region of the left frontal bone and orbit. The attending physician had attempted its removal, but failed to dislodge it. I employed every manœuvre to effect the removal of the blade, but utterly failed to change its position. Each succeeding pain served to increase the difficulty by wedging the blade still tighter. Here, indeed, was a dilemma without a parallel in my experience. We waited two hours, closely watching the case. At the end of that time no change had occurred for the better; on the contrary, the woman was becoming rapidly exhausted, with no advance of the head. We then decided upon and performed craniotomy upon a living child, which permitted the removal of the blade and delivery without further trouble. The woman made a tedious, but satisfactory recovery.

Remarks.—In my own experience, this case is without a parallel; neither does the literature of the subject, so far as I know, furnish a similar case. The factors leading to the unfortunate result are, in my opinion, the application of the forceps without a knowledge of the position of the head, and the failure to remove the instrument in time to permit the head to execute the movement of rotation in the natural way. Evidently the head entered the brim in the second position, right occipito-acetabular; in this position the application of the forceps before the head had executed the movement of flexion would most effectually prevent the brow from ascending and the occiput from descending, movements highly necessary in the rotation of the occiput under the pubic arch. As it was, however, the traction made by the forceps gave the head a new direction, forcing the occiput into the hollow of the sacrum, while the brow passed from the left sacro-iliac synchondrosis forward under the pubic arch, carrying the blade of the forceps with it. Of course a knowledge of the position in the beginning of labour, or, at least, before the application of the forceps, with a proper appreciation of the mechanism of labour, would have prevented the unfortunate result that occurred in this case.—*Dr. Rossett in American Practitioner.*

Catarrhal Diathesis in Young Girls.—A special state of the organism has been demonstrated, consti tuting what we call a *catarrhal diathesis*. We observe in a certain number of young girls, even in very early youth, general impairments of health which plainly call for that term. This peculiar form of catarrh, which often came under my observation at Mont-Dore, is in reality a constitutional affection, and is, in all the extent of the term, a diathesis. Besides, it is not conneeted with dispositions or tendencies which visibly depend on the constitution of the parents.

Etiology.—Two facts must be considered in this respect: the health of the parents, and the hygienic surroundings of the girl. (1) Most always the parents suffer from what we generally call a delicate constitution, a constitutional weakness, and suffer from some catarrhal affection or die young. In many cases they even show symptoms of adenitis, scrofulosis, or phthisis. (2) As a general rule, these young girls have been exposed to cold and dampness, either in their homes or under exposure to the influences of a cold climate.

Symptoms.—These girls have often a light complexion, are pale, and their flesh is soft; they easily take cold, and they sometimes have what we call a *fatty chest* (an increased secretion of mucus in the respiratory passages.) Although, excluding cases of more or less acute affections of the bronchi, auscultation reveals no important change, sometimes none at all. The digestive functions are often irregular. The general growth of the body is slow and laboured, as it were. The girl is said to have a delicate constitution; her menses set in late; and, in many cases, the most important point is an abundant leucorrhœa, very weakening, which may have started in early infancy.

As might be inferred, from what precedes the nervous element is found a good deal in the catarrhal diathesis of young girls. It is manifested by pains in various parts of the chest, by chokings, which take place without adequate causes, by the erratic and changeable character of the symptoms, by the frequency, obstinacy and the character of the cough, notwithstanding the negative results of physical examinations; by an abundance of expectoration, alternating or existing simultaneously with a profuse leucorrhœa. To conclude, these profuse losses from the bronchi, or from the genital passages, finally ruin the constitution. This diathesis, we are happy to say, is capable of being cured, by an intelligent observation of the laws of hygiene, by an appropriate treatment; and age may also bring a cure.—*Abstract from an Address of Dr. G. Richelot, in L'Union Medicale*, March 3.—*Medical Gazette.*

When Men are at their Best.—Dr. Beard states that from an analysis of the lives of a thousand representative men in all the great branches of the human family, he made the discovery that the golden decade was between 40 and 50; the brazen between 20 and 30; the iron between 50 and 60. (*Michigan Medical News.*) The superiority of youth and middle age over old age in original work appears all the greater when we consider the fact that all the positions of honour and prestige, professorships and public stations are in the hands of the old. Reputation, like money and position, is mainly confined to the old. Men are not widely known until long after they have done the work that gave them fame. Portraits of men are delusions; statues are false! They are taken when men have become famous, which, on the average, is at least twenty-five years after they did the work which gave them their fame. Original work requires enthusiasm. If all the original work done by men under forty-five were annihilated they would be reduced to barbarism. Men are at their best at that time when enthusiasm and experience are almost evenly balanced. This period, on the average, is from 38 to 40. After this the law is that experience increases, but enthusiasm decreases. Of course there are exceptions.—*American Practitioner.*

Catarrhal Pneumonia.—Inhalations of carbolized spray, with the administration of ammonium chloride (gr. v–xx), potassium iodide (gr. iii–v), given in compound licorice mixture (℥ ss), or elixir of yerba santa, if there is much spasmodic cough, has given decided results. Night sweats are controlled by ergot or atropia, and emulsion of cod-liver oil and extract of malt, if the nutrition is below par. A moderate amount of stimulant may be required; and if there are great daily fluctuations in the temperature, indicating the onset of pneumonic phthisis, the pill of digitalis, quinia and opium (Niemeyer) is used three times a day.

CANADA

Medical and Surgical Journal.

MONTREAL, SEPTEMBER, 1881.

THE INTERNATIONAL MEDICAL CONGRESS.

LONDON, August 10, 1881.

To the Editor of THE CANADA MEDICAL & SURGICAL JOURNAL.

SIR,—The seventh session of this body concluded last evening by an informal dinner at the Crystal Palace. The majority of your readers have no doubt already been made acquainted with many of the details through the lay press, but, according to promise, I proceed to jot down a brief account of the proceedings, which extended from the 2nd to the 9th.

Six general meetings were held in St. James's Hall, at which addresses were delivered and the business of congress was transacted. The immense assemblies which gathered on these occasions were very impressive, and the scene at the inaugural meeting was one to be ever remembered " while memory holds a seat." The sight of above 3,000 medical men from all parts of the world, drawn together for one common purpose, and animated by one spirit, quickened the pulse and roused enthusiasm to a high pitch. The presence of the Prince of Wales and Crown Prince of Prussia gave great satisfaction, and added a flavour of Royal patronage which even science—republican though it be—seemed thoroughly to enjoy. The address of the President, Sir James Paget, was the event of the meeting, and surprised even those well acquainted with his brilliant oratorical powers. Beautiful thoughts, clothed in the choicest words, and expressed with an ease and grace peculiarly his own, marked each period, and at the close all felt that they had listened to an oration worthy of the occasion and of the audience. A thrill of pride must have filled the breast of every Englishman present at the thought of having, as the representative of the nation, such a gifted man.

At the subsequent general meetings, addresses were delivered by Professor Virchow "On the value of Pathological Experiment"; "On Scepticism in Medicine," prepared by the late Prof. Reynaud, and read by Dr. Féréol; "On Medical Literature," by Dr. Billings of Washington; "On the connection of the Biological Sciences with Medicine," by Prof. Huxley, and a special one, at the request of the President, by Prof. Pasteur, dealing with the recent experiments in Animal Vaccination as a protective against certain scourges among cattle. To very many, one of the most pleasant features of the gathering was the opportunity it afforded of seeing Professor Virchow, than whom, since John Hunter, no greater name has arisen in our ranks. His extraordinary reputation as a pathologist, and the prominence of his position as a politician in his own country, made all men curious to see him. His address was most characteristic, and his arguments in favour of vivisection were most appropriate, and will, it is to be hoped, do something to lessen the fanatical outcry against its legitimate practice, which has disgraced England during the past few years. It was only natural that Prof. Huxley, who began life as an assistant surgeon in the navy, and who has, in many ways and many works, shown his continued interest in the profession, should discourse in his most lucid style on the relations of Biology to Medicine.

For working purposes the congress divided into fifteen sections, the meetings of which took place in the rooms of the various learned societies at Burlington House and of London University, and one or two other contiguous institutions. Addresses were delivered by the presidents of sections at the first meeting, after which the reading and discussion of papers followed in regular order. The committee had prepared a volume of abstracts of papers to be read, printed in English, French and German, which was ready on the first day, and greatly facilitated the working of the sections. With so much of interest in every section, it was very difficult to decide each morning which to attend. The daily programme furnished full information of the subjects to be considered at each session, and the list was usually exhausted at the conclusion of the afternoon meeting. I spent my time chiefly in the pathological, physiological and medical sections. Papers on cognate subjects were, as far as possible, read at the same meeting, and those directly bearing upon any fixed subject of discussion were taken up in connection with it.

In the Pathological section, three very interesting discussions took place on Tubercle, on Germs, and on the relations of Cardiac and Renal Disease. In each a strong array of the chief talent of the profession took part, and it was very pleasant to hear the various points discussed by men whose writings were familiar and whose names are household words among us.

The time of the Physiological section was occupied chiefly in discussing certain set topics; very few papers were read. An animated discussion on Cerebral Localization took place, in which Goltz of Strasburg, Brown-Sequard, Ferrier and others participated. In the Medical section a large number of interesting papers on Nervous Diseases were read by Hughlings-Jackson, Brown-Sequard, Buzzard, Erb and others.

In the section on diseases of children, the attendance was good and the range of subjects discussed very varied. The treatment of Potts' disease and the question of inherited syphilis brought together a large array of the authorities on these subjects.

I gathered from friends that the work in other departments was carried on with equal activity, and a glance at the published abstracts is sufficient to show the variety and extent of the papers.

One of the most instructive parts of the congress was the museum, held in the Geological Society's Rooms. This consisted of illustrations of disease in the living subject, as well as a large assortment of rare and interesting prepared specimens. Among the former, Dr. Ord exhibited a remarkable set of cases, illustrative of the disease to which he has given the name Myxœdema, from the mucoid degeneration of the connective tissues, which produces the general swelling of the skin. The cases are usually in women and the affection is progressive. The patients exhibited by Dr. Ord showed the various stages of the disorder and his lucid description left no doubt in the minds of his hearers that a definite pathological entity was before them.

Mr. Jonathan Hutchinson had a number of cases each morning, and his demonstrations on leprosy, rheumatic arthritis and inherited syphilis attracted large audiences. Rare forms of skin diseases were exhibited by many of the leading dermatologists. The museum of specimens contained about 700 examples of interesting and rare illustrations of morbid anatomy, the great metropolitan museums furnishing the larger proportion. Professor Parrot, of Paris, had on exhibition a beautiful series of bone specimens, illustrating hereditary syphilis and rickets. Prof. Politzer, of Vienna, exhibited specimens showing the normal and morbid anatomy of the ear; and other foreign members brought examples from their cabinets. The walls of the rooms in which the specimens were collected were covered with coloured drawings. Among the most remarkable of these was a set of water-colours by Sir Chas. Bell, illustrating gun-shot and other wounds seen by him after Waterloo. Mr. Hutchinson's enormous collection attracted particular attention, and illustrated most of the special departments in which he has become so famous. What struck me as most remarkable among them was a set illustrating eruptions due to iodide and bromide of potassium, particularly two portraits of a man, the subject of an extensive eruption of tuberous masses on the skin, many of them ulcerated. The iodide had been given for ten weeks in increasing doses up to 20 grains, for a swelling in one iliac fossa. The patient died two weeks after coming under observation. Several beautiful coloured drawings by Raphael of Montreal were exhibited by our townsman, Dr. Roddick. An excellent catalogue greatly facilitated the inspection of the specimens, and perhaps as much direct benefit to the working members of congress was obtained during the time spent in the museum as in any of the other departments.

The hospitality displayed by the corporations and private individuals, was of a kind that could be offered in London and probably no where else. Among the most brilliant affairs were the conversaziones in South Kensington Museum, at the Guildball and at the College of Surgeons, the Lord Mayor's dinner and the garden party of the Baroness Burdett-Coutts. On Saturday afternoon there were numerous excursions and garden parties. At Folkestone, a memorial statue of Harvey was unveiled and an address given by Professor Owen. Dr. Gerald Yeo, the Professor of Physiology in Kings College, entertained the members attending the physiological section at his residence at Staines, and took them up the Thames in a steam launch, as far as the residence of the Duke of Westminster. Many of the leading medical men kept open house, and the luncheon and dinner parties enabled visitors to meet in a friendly way and compare notes.

The General Committee carried out the various arrangements in an admirable manner, and I did not hear of a single hitch during the entire proceedings. The registration of members took place at the College of Physicians, which formed the central office of congress, and was thronged early and late. The preparation of the volume of abstracts (over 700 pages) and the museum catalogue must have entailed an immense labour on the Committee, but the general expression of satisfaction showed how much the work was appreciated by the members.

A volume of Transactions will be issued as soon as possible, in English, French and German. The members' subscriptions are expected to cover the cost. It is to be hoped that no unnecessary delay will take place in the publication, though, considering the size of the volume, and the unavoidable delays in translating papers, etc., it can scarcely be expected before this time next year. W. O.

Medical Items.

—The opening address at the Montreal College of Pharmacy will be delivered on Tuesday evening, October 4th, by Henry Lyman, Esq., on "The Progress of Pharmacy in Canada during the last fifty years." At the annual meeting the office-bearers and lecturers were re-elected. The new lecture-hall of the College, which is handsomely fitted up, is at 223 McGill street, corner of Notre Dame, and is very convenient for students.

THE FAILURE OF PILOCARPIN IN DIPHTHERIA.—We cannot but regret to announce that the more recent trials of pilocarpin, advocated so forcibly by Dr. Guttmann as almost a specific in diphtheria, indicate that it is of no use at all in that disease. Dr. Joseph Schmid, in the *Wiener Med. Press*, No. 15, 1881, says, after a full trial, he has found it "generally wholly useless, often decidedly injurious." In serious forms of the complaint, he actually believes the unfavourable termination was hastened by his use of the drug. In the lighter catarrhal forms, the symptoms were not visibly ameliorated by it.—*Cinn. Lancet and Clinic.*

THE BALLAD OF BACILLUS.—(*Dedicated to Prof. Virchow.*) —"The same *Bacillus* as that found in hay was produced. On the other hand, the innocent organism found in hay might, by a different method of cultivation, be made to acquire virulent properties. Fed on a vegetable diet, it was tame and harmless; but, transplanted to another soil and given animal nourishment, it became savage (*verwildert*) and virulent."—*Virchow's address.*

Oh, merry *Bacillus*, no wonder you lay
Quiescent and calm when at home in your hay;
You never meant evil in hayfields, no doubt,
Till cruel experiments worried you out.
An innocent germ on a sort of probation,
Oh, why did pathologists try cultivation?

We hear you were harmless and charmingly tame,
So why did our Virchow besmirch your fair fame;
Why should he transplant you, with infinite toil,
To new and to wholly unnatural soil;
When food vegetarian kept you so quiet,
Why tempt you to fury on animal diet?

"*Verwildert!*" says Virchow, who surely must know,
You are, when transplanted, and cause us much woe;
So prithee, *Bacillus*, don't travel so far
As us, but stay peacefully just where you are.
You're innocent now, and have no wish to ravage,
And we've no desire, dear, to render you savage.

—*Punch.*

"Pas Encore."—Prof. Depaul, giving an account to his class of the magnificent obstetrical clinic (constructed at the moderate cost of 12,000 fr. per bed), and stating that an amphitheatre had been provided in which remarks might be made that it would not be proper to make at the bedside, observed that it reminded him of some words which, to his infinite regret, had once escaped him when examining a poor woman who, to all appearance, had succumbed to a uterine hemorrhage. Turning to the persons who surrounded him he said: "This woman is dead." But to his great stupefaction the patient replied in a feeble voice, "*Pas encore!*" So little dead indeed was the poor woman, in spite of all appearances, that in three weeks she left the clinic perfectly well. This "*pas encore*" corresponds pretty well to what occurred to Récamier one day when he was called by a colleague to see a man, the subject of typhoid fever. Récamier complained of having been called to the case too late, saying that the patient apparently could not survive the night. The latter, on hearing him, emitted a certain noise from the lower passages, accompanying it with the words, "*Qui crepitat vivit!*" and in fact, not only did he not die of typhoid fever, but is alive at the present time."—*Gaz. des Hopitaux.*

A Novel Female Catheter.—Dr. S. C. Van Antwerp, of Vicksburg, Mich., writes: "While talking with Dr. Barnum of Schoolcraft the other day, he gave me a little of his experience, which was certainly amusing and not without interest in a practical way. Dr. Barnum said he was called one hot summer day to see a patient four miles in the country who wished his immediate attention, but he did not learn the trouble. On arriving at the house he found that his patient was a lady who had been suffering for twenty-four hours from retention of urine. She begged of him to relieve her distress at once. Most unfortunately he did not have a catheter with him, and it would take quite a while to send for one. What he should improvise for one was a question. He thought of a goose quill or piece of elder, but neither were to be had. He then thought of burning a hole through a piece of wood with a knitting-needle, but that did not work. Lastly he thought of a bent wire. And the woman in her anxiety threw the covering aside and told him not to stand on ceremony but give her relief. Pressing the bent end forward carefully, before he expected a gush of urine struck him in the face and trickled down his well-laundried summer wear, and the transition from extreme anxiety of the woman and her friends to a most ludicrous scene was the signal for a general laugh at the doctor's expense." *Haec fabula docet*, either always carry a catheter or be prepared to improvise something therefor. While on this subject I am reminded of a suggestion made by a medical friend, which is to use a gum elastic catheter in drawing urine of women, as it can, by such a length of tube, better conduct the urine into a bed pan. I most heartily endorse the use of Nelaton's Catheter in male subjects where there is much difficulty in passing a silver one.—*Michigan Medical News.*

This story reminds us of an occurrence of similar nature on one of our river boats. An elderly woman, second-class passenger, was found during the night to be groaning and suffering much pain. The watchman, after searching the list of passengers, waked up Dr. W., who happened to be on board. He found a greatly distended bladder to be the cause of the trouble. He had no catheter; finally it occurred to him that his toothpick might be pressed into the service. He borrowed a second quill from a friend, and having fastened the two together, passed this novel catheter into the bladder and received the blessings of the sufferer. It is generally believed that the doctor bought a new toothpick on reaching Quebec.

VELUTI IN SPECULO.—"The Nineteenth Century seen through the Speculum" is said to be the title of the memoirs of his time which M. Ricord has prepared as his final literary legacy. These memoirs, like those of many other public men, are not to be published till thirty years after his death. "But," says the chronicler of the *Union Médicale*, "when to a select and friendly audience he reads a few pages, it is Rabelais, Brantome, or one of the stories of the amiable Queen of Navarre, to which the hearer seems to be listening."

CANADA
MEDICAL & SURGICAL JOURNAL

OCTOBER, 1881.

Original Communications.

ANTISEPTIC SURGERY.

BY GEO. E. FENWICK, M.D., Surgeon to the Montreal General Hospital, Prof. Surgery, McGill University.

Read before the Canada Medical Association.

I desire on the present occasion to make a few remarks, and to submit the results of a series of surgical cases, which in my hands have been treated after Professor Lister's method of dressing surgical wounds.

Not long since (December 6th, 1879) at a meeting of the Metropolitan Counties Branch of the British Medical Association, held at St. Thomas's Hospital, Mr. W. MacCormack made the following remarks: "That the employment of Lister's method is not at once, or very easily acquired; it requires practice, a capacity and patience for detail, that those concerned in the management of a case shall, without reserve believe in the germ theory, or act as if they believed in it, the surgeon in charge of the case must either himself examine into and verify everything belonging to the dressing of the case, or must have some one in whom he can trust to do it for him. Less than this will not be putting Lister's method fairly to the test."

It is of no interest to us to discuss the correctness or fallacy of the germ theory and would be foreign to the object I have in hand, which is more for the purpose of bearing additional testimony to the practical usefulness of Lister's antiseptic method, than of entering into a discussion concerning a subject which, so far, rests on a problematical basis. I will admit that, for the present, the certainty of the actual presence of germs in the air is far from being proved, but in carrying out the details of Listerism I am of the number of those who act as though they believed in the germ theory. I desire simply to report, in as few words as are convenient, the details of some of the results of the last four years, during which period Prof. Lister's antiseptic method of treating surgical injuries has been adopted by me, both in private and hospital practice. The cases may appear small numerically when laid alongside of the larger number of cases reported by our brethren in the larger fields for observation, in Great Britain and on the continent of Europe. I have seen large wounds of the soft parts, wounds opening into important joints and wounds connected with fractured bones, scalp wounds in which there was considerable laceration and stripping of the bone of its periostial covering, heal by immediate union, wherein strict antiseptic precautions were adopted. These favourable consequences have been attained without redness or swelling or pain of any kind, without discharge, except a slight serosity that hardly soiled the dressings and without any or scarcely any constitutional disturbance. Such results I had never before witnessed, during the personal observations of nearly forty years, and in all honesty must admit, that the results in my hands by following strictly Mr. Lister's instructions are what I had never before seen, under any other method of treatment. I must tell you, that at the Montreal General Hospital, I have acted as one of the surgical staff during the past 17 years. After the announcement of Professor Lister's views, on the antiseptic treatment of wounds, attempts were made on various occasions, by some of the surgeons of our Hospital to treat antiseptically various forms of injury, and even in operative proceedings antiseptics were sometimes employed, and although these measures were very imperfect, as compared to the present means at our disposal, nevertheless the results were sometimes remarkable. Listerism, however, in its perfection remained unknown to us, until it was introduced by my friend and colleague Dr. Roddick, who went to Edinburgh and studied the method under Prof.

Lister himself. To Dr. Roddick then is due the credit of being the first surgeon to introduce to our hospital, in all its completeness of detail, the antiseptic method of dealing with surgical accidents as proposed by Prof. Lister.

Dr. Roddick returned from Edinburgh with a complete outfit, consisting of spray apparatus, gauze properly charged, protective, drainage and all accessories, which are essential to faithfully carrying out Prof. Lister's injunctions. It is true that a hand spray had been employed by us, on various occasions, but there had been hitherto no definite system of action, no specially prepared dressings and not altogether that enthusiasm and firm belief in the benefit to be derived by this method, if properly and faithfully carried out. Soon after the introduction of Listerism in its completeness, the very remarkable results attracted attention and the house committee of our Hospital, on the recommendation of the medical staff, sent for and supplied us liberally with all needed apparatus and proper dressings.

The practical surgeon can realize the comfort experienced from a feeling of complete confidence in the success of any justifiable operative procedure, but more than this, he will feel encouraged to undertake operations, with Listerism, that without it he would refuse to perform. Operations under Listerism can be, and are undertaken by the surgeon and carried to a successful issue, which without it would be regarded as unjustifiable, or attempted only as a *dernier ressort*, and as being the only chance of life left to the sufferer. The surgeon who adopts the antiseptic method in operative procedures, may predict a safe and successful issue in cases, which before the introduction of this method, would have been regarded as exceedingly doubtful.

Ovariotomy.—The total number of cases that have come under my own care and on which I have operated is nine. These are not the only cases that have presented at our Hospital, but are my own personal record. Of these, three were operated on by me, before the advent of antiseptics and they were all fatal. The first case dying on the third day apparently from shock, the other two fatal cases terminating within a week from general peritonitis. The other six cases recovered at different periods, all of these cases were operated on under the spray and with full antiseptic precautions.

I shall give a short synopsis of each case, noting any prominent feature which may be thought of interest.

CASE No. IV.—B. P., æt. 24 years, came under observation 29th March, 1880. A tall, well proportioned girl, was as large as a woman at full term of pregnancy. She had always enjoyed good health, and menstruated regularly; the change made its appearance about the fifteenth year of life. Six years ago had noticed a moveable growth in left groin, but it gave no pain nor uneasiness. Three years since she observed that this growth was gradually and steadily increasing in size, until it became so noticeable as to lead to observations on the part of her relatives, which obliged her to consult her physician, who pronounced it to be a multilocular ovarian cyst. The patient was brought to Montreal on the 29th March, 1880, delay was rendered necessary in consequence of menstruation coming on the day after her admission to hospital, so that the operation for removal of the tumour was performed under the spray, on 10th April. An incision four inches in length was made, from just below the umbilicus downwards towards the pubis. The tumour was freely exposed. No adhesions existed, but there was some difficulty in emptying the sac, as it consisted of a number of small cysts, filled with thick gelatinous fluid. The left ovary was engaged. The sac was with some difficulty delivered and the pedicle moderately long was secured by two carbolized hempen ligatures which were cut short off and the stump dropped back, the right ovary was likewise found diseased, it was tied in like manner by a single ligature and removed. The entire contents and solid matter removed weighed 36 lbs. This patient made an excellent recovery. The highest temperature registered was on the third day after the operation, when the thermometer reached 102°, after which it steadily subsided and became normal on the tenth day. She left her bed on the 13th day after the operation, feeling weak, and was discharged cured on the 18th day and allowed to return home. The dressings were not disturbed until the 10th day, when they were removed and the wound found healed.

I have heard from this patient quite recently, she is strong and robust in health, but has ceased menstruating. She had a menstrual period apparently at the end of the second week after the operation, which was the last seen.

CASE No. V.—Victorine V., æt. 24 years, not married, was admitted into the Private Hospital 15th March, 1881, being the subject of a large ovarian tumour apparently multilocular, with several large cysts, the following history was elicited.

She had enjoyed good health, had commenced to menstruate at the age of 14, catamenia always regular as to time and not excessive, lasting about three days, and painless.

About six years ago she noticed a swelling in the abdomen, which she declares was uniform and not situated in either groin. This gradually and steadily increased, until she became so much distended as to prevent her keeping the recumbent position. It was diagnosed to be ascites from liver obstruction. Purgatives and other means failed to reduce the swelling, and her physician relieved her by tapping; the fluid removed filled two buckets, and was thin, like water. She made a rapid recovery and on the third day was able to leave her bed. From this time, which was in March or April, 1877, the fluid rapidly accumulated, necessitating its removal every four or six weeks. So that up to the 18th February, 1881, the trochar had been used twenty five times. The fluid in quantity was on each occasion about the same as above stated, but in consistence it had changed, becoming more like gum water. She never suffered any pain or inflammatory symptoms after the tappings and with the exception of the inconvenience from distension was in good health, all the functions being regularly performed. When examined the cyst was moderately full, one month only having elapsed since the last removal of the fluid. The tumour extended to midway between the umbilicus and ensiform cartilage, there existed a well formed hymen, but with care the index finger was introduced into the vagina, the uterus was found of normal size, carried over to the left side and bulging, could be felt distinctly in Douglas' fossa, upon forcing upwards, a distinct wave was imparted to the contents of the tumour over the front of the abdomen. The last catamenial period had occurred on the 5th March.

March 19th, the operation was performed under the spray and with full antiseptic precautions, an opening of about four inches in length from below the umbilicus downwards was made, rather firm adhesions existed in front and also at the upper part and sides of the tumour, these had to be separated with great care, as the cyst wall was rather thin, all attachments having been separated the patient rolled over on to her side and a large sized trochar plunged into the sac, which contained four or five large cysts, the sac was drawn out through the abdominal wound as it became flaccid and ultimately delivered. It sprang from the left ovary, the pedicle which was moderately long was clamped and the tumour removed, the vessels of the stump were then picked up separately and tied with fine carbolized cat-gut, a double carbolized silk ligature was then introduced through the pedicle beneath the clamp and the clamp removed. No bleeding occurred, but it was thought more safe to tie the pedicle in two halves with silk; this was done and the ends cut short and pedicle dropped back. The right ovary was next examined and found to contain a number of small cysts, it was therefore removed, the stump being trusted to a medium sized carbolized catgut ligature, all bleeding points were secured by fine catgut or seared with the thermo-cautery, all clots removed and abdominal cavity cleansed, the wound was then closed with three silver wire sutures and several catgut sutures and dressed in the ordinary way with antiseptic gauze and roller. The cyst with contents weighed 28 lbs. The morning after the operation the temperature was 99°, it rose to a hundred that evening and the following the second after the operation, after which it came down to 99° and to the normal standard on the fifth day, at which it remained to the end of the case, the wire stitches were removed on the ninth day, union was complete, she left her bed and went on a sofa on the eleventh day and the day following got up and dressed. This patient returned home at the end of the third week.

Case No. VI.—Catherine B., æt. 39, eight years married,

had been three times pregnant, two miscarriages at 4th month and one child living, aged six years. Since the birth of living child has not been pregnant. Menstruation began when 13 years of age and has always been regular. In October, 1879, first noticed difficulty in micturition and found she was enlarging, supposed it was from pregnancy, although the catamenia continued regular up to April or May of last year, when the flow became profuse and occurred every three weeks. In November, 1880, the abdomen was greatly distended; she was examined by a physician, who pronounced it to be an ovarian tumour. He introduced a full-sized aspirating trochar, but without any result, as no fluid was removed. She continued to enlarge steadily, and again, in December or January, 1881, she was tapped with a large-sized trochar, and about a tea-cupful of thick glutinous material came away; this was all that could be obtained and its removal afforded no relief. She came to Montreal and was admitted into the Montreal General Hospital, on 6th May, 1881. Patient is a slight woman, rather short, greatly emaciated and abdomen enormously distended, the enlargement appears regular and uniform. Fluctuation distinct all over abdomen, with characteristic dullness, the greatest girth was on a line two and a half inches above umbilicus and gave 47½ inches in circumference.

May 11th, the operation was performed with full antiseptic precautions, an incision four inches in length, commencing just below the umbilicus, and extending downward towards pubis was made, this was carried through the abdominal parietes until gelatinous matter began to flow from the wound, as the cyst appeared to have been opened, what was supposed to be its wall was separated from the parietes of the abdomen for an inch or two, when it was found to be the peritoneum much thickened and in a condition of cystic degeneration, this was freely incised and the tumour brought into view. A large sized trochar was then introduced, but nothing came away, the cyst itself was then freely incised and an enormous quantity of thick gelatinous material removed, in quantity sufficient to fill three buckets, the cyst sprang from right ovary, with a moderately long pedicle, this was clamped, the tumour removed and the pedicle secured with carbolized silk ligatures.

The left ovary contained fluid of the same character and completely filled the pelvic basin, to which it was generally adherent by firm bands, these were stripped off and the growth removed; the pedicle, which was small, was secured by a single catgut ligature. The great omentum presented the same cystic degeneration and was greatly enlarged and thickened, this was also removed, being tied in sections, six in number, with carbolized gut, the ends cut off short. The entire mass of disease being removed, all bleeding points were secured, either by fine catgut, or the hemorrhage arrested with the thermo-cautery. The abdominal cavity was then carefully sponged out and the wound closed with three silver and eight catgut sutures. Lister's gauze dressing applied with a large pad of jute, the dressings retained by a broad roller of antiseptic gauze. The operation occupied one hour and three quarters, during all of which time the spray was kept up. The entire mass weighed 46 lbs. Half an hour after the patient was removed to her bed she became collapsed and death appeared imminent, ♏ xv of ether was injected subcutaneously, hot water bottles were applied to the surface, a second injection of ether was given, and brandy in half teaspoonful doses administered every five minutes. At the end of an hour reaction was fully established and from this time she progressed favorably. The temperature rose to 103° the evening of the operation, on the following morning it was 99° and from this time the temperature remained normal at the morning observation, with a rise to 99°.4 at night, this continued with very slight variation throughout the case. She remained in a very weak state for some time, but gradually recovered her strength and left for home on 11th June, 1881.

I have heard of this patient quite recently, September 28th, she has perfectly recovered and is in robust health.

CASE No. VII.—Hannah L., æt. 20, unmarried, a healthy looking, well nourished young girl was admitted into the Montreal General Hospital, 16th May, 1881. Has always enjoyed good health, menstruated for the first time at the age of 14 and has been regular ever since. About twelve months ago, in May, 1880, she noticed her abdomen enlarged, she did not at that time feel any distinct tumour, nor can she state on which side it first appeared. Shortly after discovering the fullness, she observed that very slight exertion induced fatigue and sometimes pain in the right side and groin. This feeling of weariness and pain has she thinks increased with the growth of the tumour.

The abdomen was found much distended, being well rounded and prominent in front. It gives a measurement at umbilicus of 35½ inches, fluctuation is distinct, the slightest tap producing the characteristic wave. The uterus was small, the fundus pushed over to left side, sound enters to the normal length.

The operation for removal of the tumour was performed on May 26th, An incision three inches in length was made in the median line commencing just below the umbilicus, the tumour freely exposed the patient was turned on her side, a large trochar introduced and the sac emptied. There was one large cyst and several smaller ones, no adhesions existed, the cyst wall was readily delivered, it sprang from the left side and had a pedicle of good length and thick, which was clamped and the mass removed. The vessels of the stump were taken up and ligatured with fine carbolized catgut, the stump transfixed and tied with strong carbolized silk, the ends cut off short and the stump dropped back. The right ovary was also found diseased and had to be removed, being tied at its peritoneal attachment by strong carbolized catgut. The peritoneal cavity was carefully sponged out and several small blood clots removed. The wound was closed with two silver wire and three carbolized catgut sutures and the ordinary gauze dressing, applied with a firm pad of carbolized jute. The time occupied was a little over half-an-hour. Weight of tumour and contents 16¾ lbs.

This patient made a rapid recovery. The highest temperature noted was on the evening of the day after the operation, when it rose to 100°.1F and throughout the case afterwards it remained at the normal standard in the morning, rising to 99½ at night. She was allowed to leave her bed on the 9th June and was discharged cured on the 15th June and left the hospital on that day.

Case No. VIII.—Jane H., æt. 40, a rather tall but spare unmarried woman, was admitted into the Montreal General Hospital, June 1st, 1881. She is from the country, and as a girl had always enjoyed good health. Menstruation set in at the age of 18 and has always been irregular and rather scanty; in 1877 it ceased for three months, and she was treated for amenorrhœa. In August of last year she took cold and was again treated for this cessation of the menstrual flow. It returned in January last, but she was never certain as to time; the last appearance was on the 16th April last.

About July or August, 1880, she observed that her abdomen was swollen, but more on the right side. Since January last this tumour had rapidly and steadily increased. In April after the last menstrual period, she found her limbs swollen and œdematous, during the past six weeks the feet and legs have greatly increased in size, the skin being white and shining and pitting on pressure. For some months has suffered from frequent miotu-rition and for the last six weeks has been much troubled in this respect. In September of last year and again in January had some pain over abdomen, lasting for over a week, this was unattended by fever. This patient is of slight build, tall, very thin and presents that haggard appearance peculiar to ovarian disease. She prefers being propped up in her bed at night almost in the sitting posture, but says she can lie down. On examination abdomen found distended with a huge tumour, which yields a dull note everywhere. A number of superficial veins apparently enlarged, are seen coursing over the tumour.

The following measurements were taken :

From Symphisis Pubis to Xyphoid Cartilage	17	inches.
" Umbilicus to right Anterior Superior Spine	9	"
" " left " " "	10½	"
" right side vertebral column	19½	"
" " left " " "	20	"
Girth of Abdomen, 2 in. above Umbilicus	41	"

Percussion gave a distinct wave at all parts of abdomen, dullness existed over the entire abdominal parietes as high as the ribs; on vaginal examination the uterus was small, the uterine sound, entering to the normal length, the organ appeared to be carried over to the left side and was quite movable, considerable fullness existed behind which pushed it forwards.

June 7th.—The bowels were cleansed by an enema and the urine drawn off, the patient placed under ether and the operation was performed in the usual way, an incision four inches in length was made, extending from just below the umbilicus downwards in the median line, the tumour was freely exposed, it was found to be slightly adherent to the abdominal wall, these adhesions were readily broken down, the patient was rolled over on to her right side, a large sized trochar introduced and the contents of a dark colour, tolerably thick flowed away. As the cyst became flaccid it was drawn out through the wound and ultimately delivered, it sprang from the left ovary.

The pedicle moderately long was clamped and the tumour removed, the vessels in the pedicle were secured by catgut and the pedicle itself transfixed and tied with two carbolized silk ligatures, the peritoneal cavity was then carefully sponged out, several bleeding points secured with fine catgut and wound closed by three silver and seven catgut sutures. From the time of commencing to give the ether up to her being placed in bed after the operation, one hour and ten minutes elapsed. She speedily recovered from the ether, one hour after she had a slight chill, ¼ gr. of morphia was given hypodermically and brandy in drachm doses, ordered to be repeated every half hour. Two hours after the operation, viz. at 4 p.m., sixteen ounces of limpid urine was drawn off, at 8.15 p.m. she again complained of pain and a desire to pass water, when twenty-two ounces of urine was again removed by the catheter, temp. 100°, pulse 98, moderately full but soft. She slept well during the night, small quantities of champagne were given occasionally. At 3 o'clock twenty-two ounces of urine was again drawn off and again at nine o'clock the following morning eight ounces of urine was removed, at twelve o'clock four ounces of urine was drawn off, making a total of seventy-two ounces of urine secreted during the first twenty-four hours after the operation.

June 8th, at the hour of visit she was very comfortable, the œdema of legs nearly altogether gone ; no pain or tenderness, pulse 108, temperature 99°. The temperature fell to the normal standard during the day, and remained at that with slight variation throughout the case. Nourishment in the form of milk and lime water, in small quantity and frequently repeated was given and champagne occasionally. After the fourth day she was more generously fed, but she preferred milk, which appeared to agree well with her. The bowels acted on the sixth day, the dressing was not disturbed until the eighth day, when the wound was found quite closed and the wire sutures were removed. from this time she rapidly gained strength and she was allowed up on the 10th June, the twelfth day after the operation.

Case No. IX.—This case is added to the series, although from the date it will be seen that the operation was performed after my return from the meeting at Halifax.

Annie McD., æt. 21, was admitted into the Montreal General Hospital, August 11th, 1881.

Previous History.—Had always enjoyed good health, the catemenia began at the 14th year of age, had never been regular as to time, five and six weeks would elapse between the periods and on several occasions three months had passed without any change, when it did occur it was sometimes profuse and sometimes scanty in amount, has otherwise enjoyed good health. Two years ago the secretion was arrested for several months and she consulted a physician, who gave her medicine, which after an interval restored the flow and she improved in health and strength. In January of this year, she noticed that her abdomen was enlarging on the right side below the line of the umbilicus. The tumour was quite distinct, movable, and continued steadily to increase in size. In March she became very ill and suffered from severe pain at the lower part of the abdomen more referable to right side, this soon spread over the whole abdomen. There was much fever, vomiting and excessive tenderness, she was actively treated and at the end of three weeks had quite recovered, but it left her very feeble. The growth has greatly increased since this attack and the menstrual irregularity remained as before.

Present condition—She is a florid complexioned girl, healthy looking although thin, has been losing flesh of late, appetite fairly good. Since March last, there has been a continual bloody discharge from the vagina, this is small in amount. The abdomen was about as large as a woman at the seventh month, the tumour could be readily made out and appeared to be made up of a number of small cysts, fluctuation was indistinct, and several hard masses could be felt. She measured 38½ in. on line with the umbilicus. By vaginal examination the uterus was found of small size, inclined to the left side and the sound entered to the normal length, the organ was slightly movable.

August 7th.—The patient was placed under ether and an incision three inches in length was made, extending downwards in the median line from the umbilicus. On entering the peritoneal cavity a large quantity of fluid escaped, the tumour was freely exposed, the patient turned on her side and a large trochar inserted, very little fluid escaped as the tumour was made up of a number of small cysts and solid matter, there were a few adhesions in front which readily broke down and several firm adhesions were found behind it, being attached to the mesentery, these were separated with care, but being unable to get the growth out through the incision it was lengthened to above the umbilicus and then the tumour was readily delivered. The pedicle was short and broad and engaged the left ovary. The clamp was applied and tumour removed, the pedicle was then transfixed and tied in two halves by carbolized silk, the ends cut short and the stump dropped back. The right ovary was found healthy, all bleeding points being secured and the cavity carefully sponged out, the abdominal wound was closed with silver and catgut ligatures and dressed antiseptically. The weight of the tumour and contents was 20 lbs. This patient made a very rapid recovery. The temperature rose to a 102° F. the night after the operation, it however gradually and steadily subsided to the normal standard. She left her bed at the end of a fortnight, the wound was not disturbed until the tenth day, when the stitches were removed and it was found completely closed. She shortly after left for home, at Gaspe Basin.

Speaking on the subject of antiseptics in surgery (*Brit. Med. Journal*, Dec. 20th, 1879, page 1003), Sir James Paget is reported to have said: "There are certain groups of surgical cases in which, so far as I can yet see, it would be absolutely wrong to dispense with any portion of the most complete antiseptic treatment. Amongst these are cases of ovariotomy." This is very strong testimony coming from a surgeon of such eminence, and one who does not appear to be thoroughly convinced of the absolute benefits of antiseptics after Lister in all surgical cases.

There are other groups of disease in which Sir James Paget speaks of antiseptics in the same strong terms. Excisions of joints are amongst the number in which he believes full antiseptic precautions should be employed. In this connection I may report the results of nine cases of excision of the knee joint treated with full antiseptic precautions, and all recovered with useful limbs; several, in a very short space of time. The splint used in these cases was that recommended by Mr. P. H. Watson of Edinburgh, employing parafine to consolidate the splints, and the antiseptic dressing was in each instance applied outside the splint. These are my own personal record.

On a former occasion I recorded eleven cases of excision of the knee joint, all my own, with one death from pyæmia and one subsequent amputation, these are to be found in the first volume of Transactions, published by this Association. Paget remarks, in connection with lumber abscesses: "Another group of cases is the opening of large abscesses. I remember to have believed, a few years ago, and I think I rightly believed, that I had never seen a patient recover who had a lumber abscess opened by free incision; I believe every one died. Since that time, I have heard of and seen a number of cases where psoas abscesses or large abscesses in any part have been opened with absolute impunity under antiseptic treatment."

In this connection I have to report four cases of psoas and lumbar abscess, opened during the past year, with full antiseptic precautions, three cases of huge peri-nephritic abscess and three cases of large empyema, all operated on under full antiseptics and all terminating favorably; in these cases free incision was practised, and a large-sized drainage-tube introduced and retained in the abscess cavity. With the exception of one case, I did not observe what has been reported by others, viz. the arrest of secretion of pus from the abscess cavity after evacuation of its contents, but then in all these in which this result did not follow the abscess cavity did not completely empty itself at the time it was opened. In the one exceptional case, that of a little girl, with disease of the spine and psoas abscess, the opening was made in the outer side of the thigh, and at the second dressing there was merely a trace of pus and subsequently serum alone flowed away until all discharge ceased and the wound closed at the end of the second week.

The delay in publishing this paper has given me an opportunity of reading what has been recently said on this subject before the International Medical Congress, held in London. Mr. Spencer Wells, in speaking on the question of antiseptics and drainage says, "what appears to me so remarkable is, that while in general antiseptic surgery drainage is so very essential, is indeed a fundamental part of the system, in my own experience of ovariotomy, and of the removal of uterine tumors, antiseptics have abolished drainage. I have not even used a drainage tube for more than three years." And again he observes, "since adopting antiseptic precautions, either fluids do not form, or if they do, they do not putrefy and they are absorbed without doing any harm, without leading to any febrile rise of temperature."

Such, indeed, was the result in all of the cases above recorded. Some stress has been laid on the sayings of Professor Lister, in connection with the use of the spray. In the September number of this Journal,* Prof. Lister is reported to have said, (referring to the use of the spray,) "I am not certain but I shall give it up, I am not at all sure but that before the next meeting, two years hence, I shall have abandoned the spray altogether." This report differs somewhat from what is to be met with in the *Lancet* and *Medical Times*. In the report of this meet-

**Canada Med. and Surg. Journal*, vol. x, page 102.

ing in the *Medical Times* of Aug. 20, page 233, it will be found that Prof. Lister, "insisted that the comparison of ovariotomy with other operations cannot fairly be made." . . . "He scarcely hoped that many of the precautions he now uses will be dispensed with; but if the time should ever come when it was proved to demonstration that no floating particles were present in the air which could cause putrefaction, he would heartily join in the now well-known exclamation *fort mit dem spray!*"

SOME OBSERVATIONS UPON THE INTERNATIONAL CONGRESS.

By R. P. HOWARD, M.D., L.R.C.P., Lond., &c.
Professor Practice of Medicine, McGill University.

(Communicated by request to the Medico-Chirurgical Society of Montreal.)

Gentlemen,—It is my intention to confine my few observations upon the great International Congress recently held in London to portions only of what I heard and saw at that meeting, selecting, more especially, topics of interest to myself, and merely glancing at, not studying, them.

The International Medical Congress assembled in St. James' Hall on 3rd August, and was opened by the President of the College of Physicians, Sir Wm. Jenner, who occupied the chair—having on his right the Prince of Wales, and on his left the Crown Prince of Germany. The vast hall appeared to be crowded with excited men, who watched with intense interest the arrivals, on the raised seats of the platform, of the distinguished men deemed to be entitled to such positions, as well as of those whose official relations to the Congress secured them places amongst the celebrities. It was soul-stirring, as well as gratifying, to hear the loud applause that greeted, from time to time, the arrival of the men whom the representatives of the medical world delighted to honour; amongst them may specially be mentioned Jenner, Paget, Virchow, Pasteur, Donders, Charcot and Lister. The distinguished chairman opened the meeting with a few well-chosen observations upon the value of the science of medicine and its superiority to other secular employments; and he dwelt briefly upon the principles which should move and regulate medical men. After the Prince of Wales had very happily paid a tribute of praise to the value of medical science to the nations of the earth, and had suggested the benefits that must result to medical science from the deliberations and discussions of the Congress, the President, Sir James Paget, delivered his inaugural address. It is quite impossible to convey any idea of the powerful impression produced on that large assembly of well-informed judicial-minded men by the address. The quiet but impassioned manner—the inspired thoughts—the eloquent words—the noble and reverent bearing of the speaker—justified the opinion that finished oratory was compatible with the highest attainments in the science and art of medicine. The address should be studied by every physician. The serious work of the Congress began in the several sections on Thursday, and was continued daily until the following Tuesday, occupying from 10 to 1 A.M. in all, and from 3 to 4 P.M. in some of the sections. It was, of course, impossible to visit more than one section at a time, and the speaker thought he would derive most instruction by confining his attention to one or two. . He selected those of pathology and medicine,—the former presided over by the distinguished pathologist, Dr. Wilks; the latter by one of the astutest diagnosticians in England, Sir William Gull.

Amongst the many topics which occupied the members of these sections, time will permit me to glance at but a few even of those which I had an opportunity of hearing discussed. Naturally, the subject of *micro-organisms* and their relations to *specific diseases*, and especially to "*unhealthy processes arising in wounds*," claimed a prolonged consideration. It was understood that Professor Lister would introduce the discussion on the latter topic, but, simply remarking that perhaps too much attention had been paid to atmospheric "germs" as causes of disturbance in wounds, he gave at some length a sort of clinical exposition of sympathetic inflammation and of the principles of counter-irritation.

Dr. Bastian, in a clear and concise speech, called in question the existence of specific germs, whose introduction into wounds interfered with their healing, and contended that minute organisms may arise in wounds, abscesses, etc., from changes in the protoplasm of degenerating or dying tissues.

Several speakers, and notably Prof. Virchow, discussed the probable intimate relations of the micro-organisms to one another, and described recent experiments which appeared to prove that the nature and properties of these lowly organic beings are largely modified by the conditions under which they are developed, the soil in which they grow, the food on which they live, etc.

On this occasion, the great Pasteur produced a sensation in the section by first confessing that his ignorance of English and German had prevented his following the arguments of the previous speakers, and by then exclaiming, in reply to Dr. Bastian, who, he was told, held that micro-organisms may be formed by heterogenesis of the tissues, "Mais, mon Dieu, ce n'est pas possible," and without advancing any argument, then sat down. The eminent man for the moment seemed unable to realize the possibility of intelligent dissent from his assertion. However, in his address on the germ theory, delivered subsequently, he vindicated his reputation as the "father" of living fungologists. In that address he confined himself chiefly to the modifications that can be produced in the virus of chicken cholera and of anthrax or charbon, by suitable treatment or cultivation of the germs of the poisons of those specific diseases. He explained the process by which the virulence of those poisons may be so attenuated that they may be safely inoculated upon poultry and sheep respectively, with the result of protecting those animals from subsequent severe attacks of cholera or of anthrax. As I remarked in my valedictory address to this Society, when vacating its presidential chair a year ago, we have here a general method of attenuating the viruses of the infectious diseases which, when completely elaborated, will place them all under our control, as vaccination has done for small-pox. Pasteur stated that within fifteen days 20,000 sheep and a large number of horses and cattle had been thus protected against anthrax in the neighbourhood of Paris.

The consideration of micro-organisms was continued next day, but from different points of view, by Prof. Klebs, Fokker and Heuter, and by Mr. Watson Cheyne and Dr. Koch. The time at my disposal would not permit me, even were I able, to relate the many important facts and theories that were adduced by the several speakers during the two days occupied in the consideration of these minute organisms, and I will be content to remark that Dr. Koch's beautiful demonstrations went far to prove that the micro-organism of each infectious disease is a *distinct species*, capable of reproducing the same disease and the same micro-organisms, and none other; and that the general outcome of the discussion went far to establish the doctrine that *specific communicable diseases* are produced by *specific germs*.

Bright's disease occupied a large attention, no less than eight papers upon that subject having been presented in the sections of Pathology and Medicine. They well illustrated the great differences of opinion that still obtain amongst pathologists as to the several alterations of the kidney which belong to that affection—the relations of these alterations to one another and to the recognized causes of Bright's disease.

While Rosenstein confined Bright's disease to *diffuse inflammation*—acute or chronic—of the kidney, and excluded the fibroid kidney of pregnancy and cardiac disease and the pure amyloid kidney, Grainger Stewart included them all under that title, which, as you are aware, is the custom with English pathologists. Again, while Saundby maintained with Weigert and Bamberger that both the large white and the small red kidney are the result of *diffuse* inflammation, involving the tubules, the Malpighian bodies, and the connective tissue, Grainger Stewart contended that the disease might *commence* in any *one* of those structures or in them *all* simultaneously, and Rosenstein held that the "red granular kidney" does not start from a *diffuse inflammation*, but from "endarteric changes" of the renal vessels with shrinking of the glomeruli.

On the vexed question of the relation of *renal diseases* to *alterations* of the *heart and blood vessels*, the opinions expressed were not at all in harmony. Sir Wm. Gull and Dr. Sutton, maintained that the thickening of the heart and vessels may precede the renal changes—that the alteration in both the renal and the vascular organs may be due to the same causes—and that the heart and vessels may be found hypertrophied and yet no changes in the kidney be discovered, *post mortem*. It is worthy of mention, that Dr. Sutton related an instance in which he knew of the existence of contracted kidney for 10 years, and yet the cadaveric examination revealed no disease of the heart or vessels. On the other hand, Dr. Grainger Stewart, Prof. Rosenstein and Dr. Broadbent had never seen a case of granular kidney unattended by hypertrophy of the heart, unless other conditions had existed to prevent the heart from suffering, and Prof. Rosenstein believed that granular kidney never exists without hypertrophy of the muscular coat of the vessels and that the thickening of the intima is inflammatory and not physiological as Dr. Johnson had taught.

Dr. Broadbent regarded excretory materials in the blood as *the* cause of Bright's, a view almost identical with the one so ably defended recently by Dr. Mahomed. He holds the arterio-capillary fibrosis of Sir Wm. Gull and Dr. Sutton to be a consequence not a cause of renal disease.

The veteran renal pathologist, Dr. George Johnson attempted, but not satisfactorily, to prove that tube casts containing white blood cells, (leucocytes) unmixed with renal epithelium occur in the urine and are diagnostic of the *glomerulo-nephritis* of Klebs. The most important paper upon Bright's disease was contributed by Dr. Mahomed who maintained that *high arterial pressure*, even in young and apparently healthy persons, if continued long, will produce the changes in the heart and vessels observed in chronic Bright's disease. Albuminuria will be absent and should death occur, the kidney will usually be red and granular. The reliable evidence of the renal affection in such cases, will be the existence of the signs of high arterial tension and of hypertrophy of the left ventricle. Mahomed's views elicited no criticism! As might be expected, a discussion on *tubercle* was amongst the orders of the day, but it was loose and erratic and unconvincing, and largely drifted into a consideration of the nature of giant cells. Dr. Creighton read a short communication, the purport of which was that *disseminated* tuberculosis is due to a *virus* introduced into the body from without, and not to a *primary focus* of disease in the body, *from which* the organs generally become secondarily infected. This *virus* theory has been favoured by Klebs and it doubtless is very acceptable to Dr. Creighton, as affording support to his recent views on the transmissability of the tuberculous affection of cows through their milk and flesh to the human subject. On this latter highly important subject, Prof. Virchow, whose opinions carried very great weight in the Congress, stated that notwithstanding the long attention that had been given to it by himself and others in Germany, there was as yet no satisfactory evidence that tuberculous disease was communicated to the human race by the flesh or milk of the cow.

Prof. Erb's paper "*on the role of syphilis as a cause of locomotor ataxy*," confirmed the very frequent occurrence of a syphilitic history in ataxic patients as had been previously pointed out by Gowers and others, but the discussion thereon left it yet to be made out what, if any, etiological relationship exists between the two affections. Certainly the failure of iod. pot. and of mercury in ataxia is a strong therapeutic argument against the syphilitic nature of the lesions found in the cord in locomotor ataxia and Prof. Lancereaux stated that those lesions do not exhibit the characters of *syphilitic* lesions of the spinal chord and other viscera.

Prof. Flint, of N.Y., read a carefully prepared communication on "*the analytical study of auscultation and percussion*," etc., the main objects of which, appeared to be to indicate the character of abnormal pulmonary sounds, by comparing them with those heard in normal chests and by analysing their component parts, so that the sounds may be recognized by their *characters* chiefly, without reference to the physical conditions under which they are produced. The many points contained in the communication and the lateness of the period at which it was read, no doubt accounted for the few remarks it elicited from those present. A committee of experts, however, was named by the chairman to draw up a uniform nomenclature for the physical signs of pulmonary disease and to submit it for general adoption at the next International Congress.

"*The value of Bacelli's sign*" was brought before the Medical Section in a short paper by Dr. Douglass Powell. Bacelli maintains that, in pleuritic effusion, if the whispered voice be well conducted and pectoriloquous on the side of effusion, the fluid is serous; if badly conducted or inaudible, it is purulent. Dr. Powell concluded that although Bacelli's sign was by no means pathognomonic, yet that in association with other signs it is of considerable value. Prof. Ewald contended that an exploratory puncture afforded the only means of determining with *certainty* the nature of pleuritic effusion.

A valuable paper on "*Ulcerative or Infectious Endocarditis*" was read in the Pathological Section by a member of this Society, Dr. Osler, the very frequent connection of which affection with lobar pneumonia he was the first to indicate and emphasize. He adduced reasons for believing that ulcerative endocarditis is less frequently associated with acute rheumatism than is supposed, and he threw doubt upon the existence of a special connection of the micrococci, found in the affected valves, with the disease. Like several other valuable communications, it was not discussed for want of time.

The last communication that was read in the Medical Section was that of Dr. C. T. Williams on "*The Treatment of Phthisis by Residence at High Altitudes.*" Nothing very important was enunciated by its author, but he had not time to read it all. The statements which specially struck me were: That all the advantages of mountain climates, without their disadvantages, can be obtained at *moderate* elevations, *i.e.*, from 4,000 to 10,000 feet; that mountain climates are generally contra-indicated in pyrexial phthisis; that the circumference of the chest in consumptives enlarges from 1 to 3 inches at these altitudes; and that, while this expansion may disappear in a few months on a return to low levels, it is, in the majority of cases, of long duration, and probably permanent. It is matter for great regret that a paper upon so important a subject should have been assigned the last place, when no adequate time remained in which to elicit the opinions and experience of so many authorities collected from various parts of the world. Only a few members spoke, and their observations were few and rather general. Dr. Herman Weber referred the good effects obtained at high altitudes to absence of matter productive of fermentation, to dryness and rarefaction. He said that wherever the air was tolerably *aseptic*, benefit might be obtained. Dr. Wilson Fox remarked that nearly all high elevations are curative, even although the climate be hot.

Besides the above, there were about thirty other communications upon many important subjects in pathology and medicine, which I did not hear, or of which I heard only parts of the discussions raised upon them. It caused me much regret not to have heard Dr. Hughlings Jackson's able exposition of his own special subject, "*Epileptiform Convulsions from Cerebral Disease*," and Jonathan Hutchinson's thoughtful observations upon "*Rheumatism, Gout, and Rheumatic Gout.*"

Of the work done in the Congress as a whole, you may, perhaps, form some idea if you bear in mind that, besides the two attended by me, there were thirteen other sections and one subsection, in most of which an equivalent amount of time and thought were devoted to their respective subjects. This large volume in my hands is made up of condensed abstracts in English, French and German, of the communications that had been promised the Congress up to the time it was published, and other communications were subsequently presented. Glancing at the table of contents, in the Anatomical Section are found the titles of 19 communications.

In the Physiological, 16 topics are specified for discussion, six of which were brought before the section. Two papers were also read, and the afternoons were devoted to demonstrations and to the exhibition of physiological apparatus. (V.) In the Surgical Section, 47 papers are acknowledged.

(VI) In the Obstetrical, 27. In Section VII—Diseases of Children, 36. In Subsection IV—Diseases of the Throat, 38. In Section VIII—Mental Diseases, 18. In Section 10—Ophthalmology, 38. Section X—Diseases of the Ear, 14. Section XI—Diseases of the Skin, 17. Section XII—Diseases of the

Teeth, 11. Section XIII—State Medicine, 25. Section XIV—Military Surgery and Medicine, 20; and in Section XV—Materia Medica and Pharmacology, 13,—making a grand total of 377 communications and discussions announced in the book of abstracts, independently of the work to be done in the physiological section. The Congress was emphatically a working one.

There were two other features of the Congress that were, I believe, new departures at such assemblies, and certainly not the least valuable methods of instructing the members. One of them was the daily exhibition of patients, suffering from unusual or newly recognised or obscure forms of disease, and the other was a temporary museum, containing over 700 illustrations of interesting varieties of disease, either in the form of drawings or of actual pathological preparations. As Dr. Osler intends describing this museum, I will confine myself to an enumeration of some of the *living* illustrations provided for our instruction. In this department that remarkable man, eminent alike as pathologist and surgeon, Jonathan Hutchinson, exhibited 2 or 3 examples of tubercular leprosy, in one of which the disease had ceased to progress, and recovery had taken place; two cases of rupture of the brachial plexus; several subjects of severe bone disease from inherited syphilis; and some cases in which rheumatic arthritis and gout co-existed.

Dr. Ord produced five patients suffering from myxœdema in various stages of progress. All were over 30 and only one of them was a male. They presented a general swelling of the skin like that of renal dropsy, but the œdema did not pit or change position and the urine was free from albumen. Other leading features were a temperature below the *norme*; a weary expression; slowness of speech, thought and movement; impairment of memory; feebleness of gait; disorders of taste and smell; loss of hair, even of eyebrows, and of teeth.

Two interesting cases of progressive muscular atrophy were shown by Dr. A. Sturge, in one of which groups of symmetrical muscles were implicated in different regions. Dr. Barlow presented a boy, the subject of inherited syphilis, and of *aphasia*, with right brachial monoplegia.

Examples of "Charcot's joint disease" were supplied by Messrs. Macnamara and Page; Mr. Treves contributed a remarkable instance of enormous varicose veins of abdominal walls, the cause of which was most obscure, and a rare deformity of the bones of the leg, in an adult, so-called "osteitis deformans."

The rare forms of skin diseases, gathered for our inspection were very numerous and diversified and in this work the following gentlemen laboured earnestly: Drs. Crocker, Duckworth, Stephen Mackenzie, Colcott Fox and Cheadle and Messrs. Jonathan Hutchinson, Startin, Morrant, Baker and Malcom Morris. Amongst the rare forms of skin disease exhibited, deserving of special mention were the following:

Three cases of diffused scleroderma, one of them undergoing cure. Three or four of morphœa, one of them involving the forehead and a portion of the scalp, and another involving almost the entire person except the face. Two females with small areas of blanched and apparently atrophied skin, symmetrically situated on either side of the neck and near the lower attachment of the sterno-cleido mastoids.

Several children in whom patches of chronic urticaria had become pigmented—urticaria pigmentosa. Two examples of pigmentation following lichen planus, and distributed all over the body. A youth presenting a miliary papular eruption, thought to be syphilitic, dating from early childhood, and scarcely to be distinguished from lichen scrofulosum.

Several examples of xanthelasma. A case, the nature of which was not agreed upon, was shown by Mr. Startin. A girl five years old, free from hepatic and other diseases, presented groups of nodules (very like the whitest nodules of xanthelasma) which were situated symmetrically on the back of the elbows, in the popliteal regions, and in the cleft of the nates. Mr. Hutchinson doubted their xanthelasmic nature.

Very many cases of lupus erythematosus were shown, and several of leucoderma. A remarkable case was that of a girl, about 12 years old, with perfectly white hair, her skin also showing a want of pigment. She had lost her hair five years previously from pityriasis rubra.

There were many other varieties of disease exhibited in living subjects, but I must bring my remarks to a close. I have avoided speaking of the valuable addresses read in the general meetings by the distinguished men selected for that duty, and in the various sections by their respective presidents, as well as of the contents of the temporary museum, and also of the social features of the Congress, with the view of leaving them for the abler handling of my companion throughout the Congress, who will now address you. But I must not sit down without bearing testimony to the abounding hospitality which was extended to the members of the Congress by the British people, lay and professional.

THE USE OF THE OPHTHALMOSCOPE IN THE DIAGNOSIS OF BRAIN DISEASE.

By W. F. COLEMAN, M.D., St. John, N.B.

(*Read before the Canada Medical Association at Halifax, Aug.* 4, 1881)

Mr. President and Gentlemen,—Our knowledge of the physiology and pathology of the central nervous system is so limited, the diagnosis of brain lesions so difficult, the well-known conditions of the eye in those lesions so unmentioned or dubiously mentioned by the text-books on medicine, as to furnish me with some excuse for urging the claims of the ophthalmoscope in the study of the intra-ocular end of a brain nerve during its structural changes and in the diagnosis of diseases of the brain and cord. Though the matter may embrace a limited personal experience, and little originality, I freely admit the testimony of such authorities and special writers as Drs. Allbut, Jackson and Gowers, and Mr. Nettleship, and, incidentally, many others. While the nature of many diseases within the chest and abdomen is revealed to touch and the ear, the maladies of that most inaccessible part of the body—the cranium—give out no certain sound, and will not disclose themselves to any wizard's touch; so it remained for the genius of VonGraefe and Sichel, the patient, skilful labours of Sæmisch, Liebreich, Schweigger, Sœlberg-Wells, Jackson, Allhut, Gowers, Hutchinson and others to illuminate with the ophthalmoscope the dawning light through which men were eagerly striving to discover the nature and situation of intra-cranial diseases.

The popular idea that the oculist has, and perchance *needs*, no knowledge of general medicine to successfully treat the eye, is no less false than the, I fear, professional belief that the general practitioner can gain little from the ophthalmoscope. With the herculean task of acquiring a fair knowledge of the structure, working, derangement and repair of the general system, it is not to be expected that even a Hercules could also keep abreast of the information and experience in regard to any special organ. Yet, since the whole is made up of all its parts, and the parts are interdependent and dependent upon the whole, any approach to a comprehension of the whole organic system must involve some familiarity with every part. No more striking illustration of this can be cited than the evidence of cerebral lesions that may be elicited by an ophthalmoscopic examination of the intra-ocular end of the optic nerve, called the optic disc or papilla. In the pre-ophthalmoscopic period (prior to the great invention of Helmholtz in 1851), there certainly had been something done to trace the connection between amaurosis and brain disease in atrophy of the optic nerve, but a meningeal inflammation propagating itself along the optic nerve as a descending neuritis had not been thought of: and the cause is not far to seek, for in brain disease, accompanied by very considerable optic neuritis, the sight may be perfect, hence disease of the optic nerve was unsuspected. It thus happens that many patients having symptoms of brain disease, with some lesion of the optic nerve, have, on account of perfect vision, no disposition to consult an oculist, and while so few men in general practice use the ophthalmoscope, one most important sign of encephalic disease will be frequently overlooked. As the optic papilla is the chief intra-ocular part concerned, and furnishes the most palpable and constant information in intra-cranial disease, let us briefly consider the anatomy of the optic nerves. Under the name of the optic tracts, they take their origin just in front of the cerebellum, in the tubercula quadrigemina or optic lobe, to which visual perception is attributed, also in the corpora geniculata; they then pass forward along the under surfaces of the crura cerebri, taking on their way some fibres of origin from the optic thalami and reaching the olivary process of the sphenoid, just under the floor of the third ventricle, unite to form the optic commisure or chiasma. The distribution of the fibres of the chiasma sometimes enable us to fix the site of lesions interfering with vision, *e.g.*, the right tract supplying optic fibres to right half of each retina, and the left tract fibres to the left half of each.

As the optic nerves pass forward from the chiasma they receive at the optic foramina a loose sheath, from the dura mater, which becomes lost in the sclera. The nerve is about $\frac{1}{8}$ of an inch in diameter, before it perforates the cribriform plate of the sclera, and contracts to $\frac{3}{4}$ of this diameter at its intra ocular end, where it spreads out to form the internal layer of the retina. The nerve is also invested by a second close fitting inner sheath, which is continuous with the pia mater, and sends processes between the nervules of the optic bundle. Between this inner and the outer sheath is the vaginal space of Schwalbe, which is continuous posteriorly with the arachnoid space of the brain, and anteriorly within the posterior part of the sclerotic opening, is by some, said to be continuous with lymphatic spaces in the substance of the optic nerve, by others to be closed. Evidently the vaginal space may become distended by subarachnoid fluid for there is *not* a reflection of the arachnoid at the optic foramen to prevent it. As the internal carotid artery emerges from the inner wall of the cavernous sinus, it gives off the ophthalmic artery, which after passing through the optic foramen gives off the arteria centralis retina, this enters the optic nerve, runs forward in its substance, perforates its disc near its centre, then subdivides and radiates to its distribution in the retina. The retinal venules, converging unite to form the two venæ centrales, which pass out through the disc near the artery and in the nerve trunk unite to empty into the ophthalmic vein, which passes through the sphenoidal fissure and empties into the cavernous sinus.

Further and most important to the subject, the blood supply

to the optic nerve and disc is according to Galizowski, independent of the ophthalmic artery (which more particularly supplies the retina) being part of the vascular system of the brain. He describes a posterior optic artery to the testis; a middle optic from the choroid plexus to the geniculata; and anterior optic from the middle cerebral to the optic tract; and capillary branches from the pia mater to the chiasma.

The appearance of the optic disc, the first time I discovered it with the eye mirror and a 2½-inch lens, struck me as resembling a cream-rose full *moon*, about the size of a large split pea, rising in a pink sky of surrounding choroid, which, by its contrasting colour, gave a well-defined sharp border to the disc. The retinal vessels radiate irregularly from the nasal side of the centre of the disc, the larger branches, passing upward and downward, completely avoiding the temporal sides.

The changes in the disc produced by cerebral and spinal diseases are—*Congestion*, *Inflammation*, and *Atrophy*. The congestion of the disc may be a simple hyperæmia; if attended by œdema, it is the stauungs papilla of Von Gracfe, the "choked disc" of Allhut, or ischæmia of the disc, or congestion papilla. In intra-ocular neuritis, or, as it is called, papillitis, the papilla alone may be affected; in other cases, the neuritis occupies the length of the optic nerve, as has been shown in autopsies by Allhut, Hulke, Virchow, &c. Atrophy of the disc may be primary or simple, or it may be consecutive as a consequence of papillitis. Authorities are in accord as to the great frequency of *optic neuritis* in intra-cranial disease. Annuske and Reich collected 88 cases of intra-cranial growths with ophthalmoscopic examinations and autopsies, and found ophthalmic changes in 75 per cent. By common consent, the most frequent cause of optic neuritis is intra-cranial tumour; next to it, meningitis. Cerebral abscess and softening are occasional causes, nnd hemorrhage a very rare one. Tumour is nearly always attended by optic neuritis (Hughlings Jackson). Allbut writes: "My own opinion certainly is that changes either of a congestive, neuritic or atrophic character may be found in the discs at some time or other in the course of almost all cases of intra-cranial tumor."

"From my own experience (Gowers) I should say that neuritis occurs in about four-fifths of the cases of intra-cranial growths." Encephalic disease may also manifest itself through paresis or paralysis of the ocular muscles, producing squint and double vision. That optic neuritis may possess diagnostic significance of brain lesion, the extra-cranial causes which produce, or are associated with, neuritis must be borne in mind, such as albuminuria, lead poisoning, the exanthemata, suppression of the menses, pernicious anæmia, loss of blood, exhausting diseases, neuralgia of 5th nerve, in rare cases secondary syphilis (Nettleship), and tumours in the orbit. It may occur idiopathically without obvious cause (Gowers). Simple *congestion* or *hyperæmia* of the papilla very commonly precedes atrophy. It is sometimes the expression of a state of congestion and degeneration of the whole optic nerve, but sometimes apparently limited to the disc (Gowers). It frequently is the first stage of tobacco amaurosis, the last being atrophy.

Choked disc, or *hyperæmia with œdema*, is the first stage of neuritis, and frequently associated with it. Its principal causes are said to be the same as produce neuritis, viz., tumours, meningitis, and hydrocephalus.

Primary atrophy of the disc is more frequently associated with locomotor ataxy than with any other diseases. Often I have seen it occur without assignable cause, and once from a blow on the eye, Galezowski gives a table of 166 cases embracing the causes of primary and consecutive atrophy.

Cerebral causes	40
Locomotor Ataxy	33
Traumatic	22
Alcoholism	13
Syphilis	12
Other causes	46
	——166

Allbut is of opinion that primary atrophy is generally due to mischief at the base (tumour), or to ventricular dropsy, which may compress and sever the nerves or tracts at some point in their course. From the evidence of Messrs. Critchett, Wordsworth and Hutchinson and others, and my own experience, I think that tobacco in excess will produce atrophy of the discs, though many deny it. To be able to distinguish between a *normal* appearance of the papilla and the inception of a pathological, much experience is required, and the attempt will soon prove the saying, "Pathology is but the shady side of physiology." A full-blown neuritis may be quite palpable to an amateur ophthalmoscopist, while an expert may be unable to decide as to a slight hyperæmia or say whether a disc is pale from incipient atrophy or simple decoloration. *The* indication of hyperæmia is an abnormal redness, which has a tendency to blur the edge of the disc. Comparing the eyes may give some help, and noting whether the redness increases from time to time. The signs of neuritis and choked disc are similar, and vary with the stage. In the first stage the disc is less swollen and red, and the edge, though blurred, may be still distinguished, while in intense papillitis the colour of the disc is so blended with that of the surrounding choroid that it can be frequently distinguished only as the points of convergence of the retinal vessels. Impairments or loss of sight is the chief symptom in intense neuritis, though there may be marked neuritis without any impairment of sight. Pain in the eye is rare. Vision usually begins to fail first in one eye, and sight may fail completely in a few days or decrease very slowly. Restriction of the visual field is common, and colour-vision may be defective. The neuritis of tumour is double, rarely unilateral. Dr. Jackson has pointed out that the neuritis often coincides in its onset with an obvious increase in the other symptoms of the cerebral tumour. It appears that neuritis is usually a late production of tumour. Dr. Jackson recorded one case in which a man had had symptoms of cerebral tumour for nine years; during the last three years his discs had been repeatedly examined and found normal; six weeks before death, neuritis was discovered.

The signs of atrophy are pallor and later depression of the disc, with shrinking or absence of the capillaries. When the atrophy is marked there is diminished vision, nearly always more considerable in one eye than the other. There is a concentric irregular marginal limitation of the field of vision. Frequently there is defect of color-vision.

The relation of papillitis to intracranial disease is still a vexed question. I shall refer briefly to the principal theories. Von Graefe gave the first in 1859. He distinguished two cases. In one the change in the disc (neuritis) was slight, with a tendency to invade the adjacent retina. In this case there was meningitis, and inflammation of the nerve trunk was found by Virchow, which inflammation was assumed to have been communicated to the optic nerve from the inflammed meninges, and to have descended the nerve to the eye. This Von Graefe designated, "descending neuritis." In other cases of considerable swelling, hæmorrhages and vascular distension of the papilla (stanungs papilla), accompanied by cerebral tumour, no signs of inflammation were perceptible on naked eye examination of the trunk of the optic nerve. This condition of the papilla he attributed to increased intracranial pressure, which obstructed the return of blood from the eye through the optic vein by compressing the cavernous sinus.

The theories of Schmidt and Manz are largely accepted in Germany. Manz showed that distension of the vaginal space around the optic nerve is frequent in neuritis, and believed the extension to be due to intracranial pressure or increase of subarachnoid fluid. Further, he found that injections into the subarachnoid space, of animals, passed into the sheath and caused fulness of the retinal veins, and in some cases transient redness and swelling of the papilla. Schmidt demonstrated that a colored liquid injected into the sheath passed into the lymph space of the nerve at the lamina cribrosa, and suggested that neuritis is produced by the irritation of the liquid passing into the lymph spaces.

A theory was put forward by Schneller, in 1860, extended by Dr. Hughlings Jackson in '63, supported by Brown-Sequard, and was formulated by Benedikt in '68. It assumes that the tumour acts as a source of irritation, which has a reflex influence through the vasomotor nerve upon the optic disc leading to its inflammation. Of these theories, that which accounts for changes in the disc by inflammation of the meninges propagated along the nerve trunk, appears the best supported by the frequent determination upon *post mortem* and microscopical examinations of the conditions upon which the theory is based. Although neuritis may occur in tumour of any size or kind, in any part of the brain, it is rare in tumour of the convexity, while it is common in that of the base and most common in that of the anterior lobes (Russell-Reynolds). Again, *meningitis* limited to the convexity is *seldom* accompanied by intra-ocular changes, while *basilar* meningitis is *usually* attended by neuritis. In many cases of tumour, a local meningitis in the vicinity of the growth and accompanied by inflammation of the optic tract have been found. Now the proximity of this *inflammation* of the basilar meninges (whether independent or the result of tumour) to the optic tracts makes its communication to the tracts highly probable, and the fact of the so common association of inflammation of the meninges and tract increases the high probability to a seeming certainty.

A case of Mr. Hutchinson's in which no distension of the retinal veins was produced, although the cavernous sinus was completely obliterated by the pressure of an aneurism, seems to go far towards destroying the theory of obstructed blood return from the eye by pressure on the sinus. The vaso-motor theory is rejected by Leber and a numerous following, on the ground that it involves a mechanism not known to exist and a complex relation of the optic nerve to all parts of the brain difficult to conceive.

In the balance of the prescribed half-hour I shall give very condensed and imperfect reports of a head case and one of spinal disease, with defective sight, under my care in the St. John General Hospital, and a head case with eye disease in the general wards:—

Jan. 31*st*, 1881.—P. G., aged 43, says his sight began to fail after cutting his thumb and profuse bleeding ten years ago, and since then could see to read only very large type. Sight has been the same for past three years as at present.

V. R. E., 15/40.	No. 15, J. 8	Not improved with glasses.
V. L. E., 15/70.	No. 18, J. 8	

There is gray atrophy of both discs. Has smoked four to five pipes a day for past 23 years, and drank pretty hard for years up to four years ago, but scarcely any since. Is very nervous. Wakes in the morning with headache and sickness. Memory bad for two years past. Gait unsteady for two or three years. Walks as though he had taken a little too much. Diagnosis—Locomotor ataxy and atrophy of discs. Treatment—Stop smoking. ℞ St. gr. 1-24; hypodermically and increase gradually.

March 4th.—Is getting gr. 1-6th Strych. Vision, right and left, increased to nearly normal, =15/16. ℞ St. gr. 1-5th. Strych. increased the staggering gait. ℞ Croton chloral grs. v, and return to St. gr. 1-6th. *15th*—Discontinue Str. ℞ Arg. Nit. gr. 1-12, and increase to gr. ½ taken daily by stomach.

April 8th.—V. R. =16/20. Discharged.

July 19th, 1878.—Mary Smith, aged 20, single, lost the sight of right eye completely and suddenly three weeks ago. Pain came on in the brow the same day, before the sight failed, and has kept her awake most of the time since. Day before yesterday, lost the sight of left eye in the same way as the right. Has no perception of light. Pupils react very slowly to light. Has *white atrophy of both discs.* Patient very nervous, and has slight choreic movements. History—For two weeks last summer had constant pain in the top of head, and vomited three or four times daily; denies syphilis. Family history—Lost three brothers and one sister in their first year. Treatment—Potass. Iodid. grs. x. Tr. Cinch. ℨi, t. d.

July 24th.—No pain in head since yesterday. Pupils widely dilated and immovable; no perception of light.

Aug. 1st.—Patient drew attention to two syphilitic ulcers on calf of leg. Diagnosis—Syphiloma at the base, implicating optic nerves. *8th*—L. E. V.: Seeing position of window. R. E., *Nil.* Stop Pot. Iodid. ℞ Hyd. Perchl. gr. 1-12; Am. Mur. grs. v.; Tr. N. Vom., ♏ x.; t. d. *20th*—℞ Ung. Hyd. ℨss rubbed into axilla and thigh on alternate days; Pil. Hyd. grs. ii twice daily.

Oct. 12th—No ptyalism. ℞ Pot. Iodid. grs. v.; Sp. Am. Ar. ℨi; Tr. Cinch. ℨi; t. d. Stop other treatment. *22nd*—Mouth very sore and mercurial fetor. Discontinue Potass. Iodid. ℞ Pot. Chlor.

Nov. 7th—V. right eye, *nil;* left eye, counting fingers 13*th*—Repeat Pot. Iod. grs. x., t. d. 25*th*—V. R. E., motion of fingers. V. L. E., fingers, two feet, and sees to get about well. Left eye diverges when right eye fixes for near point. When the eyes are at rest, both look to the left.

Dec. 21*st*, '78, *to April* 9*th*, '79—Patient had Strych. Sulph. hypodermically gr. 1-24 up to gr. ⅛, when gait was made unsteady, then gradually reduced to gr. 1-16. Had tenotomy of the right internal and left external muscles. The hands are now quiet, and patient much less nervous. V. R. E., perception of light. V. L. E., 12/200. Direction of eyes much improved, but still look slightly to left. Discharged: to take Hy. Cl. gr. 1-16, Str. gr. 1-16.; t. d.

June 5*th*, 1881.—J. B. Hansell, æt. 53, admitted into the general ward a few days ago. He is a muscular looking man, 4 ft. 10 in. high, weight about 130 lbs. Says for the past year he has had a very dizzy head and will fall any day in the road, soon gets up and walks off. The fall was always preceded by giddiness. Six months ago began to vomit about every second day, and soon after vomited every morning if he laid in bed up to 7 o'clock. When he rose earlier the vomiting did not come on. This continued up to last week, since when he has not vomited. During the past month, has had a pretty severe pain from the forehead to the back of the head, lasting an hour or two every day and has not seen to read. Memory failing for past year. Pulse 68, small and rather weak; skin normal temp. to touch; appetite good; bowels costive; sleeps well; whistles feebly; grasp of hands weak; flexion of forearms and legs strong; gait very unsteady and seems in constant danger of falling; patellar reflex normal; no lightning pains; urine normal; right ear hears the watch only at ½ in., ordinary loud voice at 10 ft.; left ear hears the watch only at contact or ordinary voice at 4 ft.; speech, broken Dutch-English, probably normal; smell normal; pupils slightly dilated by atropine; v. right eye, counting fingers, 2 ft.; v. left eye, counting fingers, 12 ft.; ophthalmoscopic examination shows intense optic neuritis with hæmorrhages and infiltration of retinal disc.

June 25th.—Right pupil half the size of left, left pupil a little smaller than an average pupil; right pupil reacts very slowly to light, left pupil reacts more but imperfect; percussion on the temples hurts a little, on the forehead less; head 24 in. in circumference.

July 15th.—Last evening and this morning refused to take his medicine, saying there was something in it to poison him. *Diagnosis*, tumour of the cerebellum involving the tubercula quadrigemina.

July 24th.—The patient was discharged at his own request.

Gentlemen, your patience must not be further tried, I shall only add if on account of any words of mine the ophthalmoscope shall aid you in the diagnosis of so obscure a class of disease, as those of the central nervous system, I shall think your time not wasted and myself more than repaid for this paper.

RECOVERY FROM A LARGE DOSE OF MORPHIA AND CHLORAL HYDRAT.

By CLARENCE J. H. CHIPMAN, B.A., M.D., Prescott, Ont.

On Saturday evening, August 27th, about 6:30 p.m., I was called to see a middle-aged lady, who was said to have taken an overdose of morphia. It appears that the lady, whose husband was suffering from partial paraplegia, and who also had the charge of a sister who had long suffered from an aggravated nervous disorder induced by the excessive use of stimulants, had herself begun to indulge in stimulants, and for a week past had eaten next to nothing, and imbibed so freely as to have been on the verge of D. T.'s. Her sister had been using the following mixture prescribed by an Ogdensburg physician, of which she took from three to four doses a day:

℞	Chloral Hydrat.	ʒiii
	Potass. Bromid.	ʒii
	Morph. Sulph.	℈ii
	Syrup Aurantii	℥iv
	Aquæ	℥viii

Dose—One teaspoonful as directed.

While another sister who had come to aid her in nursing had gone to tea, the lady whom I was called to see obtained the bottle from another room, and telling her husband that she was going to take a dose of chloral, proceeded to pour some out into an ordinary tumbler, which she swallowed. Almost immediately, as I am informed, she fell over on the bed, on the side of which she was sitting, with her face downwards.

Her sister was hastily summoned from the dining-room, and endeavored to raise her up, but the patient being a woman of large frame, rolled over on to the floor, from which she was raised with the help of a friend who happened to be passing.

I was sent for, and on reaching the house found the party lying on the bed, apparently in a state of complete unconsciousness.

The countenance was deeply livid, pupils contracted to the size of pin-heads, breathing very slow and stertorous.

Not possessing a stomach-pump myself, I went in search of one, but neither Drs. Jones or Buckley, whose assistance I called in, had one, so I obtained an ordinary enema syringe, and by tying a gum elastic catheter to one end, we at once introduced it into the stomach, and proceeded to inject warm water, which we afterwards pumped out by reversing the syringe. This we did several times till we thought the stomach was thoroughly washed out. A powerful magneto-electric battery was applied, and kept constantly going. Attempts were made to rouse her by violent shaking and slapping of the face and other parts of the body, but she seemed completely unconscious. Having brought with me a solution of atropine of ⅛ gr. to a drachm of water, I gave her 20 minims hypodermically. This soon affected the pupils, and after a time increased the breathing gradually from 4 to 12 per minute. The pulse was small and frequent, and could with difficulty be counted. During the night I gave her the rest of the atropine in two doses, and the other means were continuously kept up.

Strong tea and coffee were injected into the bowels. Frequent slapping of the face and shakings were used, but no response was elicited.

By 4 a.m. we had almost given up hope. The respiration had

again sunk to 4 per minute, and the pulse was very small. At 7 a.m. I raised her up, and sat her on a sofa, and commenced slapping the back with clothes rung out of cold water. Occasionally there appeared to be a slight movement of the eye-lids; but after a little while the face became so livid that I again placed her in a partly recumbent position.

From this time slight symptoms of returning consciousness began, and by 9 a.m. she had attempted to speak. At 12 m. (Sunday) she had spoken. At 3 p.m., with considerable difficulty, I catheterized her, and removed a considerable amount of urine, though she resisted very strongly. 8 p.m.—She had recognized those about her. 10 a.m., Monday.—This morning she seemed perfectly conscious, though she had no recollection of what had occurred.

At the time of writing, she is going about the house, and, with the exception of being weak and very sore, she is comparatively well. As to the dose taken, as far as I can make out, it was probably not less than a tablespoonful, and possibly more, which would be about 2 grains of morphia, 60 grains of chloral and 40 of bromide of potassium.

A CASE OF TETANUS NEONATORUM.

By JOHN REDDY, M.D., L.R.C.S.I., &c.,
Physician to the Montreal General Hospital, &c.

The unusual occurrence of a case of trismus neonatorum induces me to put on record the only one I have seen in this country.

On the 15th Oct., 1880, I was called to see a female infant eight days old; it was a well-nourished, healthy child. The mother gave me the following history: She had a good, natural labour, lasting about seven hours. When the child was born, the midwife remarked that she had never seen so thick a cord, which she described as being as thick as a child's wrist, and very soft, on account of which she found much difficulty in tying it. After some hours she had to be sent for again on account of a continual slow bleeding from the end of the cord, which necessitated its being tied again in two places. On the second day it nursed freely and seemed well till about 3 o'clock in the morning of the sixth day, while at the breast, it was seized with crying, as if in pain, which was quickly followed by a short fit, like a convulsion. This happened whenever the child was put to the breast afterwards. On the eighth day I was sent for.

On seeing the child, it appeared quite tranquil till the attendant began to undo its napkin, when the child became suddenly convulsed, the eyes were set, mouth rigidly fixed and jaws tightly locked, the characteristic Risus Sardonicus present and face slightly livid, the thumbs were tightly pressed into the palms of the hands, the whole body participating in the tetanic movements. The least disturbing cause reproduced a regular fit. Its bowels were opened a few times since the attack commenced, and it frequently wet its napkins.

I put it upon small doses of chloral hydrate, which, for the first two hours, appeared to alleviate the spasms, but it died in a severe tetanic spasm six hours from my first visit.

The mother fell about a month before the child was born, which, at the time, she considered had hurt it, but there was no evidence of injury at its birth. She has always been a most temperate-living woman, very healthy, and is 25 years of age. She had two children previously, and one died while teething. She lives in a very ill-ventilated and badly-lighted house. I was much struck on entering with a very bad odour. As this is supposed to be one of the most frequent causes of the disease, it may probably have given rise to it in this instance; but it may also be attributed to another cause of a traumatic character, the condition of the cord and the number of times it had been tied.

ANNUAL MEETING OF THE AMERICAN GYNECOLOGICAL SOCIETY.

REPORTED BY WM. GARDNER, M.D.,

Prof. Medical Jurisprudence and Hygiene, McGill University; Attending Physician to the University Dispensary for Diseases of Women; Physician to the Out-Patient Department, Montreal General Hospital.

Those conversant with the literature of gynecology will admit the great value of the contributions of the American Gynecological Society. They are referred to, quoted, and regarded generally as authority by workers in the special field of gyne-oology throughout the world. The transactions of the Society have now reached the number of five handsome volumes, whose contents are of interest and value alike to the practical and the more strictly scientific worker. The Society, it will be remembered, was organized in 1876, the centennial year of the American Union, with forty members. The moving spirit in its organization was the indefatigable secretary, Dr. Chadwick of Boston. The membership is limited to sixty. Candidates for election are required to submit an original paper on some gynecological subject to the council of the Society. If considered to be of sufficient merit, the council recommends the author to the Society for election, which is by ballot of the Fellows.

The sixth annual meeting was held in New York city, in the hall of the Academy of Medicine, on the 21st, 22nd and 23rd of September. After the meeting had been called to order, and in a few words cordially greeted by Dr. Reamy of Cincinnati, first Vice-President (the President, Dr. Byford of Chicago, being unable to attend from illness), he called upon Dr. Fordyce Barker, President of the New York Academy of Medicine, for an address of welcome.

Dr. Barker, in the course of his address, which was brief, but eloquent and cordial in its tone of welcome, alluded to the high character and great value of the work of the Society as embodied in its transactions. Special allusion was made to the scientific work of Dr. Dalton with reference to the corpus luteum, and to the index of the gynecological literature of all countries contained in each volume of the transactions. This index is prepared by Dr. Billings of the Army Medical Library at Washington, in conjunction with Dr. Chadwick, the secretary, and contains the title of every book, paper or article on gynecological subjects published in all countries and in every language. He further referred to the auspicious occasion of the formation of the Society—the centennial year,—and compared it to that of the present meeting, when the whole country was clouded by a national sorrow for the death of President Garfield.

A number of guests having been nominated by the council,

were elected by the Society and cordially invited to participate in the discussions and to be present at the social entertainments provided for the Society. Among these, Dr. James Bell of this city and the writer had the honour of being enrolled.

To British eyes there was the novel sight of half-a-dozen lady physicians being present, and one of them (Dr. Mary Putnam-Jacobi) taking part in the discussions. She spoke on three or four occasions. Her observations were marked by evidences of her well-known extensive professional culture and critical acumen.

The programme of sixteen papers was then proceeded with. The first on the list was on "Acute Diffuse Hyperæsthesia of the Peritoneum following Minor Gynecological Operations," by Dr. Busey of Washington. The paper was based on a case in which violent peritoneal pain and tenderness increased by the slightest motion, but without fever, tympanitis, or any other symptom of inflammation, followed dilatation of the cervix by a laminaria tent in a case of anteflexion, with dysmenorrhœa.

Dr. Busey considered the condition to be a neurosis, excited by the irritation of the terminal filaments of nerves in the lining membrane of the cervix being reflected upon the vaso-motor system, causing the pallor and coldness, and upon the pneumogastric, causing vomiting and other symptoms of this nature. The author solicited the criticism of the Fellows, in view of the frequency of such symptoms after minor gynecological operations.

Drs. Trask, Reeve, Campbell, Van de Warker, Emmet and Noeggerath took part in the discussion. Certain of the speakers welcomed the title proposed for this condition, and thought the author had done good service by calling attention to a set of symptoms rather commonly witnessed. A practical outcome of the experience thus elicited was the opinion that such symptoms passed on sometimes to genuine peritoneal inflammation, and that this might be prevented by giving opium or morphia early and in large doses. Dr. H. F. Campbell, in such cases, would give quinine in large doses. He had seen the symptoms follow vaginal injection of cold water after sexual intercourse used with the object of preventing conception. Dr. Reeve had seen it follow the application of a cold stream of water to clear away the glairy mucus from the cervix.

Dr. Emmet thought the term misleading, as tending to withdraw attention from a condition which he believed to be always present with, and usually the cause of, corporeal anteflexion, and a common complication of other uterine affections, namely, pelvic cellulitis. He reiterated his well-known views of the frequency of this cellulitis in a latent form, ready to be lighted up into the acute form by some cause of irritation of varying intensity, but occasionally very slight.

Dr. Noeggerath thought some of these cases were due to sudden expulsion of irritating catarrhal secretion from the Fallopian tubes into the peritoneal cavity. He based this opinion on appearances observed in a fatal case, in which he made an autopsy. In others he thought the condition neuralgia of the peritoneum and in others still, neuralgia of the uterus.

Dr. Garrigues of New York next read a paper on "Exploratory Puncture of the Abdomen."

This was a most exhaustive paper, of high scientific and practical value. It was based on the results of examination, chemically and microscopically of 94 specimens of fluids of all kinds, obtained from the abdomen. The results of Dr. Garrigues' investigations lead him to conclude that there are no distinctive chemical, spectroscopical or microscopical characters of ovarian fluids, but he mentioned as facts of some value, that as a rule ovarian fluids do not coagulate spontaneously, whereas fluids from uterine fibro-cysts usually do and so also ascitic fluids, to a slighter extent. There are no distinctive pathological or morphological elements to be recognized by the microscope in such fluids. The granular (so-called ovarian) cell of Drysdale, of Philadelphia, Dr. Garrigues believes to be not a cell but a fatty nucleus. It is not pathognomonic or distinctive of ovarian fluids, as it is invariably present. He has found it in cysts of the broad ligament, in cancer of the peritoneum, in renal cysts and vaginal cysts. He believes certain spindle-shaped cells to be the most valuable microscopic evidence, but their presence would not enable the observer to say more, than that the fluid was from a cyst of the ovary, Fallopian tube or broad ligament. A careful examination of a specimen fluid from the abdomen would enable a competent observer in the great majority of cases to say whether or not it was ovarian, but he did not believe that an operation in a doubtful case ought to be undertaken from evidence based on microscopic examination alone, although with other evidence he believed it to be of great value. He had found nothing morphologically characteristic of cysto-sarcoma of the ovary, but had often noticed a great abundance of cellular elements in such fluids. He admitted the danger of puncture for exploratory or other purposes, but believed that by the following precautions which he always adopted, danger would be avoided ; tapping should be done at the patient's home ; a small canula not exceeding two millimetres in diameter is to be used ; it is to be soaked in a five per cent solution of carbolic acid ; it is to be pushed in slowly, as thereby the danger of wounding a blood vessel is lessened, the artery or vein will probably be pushed aside ; the cyst is to be emptied slowly and completely except there be strong reason to suspect fibro-cyst, when it must only be partially evacuated, because of the fact that such cysts do not easily collapse ; lastly, the patient is to be kept in bed for a few days afterwards.

Drs. Drysdale, Kimball, Lyman, Barker, Emmet, Dunlap, Engelmann, Howard, Chadwick and Noeggerath took part in the discussion.

Dr. Drysdale reiterated his well-known views, maintaining the pathognomonic character of the ovarian cell. Drs. Kimball, Lyman and Barker spoke of the dangers of tapping. Dr. Barker related a case of the late Dr Peaslee, in which the patient died of bleeding into the peritoneal cavity after tapping. Emmet is opposed to puncture, as in his experience both bladder and colon may lie in front of the tumour. Dunlap disapproves of tapping, because it destroys the possibility of diagnosis, as it allows the intestines to descend in front of the empty collapsed cyst. He believed it was, however, occasionally necessary, and he had performed it on a few occasions, in desperate cases, to ward off impending death and so gain time for the performance of ovariotomy.

The other speakers conceded the dangers of tapping, but asserted its occasional necessity or expediency. Dr. Drysdale stated, however, that he had seen several hundreds of tappings in his own practice and that of his father-in-law, Dr. Atlee, and had never seen fatal results. He places the patient on her back, and causes the abdominal walls to be supported by a bandage gradually tightened. He thinks the danger increased by partial rather than complete withdrawal of the fluid.

Dr. Chadwick thinks tapping is not to be lightly undertaken; it is dangerous to leave a part of the fluid, and it is dangerous to manipulate the sac after tapping. He has not found that tapping of cysts of the broad ligament always cures them. There is decided danger in tapping uterine fibro-cysts.

Dr. Noeggerath mentioned a fact bearing on the value of microscopic examination of suspected fluids. He had sent specimens of the fluid from a cyst of the thigh to three of the best microscopists in the country. All pronounced it to be ovarian.

Dr. Lyman of Boston then read a paper on "Pelvic Effusion resulting in Abscess." It was based on 146 cases of pelvic abscess occurring in his own practice and that of his colleagues at the Boston City Hospital. This considerable mass of experience perhaps did not evolve anything very new about this condition, but it served to emphasize certain important facts in the history of such cases. 1st, That pelvic effusion is very commonly present without being recognized, the symptoms being those of fever, more or less marked, with or without dysenteric phenomena. 2nd, Early recognition of the presence of such effusion is of the utmost importance. 3rd, Early evacuation of fluid effusion, serum or pus is of great consequence, as the danger of troublesome or incurable chronic burrowing of pus in the pelvic cellular tissue is thereby prevented.

The paper elicited a spirited discussion by Drs. Albert Smith and Ellwood Wilson of Philadelphia, and Barker, Mundé and Emmet of New York.

Dr. Albert Smith agreed with the author of the paper as to the frequency with which such conditions are not recognized, and as to the necessity of early opening, through the vagina, if possible; as when the opening is into the rectum, the subsequent course of the case is often very tedious from repeated closures and reopenings of the abscess cavity, with the usual constitutional symptoms.

Dr. Fordyce Barker said that, in an extensive consultant obstetric practice, he had been much struck with the fact of how frequently physicians failed to diagnose this condition. He advocated early tapping, and related how he had often seen most remarkable results—relief of pain, fever, etc.—even when only one or two drachms of serum were removed.

Dr. Mundé is a strong advocate of early exploratory tapping in doubtful cases, and corroborates Dr. Barker's experience of the remarkably good results of removal of even small quantities of pus or serum. He had never seen any dangerous results from the practice.

Dr. Emmet spoke of the frequency of pelvic effusion—cellulitis. It may complicate every morbid uterine condition. His experience of the use of the exploratory trocar is not so favourable as that of some of the speakers who had preceded him.

Dr. Goodell of Philadelphia read a paper on "Bursting Cysts of the Abdomen." It contained reports of cases of cysts bursting and disappearing (in some cases coincidently with copious flow of urine), and occasionally reappearing, the results being sometimes spontaneous cure, sometimes death, or cure by subsequent ovariotomy.

Drs. Chadwick, Barker, Kimball, Dunlap and Marion Sims each related cases of similar nature, with varying results. Dr. Sims thought cure was most apt to result when the opening was large.

Dr. H. F. Campbell of Augusta, Georgia, read a paper on "Erysipelas in Childbed, without Puerperal Peritonitis." This was the report of a case of erysipelas of the head and face in a woman eight months pregnant, which he had attended, delivery taking place during the course of the disease, the patient recovering without bad symptoms. Dr. Campbell considered that the woman escaped ill results by the fact that she was attended in labour by a midwife and not by himself.

Dr. Mary Putnam-Jacobi suggested the explanation that as cutaneous erysipelas was now believed to be a disease of the lymphatic system, the disease in this case never came near the uterine wound which is produced, as asserted lately by Ercolani, in the human female only, by the separation of the decidua serotina.

Drs. Albert Smith, Ellwood Wilson and Lyman had each attended midwifery while in attendance on cases of erysipelas. By great care in disinfecting the hands, the lying-in patients escaped. Dr. Barker believed that there was great danger when the erysipelas was of the suppurating or phlegmonous form, but that in the cutaneous form there was no danger, or, at all events, it was much less.

Dr. Thomas of New York read a paper on "Adhesion and Expansion of the Bladder to the surface of a Tumour or to the abdominal wall, complicating Laparotomy." Dr. T. began by saying that in this paper he did not allude to simple band-like adhesions of the bladder to the tumour or other organs, but to an apron-like spread of the bladder over the tumour or abdominal wall, leading to danger of the viscus being cut into by the operator. The adhesion probably took place in the pelvis during the early stages of growth of the tumour, and was drawn up as the tumour grew. He alluded to six or seven cases which he had found on record, and then related a case that had recently occurred to himself. This was the case of a woman of 38, the subject of ovarian tumour, which he was proceeding to remove. On opening the abdomen, he was led to suspect the nature of the case. He attempted to clear up the difficulty by passing the catheter, but the instrument could not be made to pass above the pubes. He then cut through the anterior wall of the tumour and introduced one or two fingers into what turned out to be the bladder, which extended upwards over the tumour to midway between the umbilicus and ensiform cartilage. It was impossible to dissect the posterior wall of the bladder from the tumour, so he cut away its anterior wall with the bladder attached. The tumour was then removed and the pedicle ligatured and dropped. During this stage of the operation the bladder lay forwards on the thighs of the patient like an apron. The bladder was then replaced in the abdominal cavity, and the edges of the opening in it clamped by the edges of the abdominal incision. The latter was closed by the usual sutures introduced from above downwards. At the level of the opening in the bladder, the needle was made to pass through its edges as well. The patient did well. A month after the operation there was still a pin-hole urinary fistula, but this was easily closed by twirling in it a tenotomy knife and putting in a suture. Three months after the operation the patient was able to return to her home perfectly well. Dr. Thomas believes the diagnosis in these cases to be impossible before the abdominal incision, as the use of the catheter or sound is inefficient, from the size and pressure of the tumour. The operator must depend on touch and the use of the tenaculum and scalpel to open the bladder and explore by the finger.

Drs. Kimball, Engelmann and Goodell related cases of similar nature with various results.

Dr. Emmet congratulated Dr. Thomas on the masterly way in which he had successfully dealt with this rare but formidable complication, and remarked on the lesson that it taught of the necessity of care in entering the abdominal cavity.

Dr. Albert Smith, of Philadelphia, read a paper on "Axis-Traction in the use of the Forceps." The reader began by asserting that Osiander in 1799 was the first to speak of the necessity for axis-traction. Subsequently Naegele enunciated the same principle, and proposed to direct the traction in the axis of the pelvis by downward traction on the lock of the instrument by a fillet slipped over it in that position (the patient being in the dorsal position). Thirty-three years before Tarnier invented his forceps the principle of this instrument was discovered by Herman of Berne, who effected the object by attaching at right angles to the upper surface of the lock of the instrument a handle by which downward pressure was made, while traction was effected by the ordinary handles, the patient being placed on her back. Dr. Smith believes Tarnier's forceps to be dangerous and unnecessary. Other objections which, in his opinion, ought to weigh against it are its expense, the difficulty of disinfecting such a complicated aggregation of joints and screws; the compression screw, which he believes to be a dangerous method of diminishing or moulding the child's head; and, moreover, that it is very apt to rupture the vagina and perineum. He advocated, in preference, an ordinary double-curve Davis forceps, and he uses Osiander's method of directing the traction in the axis of the pelvis by making pressure on the upper surface of the lock by the palmar surface of one hand, while traction is effected by the other hand grasping the handles, and, if necessary, compressing the head. When the head comes round the pubes, the handles are of course raised. The discussion was by Drs. Lusk, Barker and Thomas of New York, and Dr. Howard of Baltimore, and Ellwood Wilson of Philadelphia. Drs. Lusk, Barker, Howard and Thomas believed Tarnier's instrument to be most valuable in a small number of cases of delay at the brim from contraction or otherwise, and in these it would enable the accoucheur to dispense with craniotomy. They admit the danger of laceration of perineum and vagina, and would always remove the blades when the head was on the perineum, and complete the delivery by the Ritgen-Goodell method. This danger has been much lessened in Tarnier's most recent model of his instrument, by an alteration of the curve and diminution of the width of the blades.

Dr. Ellwood Wilson of Philadelphia agreed with Dr. Albert Smith. He thought the Tarnier forceps undesirable and unnecessary.

Dr. Smith's paper, although not the last on the programme, was the last read. Thus concluded a very successful meeting. The social entertainments were characteristic of the profession in New York. They were lavish to a degree. Brilliant receptions were held by Drs. Emmet and Isaac E. Taylor, and lunches were provided by Drs. Barker and Thomas, Skene and Byrne, and J. Marion Sims. The Society honoured itself by the election of Dr. T. Addis Emmet to the office of President. The Vice-Presidents, Drs. Lyman of Boston and Noeggerath of New York, will meet with similar approval.

Reviews and Notices of Books.

Treatise on the Continued Fevers.—By JAMES C. WILSON, M.D., Physician to the Philadelphia Hospital: Lecturer on Physical Diagnosis, at the Jefferson Medical College. With an introduction by J. M. DACOSTA, M.D., Professor of the Practice of Medicine and Clinical Medicine, at the Jefferson Medical College, Physician to the Pennsylvania Hospital, etc. New York: Wm. Wood & Co. Montreal: J. M. O'Loughlin.

This volume is one of the series of Wood's library for this year. It will be found a sound practical treatise upon one of the most important subjects in medicine. These diseases are so common, they are so widespread, often so virulent in their character, their diagnosis not infrequently beset with such difficulty, that it is of great consequence for the general practitioner to be familiar with their every phase, and with the means which are recognised as best suited to control and cure them. The descriptions of the continued fevers here given are considerably more full than those found in most of the text books, in many of which but small space is devoted to them, and yet the author does not allow himself to be led away into a description of the many controversial points which might so readily be introduced in the course of such a treatise. This feature, and especially in a work of a professedly practical nature, is perhaps most noticeable in the chapters on treatment, where a very fair outline is found of the best practice of the present day, without unnecessary disquisitions on the various changes which have taken place and gradually led up to that which is adhered to. In speaking of the treatment of typhoid fever, it is stated that, "the expectant or rational treatment of enteric fever is that generally employed at the present time. Notwithstanding the diminished mortality following the employment of the antipyretic treatment in Germany, it has never been generally introduced in France, Great Britain or the United States, and the physicians of these countries for the most part still adhere to the expectant or the modified expectant plan." But the value and efficacy of quinine in certain cases in reducing fever is recognised, and the use of digitalis and the salicylates also recommended. The recent recommendation of Prof. Pepper to use nitrate of silver is also alluded to.

The book we find well written and think it will be well received by the subscribers and the profession generally.

Supplement to Ziemssen's Cyclopædia of the practice of Medicine. By GEO. L. PEABODY, M.D., Instructor in Pathology and Practice of Medicine, College of Physicians and Surgeons, New York; Pathologist and Medical Registrar to the New York Hospital. New York: Wm. Wood & Co. Montreal: J. M. O'Loughlin.

The object of this volume is to remove from *Ziemssen's Cyclopædia* "the few traces of time that the last few years have produced." Each special subject treated of in the original work has been carefully revised by a competent authority, and a digest made of the writings thereon, which have appeared since the date of the previous article. The work thus involved must have been very great, and Dr. Peabody is to be congratulated both upon the able staff of writers, whom he has enlisted in the service and the faithfulness with which each one has perfected the task committed to his care. Of course the additions to the text vary much in amount; in some cases it is expressly stated that it has not been found necessary to add anything to what had already appeared, as that was found to contain everything essential to completeness. Judging from an examination of a number of the sections, they all seem compiled with great care and, without being too extensive, are made to furnish any new or valuable discovery or observation, which may have been made known since the appearance of the original work. It is then an invaluable companion to everyone in possession of the great work and even to others it will prove extremely acceptable as presenting the results of recent advances in medical science in a very compact form. The general get-up and mode of division of the paragraphs, etc. is similar to that of the main volumes and it is furnished with a complete index.

A Medical Formulary based on the United States and British Pharmacopœias, together with numerous French, German and unofficinal preparations.—By LAWRENCE JOHNSON, A.M., M.D., Lecturer on Medical Botany, Medical Department of the University of the City of New York, Fellow of the New York Academy of Medicine, &c. New York: Wm. Wood & Co.; Montreal: J. M. O'Loughlin.

Some book of this kind every prescribing man must have. His pharmacopœias and dispensatories are not enough. From them he gets the official drugs, their preparations and doses, &c., and of course can, and often does, evolve from this alone his prescription for a given case. But it is not necessary for him to do this in every case. It is extremely useful for him to have put before him the combinations which, in the hands of experiencod men, have been found suitable for certain classes of cases. Thus this Formulary collects together an immense number of such prescriptions; recipes which have come into general use at some of the hospitals, or which have been brought into notice by individual physicians and surgeons. There is nothing new in all this of course, but still new remedies are always coming forward and new methods of using old drugs, and thus new formularies always contain valuable material. In looking over this book we find that the selections have been made from the best hospitals and from the published lectures and writings of the best known hospital physicians, both English and American. They seem to have been made with care and judgment, and to be in every way as complete as possible.

Medical Electricity: a practical treatise on the Applications of Electricity to Medicine and Surgery.—By ROBERTS BARTHOLOW, A.M., M.D., LL.D., Professor of Materia Medica and Medical Therapeutics in the Jefferson Medical College of Philadelphia, Fellow of the College of Physicians of Philadelphia, &c., &c. With ninety-six illustrations. Philadelphia: Henry C. Lea's Son & Co.; Montreal: Dawson Bros.

Although there are already a great many books of this kind

to be had, yet it must be confessed that there is ample room for usefulness for such an one as the present. This fact is alluded to by the author in his preface, where he says: "That there are excellent works on medical electricity is undeniable; but some of them are too voluminous, others too scientific, and not a few wanting both in fulness and accuracy. I have attempted, in the preparation of this work, to avoid these errors; to prepare one so simple in statement that a student, without previous acquaintance with the subject, may readily master the essentials; so complete as to embrace the whole subject of medical electricity; and so condensed as to be contained in a moderate compass. I have assumed an entire unacquaintance with the elements of the subject as the point of departure, for I am addressing those who have either failed to acquire this preliminary knowledge, or having acquired it, find that after the lapse of years it has become misty and confused." The object thus set before him, Dr. Bartholow would seem to have successfully carried out. Without being encumbered with numerous scientific terms and expressions, intelligible only to those familiar with the subject of electricity, this book contains complete descriptions of the various forms of electricity employed in either medicine or surgery, together with directions for their practical employment in the different affections suitable for their application. After the necessary chapters on the different kinds of batteries, galvanic and faradic treatments are fully discussed. Electrolysis finds its place as a remedial agent in tumors, aneurism and stricture. And amongst the more recent applications of electricity are the galvano-cauteries, and especially electrical lighting, full explanations being given of the numerous applications of the former in various kinds of surgical operations and the use of electrical illumination as an important aid in examination of and operations in, such concealed parts as the larynx, the nasal and auditory passages, &c. With the marvellous advances now almost daily made in electrical appliances, there can be no donbt that every year will see this agent more and more commonly used by the medical practitioner, both as a remedial agent and as a mechanical assistant; and Dr.

Bartholow's book is about the best general hand-book of the subject which we have ever seen.

An Introduction to Pathology and Morbid Anatomy.—By T. HENRY GREEN, M.D., F.R.C.P., London, Physician to Charing Cross Hospital and Lecturer on Pathology and Morbid Anatomy, at Charing Cross Hospital Medical School, etc. Fourth American from the fifth English and revised edition, with one hundred and twenty-eight fine engravings. Philadelphia, Henry C. Lea's, Son & Co. Montreal, Dawson Bros.

Green's pathology has for a considerable time enjoyed a wide spread reputation as one of the best books for the commencement of a systematic study of the subject, The reason of its popularity is to be found in the fact that it begins at the beginning and, after laying the foundation, leads gradually up towards the more difficult matters treated of under this department. It is concise and the descriptions are all remarkable for the clearness with which they are expressed. Beginning with the disturbances of nutrition and the degenerations, there follow descriptions of all the various forms of tumour; changes in the blood, thrombosis and embolism; then inflammation, with special reference to the manner in which the different structures of the body are affected by this process; tubercle and syphilis; and a special chapter on pulmonary phthisis. In its successive editions this useful hand-book has received many important additions and now in its present form contains all that it is essential to know of the morbid changes of our various organs. It is well illustrated with a large number of very useful and mostly original woodcuts.

Books and Pamphlets Received.

THE APPLIED ANATOMY OF THE NERVOUS SYSTEM.—By Ambrose L. Ranney, A.M., M.D. New York: D. Appleton & Co.

GENERAL MEDICAL CHEMISTRY: FOR THE USE OF PRACTITIONERS OF MEDICINE. —By R. A. WITTHAUS, A.M., M.D. New York: Wm. Wood & Co.

CLINICAL LECTURES ON THE DISEASES OF OLD AGE.—By J. M. CHARCOT, M.D. Translated by Leigh H. Hunt, B.Sc., M.D. With additional lectures by Alfred L. Loomis, M.D. New York: Wm. Wood & Co.

CYCLOPÆDIA OF THE PRACTICE OF MEDICINE.—Edited by D. H. Von Ziemssen. Vol. xx. General index. New York: Wm. Wood & Co.

LANDMARKS, MEDICAL AND SURGICAL. By Luther Holden. With additions by Wm. W. Keen, M.D. Philadelphia: Henry C. Lea's Son & Co.

THE MOTHER'S GUIDE IN THE MANAGEMENT AND FEEDING OF INFANTS.—By John M. Keating, M.D. Philadelphia: Henry C. Lea's Son & Co.

A SYSTEM OF SURGERY, THEORETICAL AND PRACTICAL, IN TREATISES BY VARIOUS AUTHORS.—Edited by T. Holmes, M.A. First American from second English edition, thoroughly revised and much enlarged by John H. Packard, A.M., M.D., assisted by a large corps of the most eminent American surgeons, with many illustrations. Vol. I. Philadelphia: Henry C. Lea's Son & Co.

Society Proceedings.

MONTREAL COLLEGE OF PHARMACY.

The opening meeting of this college was held on Tuesday evening, Oct. 4th, in the new rooms of the Association on McGill Street. The address was delivered by Henry Lyman Esq., upon "The progress of pharmacy in Canada for the last fifty years."

Before entering upon the subject of pharmacy the lecturer briefly alluded to the progress of discovery and the development of science generally during the past half century.

In speaking of the development of the railroad, the speaker amusingly contrasted the mode of travel of fifty years since, with its lumbering stage or mail coach, with its four or six horses and its dozen passengers, the masculine portion of whom were expected and often, in fact invited, to foot it up the hills and so work their passage; or perhaps the canal boat creeping along at a snail's pace, the luckless passengers passing the hours of darkness in a sweltering cabin, with the net work of steel that now covers the land.

After briefly alluding to the ocean steam service, the electric telegraph and the attention now given to the development of electricity for light and propelling power, the lecturer passed on to the title of his address. Fifty years since a drug shop or store in this country was a sort of *omnium gatherum*. Drugs were found in them and many other goods, also he had in his possession a copy of an advertisement, of that period in which drugs, patent medicines and surgical instruments are associated with pickled pork in *high condition*. This grouping of what every properly educated pharmacist must consider incompatibles was no doubt a feature of the times and incidental to the condition of the times. Pharmacy as an art and science had but a feeble existence in Canada fifty years ago, it was then held that if a druggist had sufficient acquaintance with his so called profession to distinguish epsom salts from oxalic acid and to judge fairly well of the value of samples of senna, rhubarb and chamomile it was all that the trade seemed to demand. For the rest the medical profession dispensed or prepared their own prescriptions and rendered their bill accordingly for attendance and medicines. From about 1831 to 1856 medical students placed themselves under the tutelage of doctors and to them appertained the use of mortar and pestle, pill tile and spatula. While pharmacy remained in this condition the medical faculty deemed it their duty and responsibility to control the druggists, and all legislation applicable to them was rather suggested by the faculty or was submitted for their approval and without any consultation with those more directly concerned. To the faculty appertained the examination of apothecaries in materia medica, pharmacy and chemistry. In due course medical schools were established and students having their choice of faculties, were no longer obliged to make pills and spread plasters, and so it came about that medical pharmacies as a rule were discontinued and the doctors sent their patients to the apothecary with prescriptions, a change beneficial to all concerned, it relieved the physician of a serious responsibility and on the whole the public were better served and satisfied. In 1867 the Montreal Chemists Association was organized and the Canadian Pharmaceutical Society in Toronto, but with no legal powers. In 1870 a permissive act was passed incorporating the Pharmaceutical Association of the Province of Quebec, but compulsory powers were withheld. It was clear the doctors were dubious whether pharmacists were capable of managing their own profession, and might be safely trusted with the powers which they claimed and freely used for themselves, but to the honor of the medical profession it should be said, that since they have seen that the druggists were both able and willing to raise the standard of their education every reasonable assistance has been rendered. In 1871 the Ontario Canadian Pharmaceutical Society was incorporated by law, and the name changed to the Ontario College of Pharmacy. Thus far the progress of the profession in the two provinces seemed to run in almost parallel lines, but it was not until 1875 that the Pharmaceutical Association of the Province of Quebec obtained compulsory powers, by which alone it could exercise the needful control of the profession of pharmacy. With a few remarks upon pharmacy in Great Britain, France and Germany the lecturer concluded by saying that when pharmacists should be thoroughly taught in the theory and practice of their profession, they would be fully able to hold their own, and when congresses are convened to discuss pharmaceutical questions of the highest importance to the profession and to the public generally they will attract the attention of the most eminent in science and literature, and what is perhaps of greater importance they will command that respect and admiration which talent and conscientiously applied industry always deserve.

Extracts from British and Foreign Journals.

Unless otherwise stated the translations are made specially for this Journal.

Mimic or Phantom Aneurisms.—Dr. Samuel West describes eight cases of temporary pulsating tumors, situated in the outer sub-clavian region, and accompanied with thrill and murmur, and sometimes dilated veins. In all, the remarkable feature was the temporary duration of these symptoms, which appeared and disappeared, usually associated with states of excitement or quietude. The prominence of the tumor, with the other physical signs, suggested aneurism of the axillary artery, but in all the cases the total subsidence of the symptoms disproved this view. Of the cases, seven were males, and came to Hospital complaining of debility or nervousness; and in four, of discomfort in the subclavian region. In half the swelling was unilateral, and in the other half more marked on one side than the other. A murmur was heard in all, and a thrill noticed in six. Dilated veins were present in five on the affected side. The signs were unaffected by position, but readily produced under excitement. With the exception of the pulsating abdominal aorta, to which Sir James Paget applied the term "mimic aneurism," this condition has not been described. Dr. West explains it as a disturbance of enervation, the sympathetic being a fault. It might "produce the required result by exciting contraction of the peripheral portion of the vessel, this being followed by secondary mechanical dilatation immediately above the constricted part."—*St. Bartholomew Hospital Reports, vol. xvi.*

A Case of Suicide by Dynamite.—This curious case of suicide is reported by Dr. Leadman in a late number of the *British Medical Journal*, and, as he suggests, may prove of interest in a medico-legal aspect.

J. H., aged fifty-six, a well-sinker, of irregular and intemperate habits, on July 12th concluded a "drinking bout" of several weeks' duration. During this debauch, one evening, when in company with other men, a man of the party lost a purse containing seventeen pounds. A statement made by H. led to the apprehension and trial of a respectable farmer, who had been present when the purse was taken. The charge was proved to be groundless. On the 13th, the day of the trial, H., though sober and perfectly rational failed to appear as a witness, making some excuse to his wife and son. About noon, at the time when he should have been in court, he walked into a garth at the back of his residence, and a neighbor in an adjoining field, observing his sudden fall, went to his assistance. He saw blood issuing from his mouth, and at once sent for me. I found the mouth full of blood, and, on examination, the soft palate torn away, the fauces rent, the tongue detached and mutilated, the teeth broken off and splintered, the superior maxillary bones separated and extensively fractured—the fractures extending to the floors of the orbits. Blood was extravasated into the eyeballs, the lower eyelids, and the upper portions of the cheeks. The inferior maxillary bone was broken into about twenty pieces.

The skin of the cheeks and lips was intact, save a few scratches on the internal surface of the latter. There was no charring of the tissues. A box of matches was found in his pocket, and one, partly consumed, close to his mouth where he fell. In his trade he used both cartridges and caps containing dynamite, and was well acquainted with this terrible explosive. One of these he had placed in his mouth, and, after igniting the short fuse attached to it, deliberately waited the result. He survived the lesions two hours, remaining unconscious the whole time The evidence given at the inquest was considered by the jury conclusive as regarded his sanity, and a verdict of *felo-de-se* was returned. Although I have both inquired of my friends and examined several works of reference I have failed to discover a similar case recorded.

Some Recent Operations by Professor Lister.—Two cases in which Mr. Lister cut down upon and sutured together the severed fragments of a fractured patella have been recently recorded. In both these cases, the fracture was of old standing. There is now in Mr. Lister's male ward at King's College Hospital a man, rather more than middle aged, on whom the operation was performed very shortly after the occurrence of the accident. The joint was laid open with antiseptic precautions by a mesial incision, the extravasated blood evacuated, and the fractured pieces of the patella brought into apposition by a strong wire suture. Up to the present time, the case has done remarkably well. In the same ward is a young man, upon whom the ordinary operation of lateral lithotomy was performed for the extraction of a large calculus from the bladder; but the curious part of the case is, that there were, in addition, several calculi in the prostate, and two, larger, in the scrotum; all these were also removed at the same sitting, and the patient since has not had a bad symptom.—*Med. Gazette.*

Advance in Therapeutics in 1880.—New remedies many, a few good, and many bad, most indifferent. Tonga valuable in facial neuralgia; sulphide of calcium in suppuration—its action marked and reliable, grain doses now admitted; the nitrites of potassium and sodium have the action of amyl nitrite, but milder; ergot (again ?) found useful in diabetes; pilocarpin useless in hydrophobia, which still defies all treatment; this last drug, tried in many directions, gave meagre results: benzoate of sodium commended in scarlet fever and gonorrhœal ophthalmia; salicylate of sodium, according to Dr. Greenhow, mitigates but litttle the complications of rheumatic fever, while it may be a positive injury to the heart; salicin is inefficacious, while salicylate is highly praised by Dr. Hewan; the value of cold baths in typhoid fever has become more than doubtful.—*Chicago Med. Journ. and Exam.*

Alopecia of the Eyebrow.—In certain cases syphilitic alopecia destroys the beard, the eyebrow and all hair-covered portions of the body. Alopecia of the eyebrow is a symptom which should at once put the physician upon the trail of diagnosing syphilis. It acts precisely as it does upon the head, that is, that sometimes it renders the eyebrow thin, sometimes removes the hair completely to a greater or less extent. When the eyebrow is discovered broken by a bald line, this single symptom is almost pathognomonic of syphilis. For the baldness which often attacks the brow, proceeds differently and denudes entirely the superciliary region.—*Fournier in Journal de Med. et Chirurg.*

The Administration of Purgatives by Hypodermic Injection.—Much attention has been directed in Germany and Italy to finding some means of replacing tartar emetic, ipecacuanha, and saline and vegetable purgatives of all kinds, by simple hypodermic injections of apomorphia and aloin (the alkaloid of socotrine aloes). Just as with a subcutaneous injection of apomorphia effects of nausea and vomiting have been obtained, so with a warm aqueous solution of aloin (one twenty-fifth) injected in the thigh or forearm, there have soon been produced true symptoms of purgation. In these cases the remedy does not act by direct contact with the gastro-intestinal mucous membrane. These, as the *Paris Médicale* says, are very singular facts which call for serious study and verification. —*Med. Press and Circular.*

CANADA

Medical and Surgical Journal.

MONTREAL, OCTOBER, 1881.

A DOMINION BOARD OF HEALTH.

Strong recommendations in favor of such an organization have frequently been made by the profession in various parts of the Dominion. The following words from the President's address S. W. Kentucky Medical Association may commend themselves to our rulers:—

"Any system of statesmanship, so called, which does not contemplate the sanitary protection and happiness of every citizen from the cradle to the grave is wanting in many elements of enlightenment. It is not justly entitled to the loyalty, confidence and obedience of good people, and should be swept away. Such a government is not worth living for, and is not worth fighting and dying for; it is a sham, and should be abolished as peacefully as possible, or made to conform to the responsibilities of its paternal duties to those whom it is in duty bound to shield and protect. If we are compelled as citizens to obey the laws and support our common country, our country must shield and succour us under all circumstances of health or disease to the fullest extent of its power."

ASSISTANT IN PHYSIOLOGY.—T. W. Mills, M.D., L.R.C.P., has taken up his residence in this city. Dr. Mills has spent more than a year in the Physiological Laboratory of University College, London, under Mr. Schafer and others, and will now act in the capacity of assistant to Prof. Osler. Dr. M. is at present at the Johns Hopkins College, Baltimore, following a short course of instruction in certain departments of practical physiology by Prof. Martin. From the zeal and ability already exhibited by this gentleman and the experience he has already had in teaching, we feel sure we have reason to congratulate the Faculty upon having added another earnest worker to their instructing staff. The readers of this JOURNAL are indebted to Dr. M. for a number of most interesting London letters, which, we have reason to know, have been much appreciated, and often quoted from by our contemporaries.

OPENING MCGILL UNIVERSITY.—The session 1881-82 at McGill University was opened on Monday, the 3rd instant, by an introductory lecture by Dr. F. Buller, Lecturer on Ophthalmology and Otology. The attendance was very large. The address, which was full of practical application, dealt principally with the great advantages possessed by the general practitioner who has acquired a fair knowledge of the essential principles of eye and ear disease, and therefore the great importance of every student devoting a share of the time at his disposal to a study of these important branches. We shall publish Dr. Buller's interesting lecture in our next number.

MCGILL MEDICAL SOCIETY.—At the annual meeting of this Society, held on Saturday, the 8th inst., the following were elected office-bearers for the ensuing year: President, W. A. Molson, M.D.; 1st Vice-President, Mr. Duncan; 2nd Vice-President, Mr. Shaw; Secretary, Mr. Loring; Treasurer, Mr. Gardner; Librarian, Mr. C. E. Cameron; Council, Dr. Buller, Messrs. Smith and Gooding. The next meeting will be held on Saturday, the 22nd inst., when Mr. Grant will read a paper on "Diphtheritic Paralysis."

COLLEGE OF PHYSICIANS AND SURGEONS OF THE PROVINCE OF QUEBEC.—The semi-annual meeting of the College of Physicians and Surgeons of the Province of Quebec was held at Laval University on the 28th ult., when the following Governors were present: Dr. R. P. Howard (President), the Hons. Drs.

T. Robitaille and J. J. Ross, Drs. Ladouceur, Comé, Rinfret, Gervais, Perrault, Belleau, Rottot, Campbell, Austin, Kennedy, Lafontaine, Bonin, Marmette, Lemieux, Hingston, Gingras, Craik, Worthington, Marsden, Laberge, Gibson, R. F. Rinfret, Rodger, Sewell, Park, Lachapelle, Rosseau and St. George. After reading the minutes of last meeting, His Honour the Lieut.-Governor moved, seconded by Dr. Marsden, and unanimously resolved:—"That this Board has learned with deep regret of the death of Dr. F. A. H. Larue, Professor in the Medical Faculty of Laval University, a gentleman distinguished alike for his medical and scientific attainments, and whose reputation extended not only throughout the entire Dominion, but to the neighbouring Republic. This College, of which he was so long a member, desires to extend to his family and relatives its sincere sympathy in their bereavement." In making the motion, His Honour paid a well-merited tribute to the deceased's memory, and was followed by Drs. Marsden, Hingston and Howard. After the ordinary routine business and the adoption of several reports, the following graduates obtained the license of the College on presentation of their respective diplomas:—

Laval University, Quebec—L. G. Phileas DeBlois, M.D., St. Henri de Lauzon; Aime Trudel, M.D., Three Rivers; Alex. Chausse, Gross Delery, M.L., St. Francois, Beauce; Napoleon Mercier, M.L., St. Jean Chrysostome; Chas. Noel Barry, M.D., St. Anne de la Perade; P. A. Gauvreau, M.L., Rimouski.

Laval University, Montreal—Jos. E. Lemaitre, M.D., Pierreville; Gustave Demers, M.D.

Victoria University—A. Gibeault, M.D., C.M., St. Jacques l'Achigan; Gilbert, Huol, M.D., C.M.

McGill University—Wm. L. Gray, M.D., C.M.; George T. Ross, M.D., C.M.

Bishops College—Frank N. R. Spendlove, C.M., M.D.; Robt. H. Wilson, C.M., M.D.

Mr. T. J. Symington, graduate of Queen's College, Ontario, obtained the license after passing a successful examination.

Obituary.

DR. J. J. HUNT.

We regret to learn of the untimely death of Dr. J. J. Hunt, of Lambeth, Ont., one of the graduates of the Class '81 of McGill University. He had gone to England to prosecute the study of diseases of the eye and ear, and when on a visit to some friends in Scotland was attacked by dysentery, which proved fatal. His death will be greatly regretted by his class-mates and friends, with whom he was a great favourite. As a student he was specially careful and industrious, and had made considerable progress in the specialities to which he purposed devoting himself.

Medical Items.

THE POETRY OF LAY-MEDICINE.—An editor of an Indiana daily paper discusses the subject of septicæmia in connection with the case of the President in the following terms: "There are sleeping organisms in the blood which fever wakes at 102° Fahr. Then death summons its drowsy cohorts in tiny legions for their ghastly work. But they have slept there since babyhood waiting for the signal. We begin to die when we begin to live. In all parts of the body are colonies of animalculæ as independent of us as we are of the stars, but no more so. As complete is their organization as ours, and with as good a reason for existence, as clear an office, and possibly as bright a future. In the crystal chambers of that masterpiece of nature, the eye, they revel or rest, living out like us their day. And more wonderful still, even they have parasites as dependent and as independent. All this we say we know, but we know it in that misty, hazy way we know the stars go round, because somebody said so, and nobody contradicted him."

VERY EARLIEST INSTANCE OF ANÆSTHESIA.—When Sir James Simpson proposed the use of chloroform in confinement cases, the religious zealots in England got up an agitation against it, on the ground of the scriptural curse, "In sorrow shalt thou bring forth children." Sir James quickly answered this party, which even comprised some doctors, with the Biblical fact that God narcotized Adam (*immisit soporem*)—"caused a deep sleep to fall upon him," when he created Eve out of his rib. It is to be hoped that the coming revision of the ancient Testament will not spoil so good an argument.

—Frequent complaints are made of the ill-odors from soap boilers, &c., in this city. Probably the reason for their continuance is the same as in New York: "The complaints against these nuisances have been so often urged that the profession and the public are familiar with them.

'No! though compell'd beyond the Tiber's flood
To move your tan-yard, swear the smell is good—
Myrrh, cassia, frankincense; and wisely think
That what is lucrative can never stink.'"

—*The Sanitarian.*

JOHNSTON'S FLUID BEEF is now extensively used in British and Continental Institutions, Hospitals and Asylums, and is prescribed by the medical faculty wherever it has been introduced. Its adaptability is general. To children it secures a strong muscular development, and for indigestion or mental overstrain, it is the perfection of known food.

WYETH'S HYPOPHOSPHITES OF LIME AND SODA WITH COD LIVER OIL.—This preparation represents in a convenient form one of the most efficient and popular remedies in cases of a PULMONARY CHARACTER, with tendency to Hemorrhage, LOSS OF APPETITE, COUGH and especially when attended with Emaciation.

The HYPOPHOSPHITES with COD LIVER OIL, may be given also with great advantage in ANÆMIA, CHLOROSIS, to NURSING MOTHERS, and in all cases of NERVOUS EXHAUSTION and GENERAL DEBILITY.

By combining the HYPOPHOSPHITES with COD LIVER OIL the latter in a finely divided state, by our peculiar process of emulsifying, and so disguised as to be inoffensive to even a delicate stomach, we are enabled to afford at the same time a stimulant to the nervous system, and a promoter of nutrition, as well as a fuel which takes the place of the wasting tissues.

We would only say further, that this preparation, like every other bearing our name, is composed of the very best materials, and made up with the utmost care. We are, therefore confident that it will fully maintain our assertions in regard to it.

JOHN WYETH & BRO., PHILADELPHIA.

CANADA
MEDICAL & SURGICAL JOURNAL

NOVEMBER, 1881.

Original Communications.

INTRODUCTORY LECTURE, McGILL UNIVERSITY.
Session 1881–82.

By F. BULLER, M.D., M.R.C.S., Eng.,

Lecturer on Ophthalmology in McGill University; Attending Physician to the Ophthalmic and Aural Department, Montreal General Hospital.

In every human life, I suppose, there are a few days fraught with a consciousness of the supreme importance, provided the holder of it retains it long enough to understand and appreciate the responsibility involved in the mere possession of life, mind, and soul. I am not here, however, to discourse upon the meaning and significance of these three wondrous monosyllables, each one of which has from the beginning, and will to the end of time, transcend the limits of human understanding. Thanks to the Faculty of Medicine of McGill University, my task is of a lighter and more agreeable nature. It is to bid the Class of 1881–82 a most hearty and cordial welcome, to wish each individual member success in the arduous work he is about to enter upon, and to assure each and all that they have the entire sympathy of, and will receive every encouragement and assistance that can possibly be rendered by, the teachers to whom they have entrusted the all-important function of guiding them for a time in their future studies. This, I believe, is for most of us the anniversary of one of those "red-letter days" to which I have alluded. For some it recalls the fading memories of the past; for others its associations seem so fresh as to blend with the busy throng of current events; to a smaller number it wears the charm of a new and not unpleasant experience. Happy are they who can look back to this, the very threshold of their career, without regret, and I will take upon myself to tell you who they are. They are the men who have started with a firm resolve to uphold the honour and good name of the profession whose ranks they have joined, and have never swerved from their purpose. They are the men who have had the strength to practice self-denial in their youth, and devote all their time and all their energies to earnest work. These are the sure foundations upon which success in life must be built. To the lack of such foundations we may trace the shipwrecks on the sands of time that are strewed on every side. Which of us is there, indeed, who cannot recall instances of blighted prospects and wasted lives in men whose early days gave promise of a prosperous and honourable future. And if we look for the causes of the disaster, we shall find they can be traced to a non-observance of the golden rule just mentioned as the secret of success.

To the young man just entering upon his course of medical studies, full of life and vigor and sanguine hopes, four years may seem a long time in which to accomplish the purpose he has in view. Some of his older schoolmates, no more intelligent than himself, have perhaps recently passed through the ordeal and, now exulting in the possession of a handle to their names, are objects of awe and veneration to their quondam associates. Be not thus deceived: the time is all too short for the work in hand. Twelve months later the most sanguine among you will freely admit I am not exaggerating when I say that if the time were twice as long there would still remain much more to learn than was ever dreamt of in your philosophy. How bitter then will be the regret if that year is wasted in idleness or pleasure taking. If any of you think to have an easy time for the first year or two, my advice would be either to abandon the fond illusion or to seek some easier route to fame and fortune. Remember always there are a dozen Professors to confront you, armed with a sum total of about a hundred dozen lectures, loads of puzzling questions, and reams of examination papers. There are weeks and months of patient toil in the laboratory, in the dissecting-room, and in the wards of the hospital; there are ponderous volumes of chemistry, anatomy, physiology, and materia medica to be stamped almost word for word upon the tablets of your memories, mere outworks as it were to the stronger fortresses of medicine and surgery. Remember that each will be judged by his merits without fear or favor, and that by men who have learned to know almost your inmost thoughts. As you become more or less familiar with each subject in turn, you will discover that each professor seems to regard his own subject as the one of paramount importance. This may be a weakness of human nature, but right or wrong it is always met with in every institution where knowledge is imparted by routine teaching. It is just possible that sometimes this peculiarity may be too distinctive a feature, and lead to spending more time over certain studies than would be the case if we could have everything equally balanced in the order of practical necessity. For my own part, knowing as I do the immense amount of work to be gone over in our medical curriculum, I should think twice before asking a student to crowd his overwrought brain with the thousand details that can be of no future use and are only crammed into the head for purposes of examination, to be studiously and resentfully forgotten as soon as it is over. There are myriads of important facts that should be stored away for future use, and these are what every student wants to grasp and retain. When the corn is cheap and plentiful who would be burdened with husks? If I were to have my student life over again, I think I could learn more in less time by searching more carefully for leading principles and striving to associate ideas. It is thus that knowledge can be retained and made available at a moment's notice when suddenly called for. Most of you will ultimately be thrown upon your own resources, and will find the physical welfare of many fellow-creatures depending upon your skill and knowledge. Most of you will become enrolled in the ranks of general practitioners, a set of men who may have their failings and short-comings, but who, on the average, are entitled to the respect and admiration of their fellow-beings. If we take the two or three thousand general practitioners constituting the great body of provincial medical men of this country, I doubt if it would be possible to find an equal number in any other class so industrious, so painstaking, and so worthy of esteem as these, often toiling day and night more for the love of doing good and for the sake of humanity than for the hope of pecuniary emolument. Where will you find any body of men who go through the same amount of worry and anxiety for so small a recompense? How few live the natural span of life! Worn out by unceasing labour or cut down by the hand of pestilence, striving to alleviate the sufferings of others when suffering most themselves, they fight the good fight to the bitter end, and we have reason to hope, receive at last their fitting reward.

Self-reliance with these men becomes a part of their very nature, without it they would be wholly unfit for the position they occupy; but to acquire this invaluable quality in its highest perfection they must have explored the whole field of medical science, and have learned to know something at least of all the ills to which human flesh is liable. Habits of accurate observation with a wide range of knowledge render these men equal to almost every emergency, and if they do not always display the grasp of detail that special study alone can give, who shall dare accuse them of ignorance or judge harshly of men who have done their best. Small wonder if mistakes are sometimes made in medical and surgical practice, when we compare ourselves with those who follow other callings. Just think of it. A man must serve five years' apprenticeship before he can be trusted to make a pair of shoes, and even then, of five hundred shoemakers, probably not five excel in their art. I might multiply similar instances, but a single sentence will suffice to express what I wish to convey. By constant practice only can the highest skill be attained. This is the true reason for the modern growth of specialism. Specialism in its best and purest form is a natural growth, and is only worthy of the name when it receives the sanction and approval of those who are best able to judge of its merits. The specialist who cannot command the respect and esteem of his confrères in the general profession is not fit for his calling; but to attain this distinction something more than a mere newspaper announcement is necessary. In addition to a thorough course of medical training, there should be a special aptitude for the particular work to be done; then long years of patient labor and a vast clinical experience of a certain kind are essential in the education of the specialist who desires to gain a lasting reputation. The extraordinary literary activity of the present day requires all the spare time even of the specialist to keep *au courant* with what is being done in his own department. I can vouch for the correctness of this statement, at least as far as the specialty which I have the honor to represent is concerned, and I have little doubt those engaged in other departments can say the same. Moreover, a knowledge of several modern languages is almost indispensable if one would keep abreast with the tide of progress. The fact that diseases of particular organs are usually more or less connected with, and dependant upon, derangements of other portions of the economy involves the necessity of a tolerably intimate acquaintance with general pathology and therapeutics, and it often falls to the lot of the specialist to supply valuable information in the diagnosis of diseases not strictly within his own province. Taking all these circumstances into consideration, there should be, and I feel confident the time is almost at hand when there will be, no antagonism between the thoroughly trained specialist and the general practitioner. On the contrary, they are natural allies and by combining their knowledge they can not only benefit each other but often render the most invaluable services to their clients.

I do not wish to convey the impression that the specialist should claim the right to treat every case of disease that occurs in the part of the body he is supposed to know all about. Such a claim would, indeed, be unjust and absurd, and with the multiplication of specialties now recognized would leave the general practitioner almost nothing to call his own; such a state of things would, of course, be intolerable, and would lead in the end to the most disastrous consequences. For my own part, I should rejoice to see a much more widely diffused knowledge of ophthalmology and otology than at present obtains. Time and again I have been told by well-educated and successful practitioners that they know nothing about diseases of the eye and ear. I am always pained and grieved to hear such a confession. Surely there is something wrong with the system of education that sends men forth by the thousand, so badly prepared, into regions where they *must* treat diseases of these organs, however ignorant they may be of the subject. Surely the organs which represent the two most important of the five senses, which are the most exquisite pieces of mechanism in the animal economy, the avenues through which almost all knowledge is gained, and the source of nearly all the pleasure of life, are worth knowing something about. What, then, can be the reason of this lamentable, this deplorable want of knowledge? It is simply this: The subjects have not been made compulsory in the medical curriculum, and most students will not study anything that does not aid them to pass their examinations. I do not blame them for this, but I know full well how keenly the deficiency is felt in after years. For some reason, which I cannot exactly define. there seems to be an idea abroad that the study of the eye and ear is too intricate and too difficult for the student to undertake. I should like to dispel this illusion, and I think I shall succeed in doing so if you will pay attention to what I am going to say:

I have no hesitation in asserting, most emphatically, that with the exception of a few points, which may safely be left to the specialist, there is really nothing either in ophthalmology or otology which cannot be readily or speedily mastered by an ordinary student during his term of pupilage. The great majority of all diseases of the eye, including most of those which commonly impair or destroy vision, are of an external character, and far more easy of diagnosis and treatment than are the diseases of the internal organs of the body. A glance at the report of the ophthalmic out-patient department of the Montreal General

Hospital, for the past year, affords a good illustration of this point. Among the total of 834 eye-patients, there were only 86 suffering from affections which could not have been diagnosticated with certainty by simple external inspection, with or without the aid of focal illumination; and of these 86, sixty were cases of error of refraction or defect of accommodation. There remain only 26 cases requiring a knowledge of the use of the ophthalmoscope to establish the diagnosis. That is about three per cent. of the entire number. In view of these facts, I say it would be idle to pretend that students are justified in neglecting the study of eye diseases on account of the difficulty of the subject. A still stronger case may be made out in favour of diseases of the ear, the vast majority of which belong to the so-called middle ear, and are associated with or dependant upon morbid conditions of the naso-pharynx, a region that every general practitioner is or should be competent to look after. The stumbling block here seems to be that only very few medical men provide themselves with the instruments necessary for examining and treating the parts affected; or if they have the instruments, they have not devoted sufficient time or attention to the subject to attain dexterity in their use, and yet there is not sufficient reason for this deficiency. Surely anyone who becomes skilled in the use of the vaginal speculum is quite well able to learn that of the aural speculum, and it is certainly not more difficult to learn how to manipulate the eustachian catheter than it is to acquire the knack of introducing the urethral catheter without occasionally making a false passage, an accomplishment I suspect rather rarely met with, even among surgeons of large experience. In any case the one thing necessary is constant practice, and for this there is plenty of material in the ophthalmic and aural department of our hospital, however it may be with the other instances mentioned. Anyone who learns to auscultate the heart and lungs can just as easily learn to auscultate the tympanic cavity, and the information thus obtainable is no less positive in the latter case than in the two former. I will go a step further, and risk the imputation of inculcating heretical maxims, by saying that in auscultation, for positive information the aurist has the advantage over his thoracic brethren. It has been stated by competent authorities that the blind asylums of the world and the institutions for deaf-mutes are more than half filled by the victims of perfectly curable diseases, and that their misfortunes are the result of neglect or improper treatment. The statement, I am certain, falls far short of the truth in regard to the blind, and is probably not an exaggeration as applied to the deaf. The most prolific source of life-long blindness is the ophthalmia of new-born infants, a disease I have never yet seen cause loss of vision when properly treated. Scarlet fever occupies a similar position in causing deafness, simply, I believe, because the ears do not get proper attention during and after the ravages of this disease. If we add to the number who become totally blind or totally deaf from these causes an infinitely greater multitude who escape with but a sad remnant of sight or hearing, we have a picture of sorrow and suffering almost too painful for contemplation. I should occupy too much time for the present occasion were I to enter into particulars concerning the preventible sources of blindness and deafness, but I may be allowed to enumerate some of the things every general practitioner ought to understand, for if he do not understand those diseases that are of frequent and general occurrence, and consequently must be treated by him, he is ignorant of his craft by his own confession, and therefore unworthy the confidence of his clients. First and before all, he should learn not to meddle with what he does not understand, for it were better far not to treat a case of eye disease at all than to use injurious remedies, or to make an unsuitable use of good remedies. To know what should not be done is often the most valuable of knowledge. But as I have already stated the great majority of diseases of the eye and ear can and should be treated by the general practitioner. All the ordinary diseases of the eyelids and conjunctiva come within this category. The same may be said of the cornea and iris. I cannot emphasize too strongly the urgent need there is of a better knowledge of the morbid conditions of these two structures among the members of the general profession. I think I am not exaggerating when I say not a week passes but I see the disastrous effect of some terrible mistake made in the diagnosis and treatment of these corneal and iritic diseases, mistakes I should feel ashamed of if made by any student who had attentively followed the out-patient ophthalmic practice of the Montreal General Hospital for the short period of one summer session.

There is one eye disease I cannot refrain from mentioning because of its infallibly destructive character if overlooked or neglected, and because I have almost never seen it recognized by the general practitioner at any stage of its progress; no, not even when the most striking symptoms proclaimed its existence more distinctly than words could describe them. Why it is that men who have learned to use [their eyesight and to know that two and two make four will persist in overlooking glaucoma in every instance, is more than I can comprehend. The one disease that most urgently calls for early recognition is the very one that seems to be never understood, and stranger still, the one disease that yields the most satisfactory results to operative surgery, is the very one for which it is the most difficult to obtain the patient's consent to an operation. There are certain cases of eye disease and many cases of injury to the eye which should, I think, be relegated to the specialist for treatment. 1st, all cases in which the medical attendant is unable to make an accurate diagnosis. 2nd, all cases requiring difficult or complicated operations upon the eyeball itself. 3rd, all cases of severe injury to the eyeball, especially if the injury be of such a nature as to involve the risk of sympathetic ophthalmia. The latter disease being of so insidious and dangerous a character, its possible occurrence requires all the watchful attention that only a thoroughly skilled observer can give. Operative ophthalmic surgery now for the most part falls into the hands of the specialist, chiefly, I believe, because the public are alive to the fact that practice makes perfect, and have a peculiar horror of bungling operations about the eye. Still, I would not wish to deter any student from fitting himself for this sort of work, indeed I would be glad if they would all try to do so, and I feel certain that some would succeed, but I would suggest this caution: that no one ever should operate upon the living human eye until he has had a large experience upon the cadaver as well as upon the lower animals. If this precaution had always been taken we should never have heard the sarcasm that "a man must put out a bushel of eyes before he becomes a skilful operator," for I am certain that with plenty of practice of the kind I have indicated anyone possessed of a fair share of natural dexterity can attain a very considerable degree of skill before touching the living eye. Another point of great importance is that no operation should be done except with perfect and suitable instruments. This of course implies the possession of a very considerable armamentum.

Much as lies in the power of the general practitioner to benefit his clients by acquiring a practical knowledge of diseases of the eye, I believe he can do even more for those suffering from the common forms of ear disease if he will take the trouble to to give the subject an intelligent attention instead of pursuing the usual "laissez faire" policy of advising the patient to syringe the ear for every ailment that presents itself, or the equally unreasonable but more injurious practice of ordering oil and laudanum as a universal panacea for deafness and earache. The first accomplishes nothing, owing to the fortunate anatomical ignorance of the public; the second does a great deal of harm twice for every time it does a little good once. It is in early life, in the catarrhal deafness of childhood or in the purulent inflammation of the exanthemata that the foundation of deafness is generally laid, and is because, forsooth, the aurist is called upon in at least two cases out of three to treat the results of ten or twenty years of neglect or mismanagement that his inability to afford relief brings down upon his devoted head the opprobrium of an ignorant and unreasoning multitude.

In an organ so inaccessible as the ear, and of such complex and delicate structure, it is too much to expect a restoration to health of parts that have undergone irrevocable morbid changes; but give us these cases in their early stages, or in early life, and we will show results more brilliant than in any other branch of medicine or surgery. If the subject were faced fairly and squarely by the medical profession, and the ear diseases of early life treated on rational principles, therapeutic and hygienic, the makers of audiphones, ear trumpets, and artificial drums would have to seek some other and, let us hope, more honest means of earning a livelihood than that of imposing on the credulity of afflicted humanity. Much might be said on the relation between diseases of the eye and ear and the various other organs of the body. It is in this direction that most of the original work going on at the present time is being done, and though the tillers of the soil are numerous, the harvest has been abundant in the past, and bids fair to be prolific in the future. Since the fertile brain of the immortal Helmholtz gave birth to that simple and beautiful invention, the ophthalmoscope, the science of ophthalmology has passed from the ravenous clutches of mountebanks and quacks, and by the exertions and untiring industry of a few of the brightest minds of the nineteenth century it has attained the dignity of the most important specialty in medicine. It has cleared up some of the darkest and most difficult points in pathology. It has added many laurels to the art of surgery. It has held up the pure light of science for the guidance of the mystified physician groping hopelessly in the dark, and shown him the kidneys, the heart and the brain of his patient by illuminating the deep recesses of the fundus oculi. It is a source of gratification to me to know that each year adds a larger number of students to the list of those who take an interest in the study of ophthalmology, and it is especially gratifying to know there are some who go out into the world with a fair knowledge of the use of the ophthalmoscope. It is an art that can only be learned by the exercise of patience and perseverance; but when once acquired I am quite certain none ever begrudged the time and trouble it had cost.

In conclusion, gentlemen, I may say that, although much has been accomplished in every branch of modern medicine, there remains much more to be done. Remember always that upon each of you a portion of the future depends, and if you will let it be your aim in life to do all that lies within your power to make the next thirty years as bright an era of progress in the medical world as the past have been, you will have no self-reproaches and no vain regrets when the sands of life have run so low that the task must be yielded to your successors just as those who are older must yield it to you.

AN ENDEMIC OF PARAPLEGIA AMONGST CHINESE COOLIES.

By H. N. VINEBERG, M.D. (McGill), Waiohinu, Sandwich Islands.

During the past six months a peculiar disease has appeared among the Chinese labourers on the several sugar plantations of these Islands. The three plantations in this district, and which I attend, employ altogether about 300 Chinese, and fully 75 have been attacked by the strange affection.

The first cases occurred at the Naalcha plantation. Some seven or eight Chinamen one day dropped down in the field, and said they were unable to stand on their legs any longer. Within a week, 15 out of a total 60 were on the sick list with the same complaint. As I cannot find anything in my limited supply of medical books which treats of a similar affection, I had better, I think, give you first a description of a typical case, and afterwards state the variations I have observed.

The overseer notices a Chinaman suddenly drop in the field, and thinking him a "shirker," perhaps, gives him a kick and tells him to go to work. The Chinaman points to his lower extremities, and by gestures endeavours to make his task-master understand that it is they who are at fault. A medical examination, I am bound to confess, does not throw much more light on the subject, and is very unsatisfactory from the nature of the circumstances. The patient's walk is not unlike that of locomotor ataxia when the ataxic muscles are beginning to show signs of motor paralysis. The leg and foot are raised high, brought forward slowly and apparently with an effort, and the whole length of the sole touches the floor at once in completing the step. He walks with his legs wide apart. The muscles feel firm to the touch, and on being tightly grasped by the hand the patient calls out with pain. Tactile sensibility is not impaired, and reflex power is normal. Pain is first referred to the region of the knees and afterwards vaguely to the thighs and legs, but most frequently to the calves only. The patient endeavours to indicate some sensation he experiences by digging the limbs with his index fingers partially closed, and which I take to be *pricking*. No pain whatever is referred to the spine, and hard knocks with the knuckles over the spines of the vertebræ elicit no cry of pain. Power over the sphincters of the rectum and bladder is retained to almost the very last. The bowels are usually costive; the appetite is good, and the tongue may be clean or slightly furred. The pulse is frequent from 90 to 110 per minute, and is rather small and compressible. The urine is clear, moderate in amount, and free from albumen. The case may terminate in one of three ways: death, recovery, or pass into a chronic state. In most of the cases ending in death, the paralysis rapidly extends upwards, invading the whole muscular frame, the muscles quickly atrophy, and the patient dies asphyxiated from paralysis of the respiratory apparatus. About 30 per cent came under this head, and in the greatest number of cases it took place between the third and fourth week. The superstitions of the Chinese about the dead is very peculiar, and I have only been able to hold one *post-mortem*. In that case the lungs, liver, kidneys, spleen, stomach and bowels appeared normal. The mitral valves were very thin and small, but showed no signs of inflammatory changes. The brain and cord were not examined.

Recovery takes place at a variable period, but most often in from three to four weeks, and is liable to be interrupted by several relapses, each of which last from three to four days. Finally, half of the cases have recovered. The duration of the chronic state I am unable to say, as some of the cases, among the first that occurred, at this day show no signs of an improvement or the reverse. The patients feed and sleep well; the muscles of the lower extremities have undergone no atrophy but the paresis remains. These, however, I think would soon improve if the plantation authorities carried out in full the course of treatment I have recommended over and over again. The following are some of the more important variations that I have observed. The attack does not always set in so suddenly as stated above; many complain for a day or two of pains in the legs before they give up work. In some cases there is complete paraplegia almost from the very beginning, and different from what one would expect; these are not always the fatal cases. I have seen some of the very worst cases recover. Marked swellings of the legs I have noticed in several cases, but do not consider the swellings as typical of the disease. In some it is due to severe heart affection, in others to a feeble circulation. Quite a large number had a murmur either over the aortic or mitral valves. A few days before death very many patients point to their abdomen and say "all burning," or its correlative in the Chinese tongue. I have not been able to make any thermometrical observations—having had all my thermometers either broken or out of gear—but judging by the feel of the hand I should say that there was little or no elevation of the heat of the body in any of the cases at any stage of the disease.

What is the causation of the disease, one naturally asks? Not an easy question to answer. Had it been an outbreak of scurvy there would be no difficulty in giving a cause. Here we have men living under conditions which are said and known to produce scurvy, and instead of swollen, spongy gums and purpuric patches we see paralysed lower extremities. The diet of the Chinese coolies on the plantations at the time of the outbreak of the disease consisted of rice, peanut oil, semi-putrified sausages and bad pork; vegetables of any kind never entered into its composition. However difficult it may be to explain the effect from the cause, it is my opinion that the above-mentioned diet is the main factor of the disease. I shall briefly state the grounds upon which I have formed my opinion, and your readers can judge for themselves whether it is tenable or not. The common method of feeding Chinamen on plantations is to allow them so much rice and beef weekly, but in many instances they are given the value of the allowance of the latter in money with which they can buy whatever they please. Their tastes run in peanut oil, greasy sausages, tainted fish and bad pork, but their delight *par excellence* is peanut oil.

The first cases that came under my notice were at the Naalcha and Hilca plantations, where that system obtained. There were none as yet at the Pahaler plantation, the only one of the three that gave their Chinamen their beef rations fresh from the commissariat. But some time after, while one of the directors was on a visit to the plantation, the Chinese laborers petitioned him to have their beef rations exchanged for its value in money, which was granted to them. In less than three weeks from that date I had no less than thirty cases on that plantation. Again, as soon as the money system was put a stop to and vegetables added to the rations we had no fresh cases. Conneeted with the plantations are several small planters who plant corn on shares. These also employ chiefly Chinese coolies, who as a rule have always some vegetables which they grow themselves, and they got their rice and beef served out to them by the planters themselves. None of the planters' coolies have been affected by the disease. The treatment which I recommended was a generous diet into which vegetables—particularly cabbage—should enter largely, better ventilated and roomy quarters, and stimulants in those cases with a feeble circulation. Stimulating liniments to be well rubbed into the paralyzed limbs, and where the paralysis showed no signs of extending I gave strychnia and ordered the application of electricity. It is no more than just to say that where this course of treatment was followed out, even if only in part, there the per centage of the cases of recovery was the highest. Any one who has had medical charge of plantations in these Islands will fully understand the meaning of the last sentence.

Before concluding this already too long communication, I would like to refer to a recent outbreak of a similar disease in the interior of Japan, mentioned by Miss Bird in her book on the "Unbeaten Tracks of Japan." The disease is known by the name of *Kak'ké*, and in a village through which she passed it carried off 100 persons out of a population of 1,500 in seven months. "The first symptoms," she says, "are a loss of strength in the legs, looseness in the knees, cramps, numbness and swelling. This Dr. Anderson, who has studied *Kak'ké* in more than 1,100 cases in Tôkyiô, calls the subacute form. The chronic is a slow numbing and wasting malady, which, if unchecked, results in death from paralysis and exhaustion in from six months to three years. Dr. Anderson describes a third or acute form in which the grave symptoms set in unexpectedly, and go on rapidly increasing." She then gives a graphic description in the words of Dr. A. of a patient in the last moments preceding asphyxia. "The opinion of the native doctors, as well as that of Dr. Anderson, is that the predisposing causes are bad drainage, dampness, over-crowding, and want of ventilation; the exciting causes the wearing of shoes, which are oftener wet than dry. In Tôkyiô two hospitals were opened, in one of which native treatment is to be tried, and in the other foreign. It has been unusually bad of late in Tôkyiô.

The predisposing causes of the endemic here, I should say, were: Chinese habits, masturbation, &c., over-crowding, and want of proper ventilation in the sleeping quarters. These latter on the plantations consist of long narrow buildings, along either side of which are arranged shelves or bunks two tier deep, much in the same way as in the forecastle of a ship. Fifty or more are housed in a building 80 by 14 feet. I have put, as you see, Chinese habits at the head of the predisposing causes. May not the too-frequent congestion of the spinal column produced by these habits make *that* the weak point in the system and the first to suffer from bad food?

I regret that my communication is of so crude a nature, and that I am not able to present you with a fuller picture of the disease.

THE PHARMACIST OF THE FUTURE.

By HENRY R. GRAY.

Nothing is so frequently insisted upon by writers on pharmaceutical matters as that pharmacists must, in order to live, combine with their profession various trades, such as fancy goods, brushes, soap, &c. Let us see if this implicit belief in a foregone conclusion is not to a great extent erroneous, and may, perhaps, have been one of the causes which has prevented pharmacy from assuming its proper rank in English-speaking countries.

We were told at the late Pharmaceutical Congress in London that pharmacists rank as professional men in France, Germany, Belgium, the Netherlands, Spain and Italy. In France it is necessary to obtain the degree of Bachelor of Science before commencing the study of pharmacy, and so far from there being any opposition to this on the part of pharmacists, Mr. Petit of Paris proposed the following resolution : "It is desirable that in all countries the literary studies required from the pharmaceutical chemist be the same as those required to obtain the diploma of a Doctor of Medicine." In speaking to his proposed resolution, Mr. Petit stated that "in France there were special institutions for the study of pharmacy, aud it was well understood that the position of a first-class pharmacist (pharmacien de la première classe) was equal to a doctor of medicine, and he thought pharmacists in general should spare no trouble to attain the same position everywhere."

In England and America the very different relations existing between pharmacy and the State has been very unfavourable to the advancement of pharmacy, and, in addition, the paucity of the reward attainable in the end is a very decided check to every effort made in the direction of high culture. It cannot, however, be denied that there are branches of scientific work adapted to the attainments of the educated pharmacist which have been hitherto entirely neglected, and unless the pharmacist of the future directs his energy to the practice of these branches, men of culture will cease to enter the ranks of pharmacy, and will join those of other professions where more honour and profit is attainable. At all events, bad as things are elsewhere, a brighter day is dawning on the pharmacist in Canada, and our medical friends are opening their eyes to the fact that we are a necessity to them, and that well-educated pharmacists and well-stocked pharmacies are coadjutors not to be despised in the successful prosecution of the practice of medicine.

The pharmacist being, by his training at college and his practical experience, a skilled chemist, why should he not announce himself as a "consulting and analytical chemist"? He is better adapted and has more facilities for doing this work than most other men. He has his chemicals and laboratory at hand. He has his clerks to do minor work, and to assist him generally. Without doubt, the physician would rather give such work as the analysis of urine, blood, &c., to his chemist, for a fee, than place himself under an obligation to any brother practitioner who happens to be more of an amateur in this sort of work than himself. Medical electricity might also be worked up into a speciality, for very few medical men can devote the time necessary to become skilled medical electricians, which, by the way, is not such a simple matter as is generally supposed. The mere applying a current at random is one thing, and its skilled application another, and it is without doubt a branch which might very well become part of the curriculum of the future pharmacist. In cases requiring this mode of treatment, the pharmacist, with all his paraphernalia at hand, could officiate under the direction of the medical attendant.

Then, again, the analytical knowledge he possesses might be of great service to the coroner in poisoning cases, and also to health departments in our great cities, where the condition of the atmosphere, the detection of sewer gases, the disinfection of houses, &c., would necessitate scientific advice and direction. The assaying of minerals, including phosphates, might also be worth attention. As a consulting chemist to the numerous manufacturing industries, a large field of usefulness lies open to the pharmacist. Very large establishments have long ago appreciated the knowledge of the practical chemist, and usually have one, whose duty it is to perfect their processes, utilize waste products, and suggest improvements generally. Numbers of smaller establishments cannot afford this addition to their staff, and are obliged to pick up information wherever they can. There is scarcely a pharmacist to-day who is not continually consulted with regard to the recipes used by tobacco manufacturers, dyers, hatters, furriers, brass-workers, gilders, &c., but his valuable hints are given gratis, and are consequently not appreciated.

In looking back, I can trace many scraps of information, given without the slightest remuneration, which have built up valuable businesses for the parties who have consulted me, and numbers of pharmacists can make the same assertion. Now the labourer is worthy of his hire, and if the pharmacist would only add to his other titles that of analytical and consulting chemist, his clients would soon take the hint, and in course of time a fair addition to the annual income would result.

Let the embryo pharmacist ponder over these things, and let him, during his pupilage, bear in mind that he should study with other objects in view than the mere obtaining of a diploma. Chemistry is, without doubt, a very difficult study, but it is at the same time intensely interesting. It can never be a useless acquirement, for no matter what position in life the student may eventually drop into, the better he is acquainted with this noble science, the better prepared he will be to avail himself of the many opportunities which will present themselves of putting it into practice. Dr. Charles Symes of Liverpool, in an address delivered at a late distribution of prizes at the Pharmaceutical Society of London, gave the following excellent advice to pharmaceutical students: "I have been urging you to strenuous efforts that you may become worthy practitioners of pharmacy, and that its professional character may receive from you, as representing *the next generation of pharmacists*, a deeper impression than is now apparent,"

Messrs. Young & Postans, of the Pharmaceutical Laboratory, Baker street, Portman Square, London, writing to the *Chemists' and Druggists' Bulletin*, published in New York, say: "We in England desire and hope for a curriculum which shall ultimately bring about and enable us to establish in this country a properly recognized Pharmaceutical University, believing that the time is coming when a large proportion of the trade element will be disassociated from the dispensing of medicine, and that the medical profession will be represented by the physician, the surgeon, and the pharmacist; yet we imagine that such consummation will not be brought about except by the united efforts of pharmacists as a body to pull themselves up to such a standard, that medical men shall feel the services of the chemist in pharmacy and science to be imperatively allied with medicine, just as we require their allegiance in surgery and general medical practice."

REPORT ON THERAPEUTICS AND PHARMACOLOGY.

By JAMES STEWART, M.D., BRUCEFIELD, ONT.

(Read before the Canada Medical Association, at Halifax, August, 1881.)

In the whole field of therapeutics, there is no subject at the present day which is so actively occupying the professional mind as that of the

ANÆSTHETICS.

Probably never since their introduction has there existed such a wide-spread desire to discover new and safer agents of this class. In regard to chloroform especially, the confidence of the profession in it is thoroughly shaken. The day of the dogmatic assertion "that pure chloroform, well administered, never kills" is past. The practical disadvantages of ether are numerous, and since its re-introduction into England there have been several instances of a fatal result from its use. Death under anæsthetics is, of course, the great and important fact connected with their use. The deaths from chloroform seem to have increased much in frequency in late years, and now amount to a very considerable number. It is very hard to estimate the exact number, as many of these cases are never published. Dr. Kappeler* says that about 300 have been published, and Turnbull gives a list of 160 as having occurred in the 10 years between 1869 and 1879. A recent writer† says that there have been as many deaths published from chloroform as there have been months since its introduction, and he considers that for every case published, two to four remain unpublished.

A very important question is, How is death caused by chloroform? If we are able truly to answer this question, we will then be placed in a position to avert it in many cases. The theories that have been advanced to account for it have been very numerous and very conflicting. The work that has been done lately in endeavouring to solve this question is of a very high scientific character, and it must be said that we have made some decided advances in this direction. Probably the work performed by the "Glasgow Committee"‡ has been productive of the

---

* Quoted by Reeve in *Am. Jour. Med. Science.*

† Reichert, *Amer. Jour. Med. Sc.*, July, 1881.

‡ *Brit. Med. Jour.*, Dec., 1880.

best results. In conducting their investigations, they endeavoured, first, to ascertain wherein the special dangers of chloroform consist; and, second, to try if some anæsthetic agent could be found which would avoid these dangers. They soon discovered that chloroform, apart altogether from its action on the respiratory centres, had a disastrous effect on the heart, while ether has no baneful influence. They now searched for an anæsthetic as powerful as chloroform, and having as little effect on the heart and respiratory system as ether. This they believe they have discovered in the ethidene dichloride. This agent was first used by Snow. He administered it in fifteen cases with good results. In 1870 it was used by Liebreich and Langenbeck. During the last year or two it has been extensively used in England. Mr. Clover* has published an account of his experience derived from 1,877 cases. In this interesting paper he gives the particulars relating to a case of death from cardiac syncope after the administration of ethidene and nitrous oxide gas, the nitrous oxide having been stopped before the ethidene was given. At the *post mortem* examination the heart was found to be enlarged, and its fibres were shown to have undergone fatty degeneration. Sauer† also mentions one case of death in a patient suffering from heart disease. In an extensive series of clinical investigations with chloroform and ethidene, conducted by the surgeons of the Western Infirmary, Glasgow, it was found that the ethidene acts quicker, but requires a larger dose than chloroform. There is a greater tendency in the case of chloroform to retardation of the heart's movements and to dicrotism. The pulse respiration ratio is apt to be more affected and oftener than with ethidene. Both chloroform and ethidene, administered to animals, have a decided effect in reducing the blood pressure, while ether has no appreciable effect of this kind. Chloroform reduces the pressure much more rapidly, and to a greater extent, than ethidene. Chloroform has sometimes an unexpected and apparently capricious effect on the heart's action, the pressure being reduced with great rapidity to almost *nil*, while the pulsations are greatly

* *Brit. Med. Jour.*, May 29, 1880.
† *Brit. Med. Jour.*, Dec., 1880.

retarded, or even stopped. Ethidene was never found to produce these alarming and sudden effects on the blood pressure. The conclusion of the Committee was that the ethidene was very much safer than chloroform.

As regards comparative danger, the three anæthetics may be arranged in the following order: Chloroform, ethidene, ether; and the ease with which the vital functions can be restored may be conversely stated, thus: the circulation is more easily re-established when its cessation is due to ether than to ethidene; and when the result of ethidene, than when chloroform has been used. The disadvantages of ether are, to a great extent, obviated by the use of ethidene, whilst the dangers of chloroform are also reduced to a minimum. Nussbaum's method of first injecting some morphia hypodermically, previous to the administration of chloroform, has lately been coming into more extensive use. It is claimed for this procedure that a much less quantity of chloroform is necessary, and that the stage of excitement, both muscular and mental, is lessened, and that thereby the dangers of anæsthesia are diminished. Mollow claims further that the morphia lessens the irritability of the air passages, and so restrains reflex action on the heart that, in this respect, its effect is similar to division of the vagus, and also that the morphia increases the blood pressure, and so is able to antagonize the deleterious influence of the chloroform for a lengthened period. Dr. Kappeler, who has had an extensive experience with this method, gives the morphia about half an hour previous to the administration of the chloroform, and in doses of about a quarter of a grain. This mixed method, he claims, is particularly suited for nervous patients, as the narcotic allays the extreme sensibility present in these cases. Dr. Crombie,* of Bengal, speaks very highly of this method also. For the prevention of cardiac failure from chloroform inhalation, Profs. Fraser and Schaefer† recommend the injection of atropine. Nitrite of amyl, turpentine, acupuncture and the application of boiling water to the cardiac region have all been recommended for the same object.

---

* *Practitioner*, Dec., 1880.

† *Brit. Med. Jour.*, Dec., 1880.

Another anæsthetic agent which has been attracting a good deal of attention on this side of the Atlantic lately is bromide of ethyl. First used and introduced by Nunnely, of Leeds, and lately extensively used by Drs. Turnbull and Levis, of Philadelphia. The latter says:* "I have used it under the most varied circumstances which could be required to test the merits of an anæsthetic, ... and in the most abnormal conditions of debility and shock of injury, in capital operations, through protracted periods of operations, in patients from early infancy to extreme old age." He is convinced that it is practically the best anæsthetic known to the profession. The two leading peculiarities of bromide of ethyl are quickness of action and speedy recovery from the anæsthetic condition. Unfortunately, this agent was not long in use before two deaths occurred from its administration, one reported by Marion Sims,† the other by Levis.‡ In Sims' case death did not take place until twenty-one hours after the operation, and therefore the fatal result was not owing to any depressant action of the anæsthetic on the heart, which is an important fact. The kidneys were found to be the seat of "Acute Catarrhal Nephritis," and it is probable that this condition was the direct result of the anæsthetic. Several cases are reported where very alarming symptoms of cardiac failure have occurred during the administration of the bromide of ethyl, but where death was apparently prevented by appropriate remedies. Wood and Reichert§ have shown that the bromide of ethyl is a direct cardiac depressant, and that it at times acts out of all proportion to the dôse administered. It has been asserted by Squibb‖ that bromide of ethyl is a loosely molecular compound, prone to undergo decomposition in the system and liberate free bromine.

Reichert,¶ in an able article, shows that it is very likely that

---

* *Amer. Jour. Med. Sc.*, July, 1880.

† *N. Y. Med. Record.*

‡ *Med. News and Abstract*, June, 1880.

§ *Philad. Med. Times*, May, 1881.

‖ *N. Y. Med. Record.*

¶ *Am. Jour. Med. Sc.*, July, 1881.

all halogen-holding anæsthetics are loosely molecular compounds, and liable to liberate their chlorine, bromine, or iodine. If this proves to be true, we are not likely to find any safe anæsthetics in this group.

The mode of action of anæsthetics on cerebral protoplasm is a subject which has lately been attracting some attention in France. Cl. Bernard,† in a series of experiments, demonstrated the fact that if chloroform blood is prevented from reaching the encephalon, no anæsthesia takes place. He compares the action of chloroform on the brain to a natural sleep, which is a slow anæmia of the nerve centres; but the diminution of blood does not reach lower than what is necessary for an organ in repose. He further states that the anæsthetics determine a coagulation of the substance of the cerebral cells. This coagulating action of the anæsthetics on protoplasm affects all the tissues. The heart of an animal placed in the vapour of chloroform soon loses its excitability, and when its fibres are examined by the microscope, they are found to be no longer transparent. If a nerve is submitted to the same influence, it is found to lose its transparency and excitability.

AGENTS WHICH REDUCE ARTERIAL TENSION.

High blood-pressure gives the earliest indications of the grave series of degenerative changes throughout the body, known as chronic Bright's disease, and may, if neglected, lead to disastrous results, both in disease of the arteries and the heart. We are able to recognize this state of the circulatory system by the sphygmograph, and this instrument gives us very valuable aid in deciding what our remedies are doing. "It is very common to meet with people, apparently in good health, who have no albumen in their urine or any other sign of organic diseass, but who constantly present a condition of high arterial tension when examined by the aid of the sphygmograph. Such people are very commonly subjects of the gouty diathesis, dyspeptics, suffer from functional derangements of the liver, indulge too freely in

† H. Duret, "Les Nouveaux Anæsthetiques et l'Anæsthesie," Charcot's Archiv., No. 1.

alcohol, or have, from one cause or another, tainted or impure blood." (Mahomed.)* When this condition of the arterial system is extreme, we can feel the "persistence" of the pulse by means of the finger alone. The artery is rigid, not from any thickening of its coats, but from a constant hyperdistension. All these facts go to show that there is present a great pathological entity, and which demands the most careful treatment, if we are to prevent those changes in the heart, kidneys and other organs which will most certainly follow in the course of time. Blood-letting is probably the most expeditious method of relieving tension in cases of impending apoplexy or in the coma of uræmia.

Hamilton† speaks highly of blood-letting as *the* remedy in the initial stage of croupous pneumonia. In this disease there is high tension, but in catarrhal pneumonia we have the very opposite conditions of the circulatory system present. The reduction of blood-pressure effected by general blood-letting is not very great, and its effect is but very temporary. We have experimental proof of the truth of this shown us by Kussmaul and Tenner, who desired, after removing the whole of the cerebrum, to take successive slices off the cerebellum. They, however, found that all their normal rabbits bled to death before they could reach the conclusion of their experiments, but they found no trouble in finishing them if they previously kept the animals on a dry diet for a period of two weeks. No deprivation of water was sufficient to bring down the blood pressure. The result of this experiment goes to show that a dry diet is superior to blood-letting as a reducer of arterial tension when we want a permanent effect. In cases of angina pectoris, due to, or accompanied by, increased arterial tension, it has long been a well-known fact that the nitrite of amyl exercises a very beneficial effect. The action of the amyl is, however, of so temporary a character that it is not adapted to those cases where we want to bring about a continuous or permanent dilatation. It has been shown by Reichert‡ that the nitrite of potassium possesses this desirable property. Its

* *Lancet*, August 18, 1877.

† *Practitioner*, 1880.

‡ *Amer. Jour. Med. Sc.*, July, 1880.

physiological actions are similar in every respect to those of the amyl nitrite, but possessing a more permanent action. This action will probably be found to be of great advantage in the treatment of those chronic conditions attended by high arterial tension. Another drug which has been experimentally found and therapeutically proved to have a considerable effect in reducing systemic contraction is nitro-glycerine. Dr. Murrell* found that one or two drops of a 1 per cent solution causes a painful sensation over the whole head, which soon extends to the entire body. It causes a glow on the face, but not the great blushing we see when the nitrite of amyl is given. Nitro-glycerine gives also a similar sphygmographic tracing to the nitrite of amyl. The amplitude of the tracing is much increased; the rise and fall is abrupt. The trace displays much dicrotism. Dr. Murrell has tested it in three severe cases of angina pectoris with very considerable success; a success quite equal to that afforded by nitrite of amyl. He gives 1 ♏ of a 1 per cent solution every three hours on sugar or in a little water. Dr. Mayo Robson† and many others have used nitro-glycerine in angina pectoris also with beneficial results. Dr. Robson‡ has also had good effects from its use in acute and chronic Bright's disease, and in the vascular tension of the aged. It has also been found of marked benefit in alleviating the paroxysms of hemicrania and preventing their frequent recurrence. Cannabis Indica is another agent of undoubted value in cases of increased arterial tension. It has been shown§ that it has a remarkable influence in ameliorating and sometimes actually curing those cases of hemicrania that have for their fundamental pathological condition a contraction of the arterioles. I am not aware of its having been used in other pathological states due to or attended by increased arterial tension, but, judging from its physiological action, it would appear to be worthy of a trial. Chloral hydrat. is another drug which possesses the power of reducing arterial tension, and on this account it is highly recom-

* Ringer's Therapeutics, Ed. 7, p. 373.
† *Brit. Med. Jour.*, April 10, 1880.
‡ *Brit. Med. Jour.*, Nov. 20, 1880.
§ The writer, in *Canada Med. & Surg. Jour.*, October, 1880.

mended by that able physician, Dr. Fothergill, in acute endocarditis. He shows* clearly how, with rest in bed and continuous small doses of chloral, the heart is placed in the best possible condition to recuperate. By these means that increase of connective tissue which is accelerated by high arterial tension is prevented. He further points out the great danger of giving what is very often ordered in these cases—digitalis ; for it is a well-known, but unfortunately not commonly recognized, fact that digitalis† contracts the arterioles and thereby increases the blood-pressure, the very condition which we should do our utmost to prevent.

This will be an appropriate place to consider the treatment of internal aneurisms by the iodide af potassium. In May of the present year Dr. Duffey,‡ of Dublin, exhibited before the Medical Society of the College of Physicians in Ireland a specimen of aneurism of the thoracic aorta, which furnished an example of the disease approaching to a cure by coagulation of the blood within the sac of the aneurism, such result being fairly attributable to persistent treatment with large doses of the iodide of potassium. It is not due to irritation of the vaso-motor centre, for Böhm and Gärtz have shown that after careful cutting of the spinal cord and both vagi, digitalis will still bring about an increase, although it is not so great on account of the previous extreme dilation of the vessels. After complete paralysis of the vaso-motor centre and spinal cord by chloral, digitalis will still raise the blood pressure. Williams comes to the conclusion that the increase is due to changes effected in the elasticity of the heart's muscle by digitalis. The aneurism was not the immediate

---

* *Practitioner*, January, 1881.

† Williams, in a very important paper (*Ueber die Ursache der Blutdrucksteigerung bei der Digitalinwerkung*) published in the *Archiv. fur Exper. Path. und Pharmakologie*, Band XIV., shows that digitalis causes the following changes in the following order in the circulation :—

(1) Increased blood-pressure with diminished pulse frequency.
(2) Continuation of high blood-pressure with increased pulse frequency.
(3) Irregularity of the heart when the blood-pressure is high.
(4) Rapid sinking of the blood-pressure as the heart comes to a standstill. What is the cause of the increased blood-pressure?

‡ *Brit. Med. Jour.*, June 4, 1881.

cause of the patient's death. In this case the iodide of potassium was administered in gradually increasing doses, until at last the patient was taking 40 grains three times daily. The effects of these large doses were most satisfactory. They produced no unpleasant effects. The patient obtained complete relief from the pains; the tumor diminished materially in size; it became quite firm and hard to the touch; and the pulsation in it, from being forcible, elastic and visible, was now barely perceptible; and he was discharged from hospital in this satisfactory condition, after being under treatment for four months. He died shortly afterwards from an attack of bronchitis, followed by pneumonia and collateral hyperæmia of the lungs. At the same meeting Dr. Duffey gave the details of another case that was then under his treatment by the iodide of potassium, and in which a remarkable change took place in the size of the sac; the pains were also greatly relieved. There can be no question whatever but what a few cases of internal aneurism have been cured by the iodide of potassium. For this we are indebted to Dr. Balfour, of Edinburgh. How does the iodide of potassium act? That it is not owing to the potash, as has been often suggested, appears probable from Balfour's experience, as a trial by him of other potash salts failed to have the least influence over the disease. The iodide produces diminution of the cardiac force and blood pressure, and for the production of these effects rest in the recumbent position is not necessary. The following appears then to be the most appropriate treatment for those cases of internal aneurism that cannot be dealt with surgically:—(1) The administration of large doses of the iodide of potassium for a lengthened period; (2) Rest in the recumbent position; (3) A dry diet. Dr. Flint* reports the case of an aneurism of the abdominal aorta, in a lady, aged 65, apparently cured by chloride of barium in doses of 2-5 of a grain continued for a period of five months.

ANTISEPTICS.

In this group of agents we have had lately some interesting work, a short *resumé* of which I will now give:

---

* *Practitioner*, July, 1879.

Klebs*, of Prague, gives an account of two cases of typhoid fever that he treated with large doses of the benzoate of magnesia. The first case, a male, aged 23, when first seen (5th day) had a temperature of 39°.6, and was in a soporose condition, and could only be aroused with difficulty. The tongue was dry and brown. He was given 10 grammes of the benzoate of magnesia during the next 24 hours, and at the end of that time it was found that the tongue was moist and the temperature down to 38°.1; consciousness had returned. On the 14th day the temperature was normal, and remained so; the benzoate was, however, continued for 12 days longer, or, in all, for 26 days, during which time 450 grammes or 28 oz. were taken.

In the second case, a male, aged 38, the temperature on the 5th day of the disease was 40°.1. He was given daily 20 grammes of the benzoate of magnesia. Eight days after the initial shivering the temperature was normal and remained so. The patient took altogether 180 grammes of the benzoate in nine days.

Such a satisfactory result in only two cases teaches certainly but little; the result, however, is sufficient to warrant the employment of this antiseptic in still more heroic doses. There is no other antiseptic at present known that can be given in such large doses without producing disagreeable and even dangerous symptoms. If the poison of typhoid fever depends on a bacillus, as Klebs† thinks he has proved, there is undoubtedly a great future before the antiseptic treatment of this and other kindred diseases. Jahn,‡ in an epidemic of typhoid fever in 1872, treated his cases with small doses of quinine, and cold baths when the temperature ran very high. He had a mortality of 23 per cent; average duration of fever 24 days. In a second epidemic (1874) he used baths alone, and had a mortality of only 8.5 per cent; average duration of fever 25 days. In a third epidemic (1875-6) he used salicylic acid, and had only a mortality of 7.1 per cent; average duration of fever 21 days. From ℈i to ℈iss of the acid or its soda salt was given daily. The use of the acid was nearly

* *Arch. fur Exp. Path. und Pharma.*, Band XIV.

† Klebs: Der Bacillus des Abdominaltyphus und der typhose process.

‡ Quoted by Klebs.

always followed by a decided reduction in the temperature, and on its being withheld the temperature quickly rose. If salicylic acid should prove to be a powerful antidote to the poisons of typhoid, we would be unable to give it in sufficient doses, owing to its producing often violent pharyngitis and irritation of the bronchi. According to both Jahn and Klebs, the salicylates have a good influence over the nervous phenomena of typhoid. Patients in a soporose condition are soon brought back to a conscious state. The unpleasant cerebral effects which salicylic acid and its salts are said to produce have not been noticed by these observers. Immerman* states that there were relapses in only 4 per cent of cases treated by salicylic acid, and 26 per cent of relapses in cases treated by all other means.

The antiseptic treatment of diphtheria has been attracting a good deal of attention lately. Chlorate of potash, which is used very extensively either locally or internally in diphtheria and other throat affections, is only antiseptic in dangerous doses. A saturated solution of the chlorate of potash in water is not antiseptic. It requires a strength of 1 to 5, and this is a poisonous solution; the chlorate acts as all other salts of potash do in large doses, by paralyzing the heart. As death in diphtheria frequently takes placc in the same way, it follows that chlorate of potash is a dangerous remedy to give in doses large enough to produce any antiseptic action. Küster† reports four cases that came under his own observation where death was in all probability brought about by the action of the chlorate of potash on the heart. Weise‡ recommends very highly a 2 per cent solution of salicylic acid in diphtheria, This is a strongly antiseptic solution, but not a dangerous one. He employs the following formula:—

℞	Acid Salicyl., - - -	1.09
	Sp. Vini Rectif.	
	Glycerine, - - - āā	25.00

At the same time he uses benzoate of soda internally.

* *Archv. fur Exp. Path. und Pharm.*, Band XIV.

† *Berliner Kl. Woch.*, No. 40, 1880.

‡ *Berliner Kl. Woch.*, No. 4, 1881.

Oertel,* of Munich, considers that he has proved that diphtheria is an infectious disease, caused by a fungus designated as "*Micrococcus Diphtheriæ*," which, localized in the mouth and pharynx, produces inflammatiou and fibrinous exudation of the mucous membranes and, after an undeterminable length of time, general infectious disease, the general infection being dependant upon and kept up by the local. If this theory is correct, all that is necessary is to destroy this organism, and remove from the affected parts the products of the disease. For destruction of the organism, Oertel employs carbolic acid in the form of spray (1 to 20). He has lately treated 27 severe cases in this manner, all entirely successful. The severity of these cases was such that Oertel believes that under any other form of treatment three-fourths of them would have been fatal. In the severest cases it was only after such impregnation of the blood with carbolic acid that olive-green coloration of the urine appeared that he observed a rapid diminution of the disease. For the separation and removal of the false membranes, he uses warm vapor locally, and the internal administration of jaborandi. As the latter remedy seems to be very useful in this disease, it will be more useful to mention what it is said to have done in diphtheria while on this subject. It was first used by Dr. Guttmann,† of Canstatt. He has used it for 16 months, and regards it almost as a specific. During this time he treated 75 cases—all recovered. It was given internally, and it was noticed that in a very short time it produced an active flow of saliva, by means of which the false membrane was loosened, the inflammatory irritation lessened, and the intense redness gave place to a more normal color. He uses the following formula:

℞	Muriate Pilocarpine, .	0.02
	Pepsine, ...	0.05
	Acid Hydrochl., . .	gtt ii
	Aq. Distil., ...	80.00

Sig. One teaspoonful every hour. For adults, double the dose. Oertel‡ speaks very favourably of this mode of treatment. He,

* *Arch. Laryngology*, January, 1881.

† *Berl. Klin. Woch.*, No. 40, 1880.

‡ *Arch. Laryngology*, January, 1881.

however, does not, like Guttmann, consider it to be a specific. Lereboullet* reports favourably of its use. Küster† reports four severe cases where pilocarpin acted very well; a fifth case died from nephritis after removal of the membrane from the throat. Weise‡ also bears testimony to its beneficial action in a few cases; and he also adds the report of a case where he considered death was in a great measure caused by the deleterious influence of the jaborandi on the heart. It is well known that jaborandi exercises a paralyzing influence over the heart, and from late researches§ it would seem that this cardiac influence resides in an alkaloid named jaborin, and not in the pilocarpine. Should this be true, we could get all the good influence exerted by a pure preparation of pilocarpine, and none of the disadvantages arising from other ingredients contained in jaborandi by using the former alkaloid. At present it becomes us to be very careful in ordering this drug in cases of diphtheria, and where there are the least symptoms of cardiac failure to discontinue its administration.

While on the subject of the treatment of diphtheria, I would like to call attention to some remarkable experiments performed by Prof. Rossbach‖ of Wurzburg on the action of papayotin in dissolving diphtheritic membranes. A solution of papayotin (1 to 20) dissolved a piece of croupal membrane (removed from the trachea and bronchi) into fine particles in an hour. In six hours the solution was perfectly clear, and no trace of any elements could be seen under the microscope. It took a lime solution three days to dissolve a similar membrane. In a bromine and bromide of potassium solution there was scarcely any change to be seen after four days immersion. Pepsine and weak acids affected no change after 48 hours. Owing to his supply of papayotin becoming exhausted, and no more being procurable,

---

* *Bulletin Général de Therapeutique*, June, 1881.

† *Berl. Klin. Woch.*, No. 27, 1881.

‡ *Berl. Klin. Woch.*, No. 4, 1881.

§ Ringer, *Practitioner*, January, 1881. Albertoni, Harnack and Meyer, *Arch. fur Exp. Path. und Pharm.*

‖ *Berl. Klin. Wochenschrift*, No. 10, 1881.

Prof. Rossbach was unable to put this agent to a practical test in the treatment of a case of diphtheria. He made use of another part of the plant known by the name of *succus*, but this is a very much weaker preparation than papayotin, requiring over a day to dissolve what the latter accomplishes in an hour. It was given to a child, aged 15 months, who had a diphtheritic exudation covering the pharynx and tonsils, and symptoms of stenosis of the larynx. Owing to the extensive surface involved, and weakness of the child, a very unfavourable prognosis was given. A concentrated solution of the "Succus Caricæ Papayæ" was pencilled on the throat every five minutes. In 24 hours the tonsils and pharynx were free from exudation. The laryngeal stenosis was, however, still present, and the local treatment was now directed to the larynx, with the result that before many hours all symptoms of the stenosis had vanished. The child, however, died from atelectasis and œdema of the lungs. On *post-mortem*, the mucous membranes of the throat and larynx were found swollen and red, but no trace of diphtheritic or croupal membrane was to be seen, except a minute patch at the anterior angle of the vocal cords. These results published by such an accurate and intelligent observer as Prof. Rossbach demand the earnest attention of the profession.

The local applications of bromide of potassium, iodide of silver and fluorhydric acid have been recommended* in diphtheria during the last year.

(*To be continued in our next Number.*)

BI-MONTHLY RETROSPECT OF OBSTETRICS AND GYNÆCOLOGY.

PREPARED BY WM. GARDNER, M.D.,
Prof. Medical Jurisprudence and Hygiene, McGill University; Attending Physician to the University Dispensary for Diseases of Women; Physician to the Out-Patient Department, Montreal General Hospital.

The Relation of Cleanliness to the Prevention of Puerperal Septicæmia is the subject of a clinical lecture by Dr. Albert H. Smith of Philadelphia in the October (1881) number of the

---

* Peyrand, Gassicourt, Brame and Bergeron, in *Bulletins et Memoires de la Société de Thérapeutique*, 30 Janvier, 1881.

Medical News and Abstract. Since it has been established beyond a doubt that the causation of the diseases classed under the title puerperal fever is absorption of decayed animal matter by open raw surfaces, all observers of note agree that these diseases are precisely analogous in their causation, pathology, course of development, urgent need of prophylaxis and treatment to septic inflammation and fever found in surgical practice; the only differences depend on the peculiarity of the tissues involved in parturition, upon their exceeding capacity for absorption and transfer of poison, and the many points likely to be presented where such absorption may take place. How to keep the genital canal clean during and after parturition is then the great question in the prevention of this horrible malady. After reviewing the various possible sources of poison and the numerous avenues by which they may enter the system of the lying-in woman, Dr. Smith speaks of an autogenetic source of infection during parturition to which he beheves attention has not hitherto been drawn, and which he believes to be one of the most tertile causes of septic fever after prolonged labour. This is the accumulation and continued exposure to atmospheric influence in contact with the warm tissues of the mother, of the natural and healthy discharge of mucus with its admixture of blood from the cervix and vagina, while the tissues are gradually relaxing for the passage of the child. This discharge is perfectly healthy when it exudes, but covering the external parts, the heat of the patient's body and the warm air of the chamber soon decompose it and sepsis results. Dr. Smith further mentions other sources of poison probably unsuspected by most accoucheurs. Such are: sores on the doctor's hands or any part of his person which may be touched by the hands; granular ophthalmia; otorrhœa; a purulent coryza; or a foul ozæna, with any one of which the finger is often brought into contact. The essential principle in the carrying out of that great indication, the prevention of puerperal fever, is cleanliness; keeping clean the tissues before and after the production of the lesions of their surface, and of everything that comes in contact with them; the purifying and removal of all morbific materials, and the prevention by suitable means, of their reproduction. Dr. Smith lays down certain rules and gives certain hints for the guidance of accoucheurs. After touching any decomposing animal matter the hands must be carefully washed with disinfectant solutions, using the nail-brush freely. This should be repeated before the person of the patient is approached. Between the washing of the hands and the examination of the patient nothing should be touched except what is known to be perfectly clean. No driving should be done, or gloves worn; nothing of doubtful character should touch the hands. The disinfectant solutions used by Dr. Smith, and which he always orders as a part of the preparation for labour, are 2½ per cent of carbolic acid, or 6 or 7 per cent of good recently-made Labarraque's solution; that is, about seven fluid drachms of a 95 per cent solution of the former, and about a fluid ounce of the latter to a pint of water. For lubricating the finger he uses washed lard carbolized to from 5 to 10 per cent. He prefers the chlorinated to the carbolized solution, as it is a more powerful disinfectant, and in such proportion as is necessary for the purpose, it does not burn the skin or obtund the tactile sense like the carbolized solution. This solution is to be used for the hands and for any instruments—forceps, vectis, catheter, or other. After a rectal enema, if the membranes be not ruptured, a vaginal injection of either is given; this is not practised if the membranes are ruptured. The external genitals are frequently bathed with one of the solutions, and from time to time a soft cloth soaked in the solution is carried by the finger into the vagina as far as it will reach. Dr. Smith believes the antiseptic spray during labour to be unnecessary and annoying to both patient and physician if carried out to the necessary extent. It chills the patient and irritates and benumbs her parts as well as the accoucheur's hands. He practises the method just described instead of it. After delivery of the placenta, he washes out the uterus at once with a syringe and hot water at 115° to 120° Fah., either chlorinated or acidulated with vinegar, about twenty-five per cent. He formerly used carbolic acid for this purpose, but within a year has seen two cases of immediate carbolic poisoning result, thus confirming Fritsch's statements on this point. For four days after labour he directs the nurse to wash out the vagina with carbolized or chlorinated water at about 110° Fah. every four or six hours. If any offensive lochia appear, with the least symptom of septic poisoning, he washes out the uterus with a ten to fifteen per cent Labarraque solution, with a double canulated uterine tube, using a syphon in preference to a forcing syringe.

Uterine Electro-therapeutics, by Dr. J. Dixon Mann of Manchester: a paper in the *Lancet* for July 9th and 23rd, 1881.—The constant current has physiological, chemical and thermal effects. The thermal effects are so slight that they may be disregarded; the chemical are of more importance. Allied to the latter are its power of promoting osmosis and absorption, and accelerating the movements of lymph in the lymphatics and lymph spaces. Its principal physiological effect is on the vaso-motor system. It first dilates the arterioles, the dilatation beginning soon after the circuit is closed, sometimes during application, and a short time after. Soon after withdrawal of the current the dilatation subsides, and there is then contraction of vessels. Thus by repetition vascular congestion is diminished. Anodyne effects of the constant current are well established.

The induced current possesses feeble chemical and catalytic effects. Its action is chiefly in producing muscular movements. The primary effect on the vascular system is to produce contraction of the arterioles. This gives place to dilatation, the result of paresis from previous excessive contraction. This effect on the vascular system is much shorter in duration than that from the constant current. An important effect of the induced current is to stimulate the muscular structure of the womb. In the treatment of amenorrhœa by electricity, a comprehensive view of uterine disorders must be taken. Electrical treatment is only useful when the causative defect is in the generative system and the organism as a whole is healthy.

The treatment of necessity must be prolonged in most instances, thus requiring patience on the part of both physician and patient. An ill-nourished or ill-developed organ cannot be immediately brought to a performance of its function. The organic defect must first be remedied. Imperfect nutrition demands prolonged use of the constant current: simple atony commonly yields to a much shorter application of the induced current. The necessary instruments for uterine electro-therapeutics are: an insulated sound (two sizes), a cervical electrode, and two or more large disc electrodes. The sound is coated with gold in its curved part, or is made of solid platinum, which is better. The stem is to be insulated to within two inches of the end by covering it with a gum-elastic catheter. The external electrode is an oval disc of flexible metal, with a layer of amadou on one side and covered with wash-leather. Dr. Mann relates three cases treated with electricity, bearing out the statements made in the first part of his paper. One of these was a case of amenorrhœa, with imperfectly developed uterus, measuring only 1⅝ in. Applications during fifteen minutes twice weekly of the constant current from twenty-five cells were made for some time. At the end of five months the uterus measured 2¼ in., and the patient menstruated for the first time. After this she was regular. The applications were now made at longer intervals, the induced current being used when the symptoms indicated approach of the menses.

The second case was one of amenorrhœa following a severe illness. Both currents were used, and at the end of two months the menses returned and continued to be regular.

Dr. Mann further relates a case of spasmodic or neuralgic dysmenorrhœa, the pain being intense for twenty-four hours before the appearance of the discharge, and attended with vomiting, successfully treated by intra-uterine applications of the constant current. In this case there was neither flexion nor congestion The sound was easily passed, but caused much pain. The applications of about eighteen to twenty cells were made three times a week. At the first period there was no vomiting and much less pain. Treatment was resumed in the interval. At the next period she was so much better that she declined further treatment. This is a remarkably satisfactory result of treatment of an exceedingly obstinate set of symptoms. Such results certainly warrant a further trial of the remedy. It is probably effectual by an anodyne or modifying effect on the mucous membrane of the uterus. Simple ovarian neuralgia or irritation without oöphoritis or peri-oöphoritis is a condition in which there is much to expect from the constant current so useful in other neuralgiæ. Simple subinvolution in its early stages, without perimetric inflammation or pelvic disease, is a condition in which electricity is likely to be useful. The author reports having treated and cured such a case in seven weeks.

Amputation of the Cervix Uteri for Chronic Metritis, by Dr. A. Leblond. (Communicated to the International Medical Congress in London, August, 1881. *Annales de Gynecologie*, Sept. 1881.)—Dr. Leblond strongly advocates this method of treatment (also practiced by Gallard of Paris) for chronic metritis which has resisted the ordinary therapeutical measures. He, however, alludes to the fact that medicines such as iron, arsenic and iodine compounds are undoubtedly sometimes of real service. Locally, at the very outset, leeching, cupping and scarification are useful, but soon a stage is reached when caustics are needed. Nitrate of silver, iodine, nitric acid, and chromic acid are useful in cases of moderate severity. In the more severe and long-lasting cases, free use of the actual cautery is necessary. If this method of treatment be selected, it ought to be thoroughly applied. A recent modification of the method of application is ignipuncture of the cervix by a filiform or needle platinum cautery heated by the galvanic current, which is made to penetrate its substance to a depth of five or six millimetres in six or eight places. The method of treatment by amputation will, M. Leblond believes, succeed when other methods fail. It will be found most useful in the early stages, when the portiovaginalis is still soft from hyperæmia and infiltration, with serum, and its surface granular and easily made to bleed. The method of amputation practiced by M. Leblond is the galvano-caustic platinum wire applied through a Goodell's speculum, and very slowly tightened so as to avoid bleeding. The subsequent cicatrization is slow, requiring three weeks or a month for its completion. The results in Gallard's and Leblond's experience have been most favourable.

The Hypodermic Morphia Treatment of Puerperal Convulsions appears to be growing in favour. From time to time favourable results of its employment are reported in the journals. Mr.

Maberly-Smith, resident surgeon at the Melbourne (Victoria) Lying-in Hospital, in the *Lancet* for July 16th, 1881, gives the results of treatment of fifteen cases in the Hospital and in the practice of physicians in the city of Melbourne. He concludes that the morphia treatment is far more successfal than that by chloral, bromide of potassium, and chloroform, which he has found to be unsatisfactory. He injects one-fourth to one-third of a grain, according to the severity of the case, and prefers the simple solution of morphia, finding it more efficacious than a combination with atropia. One large dose is better than two small ones. Patients suffering from puerperal eclampsia, whether sensible or insensible, appear to resist the dangerous effects of the drug; it appears to have no bad consequences in cases, in which, under ordinary circumstances, morphia would be strongly contraindicated. Mr. Maberly-Smith has employed it in women who were insensible, with stertorous breathing, congested lungs and faces, and contracted pupils, and in every case with the best results. After the injection the patient may have one fit before the drug has had time to act, but has no more for some hours. If they recur, they yield just as readily to a repetition of the morphia injection. No case of puerperal convulsions has ended fatally in the Melbourne Lying-in Hospital since the treatment has been adopted. Short notes of five cases are appended. Mr. Maberly-Smith's experience agrees in every particular with my own. During the last year I have seen some remarkable results from this method of treatment. Apart from, as I believe, its undoubtedly greater efficacy than the commoner modes of treatment, it has the great advantage of facility of administration. The patient is usually unconscious and unable to swallow, or semi-unconscious and resisting. It is thus difficult or impossible to give remedies either by mouth or enema. In any case the hypodermic injection is morphia or Battley's sedative, which I have used oftenest, is easily administered, and rapidly produces its effects.

The Proper Limitation of Emmet's Operation for Laceration of the Cervix Uteri.—This was the subject of a paper read by Dr. C. C. Lee, surgeon to the New York Woman's Hospital, before the Medical Society of the County of New York, on the 23rd of May last. During the discussion which followed, Dr. Emmet made some important statements with reference to the lesion and reparative operation coupled with his name. As is well known, Emmet, in his first published articles on this subject, claimed that the ill-effects of lacerations of the cervix were due to eversion or rolling out of the lining membrane of the cervix and its being pressed upon and chafed by contact with the posterior vaginal wall, and that the cause of this eversion was the increased weight of the uterus itself. At the meeting above alluded to, Dr. Emmet said that careful observation during some years past had led him to believe that the condition was due directly to the product or remains of some old inflammation in the connective tissue of the pelvis, and generally in one or both broad ligaments, by which the circulation to and from the uterus was obstructed. This would cause the parts to roll out and the erosion to form. He found this thickening always present to a greater or less degree. His study of the condition had convinced him that the operation should not be done until the parts had been brought into the best condition, for it could not be determined that the operation was necessary until this had been done. He found that in the absence of cicatricial tissue, by relieving the pelvic cellulitis and inflamed state of the cervix, he had occasion to resort to surgical measures in about one case in ten in which he would formerly have operated. A relapse of the cellulitis and of the eroded condition of the cervix was little likely to occur unless the operation involved the vaginal wall. The object in closing the laceration was to preserve what had been gained by treatment. It was to prevent a return of the erosion and pelvic inflammation. The accoucheur ought to be on the look-out for every indication of the lesion immediately after birth, and make frequent injections to keep the parts clean, and then healing of the wound without a thickened and hardened tissue would be more likely to take place. It is remarkable how much nature can do to heal such injuries, if only cleanliness be secured. He had seen at least two cases of vesico-vaginal fistula caused by labour, into which he could introduce his finger, heal up within a month of their occurrence. How much more was to be expected from such a treatment of laceration of the cervix! In case of hemorrhage, the wound ought to be closed immediately. In such cases the perineum is usually ruptured; it ought to be sewed up at the same time.—*Cincinnati Obstet. Gazette*, Sept., 1881.

Reviews and Notices of Books.

The Applied Anatomy of the Nervous System: being a study of this portion of the human body from a standpoint of its general interest and practical utility, designed for use as a Text-book and a work of reference.—By AMBROSE L. RANNEY, A.M., M.D., Adjunct Professor of Anatomy, and late Lecturer on the Diseases of the Genito-Urinary Organs and on Minor Surgery in the Medical Department of the University of the City of New York. With numerous illustrations. New York: D. Appleton & Co. Montreal: Dawson Brothers.

This comprises a course of lectures on the nervous system delivered by the author during the winter of 1880 and 1881. The following paragraph from the preface affords the *raison d'être* of the work: "The rapid strides which are being made in the interpretation of the symptoms of nervous diseases and the introduction of many new terms which must embarrass the reader of late treatises, unless he is educated up to the present standard of knowledge in this field of medicine, seem to the author a reasonable ground for belief that there is a demand for a volume which shall fit the practitioner and student to pursue his studies in this special line without embarrassment, if not with increased interest." The cerebrum and the cerebral nerves, the spinal cord, and the spinal nerves, are all described with special reference to the more recent developments concerning their anatomy and the physiological functions dependant thereon. The lectures are written in a colloquial manner, which, perhaps, often serves to render the meaning more forcible and to maintain the interest of the reader better than the more set fashion of the ordinary text-book. It is profusely illustrated with cuts from the delineations of the most noted authors—Sappey, Ferrier, Hirschfield, &c.—and many diagrammatic representations by the author, which are very useful in aiding the explanation of any difficult point. We are sure that the book will be well received, and will prove itself a very useful companion both for regular students of anatomy and physiology, and also for practitioners who wish to work up the diagnosis, &c., of cases of disorder of the nervous system.

A Practical Treatise on Impotence, Sterility, and allied disorders of the Male Sexual Organs.—By SAMUEL W. GROSS, A.M., M.D., Lecturer on Venereal and Genito-Urinary Diseases in the Jefferson Medical College of Philadelphia, Surgeon to, and Lecturer on Clinical Surgery in, the Jefferson Medical College Hospital and the Philadelphia Hospital, &c., &c. With 16 illustrations. Philadelphia: Henry C. Lea's Son & Co. Montreal: Dawson Brothers.

This is a really practical book, containing a great deal of inmation upon a subject which it is very important that physicians generally should have some correct knowledge of. It is one on which there is no doubt that very erroneous ideas widely prevail, and still the advice given in connection therewith may be of the highest value with reference to the peace of mind of individuals or the governance of their social relations. The forms of impotence are considered under the following heads: Atonic, Psychical, Symptomatic and Organic; and the conditions met with producing the disordered state in these various ways are fully described, with the treatment appropriate to each. Sterility, as is well known, may arise either from absence of the vitalizing fluid or absence of living spermatozoa in the fluid, which may be present in the usual quantity. Thus arises the division of these cases into the two classes, Aspermatism and Azoospermism. A third set of cases is described by the author under the term Misemissiom, under which he includes cases arising either from vices of conformation of the urethra or from malposition of the meatus. The subject of Spermatorrhœa is fully treated of, and all the causes of this malady are enquired into. The reality of the disease, and the fact that it is to be removed by suitable treatment, often of a local character, no physician of experience can doubt, and the chapter in this work furnishes an excellent guide for the management of such cases. But, at the same time, it seems to us that the author fails to point out the fact that an immense number of supposed cases of spermatorrhœa are purely imaginary, and arise from the ignorance of so many young men that the nocturnal evacuation of the seminal vesicles at reasonable intervals is a natural process, and one which need give them no concern. If the physician gain the confidence of his patient, this idea can soon be dissipated by him and much mental distress prevented. It is notoriously by prying on the fears of the inexperienced that the quacks gain command of their dupes, and it is the duty of medical men to protect the unwary from the wiles of these artful dodgers as much as possible. Thus every scientific treatise on these affections is a useful addition to our literature, and this book, from the pen of one having enjoyed such extensive opportunities for observation will no doubt be widely read.

The Physician's Visiting List for 1882. Thirty-first year of its publication. Philadelphia: Lindsay & Blakiston.

The above well-known Visiting List comes to hand as usual. It is, as ever, neatly gotten up, and having used it for many years past, we can recommend it to the notice of all who require such an article.

Books and Pamphlets Received.

ANTISEPTIC SURGERY: THE PRINCIPLES, MODES OF APPLICATION, AND RESULTS OF THE LISTER DRESSING.—By Dr. Just Lucas-Championnière. Translated and Edited by Fred'k Henry Gerrish, A.M., M.D. Portland: Loring, Short & Harmon.

A PRACTICAL TREATISE ON HERNIA.—By J. H. Warren, M.D. Boston: Jas. R. Osgoode & Co.

EPILEPSY AND OTHER CHRONIC CONVULSIVE DISEASES: THEIR CAUSES, SYMPTOMS AND TREATMENT.—By W. R. Gowers, M.D., F.R.C.P. London: J. & A. Churchill.

TRANSACTIONS OF THE AMERICAN OPHTHALMOLOGICAL SOCIETY. Volume V. For the year 1881. Boston: Houghton, Mifflin & Co.

TRANSACTIONS OF THE COLLEGE OF PHYSICIANS OF PHILADELPHIA. Third Series. Volume V. Philadelphia: Lindsay & Blakiston.

THE SCIENCE AND ART OF MIDWIFERY.—By William T. Lusk, A.M., M.D. New York: D. Appleton & Co.

Society Proceedings.

MEDICO-CHIRURGICAL SOCIETY OF MONTREAL.

A regular meeting of this Society was held on Sept. 30, 1881. The President, Dr. Hingston, occupied the chair.

Dr. Mills was elected a member.

Dr. Osler exhibited a portion of jejunum, presenting 53 intestinal diverticula, some of them as large as an apple, after which he read a paper on "Obliteration of the Portal Vein."

Dr. McConnell then read a paper on "A case of Ovarian Tumour, with recovery after accidental bursting of the tumour."

Dr. Ross said he knew of a case where diagnosis of cystic tumour had been made out, and while riding on horseback it was ruptured, the contents escaping into the peritoneal cavity. The patient lived for many years after. These tumours are probably unilocular.

Dr. Hingston spoke of three cases. In one, large discharge from rectum; in the second, large discharge from vagina; and in the third, where tumour disappeared and again reappeared, and then disappearing and again reappearing.

Dr. Godfrey asked if these tumours ever assumed a malignant condition.

Dr. Trenholme said he had had one case where malignant disease was seen, and thought that it had been originally a simple cyst which had become malignant. He also said he had had two cases somewhat similar to Dr. McConnell's. In one case, the phthisical condition of the patient precluded any operation, The contents of the cyst escaped through the bowels, and there was no return of the tumour. In this case the cure was effected without any severe shock to the system. In the second case, there was a large and growing cyst in connection with a solid tumour of the uterus, where the patient, after a severe fall on her buttock, passed a large quantity of fluid by the bowels. At the time of the accident she suffered from a great heat over the whole abdomen, showing that some of the fluid must have escaped into the peritoneal cavity. There have been repeated evacuations of smaller quantities of fluid, and the patient goes about with greater comfort after each discharge.

Dr. Wilkins brought forward the subject of peptonized food for rectal alimentation, stating his experience, and expressed his approbation of this form of food for enfeebled patients.

The meeting then adjourned.

A regular and annual meeting of the Society was held on the 14th October—the President, Dr. Hingston, in the chair.

The minutes of last annual and regular meeting were read and approved.

Dr. Osler presented two cases of aneurism:

The first case was from a patient of Dr. Roddick's, aged 49 years, who applied to him complaining of a cough. Did not examine chest carefully, and saw little of him till two weeks ago. He then found him almost choking, with gasping, spasmodic respirations. By stimulations externally and internally, he rallied from that attack. On examination next day, an area of dullness three inches square was found over the sternum; the left pulse was weaker than the right. This condition lasted for ten days, the paroxysms coming on at intervals, till death resulted in the end quickly. Dr. Osler said the condition was that of multiple aneurism of the aortic arch. Stretching of the trachea did not give a thrill, but this aneurism was filled with a laminated clot, which may have prevented this sign being evident.

The second case was similar. Dr. Ross said there was no alteration in speech; pulsation could be felt distinctly in this case and the other signs were evident. Dr. Osler said this sac contained no laminated fibrine.

Dr. Trenholme then read a paper on "A case of Melæna," which is of interest on account of the absence of *post-mortem* conditions accounting for death, and also because of the unusual number of diverticula of the jejunum, as well as their large size. The following history is reported:—S. S., aged 56 years, a man of medium size, well developed, active, temperate habits, and of a dull complexion. For the past 26 years his wife states she could hear rumbling or gurgling sounds in his belly after every meal, and that he was in the habit of going for a walk immediately after eating to prevent people from noticing this. The gurgling was lessened by lying down. He was also subject to frequent attacks of vomiting and sometimes purging. Generally had two or three such attacks each summer. His appetite was unexceptionally good, except at these periods. He led an active, out-door life, being almost constantly on his feet; and was in the habit of moose-hunting two or three weeks every winter. Though of a hearty appetite, he had always to be careful of the nature of his food—simple, plain, substantial food being that which best agreed with him. The sickness from which he died was of sudden onset. He went to his work perfectly well on Tuesday morning, but was seized with severe pains in the upper part of his abdomen about the middle of the afternoon, and though able to keep at his work till night, returned home prostrated with his sufferings. I saw him at 8 o'clock the same evening, and found him in a state of collapse, skin cold, and bathed with a cold, clammy perspiration; eyes sunken, voice husky, breath cold, pulse rapid, small and thready, and with great pain in the right hypochondriac region. The bowels had not been opened since the morning. Upon inquiry as to the cause of his condition, the only one he could conceive of was that the previous afternoon (Monday) he had drank a glass of iced ginger-ale. The length of time that had elapsed since the draught led me to give it little weight as the probable cause of the present alarming condition. His family history and his remarkably well-developed physique were so good as to preclude malignant disease. I was at a loss to account for the symptoms of a genuine case of cholera, less the alvine evacuations, and which were needed to complete the picture. Stimulants and hot fomentations were resorted to, together with hot bottles to feet, calves of legs, and armpits. About 1 o'clock on

Wednesday morning I was hastily called to see the patient, and found the general state much as it was in the evening, but that there had been a large bloody stool of about two quarts of blood, dark and liquid. Hot fomentations to the stomach were now discontinued, and opiates and brandy given by the mouth, and turpentine enemata administered by the bowels. During the day the condition of the patient continued as it had been. In the forenoon there was a slight effort at a reaction; but another severe hæmorrhage from the bowels occurred, and the man gradually sank and died at 7 o'clock in the evening. From the commencement of the illness till death supervened was about thirty hours. Dr. Scott saw the case with me, and while concurring in the treatment pursued, was equally with myself at a loss to account for the excessive and fatal hæmorrhage. The man's exceeding good health negatived the thought of malignant disease; while his active habits and not infrequent pains in the abdomen suggested aneurism, which was deemed hardly tenable on account of the history of the case in other respects and the course of the disease. The *post-mortem* examination was made by Dr. Osler, whose well-known ability as a pathologist made me hope that clear and satisfactory light would be thrown upon this (to me) anomalous and difficult case.

Dr. Osler then gave an account of the *post-mortem* examination. He also said the previous cases were suggestive of typhoid fever.

Dr. Gardner then read a report of the annual meeting of the American Gynecological Society, lately held in New York.

Dr. Hingston then gave a *resumé* of the year's work.

The Treasurer presented his annual report, audited by Drs. Roddick and F. W. Campbell.

Dr. Roddick moved, seconded by Dr. Osler, that the balance of amount due for furnishing rooms be paid out of the funds of the Society.—*Carried.*

A ballot was then taken, and the following were elected officers for the ensuing year: President, Dr. George Ross; 1st Vice-President, Dr. Kennedy; 2nd Vice-President, Dr. Rodger; Secretary, Dr. Edwards; Treasurer, Dr. Molson; Librarian, Dr. Gurd; Council, Drs. Roddick, Osler and Campbell.

Dr. Roddick moved, seconded by Dr. Henry Howard, a vote of thanks to the retiring officers of the year.—*Carried.*

Dr. Roddick gave notice of motion that in clause No 8 be added, " they shall also constitute a library committee."

Dr. Cameron brought up the matter of the advisability of continuing the present papers and magazines, which was agreed to.

The meeting then adjourned.

Extracts from British and Foreign Journals.

Unless otherwise stated the translations are made specially for this Journal.

Treatment of Double Talipes Equino Varus by Open Incision and Fixed Extension.—By Dr. A. M. Phelps of Chateaugay, N.Y.—Mr. President and Gentlemen of the Society: As a delegate from Franklin County Medical Society, I came to Albany expecting to take no part in the proceedings of this meeting, only so far as the duties of delegate might devolve upon me. Since my arrival I have been urged by professional friends, to whom I had previously sent photographs, to report at this session the case of a little patient suffering from double talipes equino varus, upon whom I operated by open incision and fixed extension. The patient was a little girl 6½ years old. I first saw her May 15th, 1880. The feet were rigid. The inner side was very much shortened and described a sharp curve from the heel to the great toe, which rested upon the inner side of the tibia when the weight of the body was upon them. The attempt at walking had produced large bunions upon the dorsum of the feet, which were very much inflamed. The head of the astragalus was subluxated forward, and the limbs were very much atrophied.

Fig. 1 is taken from the photograph presented at the Society, and gives a correct idea of the extent of deformity. Under an anæsthetic, and assisted by my friend Dr. Farnsworth and my student, Mr. VanVechten, I divided subcutaneously the tendo-achillis, tendon of tibialis anticus, the plantar fascia, and such contracted tendons and bands in the soles of the feet as I could safely do without wounding the artery and nerve. The feet were imperfectly restored to their normal position, and dressed with

Sayre's temporary dressing. (See Sayre's Surgery, p. 98.) After the wound had healed, and upon the seventh day, Barwell's dressing with rubber muscles was adjusted to each limb and faithfully continued for two months. Manipulations, showering of the limb, and strychnia hypodermically were used daily. Circumstances prevented the use of electricity. July 25th, 1880, the feet had not improved since the operation in May, and showed a determination to relapse when the dressings were removed.

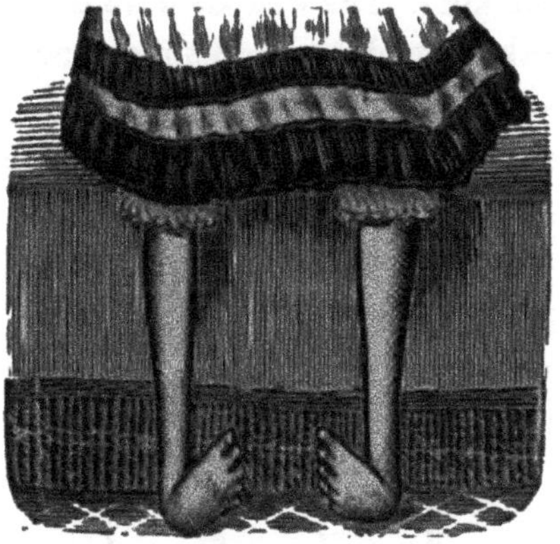

(Fig. 1.)

Dr. Alfred C. Post of New York, who was at Chateaugay a short time before, related his treatment of a case of torticollis, in which he made an open incision and divided all contracted parts upon a director, thus securing a thorough operation without the danger of wounding important blood-vessels. The case, after some thought, impressed me as being something new and thoroughly scientific. By referring to authorities, I found no mention made of an operation upon club-foot by open incision. Sayre advises the division of the skin when it offers resistance to the foot being extended to its normal position. So, with no little hesitancy, I decided to operate upon my case by open incision, and dress the foot in a normal position, and keep it so until it healed. Under an anæsthetic, and assisted by Dr. Farnsworth, I made an incision one-half inch (13 mm) in front of the ankle joint, extending across the inner side of and two-thirds the distance across the soles of the feet through the skin and cellular tissues. Each contracted part was now carefully divided as it showed itself, when the parts were put upon the stretch by extending the feet. After the completion of the operation it was found that the incision had been carried down to the bone in both feet. The artery and nerve were both divided in the right foot accidentally; but in the left they were carefully guarded. The long calcaneo-cuboid ligament was not divided, as it offered no resistance; otherwise it would have been cut. The tendo Achillis was divided subcutaneously. I would suggest the use of Esmarch's bandage in all cases of the kind. The wounds were dressed daily with balsam peru and oakum, and the feet kept extended upon a foot-rest which I devised for the purpose. A glance at the cut (*see Fig.* 2) will furnish a correct idea of its construction.

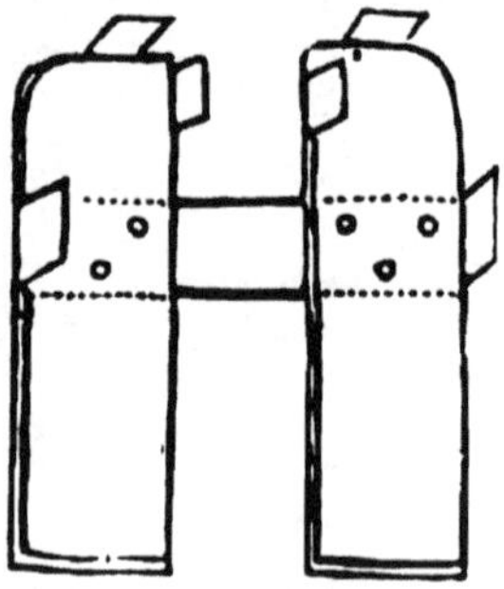

FIG. 2.

It consists of two boards the length and width of the foot, a little narrower at the heel than at the toe. screwed upon a plate of band iron one and one-half inches (38 mm.) and ten inches (25. 4 cms.) long, the ends of which are turned up, projecting two inches (51 mm.) above the board, and just in front of the external malleolus. Another piece of the same iron is attached behind the inner malleolus. A leather loop is fastened at the end of the board, through which a bandage is passed and carried over the instep to prevent the foot from slipping back. The board and projecting irons are carefully padded. A few turns of a roller bandage secures the heel between the two fixed points. Now the bandage is carried over the instep from without *inwards* under the board, then between the board and foot from without *inwards*. Turn the bandage back over the foot from within *outwards*, and the toes can be drawn outwards to the desired extent, the foot being used as a lever between the fixed points. The wound healed entirely in three weeks. The board was worn for fourteen weeks, which I think unnecessary, the patient using crutches.

Three times a *delicate point* of nitrate of silver was drawn through the bottom of the wound, which gaped one and one-half inches (38 mm.). This prevented the growth of granulations at the bottom of the wound, and allowed healing to take place from the sides by the skin gradually crawling downward into the wound. By this process, and keeping the feet constantly extended, the inner and shortened side was lengthened nearly an inch (25 mm.). The feet were flexed upon the leg by a cord passing from the end of the board to a strip of adhesive plaster secured to the leg.

Fig. 3 is from a photograph showing the result of the treatment—taken fourteen weeks after operation.

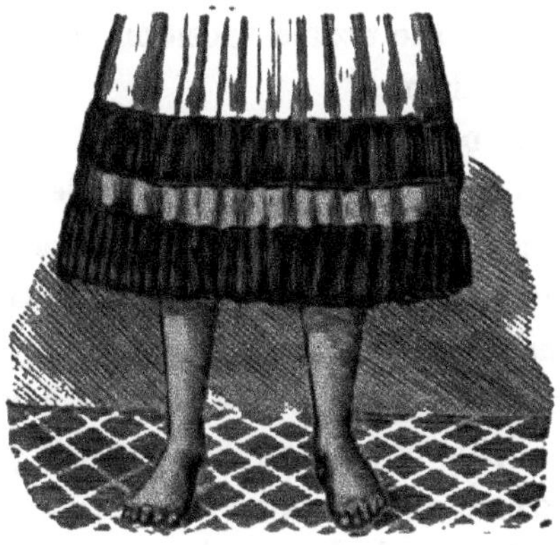

FIG. 3.

After photographing, a Sayre's shoe was put on the right foot, and an ordinary shoe with a stiff counter upon the left. The muscles are rapidly developing and sensation is perfect in both feet. The patient can walk rather awkwardly without shoes, the feet showing but little tendency to relapse. The theory that a cicatrix invariably contracts, drawing the parts to their original deformity, has, I think, been demonstrated by Dr. Alfred C. Post, of New York, to be incorrect. In his paper upon deformities from burns, recently read before this Society, the Doctor proves that if the parts divided be kept upon the stretch until the wound is thoroughly healed the cicatrix will not contract and reproduce the deformity. If this is an established fact, and I think it is, why may we not lengthen the contracted side of the club foot by keeping it constantly extended after a free incision? In this patient I am sure that I did. The result in this case and others with which I have had to do has led me to arrive at the following conclusions:—

First, That division of deep structures lying contiguous to important blood-vessels and nerves should be performed by careful open incision.

Second, That in all cases of varus, in which there is a decided shortening of the inner side of the foot from the contraction of the tissues, free division of the contracted tissues by open incision and fixed extension of the parts is the shortest and most satisfactory route to a cure.

Third, That all cases of varus should be at once extended as nearly as possible to the normal position before any appliance whatever is put on them.

Fourth, When by manipulation and a reasonable amount of force and time the foot cannot be extended to a normal position, more can be done with a scalpel or a tenotome in five minutes that can be accomplished in weeks, and often months, by all the mechanical appliances known to surgery.

NOTE. Since reading the above paper I have operated upon another case—a little boy seven and one-half years old, suffering from an extreme equino-varus of the right foot.

Fig. 4 shows the foot before and twenty-eight days after the operation. The astragalus was subluxated forward, making a serious deformity. A large and painful bunion had formed over the metatarso-phalangeal articulation upon the dorsum of the foot, making the point upon which rested the weight of the body during locomotion. All tissues excepting the artery and nerve and long calcaneo-cuboid ligament were cut. It was with great difficulty that the subluxation of the astragalus was reduced after the incision was made. Each step of the operation and after-treatment enumerated in the case of the little girl was followed in this case.

The wound, which gaped one and one-half inches (38 mm.), and extended to the bone, was entirely healed by the fourth week. At this time an ordinary shoe with a stiff counter was put upon the foot, and the little fellow runs about, the foot

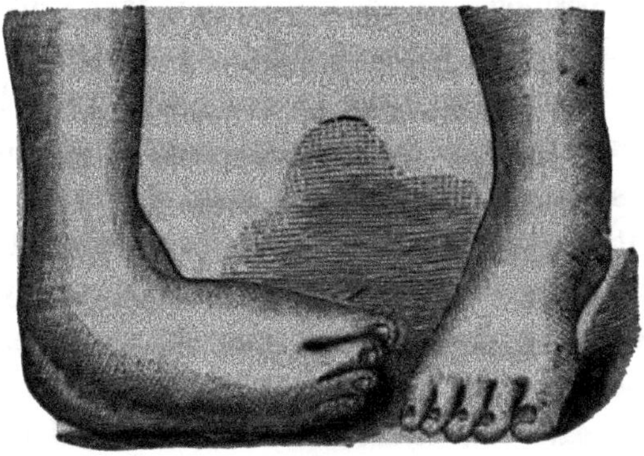

(FIG. 4.)

turning outward and being nearly free from deformity. I find that the cicatrix is somewhat sensitive, and has contracted but little. The inner side of the foot has materially lengthened. The atrophied muscles are fast regaining their normal tone and size. I had the pleasure of exhibiting this patient to Dr. Alfred C. Post, of New York, who called to this village just twenty-eight days after the operation and a day or two after putting on the stiff shoe. As to the extent of the deformity, age of the patient, mode of operating, duration of treatment, and general result, I think he will verify every statement made. In a letter bearing date April 30, 1881, the Doctor says:—

"You are at liberty to say that I have seen your patient upon whom you operated for talipes by open incision, and that I regard the result as a very remarkable success."

In another letter, dated June 14th, 1881, he says:—

"I have operated on two cases of talipes equino-varus by open myo-tenotomy. The first case was that of a child three months old. The degree of the deformity and the rigidity of the parts involved were such as I do not recollect to have seen before in so young a child. I divided the skin, the plantar fascia, the flexor brevis digitorum, the flexor longus, flexor accessorius, tibialis posticus, flexor longus hallucis, flexor brevis hallucis, abductor hallucis, etc. Having secured the vessels, I drew the foot nearly to its normal position and filled the wound with picked lint dipped in carbolized oil, ten per cent.' I then applied adhesive plaster and bandages, holding the foot nearly in its normal position. I omitted to state that I made a subcutaneous division of the tendo Achillis. I performed the operation on May 7th, and on June 11th the wound was healed, and the foot when bandaged was brought into a position of slight flexion and abduction, that is, not only as far as the normal position, but a little beyond. The result was satisfactory in the highest degree. No tractile force was employed, except normal extension followed by a roller bandage and strips of adhesive plaster. The second case was that of a little girl two and one-half years old, under the care of Dr. Jacobi, at Mt. Sinai Hospital. Dr. J. requested me to operate, and I did so, following substantially the same course as in the former case. The case is not under my own care, and I have not been able to follow it up closely; but it is, on the whole, doing well."—*Transactions, Med. Society State of New York*, 1881.

On the Origin and Cure of Scrofulous Neck.—By T. Clifford Allbutt, M.A., M.D., F.R.S. (Leeds): The purpose of the paper was to insist upon the local causation and the local development of many cases of scrofulous neck. While giving due weight to the undoubted influence of the heredity in favouring this malady, yet that such states might be, and often were, set up in young persons by local causes alone was equally indubitable. Moreover, local causes played a large—perhaps chief—part in producing the malady in those originally strumous. Artificial scrofula was at least as common as the natural. Of local causes, irritation of neighboring mucous membranes was the most common; pharyngeal and aural-pharyngeal irritations being far the commonest antecedents, and the septic kind of these the most effective. The glandular enlargements were thus bubonic, and by caseous degeneration became themselves the foci of further like mischief. After minute inquiry into possible morbid influences acting through the mucous membranes, a rapid and complete cure without disfigurement must generally be sought by surgical means. Free incision and enucleation of caseous deposits were essential. The softening mass under the jaw was usually a subcutaneous abscess with more or less thickened walls, which depended upon infection from the deeper lying caseous glands. With these it communicated by sinuous channels, often very obscure. Upon the laying open of these, and the cleaning out of the inner foci, cure and future safety depended. Many cases were given, in which Mr. Teale had co-operated with the author in carrying out those principles.

Mr. Treves (London) agreed with Dr. Allbutt that a spontaneous origin for scrofulous glands was very rare, if not doubtful. In nearly every case it was possible to make out some lesion at the periphery. Such lesion acted as the exciting cause only; and he must strongly oppose Dr. Allbutt's view, that scrofula might be due to local causes only. In every case there was, he believed, a tendency for the gland-apparatus, as well as the other structures, to react upon the most trifling irritation This might be hereditary or acquired. In no perfectly healthy person could the gland-affections of scrofula be artificially produced. The most effective exciting causes of these tumors of the cervical glands were those that involved the adenoid tissue of a mucous membrane. Inflammation of the adenoid tissue of the pharynx caused almost immediate enlargement of glands, but an eczema of the face might exist for a long time before it produced such a result. The commonest seats for scrofulous tumors of glands were the neck, the bronchial region, and the mesentery; and it was significant that the glands in these regions received lymph from the largest districts of adenoid tissue in the body, viz., the naso-pharyngeal mucous membrane, lungs, and the lining of the intestine. It was important to recognize the fact that the gland mischief extended locally, and that one gland could infect its neighbor by the lymphatic vessels connecting them. He fully agreed with Dr. Allbutt as to the treatment of certain of these glands by operation. The treatment by incision was applicable only to a few cases, to glands few in number, and not yet adherent. The treatment by scooping out the contents of the gland was apt to lead to undermining of the skin and to troublesome sinuses. The treatment he would advise was the cautery. The point of thermo-cautery was thrust into the middle of a gland in one or more directions. Through the sinus thus established the degenerate matter of the gland was gradually discharged. He had practiced this method in twenty cases with very goods results.

Mr. Teale (Leeds) could in very many cases trace the begining of enlarged glands of the neck to acute affections of the mucous membrane of the fauces, resulting from unsanitary conditions of life. The cases in which he had operated had turned out even more satisfactory that he had anticipated. These results were satisfactory; firstly, as to the effect in improving the health; secondly, as to the rapidity of healing; thirdly, as to the condition of the scar; fourthly, as to the absence of subsequent, and possibly consequent, enlargement of other glands. He had observed in the course of his operations that frequently the superficial abscess was fed through a small opening in the deep fascia, to be discovered only by careful searching by a director, and leading to a broken-down caseous gland beneath the sterno-mastoid muscle. He was also surprised how generally enlarged glands were in a caseous condition: so that in many instances he was able to eviscerate the degenerated gland-structure by Lister's scoop, leaving the gland capsule and some portion of a gland too sound to yield to the scooping-instrument.

Dr. Bowles (Folkestone) thought that, notwithstanding the graphic description of the causes of the disease by Dr. Allbutt, the causes were extremely probable only, but not proved. Confirmatory evidence was wanted. He drew attention to a class of cases of so-called scrofulous glands, which rapidly enlarged in anemic and delicate patients, and which were wholly unaffected by the usual tonic treatment, and were immediately relieved and cured by active saline aperients, followed by iron, and which left no trace behind. In these there was no evidence of local irritation.

Dr. Griffiths (Swansea) was much interested in the subject of Dr. Allbutt's paper. Nine months ago, at a local meeting at

Swansea, he expressed identically the same view as Dr. Allbutt had done, on the local causation and development of scrofulous glands in the neck. After considering the primary sources of irritaticn in decayed teeth, in the mucous membrane of the mouth, pharynx, and nares, he had pointed out that certain diseases of the ear and eruptions on the face and scalp, were frequently observed as the primary irritation in the causation of scrofulous glands in the neck. Three cases had been distinctly traced to wearing earrings. The first case, that a young woman, ended in scrofulous phthisis. The second had a chain of diseased glands of the neck below the inflamed lobe, extending to the clavicle. She persisted in wearing the earrings till the glands in the axilla became affected. She then discontinued wearing the ornament, and the primary irritation being removed, the lobe of the ear healed, and the morbid action in the glands ceased. The third case was that of a woman of forty-five similar in every respect to the last, with the exception that a large abscess formed in the axilla. He had also no doubt that scrofulous glands in the mesentery (tabes mesenterica) arose, as a rule, in local irritation of the mucous membrane of the intestines. The child, living in mesentery conditions, being "out of sorts," was dosed with various drugs, and had diarrhoea, sickness, etc. No improvement was made in the diet, irritation of the mucous membrane of the intestines was kept up, and was followed by induration of the mesenteric glands. No doubt the same law was observed in the causation of scrofulous glands in the mediastinum. The primary irritation might be in the pleura, in the mucous membrane of the bronchial tubes, or even in the blood-vessels. Not long since he traced the primary irritation of a suppurating gland at the base of the heart to an atheromatous ulcer in the aorta. Though local irritation was the main factor, hereditary tendency also played an important part in some cases. The hereditary predisposition might be a tendency to the development of a local irritation on the skin, mucous membrane, or elsewhere; or it might be a tendency to the development of scrofulous glands.

Sir William Gull (President) was of opinion that affections and enlargements of the glands of the neck were too often attributed to some defect, hereditary or acquired, in the constitution. Such a simple thing as improperly dressing the hair might give rise to enlargement of the cervical glands. When the irritation caused by improperly tying up of the hair had been relieved by a natural way of wearing the hair, the enlarged glands disappear.

Dr. Allbutt, in reply, said that there were different degrees of susceptibility to lymphatic enlargement. Some people could not, as it were, contract so-called scrofulous neck; others easily could, from very slight irritation or other cause. Again, a certain class of subjects (such as fair, blue-eyed people) could not bear peripheral irritation without secondary enlargement or inflammation, but these were not necessarily scrofulous.—*International Congress*, *Brit. Med. Jour.*

Pulmonary Cancer.—Sée (*L'Union Médicale*, January 22, 1881) claims that the following points are of value in the diagnosis of pulmonary cancer. First: A considerable amount of dyspnœa of a permanent character. Second: a sanguine-grumous expectoration. Third: considerable pain. Fourth: Dullness which does not elect any particular place, but develops and grows with the neoplasm and is found but on one side of the thorax. Fifth: The vesicular murmur is not present. Sixth: Local fremitus is not to be detected. Seventh: Slight displacement of the adjacent organs occurs. If the cancer be what Sée styles compressive, œdema, dysphagia, may occur and also variation in the radial pulses, if it presses on the subclavian artery. Phthisis is diagnosticated from pulmonary cancer in the character of the expectoration, in the lesser amount of dyspnœa, by the quantitative difference in dullness and by the difference in soufflé and fremitus. The bronchial gland affections differ from the compressive type of pulmonary cancer by giving rise to not so intense symptoms. Aneurism of the aorta differs from pulmonary cancer in the presence of aortic bruit and pulsation. While these points are of value in differential diagnosis, it is obvious their value is not absolute as the cancer must have attacked the pleuræ to have produced pain, and the other symptoms will also be somewhat varied by the position of the neoplasm. Perhaps a good way of supplementing the diagnostic points given would be by a microscopical examination of the sputa.—*Chicago Med. Rev.*, Aug. 5.

The Mosquito as a Carrier of Disease.—A correspondent inquires whether there is "anything in the newspaper statement that mosquitoes are the agents for introducing dangerous parasites into the human blood." We are pained to be obliged to say that there is good ground for this addition to the disreputable "record" of the insect. The discovery was made a year or more ago,—we cannot give the exact date,—and has since been fully confirmed by further investigation. Dr. Meisoner of Leipsic in a German medical magazine, has lately summed up what is known of the parasitic infection of the blood, and the following is an abstract from of what he says of the *filiaria sanguinis hominis* :—This parasite has been very thoroughly studied by Manson, of Amoy, China and Bancroft of Brisbane, Australia. The filiaria, while it may at times be present in the blood without giving rise to any symptoms, at other times appears beyond question to be the cause of chyluria elephantiasis, etc. The mode of its action would seem purely mechanical. The parasite in the blood or lymph channels and its accumulation at a given point gives rise to lymphorrhagia or inflammation. Two curious facts have recently come to light regarding this parasite. One is that the mosquito acts as a carrier; sucking the filaria with the blood of an affected person, it afterwards deposits the ova or embryos, which have meantime hatched, in the water when it lays its own eggs. These embryos are then swallowed in the drinking-water by another victim; and so the circle of disease is completed. Another and a very curious fact regarding the filaria was lately discovered; this is that it is a nocturnal parasite. During the day the filiariæ lie dormant at some point in the victim's circulation, but at night they sally forth and rove the currents of the blood the night long.—*Boston Journal Chemistry.*

Circulation in the Coronary Artery.—We observe a statement in some of our exchange journals to the effect that Professors Martin and Sedgewick of the Johns Hopkins University have demonstrated the synchronous circulation in the carotid and coronary arteries. The old theory is that the mouth of the latter is closed by the position which the contraction of the ventricle gives to the aortic valve, and that the blood is not thrown into it until the subsequent contraction of the aorta, by which it is then supplied. The crucial experiment of the Baltimore professors consisted in introducing a canula in the coronary artery of a dog, and another in the carotid, and connecting each with a sphygmograph. The tracings of the two instruments were found to be synchronous, which is regarded as positive proof in regard to the question.—*Pacific Med. & Surg. Journal.*

Enemata of Peptones.—M. Henninger (*Paris Médical,* No. 29) gives the following formula for enemata of peptones. Five hundred grammes of very lean meat, minced fine, are placed in a glass receiver, on which are poured three litres of water, and thirty cubic centimètres of hydrochloric acid of density 1.15; to this is added two and a half grammes of the pure pepsine of commerce, at the maximum of activity, that is to say, digesting about two hundred times its weight of moist fibrine. It is left to digest during twenty-four hours at a temperature of 45 Cent. (113 Fahr.), either in a water-bath or a stove; it is then decanted into a porcelain capsule, brought to boiling point; and, whilst the liquid boils, an alkaline solution is poured into it (250 grammes of carbonate of soda to 1,000 grammes water), until it shows a very slight alkaline reaction. About 165 to 170 cubic centimètres of this solution must be added to it. When this result is obtained, the boiling liquid is passed through a fine linen cloth, the insoluble residue being expressed; and this liquid, which amounts to about two and a half litres (three pints), is reduced in the water bath to 1,500 or 1,800 cubic centimètres. Half of it is administered every day in three enemata, adding two hundred grammes of white sugar for twenty-four hours. The whole of the meat is not dissolved; the fat, the tendons, the connective and elastic tissues, form an insoluble residue, amounting to about a third of the meat used.

CANADA

Medical and Surgical Journal.

MONTREAL, NOVEMBER, 1881.

RUDOLPH VIRCHOW.

The occasion of the sixtieth birthday of this renowned man has directed the attention of the profession and public to his extraordinary career, unexampled in the history of medicine. We have before us an address by Dr. Jacobi, delivered at the opening of the session at the College of Physician and Surgeons, in which he deals with the life and work of Virchow, and an article, for which we are indebted to the author, our friend, Prof. Ewald of Berlin, in which he treats of the influence upon clinical medicine of Virchow's work. The address of the former will be particularly welcome to English readers, as it supplies a long-felt want. In our remarks we shall draw largely from it.

Rudolph Virchow was born in Schivelbein, a small Pomeranian town, in the year 1821. He graduated at Berlin in 1843, and shortly after became Frorieps' assistant in the Pathological department, of which he obtained full charge in 1846. These early years witnessed the production of some of his most important works, as "Leukæmia," "Thrombosis" and "Embolism," the "Puerperal condition," "Septic infection," &c. In 1847 he founded his Archiv for Pathological Anatomy and Physiology and Clinical Medicine, which exists to-day in its 86th volume, the most important scientific journal in the profession. In 1848 he took part in the revolution in Berlin, and the following year edited the *Medical Reform*, a caustic publication, which brought upon him the wrath of the Government, and he was dismissed from his positions. The public and professional opinion was so aroused in consequence that he was reinstated, but shortly after accepted a call to Wurzburg, where he remained, as Professor of Pathology, until 1856, when he returned to Berlin. The occasion of the completion of his 25th year as Professor in the University is to be appropriately celebrated on the 19th of this month. The contemplation of the amount of work accomplished by him in medicine alone is simply stupifying to an ordinary intelligence. In 1856 he published his celebrated "Versammette Abbandlungen," a collection of his papers on scientific medicine. In 1879 was published "A collection of Treatises on State Medicine and Epidemics," in two large volumes, which contain numerous monographs, written between 1849-79, on "Subjects connected with public hygienic reform of medicine, epidemics and endemics, statistics of morbility and mortality, hospitals, military medicine, cleaning of cities, school hygiene, criminal law, and forensic medicine." His lectures on Cellular Pathology appeared in 1859, and were translated into English. It is worthy of remark that the two *epoch-making* works in medicine and science—Virchow's Cellular Pathology and Darwin's Origin of Species—appeared in the same year. The work on Tumours—that monument of German science, as some one has called it—was published between 1863 and 1867. In addition to these are scores of papers and monographs scattered through the volumes of his Archiv and in the Transactions of various Societies. It may safely be said that there is no single department in the whole range of medicine that has not been enriched by his keen observations. Take up any special work which possesses an index of authors, and it is surprising the length and depth of the lines containing the references to his name.

In another department of science his name is pre-eminent. As an Anthropologist and Archæologist he ranks second to none, and his studies in these subjects have been most extensive. Among the ceremonies at the forthcoming celebration will be the presentation to him of the keys of an Anthropological Institute.

Outside of his professional and scientific pursuits, he has found time to devote part of his energies to the service of his city and country. For twenty-two years he has sat as "alderman," and has been the moving spirit in all the sanitary measures which have been brought forward. Since 1862 he has represented one of the Berlin constituencies in the Prussian House, and has been one of the keenest of liberal politicians. Of his political life Dr. Jacobi says: "Bismarck has not found a more persistent and conscientious adversary than Virchow through all his parliamentary career. In regard to the latter, I will predict that among the German politicians who resisted to the utmost, lawlessness of absolutism, and claimed that law should be supreme, the rights of citizens respected, the office-holders know and live up to their duties, the constitution he carefully guarded and protected, and peace not rendered as exhausting and expensive as war, Virchow's name will, for all time, be mentioned as the first and wisest and purest." Only a few weeks ago the papers announced his return at the recent election by an overwhelming majority.

Many there are who begrudge the time he spends in these outside matters, but it should rather be a matter of pride with every member of the profession that we have in our ranks a man pre-eminent as a physician, a *savant* and a politician.

May he long be spared to adorn his profession and serve his country and humanity!

Medical Items.

—Dr. Bihaud, Professor of Anatomy in Victoria College, died on the 18th October, after a very short illness. A few days previously he had a severe attack of cerebral hæmorrhage, with paralysis, under which he rapidly succumbed.

Hôpital Notre Dame.—We have received the first annual Report of this charity. The total number of admissions during the year has been 772; and the number of out-patients was 1,609. In the Eye and Ear department 269 patients have been treated.

The Horns of a Dilemma.—Cazeaux, in speaking of craniotomy, exclaims: "What physician is there, who, driven to elect between the life of his wife and that of the child in utero, would hesitate about that of the latter?" And Dr. Dagenais, *L'Union Medicale*, replies: "What physician is there, who, driven to elect between a great *danger* to the life of the mother and the life of the child in the cradle, would sacrifice the latter? For, are we certain that the mother will die, and what difference is there between the life in utero just before birth and in the cradle just after birth?"

—M. Pasteur, it is stated, has resolved to visit the Bordeaux lazaretto to study yellow fever, and ascertain whether it be due to a parasite, and can be guarded against by inoculation.

—Mr. Wm. McCormac, the Secretary-General of the International Medical Congress, has been knighted in recognition of his services.

—The *British Medical Journal* calls upon the medical profession to take a firm stand against the obstacles thrown in the way of vivisection by the government of that country.

MORE ABOUT BIRTH MARKS.—The *Ohio Medical Journal* has the following good story, as told of a physician of Dayton, Ohio: The doctor was recently attending a case of labour in the family of one of his patrons, who, though a very excellent man, is a little slow in the payment of his medical bills. Immediately after the birth of the baby, the father nervously asked, "Doctor, is the baby marked?" "Yes," quietly replied the doctor; "it is marked 'C.O.D.'" It is needless to add that the bill for that baby was promptly settled.

—The XIXe *Siecle* relates of Dr. Nelaton that he was accustomed to say: "If you have the misfortune to cut a carotid when performing an operation, remember it takes two minutes for syncope to supervene, and as many more before death occurs. Now four minutes are four times the time required for a ligature, provided you don't hurry yourself—never hurry yourself."

—Speaking about the character of the attendants of a sick person, Dr. J. M. Fothergill says: "A pious widow, with dyspepsia and strong religious convictions, is a ghoul when illness is about. She sucks the life out of an invalid like a moral vampire. As life ebbs, she is sustained, and when the invalid has passed the p of another world, she goes away edified, strengthened ortals encouraged in her murderous mission, fully prepared to extinguish the lives of any number of relatives if ill luck should prostrate them upon the sick bed."

CANADA

MEDICAL & SURGICAL JOURNAL

DECEMBER, 1881.

Original Communications.

OVARIOTOMY.

By HAMNETT HILL, M.R.C.S., Honorary Surgeon to the General Hospital and Consulting SurgeOn to the County of Carleton Protestant Hospital at Ottawa.

About the middle of May, 1881, I was consulted by Miss G., aged 30, in consequence of an abdominal tumour, which she described had given her much uneasiness for some length of time, tracing back, as well as she could recollect, to a period of nearly four years. She was of a spare habit of body, nervo-bilious temperament, and evidently suffering from impaired health and defective nutrition, whilst her unwieldy appearance would indicate almost that she was in the eighth month of pregnancy.

On examination in the posture of decubitus, the abdomen was found much enlarged, soft and fluctuating, giving the usual wave-like feel on percussion; this softness was modified somewhat on the right side from the inguinal region upwards over a space of about 4 inches in diameter, which space gave a decided feeling of hardness. The diagnosis was "cystic ovarian tumour," with, perhaps, fibroma, corresponding with the locality where the hardness existed. This opinion, *quo ad* ovarian dropsy, was strengthened by my discovering a cicatrix below the umbilicus, for which I sought an explanation, when I learnt that she had actually been tapped so lately as the month of February, when a large quantity of glairy, sticky fluid had been drawn off, but the swelling had quickly returned, and, although painless, her existence had become miserable and wretched in the extreme. The usual treatment for such cases was explained, and she consented to put herself under my care for operation. On the 2nd of June, immediately after her menstrual period, the operation of ovariotomy was performed under chloroform at the private residence of the patient. Prior to this date I had read with much interest the valuable practical remarks on this subject quoted by Dr. Gardner of Montreal in the May No. of the CANADA MEDICAL & SURGICAL JOURNAL from a paper by Dr. Noeggerath, introducing a novelty of detail in the operation of a most useful character, namely, the evacuation of the contents of the sac by a trocar *before opening the peritoneal cavity*, a practice which cannot be too highly recommended, and of which I availed myself in the present case. The ovarian sac was found so tough and tense, that very considerable force was necessary, accompanied by a rotatory movement similar to drilling, before the trocar could be made to enter. The escaping fluid was of a peculiar character, very unlike that which I had seen in similar cases before, being usually of a dark straw colour, whereas this resembled "thickish arrowroot prepared with water"; from this cause it took at least twenty minutes to discharge itself, in quantity about three gallons. The sac was found entirely free from adhesions, arising from the right ovary, the pedicle was easily reached and secured by clamp, which was retained in position outside the wound at its inferior angle. After removal of the sac, the incision was brought together by five carbolized silk sutures, and covered with carbolized pledgets of lint. The operating table had been so arranged as to fulfil all the purposes of a bed, on which she was left for some days; 40 minims of laudanum were given as soon as she was put to rights; it was very shortly rejected by vomiting, and the same result took place on repetition of the dose; an enema of a teaspoonful of laudanum with a wine-glass of water thrown into the rectum was retained, and no more vomiting or unpleasant symptoms occurred. The urine was drawn off towards night, and at my morning visit I found she had slept comfortably and was progressing most favourably; no pain, no thirst; pulse 82, temperature about 99°. A daily record of the case would be tedious.

These favourable indications continued. Catheterism was used twice daily; the sedative enema was administered for a few nights, and then gradually discontinued. The bowels were relieved by emollient enema on the fifth day, after which the wound was dressed with carbolized pledget of lint and the patient placed on a more comfortable bed. Up to this time milk diet and gruel was the only nutriment allowed, but a more generous diet was now permitted. The pedicle sloughed away on the 14th day, and convalescence might be said to be perfected about the fourth week. The sac was found to be bilocular, without any fibroid degeneration, the hardness above referred to having been caused by a second cyst lying, as it were, on the surface of the main sac covered by a very dense membrane of about the diameter of four or five inches and about one inch in depth, and contained a fluid such as has been described above; it added so little to the size of the emptied sac, it was not found necessary to evacuate its contents prior to removal.

On visiting my patient in September, soon after my return from attending the Canada Medical Association at Halifax, I found her free from complaint and much improved in flesh and general appearance. There is, however, a most singular fact to record. On the return of the catamenial period, a very small blister, of a dark colour, appears over the cicatrix just where the pedicle was secured, and which has been perfectly healed long since; the skin gives way and enough blood oozes therefrom to stain her linen to the size of a quarter dollar or English shilling. It causes no further inconvenience, and quickly heals up again. The circumstance itself is very singular and unique, as far as my knowledge goes. Whether it will continue or increase, possibly, is a matter for future observation, and I shall endeavour to keep posted on the matter.

The following suggestions occur to me, a "Septuagenarian," which may be of some benefit to my younger *confrères*:—

1stly, I consider a private residence for this operation is much to be preferred to a hospital, as there is a largely diminished risk of septic influences in the former case, provided the locality is healthy in character, and cleanliness and comfort is the order of the day. Another important feature exists in the fact that only a limited number of assistants should be present, which again reduces to a minimum the chance of septic influence; whereas in hospitals the whole staff has a right to be present, frequently very large in number, to say nothing of students and pupils attending the surgical practice, all which *pro tanto* must increase the risk of septic contamination. In my humble opinion, four assistants—at the most, five—besides the operator are all that are required or should be allowed to be present.

2ndly, In reference to the procedure of treating the pedicle, it appears to be a matter of doubt just at present whether it is more judicious to return it well and securely ligatured into the abdomen, or leave it clamped on the outside in the wound. *Theoretically*, the latter plan would unquestionably be far superior, as sloughing must occur in either case, and this destructive process must entail the production of septic matter, which is surely better outside the peritoneal cavity; of course drainage tubes can be left in and irrigation adopted, still, it must be borne in mind that these are all foreign bodies, and not at all unlikely by their presence to produce peritoneal mischief. *Practically*, however, these unfavorable results do not appear to occur, and the latest operators seem rather in favour of returning the pedicle into the abdomen; there is yet another important matter to bear in mind, namely, the possibility of hæmorrhage from the stump, which has occurred, I believe, in some instances, and has terminated fatally.

3rdly. With respect to the new method of operating introduced by Dr. Noeggerath, namely, the introduction of the trocar into the sac prior to opening the peritoneal cavity, I think it will be considered on all hands to be a most valuable addition to surgery. It reduces the exposure of the contents of the abdomen to a minimum, entirely prevents any septic matter from the sac entering the abdomen, and also prevents cooling abnormally the contents of this important cavity, the importance of which precautionary measure has been so much dwelt on by writers on this subject. The re-inserted trocar into the canula supplies the place of vulsellum, tenaculum, hook and forceps, reducing the number of instruments very considerably, and at the same time makes a most efficient director on which the peritoneum can be opened to any extent desired, and the reduced sac immediately drawn out by simply depressing the handle towards the pubis.

4thly. Use of antiseptics. Before the operation is commenced every instrument likely to be required, sutures, needles, &c., &c., should be thoroughly anointed with carbolic oil, as also the hands of each assistant, whether his services are likely to be required or not, and each should be interrogated as to whether he is actually in attendance on any erysipelatous case, puerperal fever or any zymotic disease, in which case his absence would be most desirable. If operation takes place in hospital, carbolic acid solution should be copiously sprinkled on the floor and walls, and spray should be used ; but if at a private residence, these precautions are not so imperatively necessary ; probably the removal of all furniture, carpets, curtains, wearing apparel, pictures, &c., &c., with liberal use of scrubbing brush, and opened windows for a day or two before operation, may be all that is required.

5thly. Quietude of mind and body are essential matters of detail after operation. None but the nurse and one friend should be allowed in the room at one time for several days, and each should refrain from talking either with the patient or each other ; no other visitor should be allowed in on any pretence. As a general rule the patient would be better if left on the operating table (properly prepared before-hand) in the same apartment as that used for operation for several days. Every act like straining should be most carefully avoided ; the urine should be drawn off twice or thrice each twenty-four hours, and the bowels relieved by enema after four or five days. Milk diet, with oatmeal water if desired, as a drink. No circular bandages should ever be used, as their application and removal necessarily entail a great amount of disturbance ; a many-tailed bandage is permissible just to keep in position the antiseptic dressing over the wound, and the longer this is left undisturbed the better for the patient.

6thly. Sutures.—As to selection of material, I much prefer

silk; they are removed with little difficulty, whereas the removal of silver sutures causes much unnecessary pain, and not unfrequently a good deal of excitement. I consider it a matter of importance to have your sutures previously prepared by carbolization and 12 inches in length; insert them by transfixing the peritoneum and integuments, and extend each free end on the surface of the abdomen, but do not tie until each has been properly placed. The object of this little manœuvre is to lessen the difficulty of transfixing the peritoneum, for as the opening of the incision becomes contracted by tying each in succession, it is almost impossible to be sure that the last one or perhaps two have been properly adjusted as regards transfixing the peritoneum.

In the performance of the above operation, I must refer to the kind assistance of my *confrères*, Drs. Grant, Horsey, Leggatt, Henderson and S. Wright.

REPORT ON THERAPEUTICS AND PHARMACOLOGY.

BY JAMES STEWART, M.D., BRUCEFIELD, ONT.

(*Read before the Canada Medical Association, at Halifax, August*, 1881.)

(Continued from page 225.)

JABORANDI.

It is now several years since this drug has been employed by physicians, and although much yet remains to be discovered as to its physiological actions and uses, we are in a position to estimate in a great measure where benefit can be obtained from it. That this drug, or rather its alkaloids, are likely to come into general use as powerful therapeutic agents seems undoubted.

Harnack and Meyer* have published the results of observations which they made in Prof. Schmiedeberg's laboratory in Strasbourg on jaborandi and its alkaloids. They have found that jaborandi leaves contained not only the alkaloid pilocarpin, but also another similar body which they named *jaborin*, which was to a great extent antagonistic to pilocarpin in its action. Jaborin

---

* *Arch. fur Exper. Path. and Pharma.*, Vol. XII., page 366.

dilates the pupil, and has an action on the heart, salivary glands, the intestines and central nervous system exactly like atropine, and which is found also, like it, to antagonize the action of muscarine. Sidney Ringer* has shown that jaborandi and pilocarpin paralyze the frog's ventricle separated from the auricles, and as the ventricle contains no inhibitory ganglia, the paralyzing effect must be induced by the influence of the drug over the excito-motor ganglia or the muscular tissue, or both. In all probability the action of jaborandi on the heart is two-fold—for a heart arrested by this drug will at first contract on mechanical stimulation, but soon ceases to contract either on mechanical or electrical stimulation. As atropia antagonizes the action of jaborandi on the ventricle, it cannot act by paralyzing the inhibitory apparatus, but from its effects in the excito-motor ganglia and muscular substance, and he has suggested that this antagonism is due to chemical displacement.

The greatest value of pilocarpin appears to consist in its power of causing rapid elimination of effete material in cases of scarlatinal nephritis. It has been frequently administered in such cases, and with much benefit; and it appears likely that, if it be given with proper precaution, it may frequently be the means of saving life. It is frequently observed that oedema and uræmic phenomena are neither proportionate to one another nor to the quantity of urine passed. In some cases, uræmia occurs when a normal quantity of urine is excreted, while in others no uræmic symptoms follow several days of anuria. In the former cases, the urine contains little urea; and in the latter, the urea passes from the blood into the œdemio fluid and hence becomes harmless for a time. When, however, at the beginning of convalescence, the excrementitious materials pass back into the blood, uræmia may come on, and obviously the more rapidly they pass back, the more danger there is. In virtue of its power of producing prompt and energetic increase of the sweat, salivary and other glandular secretions, pilocarpin causes a very rapid reabsorption of the transudation, and therefore its administration

---

* *Practitioner*, January, 1881.

now applied, the action almost immediately recommences, and continues with unabated vigor. Falck* says that this is a complete physiological antagonism. From experiments performed by Ringer,† it is obvious that pilocarpin is not the chief ingredient in jaborandi which depresses the heart, for a grain of pilocarpin only slightly weakened and slowed the ventricle. On the other hand, twenty minims of the liquid extract of jaborandi, freed from spirit, stopped the heart in ten minutes. Ringer makes the following suggestion: "Pilocarpin paralyzes the heart by combining with the molecules of the excito-motor nervous apparatus and of the muscular tissue of the heart. Atropia antagonizes pilocarpin and muscaria, because it has a stronger affinity for the muscular and nervous structure of the heart than these substances, and displaces them, replacing their effect by its own."

QUEBRACHO.

First introduced by Penzoldt,‡ it has been found to be a decided palliative in many cases of dyspnœa. It is especially valuable in the dyspnœa of emphysema and chronic bronchitis. In dyspnœa depending on valvular insufficiency, its value is questionable.§ Penzoldt has lately experimented with an alkaloid obtained from this bark. It is called *aspidospermin*, and occurs in small, white, prismatic crystals. Ten milligrams of a 1 per cent solution of this alkaloid caused complete motor paralysis in frogs, with marked reduction of both pulse and respiration. Penzoldt administered it to eight patients suffering from dyspnœa due to various causes. In all there was considerable relief; in two this was very marked. According to Penzoldt, it has an undoubted influence over dyspnœa, especially that attending emphysema, but is inferior to the quebracho itself. Dr. Picot‖ of Carlsruhe used a tincture of the quebracho bark while doing some mountain climbing, with the result that he

---

* *Der Antagonismus der Gifte*, *Volkmann's Sammlung*, *No.* 159.

† *Practitioner*, January, 1881.

‡ *Berl. Klin. Wochenschrift*, No. 19, 1879.

§ *Berl. Klin. Wochenschrift*, No. 40, 1880.

‖ *Berl. Klin. Wochenschrift*, No. 32, 1879.

could climb with much greater ease and comfort. He has also used it in patients suffering from dyspnœa, and found it act well. In the same number of the *Ber. Klin. Woch.*, Berthold recommends it highly. Flint* has used it with success also.

HÆMATINICS.

Since the discovery of exact methods of estimating the number of corpuscles and the quantity of hæmoglobin, we have made some advance at least in knowing how it is that some drugs, as iron, arsenic, etc., act. We are able to estimate the changes that the blood cells and their colouring matter undergo in disease, and we can tell what our therapeutic agents are doing. Hoppe-Seyler and Preyer have shown that one atom of iron fixes two of oxygen. The following factors have to be considered: 1. The number of red cells contained in a unit of volume. 2. Quantity of hæmoglobin contained in the same unit. 3. Individual value of the corpuscles. 4. The number of white globules. 5. The number of hematoblasts.

Of all the hæmatinics, iron still maintains, as it has always maintained, the pre-eminence as a blood restorer. There are three hypotheses as to its mode of entrance into the blood: 1. Direct entrance of iron into the blood under the form of an inorganic salt and its combination with the albuminous substances of the blood. 2. Combination of the iron and the albuminates in the stomach and intestines before absorption. 3. Absorption, by these two methods combined.

E. Wild has recently shown that iron is absorbed from the stomach and intestines and then thrown out into the intestines. This explains the fact that sometimes as much iron can be found excreted through the fœces as was taken in altogether. According to Hayem† (*De la Médication Ferrugineuse*), there are two periods in the regeneration of blood by iron. During the first the iron appears to excite the formation of the globules. Then we have new globules, containing but little hæmoglobin;

---

* *Medical Record.*

† *Bulletin Général de Thérapeutique*, p. 289, 1881.

the globules are more altered than when the treatment commenced. Soon these young globules become physiological, the last being the most important part of the process. When the anæmia is slight, the first phase is very short or sometimes entirely wanting, the iron in this case causing an actual decrease in the number of red cells. Cl. Bernard considered that iron only stimulated the digestive organs and never entered the general circulation at all; but this has been disproved by Hayem, who administered in two cases for a period of two months the ferrocyanide of potassium with no effect in curing the anæmia, thus showing that an insoluble iron salt is of no use in increasing the value of the individual red cells. It is the quality of the red cells that is of so much importance. Prof. Donitz* of Japan speaks very highly of the albuminate of iron in the treatment of anæmia. He says that it can be tolerated when no other salt of iron can. It can be used hypodermically, and in this way it proved to be of great service in that disease called in India "*beriberi*." In this disease, hydræmia of a severe form is the most prominent pathological condition, especially in the early stages. Prof. Demarquay† of Paris has also found this salt of iron to act particularly well in cases where the other forms are not easily retained.

Next to iron, and in some forms of anæmia to be preferred to it, is *Arsenic*. It is the only drug that has been successful in the treatment of severe idiopathic anæmia. The following case recorded by Dr. Broadbent‡ is a good illustration of the value of arsenic in this disease: A woman, aged 42, who had been anæmic for four months, was admitted, and on examination she was found to have only 560,000 red cells per cubic millimètre, or 11.2 per cent. After taking 24 minims of arsenic daily for two months, the red cells had increased to 67 per cent. In the remarks appended to the report of the case, it is held "that there can be little doubt that it was a case of essential or pernicious anæmia; the patient had the appearance characteristic

* *Berl. Klin. Wochenschrift*, No. 35, 1879.
† *Medical Record*, Vol. XVI., p. 36.
‡ *Brit. Med. Jour.*, Sept. 25, 1880.

of this disease and the sub-febrile temperature, while the red corpuscles were not only reduced in number to an unusual degree, but deformed. Whether this diagnosis be accepted or not, the failure of iron to do good, and the rapid improvement during the administration of arsenic, are remarkable. In little more than two months the patient passed from extreme anæmia to apparently perfectly health, with wonderfully good colour of the cheeks and mucous membranes, and she continued well and strong for some months after leaving the hospital, up to the time when she ceased to present herself for examination."

Arsenic cured two cases of pernicious anæmia that were under the care of Dr. Finny* of Dublin. Whether arsenic acts in malignant lymphoma by virtue of its hæmatinic properties or not, it is a well established fact that it has proved curative in some of these eases. Several cures of this kind are reported by Billroth. Czerny has also cured cases with it. Israel† has reported the case of a woman, 65 years of age, who had a malignant lymphomatous formation infiltrating the glands of the neck, sufficient to cause difficulty in swallowing, completely cured by arsenic. The arsenic was used internally and also injected into the swelling.

Lugeois, in France, for ten years has held the opinion that mercury given in small continuous doses causes an increase in the body weight in healthy persons. Keyes‡ says "that mercury in small doses is a tonic to individuals in fair health, not syphilitic. In such individuals it increases the number of red blood corpuscles." Schlesinger§ has found that rabbits and dogs taking small continuous doses of corrosive sublimate for a year thrive better than animals placed on a similar diet, but not taking the sublimate. The red corpuscles of those taking the mercury are increased more than those not taking it. Their urine showed no change in spite of the increase of the body weight. Schlesinger concludes that mercury does not increase the amount of hæmoglobin or the number of corpuscles, but that

* *Brit. Med. Jour.*, Jan. 3 and 10, 1880.

† *Berl. Klin. Wochenschrift*, No. 52, 1880.

‡ *Amer. Jour. Med. Science*, January, 1876.

§ *Archiv. fur Exp. Path und Pharm.*, Band XIV.

it prevents the destruction of the latter. If it increased the hæmoglobin like iron, we should have an increase in the body temperature, in the pulse, and urine solids, but the latter is shown not to be the case.

FUCHSINE IN BRIGHT'S DISEASE.

Prof. de Renzi* of Genoa has used fuchsine in Bright's disease extensively. Almost after the first day there was noted a diminution in the amount of albumen in the urine and disappearance of the dropsy. The fuchsine was given in pill form 0.025 gramme twice daily. For some days the urine was coloured. In one case no result was obtained.

Dr. Brochut† of Paris has had ten cases of albuminuria cured by fuchsine. In every case the albumen rapidly decreased in quantity, and finally entirely disappeared after a longer or shorter period. The treatment generally lasted from one to six months, and the dose of the remedy varied from 10 to 20 centigrammes (1½ to 3¾ grs.) daily.

Dr. Jas. Sawyer‡ has used fuchsine in many cases of albuminuria—mostly in cases of contracted kidneys,—and says that no remedy has ever given him such good results. No untoward physiological effects have been observed from its use. The mucous membrane of the digestive organs becomes deeply coloured by its use, and also the plasma of the blood. Investigation shows this latter effect to be due not to any change in the hæmoglobin, but to the solution of fuchsine in the blood.

HOMATROPIN.

Bertheau§ has found that in frogs, in doses of 2 to 4 centigrammes, it causes motor paralysis, which affects all the muscles of the body, including the respiratory. Reflex action is first heightened and then decreased. Small doses have no effect on the pulse; large doses slow it, but do not cause any heart

* *Berl. Klin. Woch.*, Sept. 20, 1880.
† *Brit. Med. Jour.*, Oct. 11, 1879.
‡ *Practitioner*, January, 1881.
§ *Berl. Klin. Wochenschrift*, No. 41, 1880.

paralysis. In rabbits, small doses slow and large doses quicken the pulse. Electrical irritation of the vagus gives no constant result. This has also been observed by Rossbach. A few drops of a 1 per cent. solution causes a dilatation which lasts six hours. Dilatation of the pupils is produced by the internal administration of this drug, but it requires very large doses. It causes dryness of the mouth and throat. In man, doses of two centigrammes cause dilatation of the pupils. The pulse becomes slow; in no case was it observed to be quickened. This is quite contrary to what is seen in the experiments on animals, where we have first irritation and then paralysis of the vagus ends in the heart. Two centigrammes are not sufficient to paralyze the vagus ends in man, and large doses would be unsafe. Homatropin differs from atropine in requiring larger doses, and in its effects being much more transient. This last quality will make it valuable in many cases where temporary dilatation of the pupil is wanted.

JAMAICA DOGWOOD—(*Piscidia Erythrina.*)

This drug has recently been recommended as a substitute for opium. It is named the "fish-catching coral tree" by the natives of Jamaica. Dr. Isaac Ott* has investigated its physiological action very fully. He finds that it is narcotic, and without any action on the irritability of the motor nerves. Its action is on the sensory ganglia of the spinal cord, and not on the extremities of the sensory nerves. It reduces the frequency of the pulse, probably by an action on the muscular structure of the heart. The arterial tension is first increased, and then soon falls. It first contracts and then dilates the pupil. In its action on a man in health, it reduces the pulse, causes salivation and sweating, disturbance of vision, itching of the skin, sleep. It has been used in cases of neuralgia with considerable success.† I have found it to act well in the semi-delirium and sleeplessness of the very aged. It has caused in a few cases alarming symptoms.

---

* Brain, January, 1881, *Archives of Medicine*, February, 1881.

† See numerous cases reported in different numbers of the *Therapeutic Gazette*.

When better known it will no doubt prove to be a really useful addition to our lists of narcotics. For its introduction we are indebted to the ability and enterprise of Park, Davis & Co. of Detroit.

Dujardin-Beaumetz, in presenting his work, "Leçons de Clinique Therapeutique sur le Traitement des Maladies du foie et des reins," to the Therapeutical Society of Paris, made reference* to the remarkable power the liver possesses in destroying some alkaloids, such as nicotine, hyoscyamine, and curarine. Under some circumstances this destruction is not complete, and we find that alkaloids that have been fixed for a variable time in the hepatic tissue are thrown out into the intestines along with the bile. This action of the liver is one of great importance, and through it we can explain the innocuousness of some substances administered by the mouth, and the more powerful effects we obtain by hypodermic injections. It also is likely the explanation of the cumulative action of some drugs. We know that some agents, when given for a time, do not produce their usual physiological action, but suddenly we find this exercised in the most pronounced manner, and for an explanation of this, the peculiar action of the liver, above referred to, seems a very likely cause.

QUARTERLY RETROSPECT OF SURGERY.

PREPARED BY FRANCIS J. SHEPHERD, M.D., C.M., M.R.C.S., ENG.
Demonstrator of Anatomy and Lecturer on Operative and Minor Surgery McGill University; Surgeon to the Out-Door Department of the Montreal General Hospital.

[This quarterly retrospect I intend to devote almost entirely to a consideration of the proceedings of the Surgical Section at the late *International Medical Congress* held in London, Aug., 1881.]

SURGERY AT THE INTERNATIONAL CONGRESS.

Excision of the Kidney.—Several important papers were read on the above subject. Prof. Czerny of Heidelberg, in his paper, remarked that extirpation of the kidney is indicated in cases of

---

* *Bulletins et Memoires de la Société Thérapeutique Séance*, du 23 février, 1881.

wound of the kidney, floating kidney, pyonephrosis, calculous pyelitis, cysts of the kidney, and hydronephrosis, tumours, and fistulæ communicating with the ureter, as soon as the life of the individual is endangered and other methods of treatment prove ineffectual, provided that the other kidney is sound, when the kidney is fixed, or nearly so, he prefers operation by means of the lumbar incision ; but for movable kidney he prefers abdominal section. He thinks, however, that the lumbar incision is the safer of the two plans, and, therefore, is worthy of further development. Prof. Czerny thinks it best to ligature the pedicle and cut it short, adopting antiseptic precautions. In cases of fixed hydronephrosis, empyema of the pelvis of the kidney, and echinococcus of the kidney, the best plan of treatment is, he considers, incision of the cyst and stitching its margin to the skin. He thinks the plan of catheterizing the ureters of women and constricting the ureters of men, in order to confirm the diagnosis of disease affecting one kidney only, has not been sufficiently practised.

Mr. W. Morrant Baker, of St. Bartholomew's Hospital, read a paper on "The Diseased conditions of the Kidney which admit of Surgical Treatment." This paper was illustrated by three cases. The first case was that of a girl 7 years old. She had pyelitis, which had followed an attack of hæmaturia. A fluctuating tumour was found in the region of the right kidney. This was incised and a drainage tube inserted, but little improvement followed, and the kidney was afterwards removed. Three months after the wound had nearly healed and the child's general health had greatly improved. The second case was that of a lad 16 years old, admitted into hospital on account of a large fluctuating tumour in the left renal region, recurrent attacks of pain and fever, followed by the appearance of large quantities of pus in the urine. Nephrotomy was performed through a lumbar incision and thirty ounces of pale, purulent urine were evacuated from an enormously dilated kidney. A drainage tube was inserted, and two months after the patient had gained flesh and strength and had suffered no pain. Drainage is still maintained. The third case was that of a feeble woman, aged 43. She had a swelling in the right renal region, and a considerable amount of pus was always present in the urine. The swelling was punctured and 8 ounces of pus drawn off; three weeks after the tumour was explored through a lumbar incision, and was found to consist of a sacculated kidney containing a large branched calculus. The calculus was dislodged with considerable difficulty, and there was considerable hæmorrhage. The patient was much collapsed, never rallied, and died three days after the operation.

Mr. Arthur E. Barker read a paper "On some points connected with Operations on the Kidney." He only treated of questions in connection with operations on the kidney for calculous disease. He divides cases into two groups: (*a*) Early calculous disease, with little or no disorganization of the kidney; (*b*) Stone, with extensive damage to renal tissue and more or less implication of perinephritic structures. He then points out that stone may be, and has been diagnosed in the kidney very early; also, that it can be safely removed at this time by simple nephrotomy or by nephrectomy, with excellent results, compared with operations undertaken at a later stage. [The difficulty of early diagnosis is very great, and Mr. John Duncan, surgeon to the Edinburgh Infirmary, in the *Edinburgh Medical Journal* for July, has pointed out that the needle exploration is not always infallible, as in a case of his, a necrosed transverse process exactly simulated the feel of a calculus in the kidney. Mr. Barker claims to have been the first who successfully sounded for stone in the kidney by passing a needle through the loin to the kidney. It is about a year since Mr. Henry Morris read his paper on Nephro-lithotomy before the Medical Society of London. He was the first who successfully extracted a stone from a kidney by means of incision where there was no previous suppuration or sinus to guide the operator. Peters, a German surgeon, had previously, in a case of renal calculus, passed a trocar and canula into the kidney, striking the stone. Being unwilling to undertake the risk of incising the kidney, he left the canula *in situ*, dilated the wound afterwards with tents, passed in a lithotrite, and crushed the stone before removing it. Mr. Barker had previously also operated in a case of renal calculus, but the stone being branched, and difficult of removal, the patient died. He, previous to operating, sounded the stone through the loin by means of a needle, and so settled the diagnosis, which rested between renal calculus and tubercular disease. Marchetti, in the 17th century, successfully removed a renal calculus from the English Consul, Hobson, but the operation never found favour with the profession, and Charles Bernard, in 1696, says writers "ought not to have so magisterially exploded the operation." The kidney has been frequently exposed for suspected stone, and nearly every time without fatal result. The operation was generally undertaken to relieve severe neuralgia, supposed to be caused by stone. The neuralgia in every case was relieved, and in some permanently. One boy in Guy's Hospital was not only cut for stone in the kidney, but for stone in the bladder also, no stone being found in either situation. He recovered, and the neuralgic pains were temporarily relieved.]

At the Congress, Messrs. Barwell and Clement Lucas each reported a successful case of nephrectomy. In Mr. Barwell's case, the kidney was removed for nephrolithiasis, the stone having been previously detected through a sinus, and he had failed to remove it by simple incision. In Mr. Clement Lucas' case, the kidney was excised for pyelitis, in a man aged 36. The lumbar incision was used. The man is now in good health, free from pain, has gained two stone, and is able to work.

In the discussion which followed the reading of the papers, Dr. Martin stated that he had seven times removed a painful floating kidney, and once a malignant tumour of the kidney, with five recoveries in all. Three methods of removal were described: The lumbar, intra-peritoneal, and the abdominal extra-peritoneal. Dr. Martin stated that in the removal of the kidney from the front of the belly, the peritoneum falls together so completely that it does not require stitching. The precise diagnosis of the conditions of the kidney which justifies removal is a point on which more light is required.

Causes of Failure in obtaining Primary Union in Operation-Wounds, and on the methods of treatment best calculated to secure it.—This was perhaps the most interesting and important subject which engaged the attention of the Surgical section of the International Medical Congress. Mr. Sampson Gamgee of Birmingham, in his paper, said that operation-wounds heal, as a rule, directly and without complications when their surfaces and margins are placed and maintained in apposition accurately and without tension, and when effusion, air, and accumulation of liquid within and near the wound is prevented. These ends, Mr. Gamgee holds, are promoted by light manipulation, drainage, dry and infrequent dressings, pressure, and absolute rest. His views on the treatment of wounds are, from his numerous contributions on the subject, well known.

Prof. Humphry of Cambridge also read a paper. He attributes the causes of failure to (1) the delicacy and sensitiveness of the tissues in infantile and early life, which renders them liable to inflammation and ulceration upon slight irritation; (2) the deficiency of the nutritive energy requisite for the healing processes in the atonic and the aged, evinced most especially in the lower limbs, when there is disease of the arteries; (3) the presence of foreign substances in the wound, especially blood or bloody fluid, which separates the surfaces and has, further, a tendency to decomposition. The methods best calculated to secure primary union, Prof. Humphry says, are therefore those which maintain the apposition of the cut surfaces most effectually and with least irritation, and which provide against the presence of blood and bloody fluid in the wound—sutures of such material and applied in such a manner as is least likely to cause irritation, quietude of the part, gentle, uniform pressure, and fixing on a splint where that can be done. The effusion of blood into the wound after it is stitched up is best prevented by carefully securing the vessels by ligature or by torsion; the actual cautery may be freely used as an adjunct; the use of ligatures and stitches made of material which undergoes absorption; the insertion of a drainage tube and the expression of blood from the wound through it as long as it continues to flow. Prof. Humphry holds that antiseptics are an additional precaution, preventing the decomposition of any bloody-fluid which, in spite of the above-mentioned precautions, may be effused into the wound. They are especially valuable when cavities are opened. He thinks that Esmarch's bandage promotes bleeding from cut surfaces soon after its removal, but rather lessens the risk of subsequent effusion.

In M. Verneuil's paper on "Primary Union," he says, in conclusion, that the attempt to obtain primary union is sometimes essential and necessary, sometimes only a supplement to the operation, and altogether optional. Before aiming at primary union, in which it is only optional, not essential, the surgeon should satisfy himself that the patient is not the subject of some morbid state which would make it more advisable to give up or postpone the attempt. The surgeon should avoid the risk of failure, which is more or less associated with danger, and seek some of the dressings which, while offering a more rapid cure, secures greater safety to the patient.

Mr. Savory, in the discussion which followed, pointed out that primary union was most likely to occur when the fresh surfaces are brought together in their natural state and maintained so without disturbance. The chief cause of failure he believed to be "meddlesome surgery," and essential principles were rest, cleanliness, and asepsis, which admit of almost endless variation in detail. He asserted that his Cork statistics had not been surpassed, though equally good results were obtained by many different plans of treatment. Prof. Esmarch's statistics of his own practice were very remarkable. In 398 great operations (six deaths), 85 per cent of the cases cured healed by first intention with *one* dressing; in 15 per cent the dressing was renewed; and this ratio had improved of late. There were 146 excisions of large tumours, 40 excisions of mammæ and axillary glands, 14 castrations, with one death from pericarditis and old syphilis, one from apoplexy, and one from fatty heart. Of 51 major amputations (thigh, 18; leg, 27; arm, 5; forearm, 1), one died from shock and hemorrhage, and one from *delirium tremens.* There were 61 resections; 11 exarticulations; 26 necrotomies; 13 nerve-stretchings, one for tetanus, which was fatal; 8 hernias: 21 large cold abscesses; 12 large wounds; 49 compound fractures. The cases were all dressed with pads soaked in iodoform and absolute alcohol (10 per cent), fastened on by an iodoform bandage, over that a large pillow of jute and gauze, a moist bandage, and over all an elastic bandage. (Report in *London Lancet*, Aug. 13, 1881.) These statistics are certainly wonderful, and go far to confirm the confidence of surgeons in rest, support, and infrequent dressings. In fact, much evidence was offered and many opinions given which only corroborated the above, and all tending to support the views which Mr. Gamgee has so ably advocated, viz., the success of dry dressing, with support and compression, combined with antiseptics, in the treatment of wounds. A few days before, in the discussion on the recent advances in the surgical treatment of intra-peritoneal tumours, Dr. Keith had startled the section by stating that after having had a succession of eighty successful cases with Listerism, he had five deaths in the next twenty-five—two from carbolic acid poisoning, one from septicæmia, and two from acute nephritis. On account of this mortality, and of the very frequent high temperature the evening after the operation, he had *abandoned the spray* in all operations, and had had one death in twenty-seven ovariotomies without antiseptic treatment. Prof. Lister, in closing the discussion on the causes of failure of primary union in operation wounds, in reference to Dr. Keith's experience, stated that he had dissuaded him from using antiseptics in the first instance, as carbolic acid, in wounds of the peritoneum, increased the effusion and lessened absorption. He said that recent experiments showed that both blood serum and blood clot were not favourable to the development of organisms. He expressed his belief that it is "solid bits of dirt" that are the deleterious agents, and that too much attention has been paid to finest particles floating in the air. He admitted that he himself might at some future time be able to say "fort mit dem spray" (away with the spray), but that at present he could not accept irrigation as a substitute for the spray. (*Lancet* Report.) From this discussion, I should predict that the spray, and, perhaps, also the mysterious germ, are doomed, at no very distant period, to follow into oblivion many other "fads" and rituals which have before held the surgical world in bondage. The value of antiseptics is recognized by all, but many other simpler methods than Listerism are now showing as good results. We must all admit, however, that we owe much to Prof. Lister, and his name will be always remembered as one who revolutionized the surgical treatment of wounds by directing the attention of surgeons to the importance, not only of antisepticism, but of rest and support, and the possibility of preventing suppuration and the septic conditions it leads to. I have always attributed the great success of Listerism, not principally to the use of antiseptics, which answers only one of the requirements of wound treatment, but to the accurate adaptation of the wounded surfaces, the thorough drainage, the masses of stiff gauze used in dressings (make gauze a beautiful splint by its elasticity and adaptability to surfaces and parts it is applied to), also to the careful bandaging over this gauze splint and the uniform and safe compression thus obtained. The spray, &c., may be looked upon as merely ornamental adjuncts which, if somewhat troublesome, are imposing.

Recent advances in the Methods of Extracting Stone from the Bladder.—Every one must admit that Dr. Bigelow of Boston, by the introduction of his operation, has not only made one of the most distinct advances in the treatment of stone in the bladder which has taken place in the last decade, but that his operation may be considered to be one of the most important improvements in modern surgery. At the late International Congress, all were agreed as to the great value of lithotrity at one sitting, and gave Prof. Bigelow full credit for its introduction, and also for his axiom that the bladder was more tolerant of instruments than sharp fragments of stones, and that their immediate removal was the best mode of practice.

Sir Henry Thompson, in his paper, stated that he had performed the operation of "lithotrity at one sitting" 91 times, with 88 recoveries. He, however, contended that the size of the instruments should be proportionate to the size and hardness of the stone, and never larger than necessary, that risk to the patient was greatly augmented by the employment of instruments which distended the urethra beyond its natural calibre. Here his views are at direct variance with Prof. Bigelow, who believes no harm results from distending the urethra. Sir Henry advises occasionally the combination of a urethral opening in the perineum with a crushing operation in the bladder as an available means of evacuating both *débris* and urine.

In the discussion which followed, Mr. Coulson spoke of having removed 4 ounces of *débris* at one sitting. Mr. Teevan said there was complete absence of cystitis after "Bigelow's operation." Mr. Th. Anger of Paris advocated the performance of supra-pubic lithotomy by means of the thermo-cautery, when there was an enlarged prostate which was firmly wedged into the true pelvis; in other cases, the perineal incision should be preferred. In using the cautery, the operation is rendered easy, methodical and bloodless, the wound made is dry, and renders the patient less liable to urinary infiltration. Mr. Spence of Edinburgh said his experience was chiefly limited to lithotomy. In children the results of lithotomy were so successful that he would never think of performing lithotrity in them. In lateral lithotomy he used Dr. Buchanan's rectangular staff, except in the case of old men with enlarged prostates, then he preferred Listor's curved staff. In cases of enlarged prostate, where the gland is much condensed, dilatation with the finger made no progress, and it was necessary to use the knife to get room for the forceps, and in withdrawing the stone the dense prostate was forcibly wedged against the ramus of the pubis; such cases frequently died some weeks after the operation, and although the wound was not directly affected and the patient's death was spoken of as due to some intercurrent disease, they died as truly from the operation as if they had died on the operating table. Such cases, if they could be diagnosed, would no doubt best be dealt with by the supra-pubic operation. He could not, however, see the advantage of the thermo-cautery which M. Anger had so strongly recommended, as he had not been favourably impressed by the condition of the wound in cases of tracheotomy in which he had used it. Mr. Teale of Leeds said that the fatality after lithotomy had been lessened of late years by two factors—firstly, the improved sanitary condition of hospitals, and, recently, by the more gradual extraction of the stone, the surgeon taking pride, not in the rapidity, but in the carefulness of his manipulations.

Treatment of Aneurism by Esmarch's Elastic Bandage.—A number of papers were read on the above subject. Dr. Walter Reid, R.N., related the history of the original case in which this treatment was employed, and explained the principles on which it was conducted. Mr. Bellamy, of the Charing-Cross Hospital, said in his paper that he had tried the bandage in four cases; in three the treatment utterly failed. He considers the bandage quite useless in the treatment of cases in which the aneurism is of rapid development and the sac is highly compressible, and where there are heart complications. Mr. A. Pearce Gold, of Westminster Hospital, also read a paper in which he pointed out that while other methods of treatment lessen or entirely stop the flow of blood through part or parts of the main blood channel, they do not interfere with the blood current in the secondary vessels, or control the anastomotic circulation. Esmarch's Elastic Bandage, on the other hand, when firmly applied, stops the circulation in *all* the vessels of the part, and thus does not cause a deposit of fibrin, but may cause a coagulation of the blood *en masse*. Thus this mode of treatment was not applicable to all kinds of aneurisms. He insisted on the value of preparatory treatment.

From the whole discussion, it appears that the bandage is not likely to supersede the older methods of treatment, but that in certain cases, where consolidation has already commenced, it is likely to hasten the cure, and may be occasionally resorted to with success.

Excision of Joints.—M. Ollier, in his paper on the "*Comparative value of Early and Late Excisions in different forms of Articular Disease*," said that the results of resections of joints depended on the following conditions; 1. On the method of operating; 2. On the amount of existing disease. Any method may prove useless if the joint be too much disorganized. As a general rule, the earlier the excision is performed the better the result which will be obtained. Age has a great influence on the results. Antiseptic treatment makes early excision more advisable than formerly. The author then enquired into the different resections of the larger articulations, and gave an analysis of one hundred resections of the elbow performed by him. After giving some rules applicable to resection for injury, he said primary resections were apt to be followed by a too extensive deposit of new bone. He demonstrated the advantages of secondary excisions and the disadvantages of postponing the operation too long.

Prof. Kocher of Berne read a paper on the "*Results of the Treatment in Chronic Disease of the Knee Joint, including an account of fifty resections of the joint.*" The following is a summary of the paper: 1. Amputation of the thigh is indicated in cases where white swelling occurs in patients suffering from tuberculosis of the internal organs, or those whom the disease has rendered very anæmic, or who present a constant high temperature, or are reduced by prolonged suppuration. 2. In all other cases, resection is the best treatment, if contraction of the joint or considerable functional disturbance have occurred. 3. Under these circumstances, resection in every way gives better results than are obtained by conservative treatment. 4. Resection should only be resorted to in exceptional cases in childhood or advanced age. The results are as good, or better, as regards union of the ends of the bones, in adult life than in childhood. 5. Since the author has commenced the practice of resection, the mortality has only been 12 per cent, and now—thanks to recent improvements and the introduction of antiseptics—the operation has become free from danger. 6. The author's present endeavour is so to improve the method, that movable and, at the same time, firm joints may be secured.

In the discussion which followed the reading of these papers, Mr. Teale advocated subcutaneous incision of the capsule for the arrest of incipient joint disease. He considered rest of the first importance, but subcutaneous drainage of serous fluid and external drainage of pus, or trephining of diseased bony structures, necessary adjuncts. Mr. C. Heath protested against early excision when general and local treatment were available, but regarded excision as required in incurable cases; he also declared that excision in private practice was almost unknown, and not required on account of the good hygienic surroundings of the patients. Mr. MacNamara thought the majority of cases of joint disease might be cured in their early stages, and thought it wise to relieve tension of the joint where it contained much watery fluid, and after evacuating the fluid, he advised encasing the joint with cotton wool and an elastic bandage. He also mentioned that he had had recently under his care two cases which showed that acute inflammation of the epiphysis of a long bone is apt to involve not only the periosteum, but also to cause osteo-myelitis. In both these cases he had removed the whole shaft of the tibia, leaving only the epiphysis and the periosteum. In the one case the bone had been reproduced and the patient had a useful leg; in the other (referred to in last Quarterly Retrospect), after six months no such reproduction occurred, so he had transplanted some perfectly fresh and very small pieces of bone and periosteum (from the foot of an amputated limb) into a groove made in this patient's leg, in the situation of the tibia. At the present time (six weeks after the transplantation) a narrow ridge of bone could be felt in the desired situation.

Mr. Croft remarked that many patients suffering from acute articular disease did not get well without operation, but added that recent statistics showed that excision of the hip-joint diminished the average duration of the disease by one year; further, seven out of thirty-three cases of morbus coxæ, cured without excision, presented 3¼ inches shortening, which was as much as ordinarily occurred after excision. Mr. Howard Marsh pointed out that to perform early excision was to renounce the attempt to cure incipient disease and to resort to the easy method of cutting out the affected part. If this was right for joints, was it not also for the testis, which, like them, might be a source of systemic infection. He also said that in private practice joint affections were curable and excision almost unknown. Sir William Ferguson introduced excision as a substitute for amputation. This was truly conservative. He aimed at saving the limb by removing the joint. But to remove so important an organ as the knee joint for incipient disease was, surely, to turn the dial of progress many degrees backwards. Excision, like amputation, must always rank as a mutilation, and as such, he maintained, it should, if possible, be avoided. Real progress lay in the direction of insisting on the importance of early treatment by complete rest.

In the section of *Diseases of Children* there was also a discussion on the *Treatment of Chronic Diseases of Joints*. Prof. Hueter, of Griefswald, read a paper on the *Scrofulous Inflammation of Joints*. After describing what constituted a scrofulous inflammation of the joint and the results of such an inflammation, he affirmed that the early stage of scrofulous inflammation might be successfuly treated by the injection of a 3 to 5 per cent. solution of carbolic acid into the joint, and that antiphlogistic treatment (fixation, massage, compression, extension, blood letting, blistering), was of little or no value. Incisions, drainage, scraping away granulations, &c., were to be discarded, and that carbolic acid injections having failed, excision is the best treatment, especially after suppuration has set in. Excision should be total, and when practised early the results are more satisfactory.

M. Ollier, in his paper on the *Excision of Joints in Children*, said every excision of a joint during childhood interferes with the subsequent growth of the limb and that the subperiosteal method interferes less with the growth. Inequality in length becomes visible only after a time, and varies with the extremity. This arrest of growth, which is quite inevitable, should induce the use of antiseptics and the "abrasion articulaire." Where ankylosis is desired as little should be removed as possible (knee), but where mobility is essential, efforts should be made to secure a new joint (elbow.)

Prof. Sayre, of New York, believed that if these joint affections could be diagnosed early enough, resection would never be necessary. He advocated the application of an apparatus to the limb which took off all pressure from the joint and allowed the patient to get about. If the case went on to suppuration, then excision was the best operation, and often attended with wonderful success. M. Fochier advised fixation of the joint in the early stage. Mr. Benton thought with Prof. Hueter, that fixation and extension were of little use in chronic disease of the knee joint. He advocated movement of the knee; the pain, he thought, was due to adhesion, and the true way was to break down these adhesions with a sudden jerk, which snapped them in the middle; the child should then at once be made to walk about. Mr. Timothy Holmes did not understand how a disease which depends, as Prof. Hueter says, on auto-infection, can be cured by so simple a means as mere rest; yet, that it was so cured, is a very well known fact. He thought it rather too absolute a method to say inject with carbolic acid, and if that fail excise the joint. He did not feel inclined to accept this advice as final, though he had a great respect for the opinion of Prof. Hueter. He thought it necessary to give the joint rest; that it was important to achieve this end, more important even than to obtain fresh air, as was evidenced by the experience even of London hospitals. He thought the injection of joints and other violent methods unnecessary. Prof. Hueter, in reply, said he fancied scrofulous cases were more grave in Germany than in England. He did not deny that a joint might be cured without injections, &c., but he believed that it was cured by time and not by rest. (Report in *Brit. Med. Jour.*, Oct. 1, 1881.)

From the discussions in both sections it was clear that English surgeons only resort to excision in extreme cases, and all thought rest the most rational and conservative treatment in the early stages of joint disease, and deprecated the early excision of joints as a cutting of the Gordian knot. No doubt the antiseptic system is responsible to some extent for this reckless cutting out of joints; but the principal reason is that hospitals have not the space nor means to keep cases of joint disease month after month in their wards undergoing the treatment of rest, and that until more space is given by hospitals for the special treatment of joints by rest, the temptation will be to excise and so save time. John Hunter has said "to perform an operation is to mutilate a patient whom we are unable to cure; it should therefore be considered as an acknowledgment of the imperfection of our art."

Treatment of Spinal Curvature by Sayre's Method.—Papers were read on the above subject, in the section of Diseases of

Children, by Dr. Bellem, of Lisbon; Mr. Golding Bird, Mr. Henry F. Baker, Mr. Walter Pye and Mr. Arthur Barker, all of London. Dr. Bellem accepted almost to the full Sayre's views, but did not approve of the "jury-mast." Mr. Golding Bird said that in early cases of general curvature cure might be confidently expected with Sayre's jacket, but that in advanced cases little benefit could be derived from it. In spinal caries the plaster jacket gave the required "physiological rest" to the inflamed spine, and might be applied during either vertical or horizontal extension. He considered it the best form of spinal apparatus yet devised. Mr. Baker said that in angular curvature the use of the plaster jacket did not give the required rest to the spine, that it was liable to constrict injuriously the chests of growing children, and that a state of recumbency was absolutely necessary to prevent the deformity increasing in the first stage of the disease. In a very limited number of cases where the disease had been arrested and other forms of support could not be obtained, it was undoubtedly of use. In general curvature the suspension as recommended by Sayre was a useful addition to other methods of treatment, but the plaster jackets were inferior to those made of steel, which could be adjusted at any time by the surgeon. Mr. Walter Pye thought that in many cases the jacket was hastily and needlessly applied, and that its employment was often actively harmful; that it was of no use in rickety spines or simple lateral curvature. In certain cases of true spinal caries in infants in the early stages the older plan of rest in the horizontal position succeeded better, and was free from risk, but in older children the jacket might be used from the first. It might also be used from the first in cases in which the heart and lungs are affected in addition to the spinal affection, and cases in which carious spine is associated with any high degree of paralysis, incontinence of urine, &c. Many jackets he considered were too thick and strong, also badly shaped and badly fitted. He strongly disapproved of the use of the swing, and advocated, when applying the jacket, holding the child by the arms, with the feet resting on the floor He also advocated the use of the inclined plane. Mr. Arthur Barker believed Sayre's method for the treatment of spinal caries to be the best yet devised, and that failure was due to want of care in carrying out the directions of the designer.

A very spirited discussion followed the reading of these papers, in which Dr. Sayre took part. Mr. Timothy Holmes summed up as follows :—1. Nobody seriously contested the priority of Dr. Sayre as the introducer of the method. 2. The discussion had dealt almost exclusively with angular curvature, to which it would perhaps have been wiser to have altogether limited it. 3. More speakers who recommended the jacket treatment seemed to be agreed that the earlier it was employed the better, but we were unable still to say whether and how far symptoms of decided spinal irritation or inflammation should be taken as contra-indicating it. 4. Only a small minority of the speakers rejected the method ; the majority agreed that at any rate in a large majority of cases the method offered very great advantages. 5. No form of extension (by suspension or otherwise) was a necessary part of the treatment ; the jacket could be applied when the patient was suspended, or erect, or horizontal. 6. There appeared to be no evidence that any actual straightening of the spine had ever been produced. 7. Though Dr. Sayre and most other speakers appeared to prefer the plaster, there seemed no valid reason why other plastic material might not do as well. The possibility of changing the inside shirt without removing the jacket was an important practical point brought out in the discussion. [This referred to a suggestion made by Mr. Oxley, of Liverpool, viz., that patients might be kept clean by changing the undershirt. This might be done by putting on two undershirts when the jacket was first applied. When the shirt was to be changed a clean singlet was tied on to the lower edge of the singlet next the skin, and by drawing the soiled shirt off the clean one was drawn on.] 9. That there were many drawbacks in the shape of ulcers, abcesses, &c., seemed not only possible but inevitable. The extent and nature of these drawbacks should be stated, but they formed no radical objection to the treatment. 10. It seemed probable that the average length of time required for cure would be found much less than the treatment by rest in bed. 11. Finally the general opinion seemed to be that this was a real and great advance in practical surgery.—*Brit. Med. Jour.*, Sept. 24, 1881.

Few besides Dr. Sayre advocated the use of the jacket in lateral curvature of the spine, and the majority also condemned his method of extension. On the whole, however, Dr. Sayre could not but feel flattered at the almost universal acceptance of this jacket as a means of treatment for spinal curvature. After Mr. Holmes' masterly summary of the results of discussion nothing more need be said with regard to it.

Partial Excision of the Bladder.—Dr. Adolf Fischer, of Buda-Pesth, in his paper mentioned that ancient surgeons believed a surgical wound of the bladder would terminate fatally, but that in more recent times, however, comparatively large portions of the bladder have been removed on account of prolapsus without fatal result. He has made a number of successful experiments in dogs, and comes to the conclusion that in dogs at least, wounds of the bladder which are afterwards carefully united by sutures are not particularly dangerous, and that good results depend principally on the accuracy of the suture. Dr. Fischer says that the indications for partial excision of the human bladder may be brought at present under the following heads :— 1. Traumatic injuries of the bladder with contused edges. 2. Diverticula of the bladder, containing encysted calculi. 3. General dilatation of the bladder, when the cause of the disease has been removed or is removable. 4. Benign and malignant tumours involving the wall of the bladder. 5. Vesico-abdominal, vesico-vaginal and recto-vesical fistulæ. 6. Destructive ulcerations threatening rupture and withstanding other modes of treatment. I fancy that this operation is not very likely to come into fashion, especially for the diseases mentioned in the list. The diagnosis of several is by no means certain, and with regard to the others the remedy might be almost considered worse than the disease.

On the Permanent Retention of the Œsophageal Bougie.—Dr. Krishaber stated in his paper (1) that the œsophagus tolerates the presence of a bougie for an indefinite length of time, (2) that the bougie should be introduced through one of the nostrils, and (3) that the presence of a bougie leads to dilatation of stricture of the œsophagus and renders the introduction of larger bougies possible, as in the urethra. He also stated that a security against starvation is ensured and the danger of false passage avoided. It is of great use in the performance of operations about the mouth, nose, &c.

The different opinions on the variety of Chancre, by C. R. Drysdale, M.D., London.—The author said a wide difference of opinion existed on the question of primary lesions of syphilis. In France, and on the Continent, the dualistic theory was maintained, viz., that the chancre of syphilis was quite distinct from the soft sore. The former was always, the latter never, followed by the secondary symptoms of syphilis, unless the two sores coexisted on the same patient. Having shortly described the distinctive features of the two sores, both as to appearance and course, the author said he was wholly convinced of the truth of the dualistic view. But there was in England a strong school which did not hold this view, and its leader, Mr. Hutchinson, had said some years ago that "dualism was dead." Statistics collected at the Hôpital du Midi in Paris were opposed to Mr. Hutchinson's position, which was this, that soft sore was due to an inoculation with pus modified by the presence of syphilis in the person from whom it was derived. But the speaker believed that the soft chancre was a distinct disease, that it bore the same relation to syphilis as measles did to scarlet fever.

Mr. Jonathan Hutchinson said that everybody believed in the clinical difference between the hard and the soft sore, and could, as a rule, make a prognosis from the aspect of the sore, but he doubted whether it was always possible to recognize with certainty the soft sore from the hard sore, though with characteristic sores there was no difficulty. He believed that the soft sore was a sort of appendage to syphilis—an epiphenomenon. The soft sore was due to the inoculation of inflammatory secretions only, but modified, in some way which he could not explain, by the coincident presence of syphilis in the individual who yielded the pus. It was a sort of abortive inoculation. Soft chancre bore the same relation to syphilis that imperfect vaccination, which often caused much irritation and even ulceration, bore to perfect vaccination. But he agreed that the soft sore was only a transitory affection, while the hard infected the system: so that the difference between him and Dr. Drysdale was, so far as practice went, not great.

Dr. Louis Julien (Paris), in a paper on *Excision of Chancre*, believed that excision under certain circumstances suppresses all subsequent manifestations, and where it failed to do this, the subsequent disease was milder and more slowly developed.—*Brit. Med. Journal Report*, Sept. 17, 1881.

Reviews and Notices of Books.

Cyclopedia of the Practice of Medicine. Edited by Dr. H. VON ZIEMSSEN, Professor of Clinical Medicine in Munich, Bavaria. Vol. XX. General Index. New York: Wm. Wood & Co.

This is the concluding volume of this exhaustive work. The index consists of 50 pages, and seems to have been constructed with great care, so that any subject in the whole of the immense field covered by the nineteen volumes can be at once turned up. The arrangements of type, &c., to separate the various words and divisions are specially good. It is a model index, and worthily brings to a close a Cyclopedia which will long rank as one of the most valuable works of reference in the English language.

General Medical Chemistry for the use of Practitioners of Medicine. By R. A. WITHAUS, A.M., M.D., Professor of Chemistry and Toxicology in the Medical Department of the University of Vermont, Professor of Physiological Chemistry in the Medical Department of the University of the City of New York. New York: Wm. Wood & Co. Montreal: J. M. O'Loughlin.

The above belongs to the series of "Wood's Library." It embraces both organic and inorganic chemistry, but it differs considerably in its arrangement and method of treating the subject from most similar text-books. The author keeps always in view the fact that it is *medical* chemistry he is teaching, and thus special stress and most space is given to the bearings of chemistry upon physiology, hygiene, therapeutics and toxicology. It is not illustrated, as it was thought that the limited room for such an extensive subject could best be occupied by letter-press, and indeed, except with reference to technical manipulations, &c., such aids are hardly required. It is a well composed text-book, and can be recommended as a trustworty exponent of the medical chemistry of the present day.

Clinical Lectures on the Diseases of Old Age. By J. M. CHARCOT, M.D., Professor in the Faculty of Medicine of Paris, Physician to the Salpetrière, Member of the Academy of Medicine; &c., &c. Translated by LEIGH H. HUNT, B. Sc., Laboratory Instructor in Pathology in the Medical Department of the University of the City of New York. With additional lectures by ALFRED L. LOOMIS, M.D., Professor of Pathology and Practical Medicine in the Medical Department of the University of New York, &c., &c. New York: Wm. Wood & Co. Montreal: J. M. O'Loughlin.

The fact that many diseased processes are much modified by age in their course, duration and severity, renders it extremely important that we should be familiar with such modifications both with reference to the young and also the aged. The study of the pathology of the diseases met with in persons of advanced years is instructive as showing that the changes resulting from a given morbid state vary in accordance with the condition found in the structures it affects. These lectures of Prof. Charcot illustrate all these points, and will repay perusal. The first two lectures are extremely interesting, even to the general medical reader. They are upon "General Characteristics of Senile Pathology" and "The Febrile State in the Aged." The remainder treat principally of the rheumatic and gouty affections of old people as well as several other forms of articular affection to which they are peculiarly liable. The three concluding addresses are devoted to the subject of the thermometry of senile disorders. Under this head most valuable information is to be obtained, and the author clearly shows and lays much stress upon the great clinical importance of frequent and accurate thermometrical observations by those who have sick persons who are aged under their care. Dr. Loomis adds in an appendix a number of lectures upon senile affections. These are of an eminently practical character, and are composed in the happy style of this well-known writer. They include senile pneumonia, chronic bronchial catarrh, asthma, fatty heart, apoplexy, softening, chronic gastric catarrh, constipation, and hypertrophy of the prostate gland. This volume belongs to "Wood's Library," and well deserves a place in that excellent collection.

A Treatise on Diseases of the Joints. By RICHARD BARWELL, F.R.C.S., Senior Surgeon and Lecturer on Surgery, Charing Cross Hospital. Illustrated by numerous engravings on wood. Second edition, revised and much enlarged. New York: Wm. Wood & Co. Montreal: Dawson Bros.

Although this appears as the second edition of Mr. Barwell's well-known treatise on the joints, yet it will be found on examination that the additions and alterations are so numerous and extensive as to cause it to be in fact a new and modern work upon this important subject. The name of the author has long been identified with the study of this special branch of surgery, and he is well known as having introduced many novel views into the pathology of joint disease, and also many valuable improvements in the mechanical treatment of these serious disorders. The present work, besides treating very fully of all the various forms of disease to which the joints of the body are liable, is specially valuable from containing an unusually large number of illustrative cases fully detailed and with a great many wood cuts. It is thus made extensively clinical in its features, and therefore, of course, by so much the more of a practical character. As a work of reference, it will be found very serviceable for the same reasons. This addition to the library of standard authors has been a most judicious one, and will no doubt be welcomed by the subscribers and the profession generally.

Landmarks, Medical and Surgical. By LUTHER HOLDEN, Consulting Surgeon to St. Bartholomew's and the Foundling Hospitals. Assisted by JAMES SHUTER, M.A., Camb., F.R.C.S., Assistant Surgeon to the Royal Free Hospital. From the third English edition, with additions by WM. W. KEEN, M.D., Professor of Artistic Anatomy in the Pennsylvania Academy of the Fine Arts. Philadelphia: Henry C. Loa's Son & Co. Montreal: J. M. O'Loughlin.

This admirable little book of Mr. Holden's comes to us in a new form from the American publishers. The American editor has also introduced a few practical additions, which add to its value. The study of these landmarks by both physicians and surgeons is much to be encouraged. It inevitably leads to a progressive education of both the eye and the touch, by which the recognition of disease or the localization of injuries is vastly assisted. One thoroughly familiar with the facts here taught is capable of a degree of accuracy and a confidence of certainty which is otherwise unattainable. We cordially recommend the Landmarks to the attention of every physician who has not yet provided himself with a copy of this useful practical guide to the correct placing of all the anatomical parts and organs.

The Mother's Guide in the Management and Feeding of Infants. By JOHN M. KEATING, M.D., Lecturer on the Diseases of Children at the University of Pennsylvania, Visiting Obstetrician to the Philadelphia Hospital, &c. Philadelphia: Henry C. Lea's Son & Co. Montreal: Dawson Bros.

This little volume of Dr. Keating has been prepared expressly for the purpose of being put into the hands of young mothers for their guidance; and from a short perusal of it, we are satisfied that physicians in charge of families cannot do better than recommend a frequent reference to this work in order that infants in their care may be intelligently watched and judiciously managed. To a doctor caring for a sick child, it is of the utmost importance that the mother or attendant should have a reasonable knowledge of the conditions natural to early life, and should be able to recognize, and inform him of, deviations therefrom. The actual safety or the material comfort of an infant may thus come to depend upon the intelligence of those who have the immediate care of him: and the only means possible for mothers without experience to acquire such knowledge is the careful study of some book specially intended to meet their case, such as the above. It is written in plain, untechnical language; and all the directions and explanations are simple and easily understood.

We hope that Dr. Keating's manual may be widely introduced, for the inculcation of its many sound sayings and wise counsels will prove of great service amongst our infantile population.

The Physician's Hand-book for 1882.—By WM. ELMER, M.D., and ALBERT D. ELMER, M.D. New York: W. A. Townsend.

In this hand-book the compiler has endeavoured to bring together, condensed into as small a space as possible, a large amount of general information and useful facts which may be called for at any moment. It is a combination of a visiting list, abbreviated ledger, and practitioner's *vade mecum*, all in one, and yet the size does not exceed that of an ordinary pocket-book. It has been in use for a number of years, and is extensively used by physicians in the United States and in this country.

The Medical Record Visiting List for 1882 (Wm. Wood & Co., New York), is again to hand, and fully equals its predecessors from this well-known publishing house. Two varieties are printed this year for 30 or 60 patients, the volumes being handsomely and at the same time strongly bound (a great desideratum for a physician's diary) in red leather. We have much pleasure in recommending this book to our *confrères*, and feel assured if they once begin its use, they will not care to make any change.

The New England Medical Monthly.—We have received the first number of a new journal bearing this title, and published at Newtown, Conn. It is a handsome, 50-page, double column sheet, and contains some very good original articles from known writers, along with editorial and other matter of interest. It will, no doubt, find a field for usefulness, and, as its editor says, "it has come to stay," we hope to find it a regular visitor, and wish it cordially a successful career.

Books and Pamphlets Received.

ESSENTIALS OF THE PRINCIPLES AND PRACTICE OF MEDICINE: A HANDBOOK FOR STUDENTS AND PRACTITIONERS.—By Henry Hartshorne, A.M., M.D. Fifth edition, revised; with 144 illustrations. Philadelphia: Henry C. Lea's Son & Co.

PHOTOGRAPHIC ILLUSTRATIONS OF CUTANEOUS SYPHILIS.—By George Henry Fox, M.D. Nos. X, XI and XII. New York: E. B. Treat.

THE DIAGNOSIS AND TREATMENT OF THE DISEASES OF THE EYE.—By Henry W. Williams, A.M., M.D. Boston: Houghton, Mifflin & Co.

A TREATISE ON THE DISEASES OF CHILDREN.—By J. L. Smith, M.D. Fifth edition, revised; with illustrations. Philadelphia: H. C. Lea's Son & Co.

THE PHYSICIAN'S CLINICAL RECORD FOR HOSPITAL OR PRIVATE PRACTICE. With Memoranda for examining patients, Temperature Charts, &c. Philadelphia: D. G. Brinton.

ECZEMA AND ITS MANAGEMENT.—By L. Duncan Bulkley, A.M., M.D. New York: G. P. Putnam's Sons.

A MANUAL OF OPHTHALMIC PRACTICE.—By Henry S. Schell, M.D. With fifty-three illustrations. Philadelphia: D. G. Brinton.

A TEXT-BOOK OF PHYSIOLOGY.—By M. Foster, M.A., M.D., F.R.S. Second American from the third revised English edition. With extensive notes and additions by Edward T. Reichert, M.D. Philadelphia: Henry C. Lea's Son & Co.

A SYSTEM OF SURGERY, THEORETICAL AND PRACTICAL, IN TREATISES BY VARIOUS AUTHORS.—Edited by T. Holmes, M.A., Cantab. First American from second English edition. Thoroughly revised and much enlarged by John H. Packard, A.M., M.D., assisted by a large corps of the most eminent American surgeons. Vol. II. Philadelphia: Henry C. Lea's Son & Co.

Society Proceedings.

MEDICO-CHIRURGICAL SOCIETY OF MONTREAL.

This Society held its regular meeting on October 28th, 1881. the President, Dr. Geo. Ross, presiding, who delivered the following address:—

Gentlemen,—Before introducing the regular business of the meeting, will you allow me to say a few words upon our beginning a new year. In the first place, I have to thank you very sincerely for my election as your President for the year. I can assure you that I deem it no small honour to occupy the first position in the Medical Society of our metropolitan city, and I shall endeavour to perform the duties of that office with such efficiency as I can, trusting always to the kind consideration which your Chairman has invariably met with at your hands. The fact confronts me at once that I am succeeding in this chair a series of men, the acknowledged leaders of the profession in this city for many years past—men whom age, experience and prolonged opportunities for observation, have rendered ripe for evolving wisdom and counsel for their juniors. I cannot fail to see the disadvantage under which I thus labour; but I hope that an earnest desire and attempt to serve faithfully the interests of the Society may to some extent remove these deficiencies on my part.

With your permission, I will make a few remarks upon the work already accomplished and still to be done by this Society. At our last meeting the retiring President gave us an account of the work done by this Society during his term of office; and when we consider the number of our members and our comparatively limited opportunities, I think that we have reason to congratulate ourselves upon the result. The aim of this association is chiefly to promote by mutual intercourse and by friendly criticism the mental furnishings of every individual member. This object has been constantly kept before us, and the interest taken by the members has been shown by the large number of original papers read and discussed—by the fact that nearly at every meeting men have brought forward facts of general interest coming under their own observation, or points in actual cases either difficult of explanation or presenting some anomaly important to be made known, or some peculiarity which rendered them worthy of note. These short communications are, to my mind, a valuable feature of our gatherings, and one which we should in every way encourage, especially because it is a part of the proceedings in which even the youngest member can take an active part. He is just as likely as any of his seniors to meet with cases of the greatest medical interest, and with more time at his disposal is able to observe all the more carefully the peculiarities of a case. Already several of our most recently acquired members have thus added their quota to the general stock. Cases, apparently affording little prospect of instructive debate, have sometimes proved most useful as bringing out the ideas, experiences, failures and successes of many who have thus been led to participate in the discussion following. I would therefore ask the members in their daily practice to think often of the Society and not to wait for a case of great rarity or unusual interest, but to bring to us the thoughts on even very common cases which have occurred to themselves, because these often make a text from the working out of which great profit may ensue.

Another function of this Society, and one which it has on several occasions made worthy efforts to perform, is that of taking cognizance of prevailing or epidemic diseases, and offering such expressions thereon to the local authorities as may be of service to them in promoting the health of the city and of the public generally. I might mention the action taken by the Society with reference to the scourge of small-pox, which so long made our city a by-word and a reproach. That action went a long way to assist in forwarding the plans of the sanitary authorities for the general enforcement of vaccination. Our discussions here may also be said to have been influential in securing the adoption of animal vaccine in place of the old, deficient, humanized virus or imperfectly preserved crusts. A member of this Society has also recently still further advanced the cause of vaccination by showing that children with eczema, and probably many other kinds of skin disease, may not only be vaccinated with impunity, but that, in many such cases, the performance of the operation has a curative effect upon the cutaneous complaint. By such means it is to be hoped that we have done our share towards promoting correct views upon these important matters.

Here also was first pointed out, with tolerable certainty, the fact that the milk supply in this city, as elsewhere, is sometimes to be taxed with being the vehicle for the conveyance of typhoid fever; and the facts laid before us led to important recommendations to the Sanitary Board concerning inspection of milk and dairies. This disease is again very rife amongst us, and it is to be hoped that some one may investigate and report to us the probable causes of its undue prevalence this year.

There is also, at the present time, a scheme in the hands of the Municipal Health Officer looking towards the extension and improvement of the sanitary by-law for the city of Montreal. Many clauses of this by-law affect the medical profession very closely, and it behoves their representatives here to see that the views of the profession are properly represented to the framers of the bill. This scheme contemplates also the possible inauguration of a general Act for similar purposes to govern the entire Province of Quebec. In this connection it is to be noted that the profession in Nova Scotia have this year moved in the same direction, so as to secure sanitary legislation for that Province. The ultimate aim of this should undoubtedly be the establishment of a permanent Health Department for the Dominion at Ottawa, which would govern and unify the results and actions of the combined Provincial Boards. This Society, as you are aware, named a committee, which has been in conference with the Medical Health Officer and Aldermen on the subject. Affairs of this kind move but slowly, and the committee have not yet reported any definite action, but no doubt before long their united efforts will have produced some good results.

The Council of the Society, by consent of the members, has committed to its care the examination into all ethical disputes which may chance to arise between members—an important office, and one which it has always hitherto fulfilled in a fair, judicial spirit, and in a manner which, by giving satisfaction, has been the means of averting strife, promoting harmony and preventing the continuance of heart-burning. I think those who best know the condition of the profession in Montreal, as compared with that in other Canadian cities, will agree with me in saying that in no other is there so little of professional jealousy, so little tendency to underrate the abilities of a rival, to grudge the good fortune or envy the success of a *confrère* as there is here; and it is but right to recognize the undoubted fact that one reason for this satisfactory state of things is the existence of this Society, where all are equal—where a professional injustice or breach of ethics is met by a suitable rebuke, and where nothing so tends to give a man the respect of his fellows as the knowledge that all his actions are fair, above-board, and invariably governed by a gentlemanly instinct. It is to the credit of the profession that the work of the Council in this respect during the past year has been almost *nil*. Let us hope that they may continue in the future to enjoy prolonged immunity from such tasks.

The exhibition of morbid specimens is, without doubt, one of the most important parts of our proceedings, and we are extremely fortunate in having such a large and varied assortment of pathological illustrations and curiosities presented to us annually; and we fully recognize the debt we owe our Pathologist for his labours in this direction. There is just one suggestion which I would make. It has appeared to me that if the member who reports a case with fatal termination and autopsy were himself to describe in a general way the morbid appearances whilst presenting the specimen for the inspection of the Society, it would be more advantageous than our present method, whereby the descriptions are all given by the gentleman who performs the examination. I think this would lead to a more careful and thorough personal study of the parts dissected, and further familiarize some with the technical anatomical delineation of diseased viscera and structures. At the same time also the connection between what is observed in the organs and what was noticed during life could be simultaneously pointed out for our instruction. Nor would this at all interfere with our having the benefit of Dr. Osler's views upon the pathology of the case, for I think in nearly every instance he would be expected to add further observations of his own to what the reporter may have previously brought forward. It appears to me that some arrangement of this kind would tend to increase the interest taken by our members in the work of the Society.

I might enumerate a number of matters of general professional interest which have been discussed by us, and some of which will no doubt come up again,—such as the general tariff of fees, insurance fees, registration of births and deaths, coroner's inquests, and many others which will occur to every one. The views expressed here on these important subjects always carry weight, because the general consensus of opinion is pretty sure to be a reflexion of the ideas of the profession at large.

It is to be remembered also that the usefulness of the communications and discussions in this room does not cease with ourselves. They are published in the local journals, and are read by great numbers of our fellow-practitioners throughout the country: and I have reason to know that a very widespread interest is attached to these published proceedings. The transactions of the Toronto and other local Medical Societies are likewise published in the journals of that city, and it should be matter of pride to every member here to add his share to the interest of the meetings in order to show that this Association is fully able to hold its own, at the very least, with any other in the value of the papers placed before it, and in the keenness of criticism and debate.

Quite enough, gentlemen, has been said to show that there is plenty of work to be done by this Society. It has been steadily growing in favour, influence and numbers. It has done very good service for several years past, and I sincerely trust that each year will see it becoming more important, more active, and more respected.

Dr. Osler then exhibited a specimen of extreme dilatation of the bile ducts without suppuration. The patient, a woman, aged about 40, was admitted to Hospital in September, 1880, with symptoms of jaundice, believed to be catarrhal, but the jaundice deepened and the liver rapidly enlarged. She remained in Hospital several months, and the enlargement of the organ, the continuance of the jaundice, and the loss of flesh, suggested the probability of cancer. She was admitted again in the spring of this year under Dr. Osler, with symptoms materially unchanged—intense jaundice, enlarged liver, smooth, no nodules, no fever, no sweats, moderate emaciation. She lingered until June. At the inspection, which was made in the dissecting-room, great narrowing of the lower two inches of the common duct was found, and dilatation of the main branches in the liver, which formed large sacculi filled with a clear fluid. There was no inflammation of the wall. The gall-bladder was very much distended and contained several small calculi; walls roughened; orifice of the cystic duct closed. Dr. Osler remarked that the narrowing might have been due to inflammation caused by the passage of a gall-stone. Dr. Ross thought it more probably succeeded catarrhal inflammation, as the woman had never had any symptoms of gall-stone.

Dr. Ross showed a case of Ulcerative Endocarditis. He said the patient was sent to Montreal General Hospital in September, supposed to have typhoid fever. Suspicions were first aroused by the marked remissions of temperature—in the evening, 104°, and morning normal, which continued with occasional chills. General condition was typhoid, the patient being weak, heavy, and listless. Previous to admission, had severe pains in joints. On examination, found a mitral murmur; spleen enlarged; entire absence of abdominal symptoms of typhoid fever. It was at first doubtful whether the case was not one of pyæmia from deep-seated suppuration, but observation for a short time resulted in a positive diagnosis of ulcerative endocarditis. There was a large fungoid growth both on the mitral and aortic valves; no disease in the lungs.

Dr. Hingston exhibited a patient, a young man, on whom he had operated for a firm, broad-based, fibrous, naso-pharyngeal polypus, at the Hotel-Dieu Hospital, a fortnight before. He had followed the method advised by Professor Bruns of Tabingen, consisting of a temporary resection of the bony skeleton of the external nose, and turning aside the bony and cartilaginous portions in connection with soft parts. He made an incision below the edge of the left alæ nasi, carried it to the right across the upper lip without wounding the mucous membrane of the mouth; a second incision over the root of the nose at the naso-frontal suture, and a third joining these two on the left side. With saw and bone forceps the hard parts were then divided. The vertical section of the septum was cut through from above and below, and with Langenbech's osteotomes, the nose was thrown over till its tip touched the right cheek. Room obtained in this way was found to be insufficient, and the periosteum, for some distance on the left superior maxilla, was raised and the subjacent bone removed. A piece of cord was then passed through the back part of the tumour, above the soft palate, passed out at the mouth, and entrusted to an assistant. The tumour was detached with periosteum. The hæmorrhage was alarming, and at one moment threatened suffocation and fatal syncope. The operation was concluded with patient's head and shoulders hanging down. The nose was then placed *in situ*, and has united without any displacement or deformity. Dr. Hingston thinks this method preferable to that recommended by Mr. Syme (excision of superior maxilla), or that through the antrum, as, although it is more difficult, from having less room to work in, the results are better, in an entire absence of deformity, without a scar across the cheek, and with no interference with the lachrymal passage, and therefore without epiphora.

The meeting then adjourned.

Extracts from British and Foreign Journals.

Unless otherwise stated the translations are made specially for this Journal.

Antiseptic Inhalation in Pulmonary Affections.—J. G. Sinclair Coghill, M.D.,F.R.C.P. Ed., in *British Medical Journal*: The objects of treatment are: 1. To lessen secretion; 2. To promote evacuation of what secretion is formed; 3. To disinfect the air which may pass into surrounding or deeper healthy portions of the lungs. Again he says, "Besides acting as disinfectants, antiseptic inhalations promote expectoration by increased energy of expiratory acts." Dr. Burney Yeo also recommends antiseptic inhalations, "if they have only the effect of temporarily cleansing, as it were, the pulmonary surface. It is a process analogous to that of washing away the decomposing discharges of a foul superficial ulcer." Dr. Clifford Albutt has broadly stated, and as truthfully, that "most phthisical patients die of septicæmia; and the arrest of this daily repoisoning is a primary object of treatment." Antiseptic inhalations again assume a still more important position, if the latest pathological theory of the contagiousness of phthisis through the respired air be well founded. . . The apparatus is extremely simple. It consists of a space for a pledget of tow or cotton wool, inclosed between the perforated surface of the respirator and an inner perforated plate, which can be raised so as to permit the tow to be saturated with the antiseptic solution. Elastic loops are attached to pass over the ears and retain it in position. The inhaler may be procured either plain or of a slightly smaller size, and covered with black cloth for wearing out of doors. The pledget of tow, which may be changed once a week or so, sprinkled with from ten to twenty drops of the antiseptic solution, from a drop-stoppered vial, twice a day at least, according to the extent to which the inhaling may be carried on. Of this the patient is the best judge, and the length of time and quantity of solution should be regulated by tolerance and effect. The most important times for inhaling are for an hour or so before going to sleep at night, and after the morning expectoration, which leaves the suppurating surface or cavity dry to be aeted upon—disinfected, so to speak—by the antiseptic vapor. A great many of my patients have of their own accord come to use the respirator almost continuously day and night from their experience of its good effects. I attach the utmost importance to the mode in which the respiration is conducted while inhaling. The patient should be carefully instructed to respire through the mouth alone, and expire through the nose. In this way the breath is drawn through the saturated tow in the perforated chamber of the inhaler, and passes directly into the lungs laden with the antiseptic materials. Expiring through the nose only, necessarily involves a complete circulation of the medicated air. The breathing should be short at the beginning of the inhalation, but gradually deepened, so as to displace and effect the residual air in the more distant portions of the lungs. This form of respiration itself is not only of great use in favoring the circulation of the blood in the lungs, and thus aiding local and general nutrition through that fluid, but it helps very much the expulsion of the sputa by means of the increased energy and thoroughness of the expiratory acts.

After many trials of the now formidable list of antiseptics, I find that carbolic acid, creasote, and iodine, in combination with sulphuric ether and rectified spirits of wine, are the most efficacious and satisfactory. The want of volatility in boracic, salicylic, and benzoic acids, and their salts, proves a bar to their employment by this method. Dr. Horace Dobell, who has had a very favorable experience of this treatment, writes to me that he has found thymol, in the form of Shirley's thymoline, very grateful and efficient in many cases where the smell of carbolic acid and creasote was intolerable either to patients or to their friends. Of the three antiseptic agents I chiefly use, I find iodine most useful in the second stage of phthisis, when the expectoration is passing from the glairy into purulent character. I use the tincture for inhaling purposes made with sulphuric ether instead of spirits of wine, and this etherial solution has a singularly soothing effect on the cough and pulmonary irritation. In combination also with carbolic acid as carbolized iodine, or iodide phenol, it is extremely useful in the purulent expectoration accompanying the resolution of pneumonia, both catarrhal and croupous. In the stage of excavation, whether tubercular or pneumonic, the combination of iodine with carbolic acid and creasote is most potent. The acid seems to have the greater influence in checking the amount and purulent nature of the sputa; while creasote acts merely as a sedative in the cough, apparently by reducing the irritability of the pulmonary tissues. The addition also of varying proportions of sulphuric ether and chloroform greatly assists in soothing and allaying irritation. These combinations also act frequently like a charm in the profuse expectoration of purulent bronchitis, as also in bronchial asthma.

The Diagnostic Importance of Odors.—In a recent lecture Dr. Julius Althaus, of London, says—: I must say a few words on the diagnostic importance of certain smells in the sick room, which was formerly much insisted upon; indeed, whole treatises have been written on the recognition of disease by sniffing. Dr. Heim, who was the popular physician of the day at Berlin some fifty years ago, recognized measles, scarlet fever, small-pox by their peculiar smell on first entering a house, and before having seen the patient. Mr. Bernard, of Upton Park, has recently recorded in the *Lancet* two cases of small-pox in which the patients themselves perceived a dreadful smell, apparently just at the moment of being exposed to contagion; and one of them, when suffering from the eruption, said that his perspiration had the same smell as that which made him sick before. When attending Skoda's clinique in Vienna, twenty-five years ago, I noticed that this celebrated teacher was in the habit of sniffing when approaching the bedside of patients from the last stages of pneumonia, phthisis, typhoid fever, etc., and he would give a bad prognosis when he perceived what he called the "cadaverous smell." Mr. Crompton, of Birmingham, has noticed a peculiar earthy smell from the body, a week or a fortnight before death, which, he says, has never deceived him; an appropriate illustration of the saying, "Earth to earth." Dr. Begbie distinguished typhus and typhoid fevers by the sanguineous (others call it "mousy") smell of the former. Prof. Parkeshas noticed a peculiar order in the skin of cholera patients. A pungent smell in the chamber of a lying-in woman shows that lacteal secretion is well established, while an ammoniacal smell has been said to indicate the approach of puerperal fever. Many women emit a particular odor while menstruating, which resembles a mixture of blood and chloroform, and that is believed to arise, not so much from the discharge, as from the more pungent character of the sweat secreted in the axilla. Persons of costive habits have a fecal smell; and this is also often noticed in hypochondriacs and lunatics. In uræmia, whether owing to kidney disease or to severe retention of the urine, a urinous odor is emitted by the body, and the presence of pus in some part of the body has been recognized by a peculiar warm, milky smell of the patient.

Apart from the odor of the sick room and the body generally, the smell of the sputa, urine, fæces, sweat, ulcers, etc., was carefully noted by the older practitioners and utilised for prognosis and treatment. Unquestionably there was much that was fanciful in such ideas; but occupied as we are at present with the study of more precise and definite symptoms, we have perhaps gone to the other extreme in neglecting such signs altogether. Everybody has his own special odor, and this varies according to the circumstances of life, the food taken, and the state of health in which he happens to be. That it should be altered in disease, and that special diseases should have special odors, is only what one would expect; yet the increase of cleanliness and ventilation has no doubt done away with a large variety of smells which formerly used to assail the nostrils of the physician.—*Mich. Med. News.*

New Treatment of Abscesses.—Dr. Steven Smith, of Chicago, has inaugurated a new treatment af abscesses, which he affirms to be very successful. It is thus described in the *Chicago Medical Review*: —"When the abscess points it is opened and the contents evacuated. The cavity is then injected with carbolised water, and over-distended for two or three minutes. The water is then pressed out, and over the whole area undermined by the cavity, small, dry, compressed sponges are laid and bound down with a bandage. Carbolised water is then applied to the bandage and injected between its layers until the sponges are thoroughly wet, after which a dry bandage is applied over all. The sponges by their expansion make firm and even compression upon the walls of the abscess, and hold them in perfect apposition, thus favouring a union. The dressing is left on for five or six days, unless there is a constitutional disturbance, or pain in the seat of the former abscess. It is found, in most cases, when the bandage is removed, that the abscess has completely closed by an approximation of its walls, and the external wound heals readily under a simple dressing of carbolised oil. A case was recently seen where this admirable result was secured in a child, although the abscess was a large one, originating in caries of the head of the femur, and opening on the outside of the thigh. No constitutional disturbance, no discharge, no reaccumulation, and no pain followed its use. Mammary and submammary abscesses have been treated by this method with excellent results."

Precautions in Thoracentesis.—M. Raynaud (*Journal de Médecine*) insists on a certain number of precautions which he considers it important to observe in thoracentesis. To avoid severe attacks of coughs, which often occur in the course of the operation, and are extremely painful and inconvenient, he recommends the subcutaneous injection of a full dose of

Drs. Fenger and Hollister of Chicago, in a paper on this subject in the October number of the *American Journal of the Medical Sciences*, state that thus far only six cases of this form of interference with cavities have been reported, and only one, their own case, was successful, in so far that it terminated in complete recovery. The clinical histories of these several cases are communicated in this paper, the original case being one of suppuration around a large echinococcus cyst in the lung of 12 years' standing. An incision was made in the third intercostal space anteriorly, through which the large cyst was subsequently removed. A counter opening being made between the fifth and sixth ribs, a drainage tube was introduced, and daily injections of carbolic acid practised. The authors conclude that "the operation is justifiable in any case where the presence of a gangrenous or ichorous cavity having been ascertained, it is found that, notwithstanding an outlet through the bronchi for a portion of the contents of the cavity, it steadily fills up again, the partial evacuation does not relieve the patient, who gradually loses strength and progresses towards a condition of collapse, a steady or intermittent rise in temperature continues; the infection of the healthy portions of the lung from the decomposed contents of the cavity has commenced, or is evidently about to take place; the breath and expectoration continue fetid; absence of appetite; increasing weakness, with or even without fever, etc. These indications will enable any medical man of some clinical experience to determine, in the majority of such cases, when the disease has reached a point from which spontaneous recovery is impossible." At the same time it is observed that any cavity covered by the scapula, or situated within the supra-clavicular and infra-clavicular regions may at present be regarded as inaccessible. The immediate indications and details of the operation are fully discussed in this paper, as well as the methods of after-management of an interesting class of cases otherwise not amenable to treatment.

Treatment of Typhoid Fever by Salicylate of Soda.—M. Caussidou made a communication to the French Association for the Advancement of Science at the Congress of Algiers, which was based on thirty-two cases of typhoid fever treated by salicylate of soda, and in which the rise of the temperature and the influence of this drug on the febrile process had been registered with the greatest care, as attested by numerous tracings shown by the writer. M. Caussidou arrived at the conclusion, in opposition to the facts observed in several wards of the Paris hospitals, that salicylated medication gives larger, more certain, and more permanent effects than refrigeration. M. Caussidou has even been in doubt if, by administering salicylate of soda from the outset of typhoid fever, it would not be possible to limit the duration of the disease to the first week (?), and if, at least, it would not be possible to obtain a number of cases belonging to the abortive form. Nevertheless, M. Caussidou does not conceal the dangers of salicylate medication. Like other observers, he has noted dyspnœa, precordial trouble, and exhaustion in patients where the salicylate of soda brought on a too sudden apyrexia. To avoid these objectionable results, he proposes to administer salicylate of soda in fractional doses of one gramme given every two hours, and to stop as soon as the temperature falls below 38° Cent. (100.4° Fahr.) In a complicated case of erysipelas, the salicylic medication was powerless to produce a febrile recrudescence brought on by this complication. M. Hérard declared that he had nothing but commendation for the use of antiseptics, such as carbolic and salicylic acids, in the treatment of febrile diseases.—*London Medical Record*, July 15, 1881.

Viburnum Prunifolium.—The black haw bush, or small tree, everybody knows; but medicinally, very few know that the profession have in it a real remedy in threatened abortion, or flooding after it. I was called to a lady in her seventh month of pregnancy, with violent pains coming on every five minutes, and which had been increasing for several hours. I gave her at once one drachm of the fluid extract, with thirty grains of hydrate of chloral. In an hour the pains moderated somewhat, and I repeated the viburnum, with twenty grains of chloral. Two hours after, I gave the same and the pains subsided.

Harry read this - Thus talking with

The patient slept several hours. In six or seven hours the pains returned again, and I again gave one drachm of viburnum and twenty grains of chloral; I gave three doses, subduing the pains. Being called away to a labour case, I was absent twelve hours, and being sent for hurriedly, I found my patient, as before, with more violent pains, and the os uteri opened three-fourths of an inch. I repeated the same doses four times, and the pains subsided. This condition continued about eight days, but required less chloral each day. Every three or four hours I gave milk freely, keeping the bowels open by enemata. The patient bore the medicine well, and made a good recovery; and two months afterwards went through her labour satisfactorily.

I had often tried hydrate of chloral and other medicines vainly to check abortion or miscarriage after the womb commenced opening.

Two months afterwards I was called to a similar case in threatened abortion, with flooding. I gave the viburnum alone, as I desired the patient to be awake in order to report hæmorrhage. In two hours the pains and hæmorrhage both ceased, with good recovery.

I was called last year to another patient, flooding dreadfully, and the contents of the womb were partially removed. I gave viburnum and ergot, and used hot-water injections with the bag syringe (otherwise called fountain syringe), a great improvement on the rubber bulb. The flooding was violent, and required continuous use of the syringe and medicine for two days before the hæmorrhage ceased. The abortion was complete.

A short time since I was called again to the same lady, in her seventh month of pregnancy, with violent pains every seven minutes, but no flooding. I gave viburnum and chloral, as before; but the stomach rejected three doses in succession. I then gave four drachms of viburnum and eighty grains of chloral by enema. In one hour the pains moderated somewhat. I gave half the quantity for the second dose, and the pains gradually stopped without further trouble. I used the fluid extract prepared by Parke, Davis & Co., Detroit. If this preparation is not accessible, I would use the decoction of the fresh bark.

The profession can rely on this remedy, and doubtless many lives will be saved by its prompt use.—*Dr. Cullen in American Medical Bi-Weekly.*

Accidental Ante-partum Hemorrhage.—Dr. E. L. Partridge of New York contributes an article in which, after briefly reviewing the current doctrines concerning so-called accidental hemorrhage preceding the birth of the child, he boldly challenges the expediency of the practice of rupturing the membranes. He believes that rupture of the membranes does not meet the indications—*i e.*, it does not in itself or in its results offer any reasonable probability of checking the hemorrhage—and that the method is highly dangerous from the increase of facilities for loss of blood, and because it adds to the difficulty and danger of proper subsequent steps in treatment. As to whether it really does check hemorrhage, it cannot do so unless a decided decrease in uterine bulk can be secured and maintained thereby. There must, therefore, be a considerable number of cases in which, a small amount of liquor amnii being present and the reduction in size being very slight after its escape, no benefit can accrue. In cases which present an average amount of amniotic fluid, after its evacuation the uterus is decidedly, though not greatly diminished in size. What is to show, however, that this decrease is sufficient to close the mouths of bleeding vessels? There is no practitioner who cannot affirm that alarming hemorrhage does often threaten after the birth of the child, and before or after the complete separation of the placenta, when the uterus is *greatly contracted.* Even this degree in the reduction of bulk fails to close the uterine sinues in the intervals of contraction. All those writers who advise rupture of the membranes couple with this advice the information that there is danger of continued hemorrhage. One says, "Of course there is risk," while all suggest methods by which they think a loss and a large accumulation of blood can be prevented after the escape of the amniotic fluid—these suggestions looking toward the maintenance of contraction. Accidental hemorrhage usually takes place prior to or during the occurrence of infrequent and slight early uterine contractions, when the os is slightly dilated or not at all. Superadded is the condition of collapse. If the liquor amnii is now permitted to escape, can any candid, practical obstetrician admit, the author asks, that there is any known way by which a momentary reduction of uterine bulk can be maintained for a period which will check an alarming hemorrhage? The uncertainties and tediousness of efforts at excitation of the uterus in cases of induction of labour afford a good illustration of the difficulties which would be encountered. Ergot is uncertain and almost valueless, for the stomach will either reject or fail to absorb it; or, if absorption does take place, or if the drug is given by the hypodermic method, its action is imperfect when there has been a great drain upon the vital powers. The abdominal binder cannot be applied in a way to crowd the resilient uterine tissue into contraction. Manual efforts cannot be kept up with any precision or efficacy during a period necessary to check the hemorrhage and keep it in control. Good uterine action cannot be excited when the uterus is surprised into labour. Good labour pains will not occur when the patient is exsanguinated. The suggestion of Leishman, to the effect that the placenta will be compressed between the uterus and the child after the escape of the liquor amnii, and hemorrhage thus be checked, is, Dr. Partridge thinks, fanciful; for no sufficient uterine action will take place to effect this. There are a great many chances also that the part of the child nearest the placenta would not be one which could make an even, perfect compression, if suitable uterine action did take place. Far from meeting the emergency, the method greatly increases the dangers. If the uterus does not contract promptly and permanently after the escape of the liquor amnii, an ample space is afforded for a further extravasation of blood. A very limited space will afford room for a dangerous extravasation. Another danger is from a more extensive detachment of the placenta when the uterus is even temporarily contracted. Another objection to the early removal of the liquor amnii in accidental hemorrhage is, that an obstacle is created to the use of the most efficient method for securing dilatation of the os—*i.e.*, by the dilators. Their use would be improper, lest, acting also as a tampon, they should prevent egress of diffused blood, and add to the accumulation.

A fourth danger will be from the increased difficulty encountered in the performance of version if the child is not surrounded by liquor amnii. This operation is often imperatively demanded in the treatment of accidental hemorrhage, under circumstances, too, when its ease of performance is of great importance. There is one class of cases of accidental hemorrhage in which the amount of blood lost does not fully explain the degree of shock. In these the factors in the production of collapse are the over-distension of the uterus and consequent irritation of the peripheral nerves of that organ, as well as the abstraction of blood from the circulation. Here, then, we might believe, was found sufficient ground for the treatment by early rupture of the membranes, relieving thereby uterine distension and the resulting irritation to the nervous system. Upon consideration, however, we find, first, that it is impossible to prejudge in these cases. It is only *after* delivery, when the amount of effused blood can be estimated, that we discover that the shock was proportionately greater than the hemorrhage. Again, collapse brought about in this way does not obstinately refuse to yield to treatment, but will be remedied usually by the customary measures, such as stimulants, the application of external heat, etc., without the need of any decided local interference. Finally, this variety of the accident is not very common, as indicated by clinical records, the possibility of its occurrence being so lightly regarded as hardly to be mentioned by writers. What, then, should be the treatment looking toward the safety of mother and child when immediate delivery cannot be resorted to, owing to incomplete dilatation of the os? By all means *preserve the membranes intact*, and thus tampon the uterine cavity with liquor amnii. Then, in the great majority of cases, employ Barnes's dilators until the desired result is obtained. Of course, this or any similar treatment must be employed at a suitable time. It must not supersede efforts for the relief of collapse, and it may be necessary to defer all operative measures until the patient can be rallied from the alarming constitutional symptoms. The os being sufficiently dilated to enable delivery to take place, rupture of the membranes is proper, and should be followed by manual efforts to compel the uterus to descend upon the child, whose expulsion should be immediate. Version fulfils the indications better than the forceps, as by the former operation there is less danger from delay during delivery, and because it can be successfully resorted to at an earlier period in the dilatation of the os than the forceps can. Bimanual version should not be considered for a moment, as in cases apparently most favourable it cannot always bv accomplished, while in this accident the irregularity of the internal uterine surface caused by the collection of blood would certainly interfere with the change of position of the child. During the entire time stimulants must be freely used and warmth to the surface, and in exceptionable cases, when the hemorrhage does not appear to be continuing, it is proper to wait for returning vitality before operative measures are undertaken, lest the condition of collapse be aggravated. The danger is not necessarily over after delivery, for it is often difficult to bring about reaction from the dangerous condition, and convalescence will often be slow.—*N. Y. Medical Journal and Obstetrical Review.*

For Night-Sweats in Phthisis.—Köhnborn recommends the dusting of the body every evening with the powder used in the Russian army for sweating feet (*Medical Bulletin*):

Acid. salicylic, - - - - - - - -	3	parts.
Amylum, : - - - - - - - - - -	10	"
Powdered talcum, - - - - - - -	87	"

If the skin be very dry, it may be rubbed with bacon, alcohol, or tannin, which will cause the powder to adhere to the body. The patient should hold a cloth to the mouth and nose during the dusting, that bronchial irritation from the salicylic acid may be prevented. Success has attended this method of treatment after quinine, atropia, digitalis, boletus laricia, cold sage tea, and frictions with alcohol, tannin, and bacon had failed. Waldenburg holds that the action of salicylic acid, when given internally in night-sweats, is similar to atropia, but far more effectual.

CANADA

Medical and Surgical Journal.

MONTREAL, DECEMBER, 1881.

MONTREAL VETERINARY COLLEGE.

The fifteenth session of this institution was opened on Tuesday, 4th Oct., at eight o'clock in the evening. The opening lecture was delivered by Principal McEachran, and a large number of citizens and students listened to his most interesting address.

We learn that this institution is still making progress. The number of students is larger this session than ever before, and from the fact that a matriculation is now required, the standard of education has advanced. The number of students attending the classes this session is about forty. The following students passed successfully in the matriculation examination held by Mr. A. Shewan, M.A., viz.: Messrs. H. C. Kingman, Middlebro', Mass.; Geo. Rennicks, Huntingdon, P. Q.; J. E. Gardner, Springfield, Mass.; T. A. Bishop, Montreal, P. Q.; E. P. Balls, Stanstead, P. Q.; W. P. Robins, Montreal, P. Q.; Villade Seguin, Rigaud, P. Q.; Joseph A. Levis, St. André, P. Q.; A. P. Belair, St. Rose, P. Q.

The following extracts are taken from the Principal's address:

The importance of veterinary science and the necessity for both governments and individuals according to this profession the aid and influence necessary to enable us to prosecute those researches which are now found to have so much influence on the prosperity of a country, is becoming more and more felt; never was this more felt than at the present moment. European countries were slow to see the importance of encouraging the educational development of this profession, but the destruction of their herds, the injury to their agriculturists by contagious diseases, led them at the close of the last century to expend large sums of money on their veterinary colleges, to organize regular systems of veterinary sanitary science, and police controlled by the Government, and in this way gave the profession a social status which slow England has not yet awakened to the necessity for. What is the consequence? When contagious diseases of cattle were imported from the Continent, where they had worked havoc among their herds for generations, few among the members of this neglected profession, which had been left by their Government to drag along uncared for and unencouraged, without means to pay competent teachers (most indeed of the pupils requiring to work for their existence while they struggled at their studies), recognized the enormity of the danger, and while they discussed the question of the contagiousness of the disease, and the Government turned a deaf ear to their warning voice, pleuro-pneumonia and foot and mouth disease rapidly spread, and soon gained a permanent foothold in the country. Again, when from neglect of quarantine regulations, the dread rinderpest reached the shores of England, the same blundering took place, and the profession, with a few exceptions, notably Prof. John Gamgee, proved themselves incapable, from the same cause, of dealing with the question, and the Government maintained the same masterly inactivity. The disease meanwhile spread from end to end of the land, decimating the herds and completely paralyzing the agricultural community, producing death and starvation among the labouring classes, and causing the destruction of over a qaarter of a million head of cattle. Who will hold a Government blameless which would trifle with such a weighty matter? Who will deny that the persistent neglect of veterinary science by the British Government has a very direct and important influence on the condition of her agriculturists to-day? Their means destroyed by cattle disease, which ruined many and seriously crippled the majority, could they be prepared to stand a few bad years of indifferent crops and low prices from American competition? Who will deny that the neglect of veterinary science in Britain will indirectly lead to the emigration of large numbers of her best farmers to make homes in Canada? Does it not astonish the world that a country like the United States, foremost in the invention and adoption of everything for the benefit of the farmer, celebrated for intelligence and all that tends to progress, with all the above facts before them, has followed the unfortunate example of the mother country, has turned a deaf ear to the pitiful wailings of thousands of ruined farmers in England, and failed to see the black spots on their sanitary maps which mark their Atlantic states as infected places and hells of cattle disease? It seems inexplicable that men of intelligence can shut their eyes to the fact that they are in the most imminent danger of having the most destructive of all scourges, pleuro-pneumonia, introduced among the countless herds in the vast cattle regions of the West.

Those who slight our profession do so in ignorance; there is none more important, none more honourable, none more independent. Whether you will succeed in occupying influential social or professional positions, will depend on yourselves. If you are proficient in your profession attend to your business, conduct yourselves like honourable men and gentlemen; your profession holds out high and honourable positions for you. It is not a profession that makes a man respectable or respected, but the man the profession.

At the outset, therefore, I beg of you to aim high, have high aspirations, feeling proud to belong to what, to my mind, is the most noble of all professions, whose object is the relief of suffering and curing of disease in those poor dumb companions of our earthly pilgrimage. You should cultivate a love for animals, their care and comfort should be your constant thought, you should never inflict unnecessary pain yourselves, and you should under all circumstances discountenance it in others.

I am happy to be able to inform you that since we last met, important changes have taken place, all tending towards the advancement of the profession. Valuable scientific discoveries have been made, notably the artificial propagation of bacteria: and the value of inoculation by ameliorated virus as a protection of the system against the otherwise fatal influence of the unmodified virus, which has been demonstrated by M. Pasteur, may prove of incalculable value to medical science generally, as has already been demonstrated by him, in preventing the dread malady, anthrax.

During the past summer, following the example of the medical profession, the veterinary held a congress in London, at which this College was ably represented by Dr. Osler, where subjects of great importance to the profession were discussed, and from which great good will no doubt result. On the American continent, in which we are after all most interested, we find that important strides have been made. A regular Veterinary Department has been created at Washington, with Mr. C. Lyman at its head, in connection with the Department of Agriculture, by whom investigations have been conducted and reports published on all reported outbreaks of disease. Besides this, the Treasury Department have appointed a separate commission, consisting of Prof. Law, Mr. Shayer and Mr. Saunders, to enquire specially into pleuro-pneumonia and other contagious diseases. Veterinary surgeons are now appointed to the United States army, port inspectors are about to be appointed, and this year will see that the profession is at last receiving that recognition which is its just due, and which it ought to have received long ago.

It is gratifying too to know that the service of the profession in Canada continues to be appreciated, and has a just claim to the credit of being of some value to the country. It is gratifying also to see that each year a number of our young men graduate in both professions, and, thus acquiring a knowledge of both sciences, place themselves on the same professional and social footing as medical practitioners. The introduction too of practical work in comparative pathology and comparative anatomy into medical courses tends greatly to elevate veterinary medicine, for the comparative pathologist is essentially a student of veterinary science.

I have mentioned that at the beginning of the present century dates the establishment of a few veterinary colleges in Europe and Britain, and I may add that these few existed under great disadvantages, especially in the quality of students who were found to enter the profession. Now all that is changed. Veterinary colleges now form important institutions in almost every state in the civilized world, and most of them have adopted a moderately high standard of education; the courses delivered at most of them are equal in all respects to those of medical colleges.

OUR REPORTS.—We devote a considerable amount of our space this month to reports upon Surgery and upon the progress of Pharmacy. The former gives a condensed account of all the most noticeable features of the discussions in the Surgical section of the great International Congress of last summer. The latter is the completion of a very able report presented by Dr. Stewart to the Canada Medical Association last August at Halifax. Although the space thus occupied precludes us from presenting the usual number of pages of selected matter, still we have every reason to believe that the substitution therefor to some extent of periodical reports, is appreciated by the readers of the JOURNAL. We have communications from numbers of our friends in various parts of the country stating the value which they attach to the Gynecological reports we have been publishing, and we have no doubt the same feeling is entertained towards these others. The system has the advantage of presenting at stated times a *resumé* of all important work done in that department, and if these be preserved, they form at the end of the year a compilation extremely useful for future reference.

Medical Items.

PERSONAL.—James Ross, M.D., and James L. Foley, M.D., were admitted L.R.C.P., London, on 27th October. William Cormack, M.D., has obtained the double qualification of L.R.C.P. and L.R.C.S. We have learnt that on this occasion 60 per cent. of the candidates were rejected.

—Erasmus Wilson has been knighted on account of his munificent gifts for the support of hospitals and the encouragement of medical study.

—L. D. Mignault, M.D. (McGill), has been appointed as Lecturer on Anatomy in Victoria Medical College, in this city, *vice* Dr. Bibaud, deceased.

—Lawson Tait speaks of Listerism as "one of the largest, best-blown and most attractive bubbles ever diplayed to a surgical audience."

—In Maine they have a law that no medical student shall be allowed to graduate and practice medicine who has not had regular practice in the dissecting-room. Then they passed a law that no bodies, save only the bodies of executed criminals, should be cut up in dissecting-rooms. Then, as a climax to all this, they abolished capital punishment.—*St. Louis Globe-Democrat.*

ANOTHER MRS. PARTINGTON.—"How flagrant it is!" said Mrs. Mixer, as she sniffed the odor of a bottle of Jamaica ginger. "It is as pleasant to the oil factories as it is warming to the diagram, and so accelerating to the cistern that it makes one forget all pain, like the ox-hide gas that people take for the toothache. It should have a place in every home where people are subject to bucolics and such like melodies; besides, a spoonful is so salubrious that when run down like a boot at the heel in walking, one feels like a new creature."—*The Druggist.*

THE FUTURE OF INNOCULATION.—*Customer*—"My nephew is just starting for Sierra Leone, and I thought I could not make him a more useful present than a dose of your best yellow fever. Would you tell me the price, please?" *Chemist*—"Well, ma'am, the germs are so difficult to cultivate in Europe that I would advise your waiting for the next West India mail, when I am expecting a nice, fresh consignment from St. Thomas. Meanwhile we would recommend our half-guinea travellers' assortment of the six commonest zymotics, and could add most of the tropical diseases from stock at five shillings each. We have some nice Asiatic cholera just ripe, but they are more expensive."—*Punch.*

CANADA MEDICAL & SURGICAL JOURNAL

JANUARY, 1882.

Original Communications.

ON ERYSIPELAS.

By R. W. POWELL, M.D., Ottawa.

(Read before the Ottawa Medico-Chirurgical Society.)

We are fortunate, I think, in having chosen erysipelas as a subject for discussion, because it is a disease with which we all ought to be intimately acquainted. It crosses us at times, no matter what branch of the profession we are engaged in—as physicians, surgeons, or obstetricians,—and though, under these altered circumstances, it may wear different aspects, yet we have to deal with one and the same poison.

To the physician, it constantly assumes a severe character, either by its being prolonged from day to day, perhaps with a discharge and an elevated temperature, thus tending to exhaust the patient; or frequent relapses may bring about a similar result; or, again, its frequent repetition in the same patient leaves both himself and his physician in a state of uncertainty as to its cause, its prevention, and its consequences.

To the surgeon, it is a continual source of anxiety, often marring the effects of an otherwise successful operation, always an interference with nature's efforts at repair, and occasionally placing a patient in jeopardy who has sought the surgeon's aid to rid him of perhaps some slight disfigurement or deformity. Following an operation, it lends a totally different complexion to the case at once, and though it may not actually cause death, yet it seriously impairs the result, as well as retards recovery.

The danger of this, however, is now reduced almost to a minimum by a strict observance, on the part of the surgeon, of proper antiseptic precautions, cleanliness, and well-directed drainage.

To the obstetrician, it is, perhaps, a still graver complication when it occurs; but, I believe, in this country it is a rare sequel to parturition, mainly, I daresay, owing to the few maternity hospitals and few centres of dense population, and thus overcrowding is avoided and the chances of contagion much reduced, but partly, let us hope, our immunity to be due to the precautions and cleanliness observed by Canadian surgeons.

Though some periods of life are less obnoxious to this disease than others, and though it may be more frequent at certain seasons of the year, yet it will occur at all times of life and in every month in the year. It will, at times, attack the new-born as well as the octogenarian, the rich and well-to-do as well as the pauper. The gouty system due to the effects of high living and sedentary occupation will be as prone to it as the system broken down by intemperance and bad hygienic surroundings; and, lastly, the sexes serve to divide the palm about equally.

These considerations, then, should teach us to watch closely for its premonitions, to observe carefully its clinical varieties and peculiarities, to take reasonable precautions against its occurrence when we are aware of its close presence, and, more than all, to be careful, in our own dealings with the disease, not to convey it by any means from patient to patient. Though erysipelas has been recognized since the earliest times as a specific disease, and has received the attention of the most able in our profession, there seems yet to be some difficulty in accurately defining it so that we may place it in its proper class. The earlier writers believed it to be due to a poison generated in the body itself, and finding a local expression in the skin whereby it was thus excreted from the body. Later on, it was supposed to occur in consequence of a stoppage to the escape of acrid materials from the blood through the pores of the skin. The theory that it was, in fact, a lymphangitis first emanated from Germany, and this was followed by another, which classed it as a simple dermatitis.

The later theory, and the one acceptable to the greater number, places it among the acute exanthems. It has, however, some marked differences from these diseases, among which are the following: The short invasion, the indefinite course, the liability to relapse, the definite starting point (usually from that part which happens to present a broken surface), its occasional protracted course, and, further, the first attack, instead of being a protection against subsequent invasions, often renders the patient peculiarly sensitive to the action of the poison for ever after. To these may be added, its occasional apparent tendency to attack certain families, *i.e.*, to be hereditary, though this is not established. On these grounds Trousseau opposed the view of is being an exanthem, and he therefore makes no distinction between idiopathic and traumatic erysipelas, and, in fact, regards every erysipelas as traumatic, believing that, if looked for, a wound in the surface will always be found as a starting point. There can be very little doubt, at any rate, that erysipelas is due to a specific poison, but that it comes fairly under the category of the exanthemata is open to grave question. It would appear, also, that, according to some observers, the varieties of the disease depend in great part upon the mode in which the poison enters the system, all not holding with Trousseau that it invariably enters by a wound ; and, in fact, many close observers acknowledge that it may arise spontaneously (that is, not due to a previously existing case.)

More recent investigations into the nature of this poison have discovered a bacterium or a microphore, and it would seem that this growth constitutes the true *materies morbi* of erysipelas.

However produced, when once it attacks the skin it seems to be endowed with great powers of reproduction, and thus the disease is extended by actual contact, and the resulting dermatitis is the effect of the irritation produced by this minute foreign body in countless myriads. They would appear to be endowed with only a brief existence, but, as I said before, having great powers of reproduction, so that by their rapid multiplication the disease is extended from part to part. The experiments of Lukomsky go to shew that the micrococcus is only present during the dermatitis and disappears as it subsides. This observation explains itself better I think, and is more consistent with the theory, if we say that the dermatitis subsides when the term of life of the micrococcus ends.

This theory to my mind fills the gap in the pathology of erysipelas and fully accounts for the symptoms and clinical history of the affection. The varieties met with will depend first upon the virulence of the poison when it attacks the system—*i.e.*, with its state of dilution as it were—and the degrees of severity in different cases will depend in a great measure upon the fertility of the soil upon which the poison is sown. This accords with what we actually observe. Subjects in fair health and with their secretions all in a normal state, do not seem to take on the morbid action even when exposed to the contagion, and if they do it will occur as a rule, mildly. As we descend the grade of health we observe the disease attacks in a more severe form, and especially is this observed in those living in bad hygenic surroundings. This disease, then, usually confines itself to the skin, but it is agreed that the mucous membranes will sometimes take on the morbid action as well, and, indeed, it very frequently begins near one of the orifices of the body where skin and mucous membrane seem to merge the one into the other. Trousseau says it is this fact that sometimes leads one to believe that it arises spontaneously and without a break of surface because the swelling and inflammatory action that at once ensue on its introduction mark the probably small and insignificant wound in the soft mucous membrane.

As to its affecting internal organs it never does so primarily, but if lungs, stomach, intestines or other viscera become affected it is due to the spreading of the poison by actual continuity of surface. I have contented myself, then, with these few observations on the pathology of the disease in the hope that others here may offer remarks upon other branches of the subject. To go into the symptomatology, clinical history, terminations and varieties of the disease would occupy too much of our time for one evening. With regard to the treatment of this affection I think our knowledge is yet very imperfect. If the pathology hinted at above is correct, then we may hope for some specific treatment to arise in the near future. Now that animal and vegetable chemistry is assuming such an important place in our therapeutics we must hope for an antidote to this erysipelatous germ, if I may use the word. In the meantime, we must content ourselves with rational orthodox treatment. I would like now to ask those present to state shortly their method of treating this affection, taking a moderately severe case and standard. Whether they have found Tr. Ferri Chlor. sufficient to meet the symptoms. If so in what doses is it prescribed in the case of children and of adults? Lastly, whether any benefit can be expected from local applications? If used, what variety seem to be the most beneficial? Do they ever check the onward march of the disease?

SOME CASES OF GUN-SHOT WOUNDS.

By W. H. BURLAND, M.D., Montreal.

(Read before the Medico-Chirurgical Society of Montreal.)

Mr. President and Gentlemen,—The paper I am about to read to you this evening is not a dissertation upon gunshot wounds, but simply a synopsis of several severe injuries of this class, whose course I had an opportunity of watching, as they were treated in the practice of the Montreal General Hospital during my residence in that Institution.

Our attention has been but lately called to the sad results of a wound of this nature in depriving the neighbouring Republic of its chief magistrate; and, although the cases I have to recount to you on this occasion did not terminate in such a lamentable manner, yet, several of them came so near doing so, that I hope they will interest you sufficiently to bear with me during their rehearsal; but before reading their histories, it will not, I deem it, be out of place to make a few general remarks on injuries of the nature under consideration.

Gunshot wounds belong to the class of wounds called *Contused*, when penetration of the body does not take place; and to that of *Lacerated*, when it is entered or traversed by the shot. They are, in fact, the most complicated of wounds, combining, as they do, contusion, attrition, and laceration to a high degree, occasioning all kinds of fractures, introducing extraneous matter into the body, and often giving rise to such complications as hæmorrhage, inflammation, septicæmia, erysipelas, and even gangrene. These injuries are produced by all sorts of missiles—such as small shot, bullets, grape or canister, chain or bar shot, shells, slugs, and even the powder itself, as well as fragments of wood, stone, clothing, buttons, portions of another person's body, &c.,—but as the cases to which I wish to draw your attention to-night were all produced by the ordinary cylindro-conoidal ball of common use, I will refer principally to wounds inflicted by such means. We do not now see, since the introduction of this modern form of bullet, the wonderful, yes, extraordinary, courses taken which were sometimes seen in injuries caused by the old spherical ball, such, for instance, as that spoken of by Heunen, who relates the case of a man in whom the ball, which struck the Pomum Adami, was found lying in the orifice of its entrance, having gone completely around the neck. The works on military surgery, written during the last century, abound in examples of just as strange deviations, but at present such instances are exceedingly rare, for it is now usual to find the missile traverse the body in the same line in which it entered, unless deflected by some of the heavier osseous structures; in fact, the conical ball is not influenced by the tissues through which it passes, and, if it has not passed entirely through, is generally found immediately under the skin at a point directly opposite to that in which it entered, or rather in the line in which it was travelling when it struck the body, and this fact is useful, from a clinical standpoint, as a guide to locating the bullet. Sometimes the place where the ball lies is plainly enough indicated by a slight reddish discoloration; generally, however, it can only be discovered by passing the hand carefully over the skin, when a hard substance will reveal its presence. (F. Hamilton.) The ball, having been grasped by the thumb and first finger of the operator, or by an assistant, is best removed by a free incision. If the above precaution is not attended to, the bullet may slip back into the track of the wound, or to one side, and render its extraction difficult. It is usually necessary to free the ball of its entanglements before removal, and this can be done by a few cuts with the point of the knife, or by cutting firmly into the lead from end to end. As to the differences between the point of entrance and that of exit: in the old spherical ball these were tolerably distinct, as the aperture of entrance was usually round and clean, with inverted edges, while that of exit was everted and jagged; on the other hand, the wound of entrance made by the conical bullet is generally larger than the diameter of the missile, and its form much less regular, being sometimes oval, sometimes linear or crucial, and even triangular in shape, while the point of exit is very much larger and still more irregular in its outline, but, as a rule, the two wounds are much of a size, and hard to be distinguished between. Probes of various makes and some very ingenious instruments have been devised at different times to aid in the detection of bullets and their removal, but time will not allow of my referring to them. In the primary local treatment of a gunshot wound, water-dressing at or below the temperature of the patient's body seems to be generally accepted as the most suitable application.

Having given these few hints concerning the injuries of which I am about to speak, I would crave your attention to the following cases:—

CASE I.—William E., a tall, well-proportioned young man of 21, was admitted to Hospital under Dr. Drake's care on the 16th July, 1877, having received a bullet wound in the back. It appears that the patient had come to town to attend the funeral of young Hackett, who was murdered on the 12th July, 1877, and as he was going to a friend's house in the evening, was deliberately shot at, a ball entering the right side of his back. Upon examination, it was found that the bullet had pierced about 3¾ inches to the right of the spine, and about 1¾ inches below the angle of the scapula. The ball had struck a rib in its course and passed forward in a slightly downward direction, but it was not located. There were no signs of wound of the lung, but the injury was followed by a severe attack of pleurisy, which pulled the patient down in strength. He was, however, able to leave

Hospital eight days after admission, and when discharged on July 24th the wound of entrance had healed. The ball, although not discovered in this case, must have been a small one, as the orifice of admission was not over a ¼-inch in diameter. He states that he was glancing over his left shoulder when he received the wound, so that the ball entered in an oblique direction, although the party who fired it was directly behind the patient. This was corroborated by the hole in his outside coat, which was only 2⅛ inches from the centre seam, while the wound in the body was about 3¾ inches from the spine. I have since had an opportunity of learning that this patient has felt no inconvenience from the lodgment of the ball. From a medico-legal point of view, this case is interesting, for this reason, viz., that the party wounded is confident that he could recognize the person who fired the shot which wounded him, as he was glancing over his shoulder at the time. The injury being in the back, some doubt might arise upon this point.

CASE II.—John G. B., a well-built young man of 22, evidently very muscular and of good constitution, received a bullet wound in his back on Sunday evening, 10th March, 1878, at about 9 P.M., and at 10 P.M. he entered Hospital under Dr. Roddick's care, at which time he was suffering some slight inconvenience from the injury, but had spat no blood, had no cough, nor did deep inspiration produce much distress. The wound was situated about 3¾ inches from the spine, and about 5 inches below the right shoulder-blade; it could be probed for about 3 inches directly towards the spine, but the ball could not be felt, nor was it discovered at any time during his stay. The injury was not followed by any bad symptoms, and the patient was discharged in twelve days, with the point of entrance completely closed. This case is interesting from the small amount of (if any) local or constitutional disturbance which followed the lodgment of such a foreign body as a bullet. As to the direction which the ball is supposed to have taken, it might be well to state that the hole in patient's coat was 4¼ inches from the centre seam, while the entrance made in his skin was only 3¾ inches from the spine.

CASE III.—Solomon W. was admitted to Dr. Roddick's wards

Jan. 3rd, 1878, having received a bullet wound in the back part of his right leg. As the injury was incurred at the Back River, in some hotel quarrel, the leg was very much swelled before he arrived in Hospital. Upon examination, a small, somewhat circular, wound was found to exist in the central part of the posterior aspect of the right thigh, a short distance above the flexure of the knee. Having satisfied himself that the ball was lodged against the bone, Dr. Roddick cut down under complete antiseptic precautions, and removed the bullet, which I now present to you for inspection, it having been found somewhat imbedded in the femur. I have drawn attention to this case, though simple in its aspect as a gunshot injury, from the fact that the wound was very near a large joint, and that inflammation, with its accompanying swelling, prevented the surgeon locating the ball for two or three days after its lodgment. This patient made a rapid and complete recovery, being discharged from Hospital in about three weeks.

Case IV.—James H., a robust, muscular carter of 19, having been wounded by a bullet in the upper part of the left side of his chest, in a street brawl, on the 25th April, 1878, was brought to Hospital soon after being shot, in a semi-comatose condition. Upon admission, he seemed to be suffering from intense shock; pulse weak, face pale, lips anæmic, and he could with difficulty be aroused. As the case was evidently a very serious one, I at once sent for Dr. Roddick, the attending surgeon, and a magistrate, as the affair was fraught with legal difficulties as well as vital ones. On closer examination, it was found that a bullet wound about $\frac{3}{8}$ to $\frac{1}{2}$ inch in diameter existed in the left infra-clavicular region, over 3rd rib, about 4 inches from the sterno-clavicular articulation, and $3\frac{1}{2}$ inches above the nipple. A probe could follow the track of the bullet in an oblique direction from left to right as far as the intercostal muscles, but farther it was not deemed advisable to go. Very little blood, if any, had been lost externally, and none had been spat up, nor had cough occurred. No evidence of any kind was obtained from auscultation at this time. The taking of his deposition seemed to prostrate him exceedingly, and it was with difficulty that answers could be obtained from him. Next day, April 26th, was still semi-comatose. Breathing short and rapid. Temperature in the evening, 101°F.; pulse, 100 ; respirations, 44. He complained of pain about the wound, which was increased by moving him or by deep inspiration; but neither cough nor expectoration were present. A pericardial friction sound, accompanied by great dyspnœa and pain, now developed itself, having its greatest intensity about 2 inches to left of sternum, and râles, supposed to be pneumonic, were detected near the wound. The necessity of keeping the patient absolutely quiet prevented an examination of the back parts of his chest at this time. Leeches were applied to the precordial region and cold to the wound.

April 27th—Pericardial friction most marked at left edge of sternum ; pain less severe. Morning : temperature, 100° F. ; respiration, 22 ; pulse, 102. Evening : temperature, 102°.4 F.; respiration, 28 ; pulse, 104.

April 28th.—Pleuritic friction was noticed to-day in left side, accompanied by severe pain. Pericardial murmur has descended and is more diffuse. Temperature, 102°F.; râles have disappeared from upper part of chest.

April 29th.—Pericardial effusion has supervened; pain in left side more intense. Ordered calomel gr. i, with pulv. opii gr. ½, 3 q. h. Morning: temperature, 98°.2 F.; respiration, 22. Evening : temperature, 100°.8 F.; respiration, 22.

April 30th.—Pleuritic pain still intense. Precordial bulging diminished. Pericardial friction again intense at point where it commenced.

May 3rd.—An opportunity occurring for examining the back, fluid was discovered in the left pleura, which proved to be a bloody serum—this fact being ascertained by the use of a hypodermic syringe. Some suppuration now took place about the wound. His temperature ran up to 103° F., and dyspnœa became a marked symptom, while pain and pericardial friction again set in, pulse being weak and irregular. Sherry wine was given. By 7th May these severe symptoms had slackened off, dyspnœa having given way to fairly natural breathing, unaccompanied by pain. Pulse much improved, but dulness persisted over the pleuritic effusion. Wound almost healed. Was allowed a better diet. About 19th May patient had a bad turn; temperature in the morning was up to 103°F., which before had ranged below 100°F. At this time constipation seemed to be an important factor. Aspiration with a hypodermic needle again detected a bloody serum. Ordered a tonic of iron and quinine. From this time rapid improvement followed, and spontaneous absorption must have supervened, for when discharged on the 13th June, after a stay of 49 days in Hospital, the dulness had almost entirely disappeared, and his breath sounds had regained their normal properties.

I have abstained from giving too full a report of this most interesting case for fear of tiring your patience, but if you have been able to follow from my description the severe and alarming complications by which this patient's life was jeopardized, I will feel sufficiently repaid for taxing your kindness even to the extent I have.

Case V.—Louis P., aged 32, a strong, muscular, labouring man, was admitted to Hospital under Dr. Roddick's care, suffering from the effects of a bullet wound in the left side, December 18th, 1877. Patient was one of the men engaged in a strike on the canal, and on the day on which he was wounded, he, with a number of others, assembled near the contractor's office. An altercation ensued, and one of the occupants of the office rushed out, and, while standing on a slight elevation, shot down at the patient, who was near him, but on a lower level. Patient, feeling that he was wounded, ran about two acres, and sat down. Immediately after being shot, blood had gushed from his mouth and nose, and a large quantity had escaped also from the wound. He soon felt weak, and complained of pain and faintness, but retained consciousness throughout. He was taken to a house in the vicinity, where he received temporary medical treatment, but was soon after removed to Hospital. On examination, it was found that the bullet had entered the chest in the 6th interspace, about one inch to the left of, and a little below, the left nipple. It had taken a direction downwards towards the left side, and had evidently struck the 6th rib in its course. The point of entrance was about ⅝ of an inch in diameter, circular, and somewhat inverted. Blood still escaped from the wound, but only in a slight degree. He had expectorated a large quantity of blood, while cough and deep inspiration caused pain. The wound was dressed, his chest strapped on both sides to restain movement, and ice applied. Pb. acet. and opium were given, as well as a daily hypodermic injection of grs. v ergotine. Extensive emphysema of the tissues was noticed over the left side. The position of the ball was not made out at this examination.

Dec. 19th.—No blood oozed from the wound to-day; experienced pain in left side, but not of a severe character, also some distress upon coughing. There were no evidences of pneumonia, although carefully examined for. Same treatment continued. Temperature 101°F. Has great anxiety of mind, and had not slept well. Emphysema of tissues has almost disappeared.

Dec. 20th.—Has expectorated much less blood to-day, and coughing does not distress him much. Temperature 99½° F.

Dec. 21st.—Still spitting some blood. Was ordered—℞ Acid Hydrocyan. dil. B.P. ♏ 80; Liq. Morphiæ ℥i; Ext. Bellad. fld. ♏ 24; Aquæ ad ℥viii; ℥ss t.i.d. Continues to improve.

Dec. 23rd.—The position of the ball was discovered; it was found lying posteriorly between the 9th and 10th ribs, in a line with the inferior angle of the scapula, having evidently, from the above symptoms, passed through the left lung. The patient is still doing well. Temperature low. Ice was removed to-day and carbolic lotion applied to wound. Is still expectorating some blood.

Dec. 24th.—Without any evident cause, or any great rise in temperature (100°F.), the patient suddenly became delirious, with a strong, bounding pulse. This change seemed to depend upon his anxiety about the strike. The ball was extracted to-day by Dr. Roddick, under complete antiseptic precautions. When removed, it was found to be split and flattened on one side, which can be accounted for by its having struck a rib in its course. Was ordered—℞ Pot. Brom. ʒss; Chloral Hydrat. grs. x; Tinc. Hyosc. ʒss; 4 q. h.

Dec. 25th.—Delirium has not abated; in fact, he has torn the dressings off his wounds, and it is difficult to keep him in bed. A blister was applied to the nape of his neck. No blood in the sputa to-day.

Dec. 26th.—Delirium passed off to a considerable extent. Some pus, but not of a fœtid character, appeared on the dressings to-day. Wound of entrance almost closed.

Dec. 27th.—Complains of pain in left side from wound to base of lung. Temperature 99°F. *29th*—Seems to be improving generally. *30th*—Some pain still persists in left side. Temperature 98½°F.

Jan. 2nd.—Patient was allowed up, feeling no pain, but well and hearty.

With the exception of a return of the pain in his side for a short time, the patient continued to improve until discharged on the 15th January, after 28 days' stay in Hospital, wound of operation having healed some time before.

Case VI.—D. C., aged 20, a powerful young man of good constitution, was admitted to Dr. Fenwick's wards on 13th March,'78, suffering from two bullet wounds received as he was entering a dark gateway leading to his home. One ball had pierced his nose, the other his right leg. The shots, to my mind, were fired with intent to kill, as one of the balls, which was subsequently extracted, was of a size which no person would have used for the mere purpose of giving a fright; and as both bullets, evidently shot from different weapons, took effect, it is likely that more than one person perpetrated this outrage. The wound in the nose was followed by some hemorrhage; that in the leg was not, but the patient experienced a pricking sensation on its receipt. The nasal wound was situated a little above the centre of the left side of the nose, seemingly produced by a small ball, and was about a ¼-inch in diameter. The probe could be passed directly back to the pharynx in a slightly downward direction, but it was impossible to trace the bullet farther. Considerable bleeding followed this exploration. From the size and direction which the ball had taken, I happened to say one morning, in making my usual rounds, that probably he would spit it up; and strange to say, on the morning of St. Patrick's day, the patient did cough up the very much distorted bullet which I now present to you.

The wound in the leg was situated about 1 inch to the outer side of the centre of the thigh, 7 inches below the anterior superior spinous process of the ilium, and about 10 inches above the patella. The track could be probed for about 4 inches, but the ball was not detected until some time later, when it was found lying in the outer aspect af the leg. It was removed by Dr. Roddick, under whose care the patient was at the time. The bullet, which, as you can see, was of considerable size, was very much flattened on one side, where it had evidently come in contact with the bone, but no splintering of the femur was made out at any time. The case progressed rapidly, so that the patient was discharged in 28 days.

BI-MONTHLY RETROSPECT OF OBSTETRICS AND GYNÆCOLOGY.

Prepared by WM. GARDNER, M.D.,

Prof. Medical Jurisprudence and Hygiene, McGill University; Attending Physician to the University Dispensary for Diseases of Women; Physician to the Out-Patient Department, Montreal General Hospital.

From the character of the International Medical Congress held in London during the past summer, it was to be expected that in the Obstetric section all the more exciting gynecological topics of the day would be discussed. Improvements in the construction and application of the Forceps; Oöphorectomy—Battey's operation—Spaying—Castration of Women, as it is variously termed (a good name for the operation is still wanting); Diagnosis of Ovarian Tumours; Operative Treatment of Extra-uterine Pregnancy; the Treatment of Puerperal Hæmorrhage; the Reparative Surgery of the Genital Tracts; Antisepsis in Midwifery; Laceration of the Cervix Uteri; Total Extirpation of the Uterus; the Mechanical Treatment of some of the Displacements and Diseases of the Uterus, were the more important of the subjects under consideration. Space will not permit more than a brief allusion to the most important of these.

Prof. Tarnier of Paris presented his forceps, and made some

remarks on improvements in its construction. The discussion which followed shewed that he has a most respectable following of eminent names who approve of his improvements to the instrument. Among these, Dr. Fordyce Barker of New York, Prof. Simpson of Edinburgh, Dr. Budin of Paris, and Dr. Robert Barnes of London, may be mentioned. Dr. Matthews Duncan (London), Prof. Stephenson (Glasgow), and Dr. Lombe Atthill (Dublin), were opposed to it chiefly because of its continuous compression of the head.

The ever-interesting subject of the treatment of puerperal hemorrhage had a due share of attention. Dr. Robert Barnes of London reiterated his well-known views. In the course of his address he spoke of physiological puerperal hemorrhage, viz., the loss of the excess of blood, which, having served in the nutrition of the fœtus, is expelled from the uterus during and after detachment of the placenta. Any loss beyond this is extra-physiological hemorrhage, and is to be checked by the assistance of the physician. He concluded by asserting that in a certain number of cases, when uterine contraction fails, we have no reliable alternative but the intra-uterine injection of perchloride of iron, the peculiar dangers of which over other intra-uterine injections he believed to be few and mostly avoidable.

Dr. T. More Madden of Dublin read a paper on the same subject. He beheved death from post-partum flooding to be generally preventable, and thought that in the future it would be unknown. We may almost always obviate, though we cannot yet always arrest, flooding. The more children a woman has borne, the more likely she is to flood. When we have reason to anticipate hemorrhage, he had firm belief in the efficacy of a course of any astringent preparation of iron during the last months of pregnancy. In such cases in labour he would rupture the membranes early to allow the uterus to contract, and would give a dose of ergotine or fluid extract of ergot hypodermically before the head comes to press on the perineum. He beheved injection of both hot, cold and iced water to be unreliable. Injection of perchloride of iron was effectual, but dangerous. He strongly recommended the introduction of a sponge soaked in the solution of perchloride of iron to the uterus, and there retained till it and the hand in which it is held are expelled from the uterine cavity. When collapse had come on, he had little faith in transfusion, as now practised, but advocated instead hypodermic injection of ether in large doses, as recommended by Von Hecker of Munich. He believed he had seen it save a number of hopeless cases. The value of ether was also affirmed by Prof. Winckel of Dresden and others. The iron injections had a number of advocates in the Dublin School of Midwifery, and amongst others. All admitted its dangers, but considered that desperate cases justified its employment. Dr. Matthews Duncan regarded intra-uterine injection of perchloride of iron as more dangerous than the condition it was intended to obviate. Dr. McClintock thought that promptitude and energy in applying the remedies were of the greatest value. He admitted the danger of the perchloride of iron injections, but desperate cases required desperate remedies. He believed that chloroform to a considerable extent predisposed to hemorrhage. As a preventive, he had seen great benefit from gallic acid given a few days before labour. A number of the speakers emphasized the importance of preventive treatment by proper management of the third stage of labour. The great object is to keep the uterus duly contracted by pressure and friction during and for an hour after the expulsion of the placenta.

The celebrated Prof. Otto Spriegelberg of Breslau had prepared a paper on *Antisepsis in Midwifery*, but as he was unable to be present from illness (he has since died), it was read in abstract. He began by stating that the great reform in surgery brought about by the antiseptic treatment could not fail to have a deep influence upon the treatment of the complications in childbed, as it was well known long ago that the latter are the same as those which arose from wounds. If, however, scrupulous cleanliness, which had been advocated long ago, favoured a normal course of the puerperium, the practical gain was not very great. The idea that the puerperal wounds are infected, and the inflammations of the genital organs are initiated by germs coming from outside, became more in vogue, and in consequence, the idea that phlogogenous matter might be produced spontaneously within the genital tract was almost abandoned. The consequence of this idea was, recommending the most scrupulous cleanliness of hands and instruments; forbidding practitioners of midwifery to attend other patients; forbidding students who dissect from attending midwifery cases; and forbidding nurses attending cases of puerperal fever to attend normal cases at the same time. But these measures had but little effect in reducing the number of bad cases. This fact originated the idea of secondary antisepsis. Intra-uterine irrigations and drainage came into use, but without much avail. The failures can be understood. Lister's system is founded on the view justified by experience, that infection of wounds is caused by germs floating in the air around a wound, and falling on the recently made wounds. It is therefore necessary to clean the surroundings from germs; if that cannot be done, then to destroy the efficiency of these germs while the wound is open, and to keep the wound subsequently closed as much as possible. The application of these rules upon the puerperium means the strictest cleanliness and antisepsis during the time in which the puerperal wounds arise—that is, during birth—as well as from the part of the persons attending the mother as from the mother herself; prevention of air entering the genital tract, and as this cannot be done absolutely, disinfection by frequent vaginal irrigation with antiseptics during birth. After birth, care is to be taken to secure perfect rest for the genital tract, to encourage involution, avoiding every intra-vaginal or intra-uterine manipulation not absolutely necessary. If such be necessary, it must be done under antiseptic precautions. Antisepsis after the infection has taken place is not of much use. It is only directly useful in processes of decomposition, so long as they have not passed the surfaces of the tract, and not yet attacked the parenchyma of the organs. If this have occurred, antisepsis is not a trustworthy remedy, it is only palliative, since drainage and irrigation do not touch the deep seats of the disease, and do not remove or destroy the germs.

Prof. Winckel said that all the midwives under his direction were under instructions to keep all catheters, vaginal tubes, diapers for washing the genitals, &c., lying in a two per cent. solution of carbolic acid. Two per cent. carbolic oil is used to lubricate the finger.

Dr. Fancourt Barnes said that in the British Lying-in Hospital all his patients were delivered under the carbolic spray. The vagina was syringed with a one-to-forty solution. A one-to-eighty spray was always playing in the wards. All washings of the genitals were done with a one-to-eighty solution. The results showed great diminution of feverish attacks.

Dr. Graily Hewitt said that as regards prevention of introduction of septic matter from without, the rule should be to use the nail-brush assiduously in all midwifery cases. Many cases he thought were due to septic action from within. Some cases resulted from too complete rest on the back during the first few days after labour. Septic fluid collected in the vagina and was absorbed through lacerations that might exist. Dr. Goodell had done good service, he thought, by insisting on the necessity for drainage of the vagina by changing the position of the patient. An important point was to secure good uterine contraction. To secure this the patient's strength must be kept up by food of good quality.

Dr. Edis followed somewhat in the same strain.

Prof. Tarnier had made an experiment with reference to disinfectant solutions. He had placed pieces of placenta in the following solution: Liquor of Van Swieten (bichloride of mercury at one-thousandth), boric acid (forty grammes per litre), and in others. In all except the mercury and boric acid solutions, living organisms appeared in a few days. He had great confidence in the parasiticidal action of bichloride of mercury solution. Whenever he had reason to think his hands "suspicious," either at the hospital or at home, he washed them in the bichloride solution. His pupils did the same. No instance of mercurialism had occurred. To prevent implantation of the germs in the air into wounds produced at the moment of expulsion, he made the midwife anoint the fœtal hand with a one-tenth solution of carbolic acid each time it appears at the vulva. He thought this better than the spray, which was too cold for the patient.

Dr. J. Henry Bennet (Nice) read a paper on *Laceration of the Cervix Uteri: its causes and treatment.* Dr. Bennet agreed with Drs. Emmet and Pallen of New York and others as to the frequency of this lesion during labour. He had himself pointed out the fact so long ago as in 1849. He then stated that the principal cause was previous inflammation and induration of the cervix, non-softened during the latter period of pregnancy. This condition during labour gives rise to rigidity of the cervix, and subsequently to laceration. He had attended to many hundreds of such cases, slight and severe, and had never operated. He always found that under the treatment of the inflammatory state which attended them, the ulcerated edges healed, and all that was left was a mere notch.

Dr. Playfair (London) believed in the operation, and regretted that it had received so little consideration at the hands of British obstetricians. The fact that men like Emmet, Thomas, Pallen, Sims and Goodell performed it from deliberate conviction of the serious uterine disease it led to, spoke strongly in its favour. He had performed the operation himself with success.

Dr. Goodell had operated 107 times without a death, and with great benefit to nearly all the patients. Ectropion of the cervix could be cured by nothing but operation. He believed cancer of the cervix started from the raw irritated surface of a cervical rent. Acting on this knowledge, he had operated on a lacerated cervix when no constitutional symptoms were present, simply because cancer was hereditary in the patient's family.

Dr. J. Braxton Hicks (London) made some further remarks on the "Use of the Intermittent Contractions of the Pregnant Uterus as a means of Diagnosis." He referred to his paper published in the London Obstetrical Transactions for 1871, vol. xiii., p. 216, in which, after showing that the uterus contracted usually at intervals of from five to twenty minutes during the whole of pregnancy, and that these contractions were readily recognizable by the hand, he wished now to emphasize what he then said as to the value of the fact as a means of diagnosis. He gave difficult cases where the diagnosis had been set at rest. 1. Suspected extra-uterine pregnancy. 2. In hydramnios, where ovarian cyst was supposed to exist, and paracentesis abdominis had been performed through the uterine wall. 3. In cases of pregnancy where tumor was supposed to co-exist. 4. Hydramnios with twin conception. Dr. Matthews Duncan pointed out that the value of this sign as a diagnostic one was diminished by the fact that soft fibromas contracted quite as marked as the gravid uterus. Prof. Hennig (Leipzig) said the diagnosis was still more difficult when fibroma and pregnancy co-existed.

Dr. Robert Battey (Rome, Georgia) read a paper on Battey's Operation. He said: "The operation is peculiar, in that it has for its primary object, not the removal from the body of a diseased organ, but the abrogation of a physiological function. Whilst it is undoubtedly true that the ovaries extirpated, in the majority of instances, are structurally diseased, the end aimed at is not the removal of diseased ovaries, but it is the production of the change of life by art." He had foreseen the wide sphere of the operation in exceptional cases. To cover the ground fully, and give a key for the selection of suitable cases, it was proposed: "Ovariotomy to determine the change of life; and the change of life for any grave disease, which is incurable without it and which is curable with it." He thought the safest rule was embodied in the three questions: Is this a grave case? Is it incurable by any of the resources of art short of the change of life? Is it curable by the change of life? If all these three questions can be answered in the affirmative, the case is a proper one; but if not, the operation is not to be justified. The operation opens a door for wide-spread abuse. It is in no case to be received as an alternative for any other means of cure, but as a *dernier ressort*.

Operation—Mode of Access.—In America, both vaginal and abdominal methods are in use; in Europe, the abdominal alone finds favour. For the vaginal it is claimed (*a*) the mortality is less; (*b*) it favours perfect drainage; (*c*) less air is admitted to the peritoneal cavity; (*d*) the intestinal mass is but little exposed to mechanical irritation. The objections are the frequency of adhesion and the difficulty of dealing with them, and completely removing the ovaries. This, however, is an excellent method, and not to be abandoned in properly selected cases. *Dealing with the Pedicle*—The ligature, simple or carbolized, with ends cut short, is well-nigh universal. The author has in 13 instances severed the pedicle with the ecraseur alone; in no case was there troublesome hemorrhage. *Proximate results*—1st, Mortality—In the cases collected, the death-rate has been 22 per cent. for the complete operations and 9½ for the incomplete. 2nd, Menopause—It is well known that exceptionally after double ovariotomy the menses have reappeared, not occasionally only, but regular in occurrence and normal in characteristics. In none of these cases, however, has it been shown that a third or supplementary ovary did not exist, or that fragments of ovarian stroma were not left behind. In the author's cases, even when small fragments of the ovaries were left, the menses invariably continued, and in one instance a child was born. *Ultimate results*—1st, Aphrodisia—Patients on whom the operation has been performed have in no case complained of the loss of this power, but, on the contrary, have, in a number of instances, borne testimony to their full competency. 2nd, Female graces—These have not been impaired in any case, but a positive gain has often been noted. 3rd, General health—As the operation is proposed as a *dernier ressort* and in desperate cases, whatever of benefit is to be secured must be accounted actual gain. In a number of cases there was no benefit for a few months or a year or more, after which were much improved, and in some instances quite cured.

Dr. Savage of Birmingham also read a paper on the same subject. He gave a record of thirty successful operations during the last two years, for various conditions, which were detailed; ten were for long-standing and painful ovarian prolapse, and four for myoma. In these last-mentioned conditions the author thought there was a good field for successful and beneficial practice. In ovarian dysmenorrhœa, it is more difficult to come to a conclusion as to the cases where it will be most useful.

Dr. Priestley (London) thought favourably of the operation, especially in cases of myoma with hemorrhage. Mr. Knowsley Thornton had not had much experience; his results had been various. He thought there was a good field in the direction of the checking of hemorrhage by the operation. Mr. Lawson Tait (Birmingham) had operated 70 times, with a mortality of from 3.1 to 14.7 per cent., according to the class of cases. In two cases of epilepsy the results are extremely satisfactory. The secondary results, in the great majority of his cases, have been very satisfactory. He believes that complete removal of the Fallopian tubes, as well as of the ovaries, is most important in completely arresting menstruation. Drs. Pallen of New York and Goodell of Philadelphia had each performed the operation a good many times. Dr. Goodell believed the operation would be useful in insanity, with monthly exacerbations. Dr. Matthews Duncan differed from the general tenor of most of the speakers. He regarded the operation as being in the earliest experimental stage. He pointed out, with reference to oöphorectomy for bleeding uterine myomata, that a series of cases had been laid before the meeting by Mr. Lawson Tait, with five deaths in twenty-six cases. He knew of no such bad results in fibroids under any kind of treatment, and was sure that such disasters were unequalled in the history of the subject. As regards pain, for which the operation is sometimes performed, the sufferings of neurotic women were often exaggerated. He had seen patients by whom indescribable agonies had been endured during the day go to concerts and balls in the evening. He knew of no death from ovarian pain.

Dr. Graily Hewitt (London) read a paper on "The exciting cause of attacks of Hysteria and Hystero-Epilepsy." The object of the paper was to show, by the results of clinical observation, that in cases of hysteria and hystero-epilepsy, the exciting cause of the attacks is distortion of the uterus, produced by anteflexion or retroflexion. Irritation consisting in the physical compression and tension of the uterus, consequent on forcible bending of the organ, is reflected, and results in the attacks. The flexion further causes congestion of the whole organ from interference with the circulation. As evidence in support of his statements, the author recited eighteen cases of hysteria and hystero-epilepsy. In all, the uterus was markedly distorted. Complete relief from the attacks and hysterical symptoms was obtained by treatment directed to a removal of the uterine distortion· Of 18 cases, perfect relief is known to have been obtained in 17 cases. Of the 18, twelve were anteflexions and six retroflexions.

Dr. A. W. Edis (London) read a paper on "The Influence of Uterine Disorders in the production of numerous Sympathetic Disturbances of the General Health and Affections of Special Organs." Dr. Edis directed attention to the frequency of sick headache, often extending over many consecutive years, due entirely to some uterine disorder. This was shown by headaches of many years duration disappearing when some unsuspected uterine disorder was removed, other more general remedies having failed to give relief. The morning sickness of early pregnancy was shown to be frequently dependent upon some flexion, inflammatory condition of the body or cervix of the uterus, or some well-recognized uterine disorder. Relief was obtained by directing appropriate treatment to this latter condition. Uterine epilepsy frequently depended upon ovarian irritation, flexion producing dysmenorrhœa, or other well recognized form of uterine or ovarian disorder. Other neurosal affections, such as asthma, neuralgia, and chorea were not infrequently dependent on some overlooked uterine disorder. Amaurosis, asthenopia, and many other pathological conditions of the organs of vision, were often found to be due to morbid conditions of the uterus. Aphonia, spasm of the glottis, sensation of choking, and other similar reflex phenomena, were often traced to alteration in the position or condition of the uterus.

Dr. Mundé (New York) said it could hardly be doubted that displacements and flexions of the uterus often produce reflex nervous and neuralgic affections of different parts of the body, and more or less pronounced mental aberrations. But other diseases, such as areolar hyperplasia or choreic metritis, played quite as prominent, perhaps a more prominent part than flexions and displacements. He related a case in which laceration of the cervix appeared to be the cause of syncope during coition and digital examination. Compression of the ovarian region (Charcot) always roused the patient from her paroxysm, This and other hysterical phenomena were removed by Emmet's operation.—*American Journal of Obstetrics*, October, 1881, and *British Medical Journal*, Sept. 3, 1881.

Hospital Reports.

MEDICAL AND SURGICAL CASES OCCURRING IN THE PRACTICE OF THE MONTREAL GENERAL HOSPITAL.

MEDICAL CASES UNDER THE CARE OF DR. GEORGE ROSS.

Two Cases of Tubercular Meningitis.

CASE I.—A. R., female, aged 25, admitted into Hospital to be treated for headache, which had lasted two weeks. Family history good. Was a healthy girl till one year ago, when she began to ail; nothing definite about her illness at this time. Had a child six weeks ago.

No definite history can be obtained of her present illness, except it has lasted two weeks. At present she lies in bed with her eyes closed, moaning lowly as if in pain. When questioned, rouses up and answers apparently in a rational manner, but makes contradictory statements. Says she has been ill fourteen days, with pain in head, back and limbs, and unable to move in bed. As she lies in bed moaning, her hand is frequently raised to her head, as if in pain. During the night was very noisy and restless, and made frequent attempts to get out of bed. By turns she would cry, laugh, or scream out as if frightened. Toward morning, slept for four hours.

Patient is a thin, sallow woman, with sunken eyes. Lies principally on right side, with eyes closed, though, when told to, will open them readily, when it is seen that the right lid does not open quite so wide as the left. Pupils equal and about normal size; respond readily to light. Tongue heavily coated. Abdomen retracted. Bowels constipated. No vomiting. Patient asks for anything she wants, and swallows without difficulty. Tache cerebrale well marked. No paralysis except that noticed in right upper lid. Appears to be general hyperæsthesia. Temperature 100°F.; pulse 96, regular, small and weak; respirations 24. Nothing abnormal found in lungs or heart. Urine throws down a very small deposit containing pus; no casts; slight trace of albumen.

Dec. 9th.—The hyperæsthesia spoken of above is perhaps not correct; her cries when touched appear to be due to great nervous irritability. No further evidence of paralysis. No change in delirium. To have Potass. Iod. gr. v; Potass. Bromid. gr. x; 4 q. h. *11th.*—For last few hours has been quiet, evidently becoming comatose; up to that time delirium remained as on first day. Bowels well moved by a purgative; stool passed in bed. Urine retained to-day for first time. Pulse very weak and small, 126; temperature 100°F. *12th.*—Becoming more comatose; cannot now be roused. Pupils equal, dilated and oscillating. Pulse 150; temperature 103° F. Lungs normal. Sinking rapidly. *13th.*—Died early this morning.

Autopsy.—Brain: Membranes at base much infiltrated, turbid and œdematous. Matting and some thickening of pia in Sylvian fissures, and numerous small, grey granulations could be seen scattered over the membrane. On removing the arteries and washing in water. many small fusiform enlargements could be easily detected with the naked eye, and with the microscope presented the usual appearance of miliary tubercles. A considerable quantity of fluid in ventricles; marked central softening; fornix and septum quite diffluent. *Lungs* crepitant throughout; no tubercles. One small cretaceous nodule in middle lobe of right lung. *Heart* normal. Abdominal viscera presented nothing special; no miliary tubercles. *Kidneys* enlarged, and presented many greyish-white elevations beneath the capsule. On section, presented (1) localized caseous abscesses; (2) extensive areas of disease in the apices of pyramids; (3) pyelitis; a large part of the mucosa on each pelvis presented a thickened infiltrated appearance and a rough, caseous surface. Each ureter was in much the same state. Bladder normal.

Case II.—C. M., aged 37, admitted to Hospital Dec. 5, 1881. Present illness began November 25th with a chill, followed by severe vomiting and headache. Vomiting lasted four days; headache continued bad till December 2nd, when he began to wander a little in his mind, but would still give an intelligent answer when spoken to; bowels very constipated. Since admission lies almost constantly quiet in bed with closed eyes. On being questioned answers rationally, but slowly and hesitatingly, and cannot depend on his answers to questions about his previous history. Makes no complaint of pain anywhere; says he has no headache, no evidence of paralysis. Urine obtained by catheter is very scanty, sp. gr. 1024; no sugar or albumen. Right lung, nothing abnormal found. At base of left lung from lower angle of scapula down is dullness, with feeble breathing. Front and axilla normal; tongue dry and heavily coated; abdomen retracted.

Dec. 7th.—Not much change in condition since his admission except that he is rather more delirious. Can still be roused and will answer questions though in a dull, dazed manner. Temperature, 100°F.; pulse, 84, small and weak; respiration, 28; optic disks slightly congested.

Dec. 8th.—Was very delirious last night, talking continually and attempting to get out of bed. If allowed to walk, staggers always to right and is inclined to fall backward and to right. No paralysis of face or extemities; ancle clonus well marked on left side; not present on right. Bowels not moved since admission; urine has to be drawn off; no change in condition of lungs; pulse, 88; respiration, 32; temperature, 99°.

Dec. 9th.—Continued delirious during night but this morning became suddenly cyanotic and inclined to coma. Respirations increased to between 50 and 60; pulse so small that could not be counted, about 150 to minute; large bubbling râles all over front of chest; right pupil dilated more than left. Patient is quite unconscious and evidently sinking fast. Died at 10 P.M. quite comatose.

Autopsy—Brain: Much sercsity escaped in removal. Base infiltrated; membranes turbid and present many small miliary tubercles, particularly in the Sylvian fissures. There was no congealed lymph or purulent exudation. Ventricles were dilated and septum very soft. *Lungs.*—Universally adherent. At base of left lung pleura was much thickened, and there were numerous flakes of yellowish white lymph, dry and firm. The base of this lung was collapsed, the rest of it and the right one crepitated. On section both are thickly studded with small grey tubercles, chiefly isolated but here and there in groups. No cavities and only two small cheesy masses in the apex of left lung; heart normal. No tubercles in abdominal organs; *spleen* a little enlarged; kidneys healthy.

Reviews and Notices of Books.

Photographic Illustrations of Cutaneous Syphilis.—By GEORGE HENRY FOX, A.M., M.D., Clinical Lecturer on Diseases of the Skin, College of Physicians and Surgeons, New York. Surgeon to the New York Dispensary, Department of Skin and Venereal Diseases. Nos. X, XI and XII. New York: E. B. Treat.

These three numbers complete this admirable and original work. The high artistic merit which has characterized the previous numbers is maintained in these. They illustrate the following conditions, viz.:—Syphiloderma Ulcerativum, Chancre, Chancroid, Periadenitis, Condylomata lata, Syphilis hereditaria, and Dactylitis Syphilitica. In concluding our notice of this atlas of cutaneous Syphilides we can only once more congratulate the author upon the excellence of the work, which furnishes a far more real and reliable illustration of these disorders than any other similar set of plates extant, and we would advise every one interested in these highly-important affections to furnish himself with a copy.

Essentials of the Principles and Practice of Medicine: A Handbook for Students and Practitioners.—By HENRY HARTSHORNE, A.M., M.D., lately Professor of Hygiene in the University of Pennsylvania; Editor of American Edition of "Reynolds' System of Medicine," &c. Fifth edition, thoroughly revised and improved; with 144 illustrations. Philadelphia: H. C. Lea's Son & Co. Montreal: Dawson Brothers.

This is a concentrated extract of a text-book upon medicine.

to be carefully traversed in this treatise. Although the scientific descriptions of the development of the ovum and the changes in the uterus are very thorough and complete, it may, perhaps, still more interest the practical physician to know that its greatest excellence consists in the admirable manner in which the chapters on the art of successful delivery are conceived and written. Nothing which it is useful for the practitioner of midwifery to know is lost sight of in the directions for managing labour of all kinds, as well as those troublesome accidents, abortions. Not only so, but copious references are given to native and foreign authors for all important statements made, so that any one may for himself refer for confirmation and further information to these authorities. We know of no modern work which can be more conscientiously recommended both to students and to physicians.

Transactions of the American Gynecological Society. Vol. V. For the year 1880. Boston: Houghton, Mifflin & Co.

This elegantly-prepared volume comes to hand containing as usual an immense amount of carefully elaborated matter. The papers are many and of varied interest, covering great part of the ground of all the questions at present occupying the minds of those specially occupied in this particular branch of Medical Science. Amongst the numerous articles we can only select a few for special mention: "What is the proper field for Battey's operation?" by Dr. Robert Battey. This question of course is one of the unsettled ones of the day. The author endeavors to explain more fully the boundaries of suitable cases which he had hitherto limited by insisting upon affirmative answers to the three following questions: (1.) Is this a grave case? (2.) Is it incurable by other means? (3.) Is it reasonable to expect a cure by this method? The treatment of uterine enlargement by massage applied to the womb is introduced by Dr. Jackson, of Chicago, and is made the subject of considerable discussion. Dr. George J. Engelman, of St. Louis, contributes a paper on "Posture in Labour," in which he studies with much minuteness and after great research the various positions habitually assumed by the women of different races during the act of parturition. This treatise is illustrated by a large number of outline woodcuts. It is of interest in many respects and leads the writer to the conclusion that the decubitus usually adopted in England and Continental countries is wrong and should be modified. Some curious stories were related by those who joined in the discussion. Amongst others, this one: A woman in her 60th year was to be confined of her 18th child. She declared she would not be delivered till she was in the lap of her husband. She weighed 250 lbs. and her husband only 95 lbs. The Doctor insisted that she should have her baby without the aid of the old man and like other women. At the end of sixty hours he was obliged to give up and the little old crooked-back husband was brought in and put into a chair, and the old woman was put into his lap, and they had the baby in a trice! Dr. Chadwick's observations on the value of the hot rectal douche are already widely known. The volume concludes, as always, with a complete list of Gynecological and Obstetric Journals, and a "Gynecological Index," giving references to the whole of the world's literature on this branch for the year. This volume is fully equal in every respect to any of its predecessors. We can only regret that it is not possible to have it appear earlier in the year succeeding the annual meeting.

A Text-book of Physiology.—By MICHAEL FOSTER, M.A., M.D., F.R.S. Second American from the third and revised English edition; with extensive notes and additions by E. T. REICHERT, M.D., Demonstrator of Experimental Therapeutics, University of Pennsylvania. Philadelphia: Henry C. Lea's Son & Co. 1881.

It is gratifying to see that Dr. Foster's work is being appreciated in America. Let us hope that the exhaustion of a large edition within a year means the acquisition of a solid knowledge of the laws of life by many hundreds of the young students throughout the country. Praise of the book is at this date superfluous. Dr. Reichert's additions are just such as were needed for the general wants of the American student who wishes to have the histology and physiology in one volume. On the whole, his part is well done. There are not many changes of importance in this edition, though in places we notice the sections have been rearranged and new woodcuts inserted. Why Pfluger's figure of termination of nerve fibres in cells of salivary glands? Who believes it? We should like to have seen the sources of the drawings more generally acknowledged. McMillan & Co.'s American edition from their New York house has evidently been run off the field. It was a foreign bantling, and no wonder it could not thrive in the absence of the gentle touch of a native editor. Let us hope that Dr. Foster will receive something more substantial than praise to remind him of the success of his book in America.

Books and Pamphlets Received.

ON SPERMATORRHŒA: ITS PATHOLOGY, RESULTS AND COMPLICATIONS. By J. L. Milton. Eleventh edition. London: Henry Renshaw.

THE OPIUM-HABIT AND ALCOHOLISM. A treatise on the habits of Opium and its compounds, Alcohol, Chloral-Hydrate, Chloroform, Bromide Potassium, and Canabis Indica, including their therapeutical indications. By Dr. Fred. Heman Hubbard. New York: A. S. Barnes & Co.

THE PREVENTION OF STRICTURE AND OF PROSTATIC OBSTRUCTION. By Reginald Harrison, F.R.C.S. London: J. & A. Churchill.

FAVOURITE PRESCRIPTIONS OF DISTINGUISHED PRACTITIONERS. With Notes on Treatment. By B. W. Palmer, A.M., M.D. New York: Bermingham & Co.

A STUDY OF THE TUMOURS OF THE BLADDER. With original contributions and drawings. By Alex. W. Stein, M.D. New York: Wm. Wood & Co.

Extracts from British and Foreign Journals.

Unless otherwise stated the translations are made specially for this Journal.

Uterine Chloasma, in Contrast With Addison's Disease.—GENTLEMEN—I will call your attention to-day to an obscure case sent to us for diagnosis, a case which has been very perplexing, and which, I am sure, will be of great interest to you. The patient, Jennie C——, is forty-one years of age, of Scotch extraction, and married. Her family record is good, free from any syphilitic, tuberculous, cancerous, or other taint; and there is no history of any exposure to unusual hardships or anxieties. She has never had any children. She always enjoyed good health until the outset of the present illness, which began twenty-one years ago, or one year after marriage, and without any apparent cause. It commenced with a feeling of general weakness, pain in the back and abdomen, and a profuse muco-purulent discharge from the vagina. The weakness did not cause her to go to bed, but made her indisposed to perform any active household duties. There was decided loss of flesh. Ten years later, the symptoms still continuing, but subject to periods of improvement and relapse, she noticed, for the first time, an arched band of bronzed skin on the forehead, and shortly afterward patches of the same color appeared on the cheeks and abdomen. With the appearance of this discoloration there was no alteration in the other symptoms, for the pain in the back and the sense of weakness were still felt, and the loss of flesh had not been regained. During the last ten years her condition has gradually grown worse. The weakness and emaciation have slowly progressed, the discoloration of the skin has become more marked, and the pain in the back more intense. In addition to these, she has suffered during the last eight months from several attacks of palpitation of the heart, and has fainted a number of times without any apparent cause. The weakness complained of has been greater at some times than at others, and has presented remarkable fluctuations, but always with a tendency to become worse. The periods of weakness would come on without any evident cause, and would generally last three days.

The emaciation has been subject to no fluctuations, but has been steady and progressive. The appetite and digestion have been poor, the bowels occasionally loose, but not sufficient to produce the weakness and wasting.

Careful examination of the patient yesterday disclosed no disease whatever of the nervous system, nor any sign of any pulmonary lesion. The heart is healthy, the pulse moderate in frequency and strength. The lymphatic system presents nothing abnormal, and the liver and spleen are of natural size.

The urine is acid in reaction, and a special gravity of 1·017, and is free from either albumen, sugar, or any deposit. The uterus is enlarged, congested, and retroverted. Its cavity measures three inches in length. The left ovary is prolapsed, and lies behind the body of the uterus. The catamenia are regular, last three days, but are attended with pain. The blood, as drawn from her finger and examined by my assistant, is paler than usual, from diminution of its colouring matter; but an enumeration of the blood-corpuscles with a hemacytometer, shows one cubic millimetre of blood to contain 4,450,000 red cells, and 1 white cell to 224 red ones, which, you know, is about normal. The discoloration of the skin is quite evident. There is a bronzed arch on the forehead and patches of like colour on the cheeks. The backs of the hands and forearms are also discolored. These patches, the patient says, vary in shade from day to day, and are separated, you see, from the naturally coloured skin, by a distinct line of demarcation. There is no discolouration of the axillæ, nor around the nipples, nor at the flexures of the joints. Lastly, there is decided weakness and emaciation.

I have been especially particular in detailing these symptoms, gentlemen, because you will appreciate their value and importance when we endeavor to arrive at a diagnosis. The case is, as you no doubt perceive, an obscure one, and yet upon its correct diagnosis will, of course, depend the treatment to be pursued, and the amount of good that we can do our patient.

The discolouration of the skin is the sign that would first attract your attention, and this, in conjunction with the progressive weakness and emaciation, would immediately raise the query: Have we to deal with a case of Addison's disease? But you should be aware, gentlemen, that a like discolouration of the skin sometimes occurs in chronic diseases of the liver, spleen, stomach, uterus, intestines, or peritoneum, due to long-continued irritation of the abdominal sympathetic centres. Hence, in a case such as the one before us, we should be careful to search for the existence of any local irritation of the abdominal organs, to study the progress of the disease, and to analyze most minutely the various symptoms present. Addison described the disease which now bears his name, as a progressive, idiopathic anæmia, accompanied by a general languor and extreme debility (but without much loss of flesh), and by a bronze discolouration of the skin. The heart's action he stated to be remarkably feeble, the pulse weak, much shortness of breath to occur on the slightest exertion, and death to result from asthenia in the course of from one to several years. It is a disease essentially of the suprarenal capsules, bodies without any definitely known function. They become the seat of a chronic inflammation, are enlarged, and later undergo a cheesy degeneration, and their capsules thicken.

Lying in close contact to the semilunar ganglia and their nerve-prolongations, a constant irritation of these great centres is produced; it is by reference to the long-continued irritation of their numerous and varied plexuses that the different symptoms, such as pigmentation of the skin, palpitation of the heart, dyspepsia, breathlessness upon exertion, etc., are to be explained. The cheesy mass may also act as a centre of infection, and occasionally tuberculosis may result.

Having given the symptoms of Addison's disease, let me again direct your attention to the case before us, so that we may compare the two, and see in what they differ. The bronzing in the patient here is not uniform or diffused, but is separated from the naturally coloured skin by distinct lines of demarcation; it has not progressed, and there is no discolouration around the joints, umbilicus, genitals, or armpits. It is true that, in cases of discolouration of the skin due to chronic disease of the abdominal viscera, it is usually limited to the face and abdomen, and does not, as in this instance, occur on the hands. But this is not a constant rule. I have known almost universal bronzing of the skin to attend chronic peritonitis, without any disease of the capsules; while, on the other hand, in the present case there are no purplish spots on the mucous membrane of the mouth, and no bronzing about the genitals or flexures of the joints. The latter points are of value as being unlike what are apt to occur in true Addison's disease.

The feeling of debility has not been so extreme as in the latter disease; the tendency to palpitation of the heart has been very slight; and the gastric disturbances have been very mild. Lastly, the patient has chronic endometritis with prolapse of an ovary, with which condition there is often associated such irritation of the abdominal sympathetic ganglia as to prove the source of weakness and debility.

Progressive, causeless, and irregular debility (not accompanied with marked loss of flesh) is the most prominent symptoms of this peculiar disease of the suprarenal capsules. The prostration and loss of muscular power cannot be explained by any functional disturbance that a patient may present, nor will diligent inquiry find any special lesion as a cause of the constitutional change. It seems that in the case before us we can develop a debility not due to any organic disease except a chronic endometritis with prolapse of an ovary. Now, in some women, a slight uterine catarrh will produce marked debility and disturbance of health, whereas in others a more serious disease of the womb will cause no bad symptoms whatever. Again, we have the weakness in our patient accompanied with emaciation, while in Addison's disease the latter is not at all commensurate with the former. In Addison's disease we usually have vomiting, dyspepsia, or other symptoms of a disordered condition of the stomach; but in this case, although there has been some irritability of the stomach, it has been very slight, and the uterine condition is sufficient to explain it. Palpitation of the heart, feeble pulse, and breathlessness upon exertion, have not been at all prominent in the present case, as they are in disease of the suprarenal capsules; and those attacks which have occurred the morbid state of the uterus could readily produce. I would ask especial attention to the analysis of the blood in this case. The state of this fluid differs greatly in different cases of Addison's disease. As will have been seen, Addison regarded the disease as essentially one of progressive anæmia; and so in some cases there is a very marked degree of anæmia, probably due to some deteriorating influence by the focus of degenerating exudation and to the reflex disorders of digestion. But in other cases the force of the disease expends itself on the nervous connections of the suprarenal bodies, and the composition of the blood undergoes but little change. Hence it is evident, that no diagnostic importance can be attached to the absence of anæmia in the present case. Lastly, the course of Addison's disease extends over a period of from two to five years. while the woman before you has been ill twenty-one years.

The case, gentlemen, you perceive is not clearly defined, but lies, as I may say, on the border-line. I think, however, that from the careful analysis and differentiation of its history, symptoms, and progress which have been made, we are safe in considering it as one of uterine chloasma with debility, due to chronic endometritis and prolapse of an ovary.

The prognosis, therefore, is favourable, and the woman will be benefitted by local treatment applied to the womb, for which purpose she will be placed under the care of my colleague, the Professor of Gynecology. In addition to this, careful attention must be paid to her diet and mode of life, and internally a course of ferruginous tonics must be directed. Among the best of these would be:

℞. Acid. phosphorici diluti,
Tr. ferri chloridi - - - - - - āā f. ℥j.

M. Sig.—Twenty to forty drops in a wineglassful of water, through a glass tube, three times daily, after meals.

Or,

℞. Elix. ferri pyrophosphat., quiniæ et
strychniæ - - - - - - - - - f. ℥ ij.

Sig.—Teaspoonful after meals, in water.

Hence you see the importance of a direct diagnosis in such cases.

In Addison's disease there is no direct line of treatment, as we have no means by which we can influence the morbid process in the suprarenal capsules, and our remedial measures are consequently only palliative. I will merely indicate the leading ones. They are as follows: 1st, Rest. Especially during the periods of intense weakness, which occur at irregular intervals during the course of the disease. 2nd, Regulation of the diet; only nourishing and easily assimilated food, such as milk, soups, eggs, farinaceæ, and oysters, should be allowed. 3rd, Counter-irritation over the region of the suprarenal capsules by irritating liniments and dry cups; but, best of all, by the actual cautery. 4th, Electricity—either the faradic or galvanic current may be used. 5th, The use of alteratives. Minute doses of bichloride of mercury, iodide of potassium, nitrate of silver, and arsenic, have seemed to do good. Cod liver oil, iron, extract of malt, and the hypophosphites, may be used to influence nutrition, but exert no influence over the morbid process proper. 6th, All specifics are without value.—*Dr. Pepper in N. Y. Medical Record.*

Frothing Urine.—Dr. Southey, in his valuable Lumleian lectures on Bright's disease, has quoted the aphorism of Hippocrates, to the effect that "bubbles maintained upon the top of the urine signify a disease of the reins, and likewise its long continuance," a fact, Dr. Southey remarks, which remained "unimportant until the end of the last century, when it was ascertained that albuminous urine held a froth of bubbles on its surface." That the persistent presence of air-bubbles on the surface of urine may be noted in most cases of albuminuria is undoubted; but, since the same condition occurs in a variety of other cases, it cannot be relied on as a test of the presence of albumen in urine; and, when so interpreted, it will in many cases prove misleading, and give rise to unnecessary alarm. I have frequently met with urines which have retained a froth on their surface, from the moment of being passed for 12 and even 24 hours, and which have not contained a trace of albumen. I have at the present time two cases under my care in this town (San Remo); the one of diabetes, and the other of dyspepsia. The froth in the diabetic case is certainly not due to decomposition of the sugar, since the froth forms upon it immediately it is voided; while the only noticeable features in the second case are, that the urine contains an excess of earthy phosphates, and its acidity is beyond the normal standard. I believe that the occurrence of retained and persistent air-bubbles on the surface of urine is always of pathological significance;

and that their presence, when rightly understood, is capable of affording valuable practical information, although, so far as I am aware, the subject has not hitherto been followed out with the requisite care and minuteness. In some cases the frothing appears to be connected with the high density of the urine; in others, with its feeble acidity or alkalinity; and again, in others, with an excess of mucous.—*Arthur Hill Hassall, M.D., in the British Medical Journal.*

Aural Affections in Exanthematic Diseases.—In the *Archiv fur Ohrenheilkunde*, Vol. XVI, Dr. Gottstein has a paper on this subject. He refers to the rarity of observations, by competent observers, of the earlier stages of the ear diseases which occur during the exanthemata. From the statistics of Burckhardt Merian it is seen that of all the cases of ear disease which were referred to the exanthemata, but 16 to 18 per cent. were seen within the first six months of their development; and Gottstein's own statistics are not any more favorable for the observation of the acute stages of disease, and for the determination of the question of how the great destruction which is so often seen in such cases occurs. Wreden, of St. Petersburg, from his connection with the large children's hospital of that city, had most unusual opportunities for early observations. He has reported diphtheritic inflammation of the middle ear as very common in scarlet fever, but his observations have not been confirmed by others, as Gottstein thinks, owing to the ear disease being seen only in its later stages. According to Wreden, the diphtheritic exudation continues only fourteen days, and is succeeded by suppuration, the stage in which the disease usually comes under treatment. As contributions to this subject, Gottstein narrates three cases—one of croupous inflammation of the velum, pharnyx, nose, and both middle ears, in the second week of scarlet fever; one of diphtheria of the throat, with diphtheritic inflammation of the left tympanum, in the second week of measles; and one of acute desquamative inflammation of both tympanic membranes, with perforating tympanic inflammation, in the course of measles. In the first case, two days after the appearance of diphtheritic membranes in the pharnyx and nose, great deafness was noticed, and examination showed diphtheritic membranes over both drumheads, which were already perforated, and the same exudation covered the tympanic mucous membrane. From the history, the presence of membrane first in the nose and later within the tympanum, Gottstein concludes that the exudative process extended up through the Eustachian tube to the tympanum and produced the destruction from within outward. In the second case, soon after the appearance of diphtheritic membranes on the uvula, palate, and tonsils, great deafness, without pain or discharge, was noticed in the left ear, and the deeper meatus was found to be covered by similar membrane. After removal of this, the membrana tympani was found perforated and the tympanic cavity in a state of suppuration, but without any membranous deposit, and Gottstein feels uncertain whether the exudation of the ear was an extension from the pharnyx or was an independent deposit. In regard to the treatment of diphtheria, Gottstein has never seen the diphtheritic process shortened by cauterization, and considers that therapeutic efforts should be directed to removal of the exudation and to disinfection of the mucous membrane. He advises prolonged baths in aqua calcis, and powdering the diseased surfaces, after removal of the membranes, with salicylic acid.—*Medical and Surgical Reporter*.

Suprapubic Lithotomy.—Langenbuch of Berlin advocates this method in preference to all others in removing stone, claiming that the risk of wounding the peritoneum is not so great as is supposed, and that the antiseptic method is applicable, whereas in perineal lithotomies it is hardly possible to carry out the details of that method vigorously, in consequence of the anus being so near the wound. Of 478 cases of suprapubic lithotomy, collected by Dr. Dulles, only 13 were complicated by a wounded peritoneum, three of which were fatal. The author showed that a stone weighing more than two ounces could be extracted with less risk by the high than by the perineal method. The comparative advantages of perineal and suprapubic lithotomy are considered by the author, who states that urinary infiltration of connective tissue, it is pointed out, is a danger common to both operations, which, however, in the high operation can be prevented. The danger of this infiltration when it has occurred is much less after the high than after the perineal operation, since the epicystic is more accessible and less confined than the periprostatic and circumrectal connective tissue; can be more readily incised and disinfected, and, as it is not connected with any large venous plexus, is less likely, through its decomposition, to set up general septic infection. In the high operation the incisions can be made carefully and precisely, and through structures that are freely exposed to view, and there is no necessity for forcible laceration and contusion of connective tissues and other soft parts. It may be said the author suggests that it is as difficult to set up urinary infiltration after the high operation as it is to prevent such infiltration after lithotomy by the perineum. For the removal of a large stone—one with the maximum diameter of about two inches—the safest proceeding, Langenbuch thinks, is the high operation performed in two stages and under strict antiseptic conditions. To meet the case of a monster stone, measuring from 4 to 7 inches in diameter, the extraction of which in the second stage of the high operation would probably cause much laceration of the recently healed superficial parts, and also of the peritoneal fold, he proposes a complicated proceeding. In the first stage, the anterior surface of the bladder is freed to some extent of its layer of peritoneum, and a plastic operation is performed on this membrane. In the second stage—that of extraction performed after an interval of from five to eight days—elaborate preparations are taken to disinfect the bladder.—*Boston Med. & Surg. Journal.*

A New Theory of Uræmia.—MM. Feltz and Ritter have recently announced that the real cause of uræmia is a change in the proportional quantity of potassa in the blood. The amount of the potassic salts in the blood, as in the urine, varies with the quantity and quality of the food. A special alimentation, in which the sodic salts preponderate, long-continned, has the same effect upon the quantity of the salts of potassium, as a poor and insufficient diet. The quantity of the salts of potassium contained in the blood influences in a certain degree the amount of urea necessary to produce grave or fatal results. Suppression of the renal function by the simultaneous ligation of the ureters determines in the blood and in the serum a sensible increase in the potassic salts except the supplementary gastro-intestinal excretion. In this respect the alkaline salts obey the same law as urea and extractive matters, which increase in the blood under the same conditions. The most serious results of experimental uræmia are not connected with the retention and accumulation in the blood of the urea or extractive matters of the urine, but, on the contrary, are produced by the injection of fresh, normal urine,.or of equivalent solutions of the salts of potassium in distilled water. We think it must be admitted that the real agents of the toxæmia are the salts of potassium which accumulate in the blood.—*Bull. Gèn. de Thèrap.*, *Sept.* 15, 1881. *Medical News.*

Acute Diabetes Mellitus.—Dr. George Harley states in his work on the urine and its derangements, that "there are such things as *acute*, as well as *intermittent diabetes*," and quotes briefly from a report made by Dr. Noble in the *British Medical Journal*, January 17, 1863, of two cases of the former: one a boy of seventeen years of age, who died three days after the disease was discovered, and only a few weeks after he first felt ill; the other, a young lady, who died on the tenth day after the nature of her malady had been diagnosed.

Dr. Brunton, in Reynolds' "System of Medicine," says: "Cases have been recorded in which the disease seemed to run a course of only a few weeks before phthisis set in," but Dr. Noble's report is the only one I can now find in several treatises on diabetes mellitus, where the disease ran its course with such shocking celerity. This being so, it must be of interest to the profession to hear one other detailed, which came under my notice last Thursday, and terminated fatally within sixty hours.

M. C——, a young man thirty-two years of age, tall and stout, weighing in health 240 lbs., came to my office for treatment an the afternoon of December 8th, complaining of what he called malaria, and for which he said he had taken quinine without benefit. He was then in a state of exhaustion, with a tongue dry and irritant as a rasp, and tortured by fiercest thirst. Upon inquiry, I learned his health had been excellent to within three weeks, when, without apparent cause, he began to pass enormous quantities of urine, and consume an extraordinary amount of liquid. He had lost 25 lbs. in weight in about fifteen days. His appetite had not failed him until two days before, when the bowels had been moved copiously, after taking repeated cathartic doses to overcome an obstinate constipation, since which time he has lost all desire for food, and felt more than usually wretched. His breath had an odor of hay. He stated that, when voiding urine, if a drop should fall upon his boot or clothing it would leave a white spot, and showed me several recent spots on a corner of his overcoat.

I found the urine to have a specific gravity of 1040, and with the copper test to show a large amount of sugar. Examined since, under the microscope, abundant crystals of diabetic sugar have been exhibited.

My patient called at the office on Friday, but was now in an almost incoherent condition, skin hot and dry, heart labouring hard, nausea, constipation, excessive diuresis. He told me he had probably passed twenty pints of urine, as nearly as he could estimate, during the past twenty-four hours. I directed him to return home at once and remain there, continuing the prescribed treatment, with supporting measures added, when I would call and see him the next morning.

During the night he ate ravenously of ice, and, ascertained by subsequent measurement, passed about a pint of urine every hour until 3 A.M., when, being hastily summoned, I found him vomiting, breathing heavily between whiles, sighing, and in great apprehension of mind. He complained of gastric pain, probably caused by the ice, which, with the vomiting, was soon ameliorated. Calling again at 9 A.M., I found he had taken hourly doses of medicine, and, in answer to my questions, stated he felt better. No more urine had been passed. At 2 P.M. Drs. Arrowsmith and Hodges met me in consultation. The patient was in profound coma when we reached the house, and died in that condition at 3 A.M. on Sunday, the 11th inst., sixty hours after his disease was first diagnosed. His system did not respond to galvunism, revulsives, or hypodermic measures after coma began. I introduced a catheter into the bladder, but drew off only about eight ounces of urine, and a subsequent use of the catheter some hours afterward did not bring so much.

Any intelligent physician will see that, in a case sliding so rapidly into the grave, scarcely any of the remedies appropriate to saccharine diabetes could be used. The appetite being gone entirely, it was useless to speak of diatetic measures, and beyond tonics, acids, and supporting measures, there was scarcely time to look about one before life had hurried away. No autopsy was obtainable.—*Dr. Welch in N. Y. Med. Record.*

Primitive Physic.—It is curious to think of a whole religious organization medicinally treated according to the notions of the founder of the sect. Yet this is precisely what happened to the English Methodists. John Wesley was not content with caring, as he only could, for the souls of his followers, but he thought that it was within the line of his duty to care for their bodies. He therefore prepared and published his "Primitive Physic: or, an Easy and Natural Method of Curing Most Diseases." The book had a tremendous sale among the connection. My edition, dreadfully shabby, looking as if some of the reverend man's medicine had been spilled upon it, is the twenty-fourth; it was published in London in 1792, and it was "sold by George Whitfield, at the Chapel City Road, and at all the Methodist Preaching Houses in town and country." Wesley takes care to assert in his preface that "love of God, as it is the sovereign remedy of all miseries, so in particular it effectually prevents all the bodily disorders the passions introduce, by keeping the passions themselves within due bounds." Wesley had gathered together from old wives and highly religious old valetudinarians, a quantity of the most hopeless prescriptions which were ever entertained by the votaries of dosing. He is good enough to omit from his list of remedies "the four Herculean medicines—opium, bark, steel, and mercury, together with antimony." So much the better, it may have been, for the Methodists of the period, and of subsequent periods, down to those who bought the twenty-fourth edition of the "Primitive Physic."

His prescriptions, as a rule, are singularly speculative. For the ague he orders "a large onion, slit, to be applied to the stomach." For the tertian ague, he directs that a plaster of molasses and soot shall be applied to each wrist; for apoplexy a handful of salt in a pint of cold water, poured down the throat of the patient. This remedy is also sovereign "for one who seems dead by a fall." "For a convulsive cough, eat preserved walnuts; for deafness, put a little salt into the ear; for dropsy, drink six quarts of cider every day; for the falling sickness (epilepsy ?), drink half a pint of tar water, morning and evening; for the gravel, eat largely of spinach; for the headache, take a little of the juice of the horse-radish." Wesley even prescribed for lunacy. The patient, however crazy, had only to take "a decoction of agrimony four times a day." If this did not collect his scattered wits he was to rub his head several times a day with an infusion of ground ivy leaves and vinegar. For "raging madness," the patient "was to be set under a great water-fall as long as his strength conld bear." This is varied by a recommendation to "pour water on his head out of a tea-kettle." The most wonderful of Wesley's prescriptions are those which he gives for old age, a disease which has not usually been regarded as curable. The octogenarian is to drink tar water morning and evening: he is to chew cinnamon daily; he is to swallow a decoction of nettles. Much of what he recommends would either prove inert or injurious.—"*Recollections of a Reader,*" *in N. Y. Tribune.—Coll. and Clin. Record.*

Milk.—Dr. Dyce Duckworth, in the *Popular Science Monthly*, says: "Milk is a food that should not be taken in copious draughts like beer or other fluids, which differ from it chemically. If we consider the use of milk in infancy, the physiological ingestion, that is, of it, we find that the sucking babe imbibes, little by little, the natural food provided for it. Each small mouthful is secured by effort, and slowly presented to the gastric mucous surface for the primal digestive stages. It is thus regularly and gradually reduced to curd, and the stomach is not oppressed with a lump of half-coagulated milk. The same principle should be regarded in the case of the adult. Milk should be slowly taken in mouthfuls, at short intervals, and thus it is rightly dealt with by the gastric juice. If milk be taken after other food, it is almost sure to burden the stomach, and to cause discomfort and prolonged indigestion, and this, for the obvious reason that there is insufficient digestive agency to dispose of it. And the better the quality of the milk, the more severe the discomfort will be under these conditions. Milk is insufficiently used in making simple puddings of such farinaceous foods as rice, tapioca, and sago. Distaste for these is engendered very often, I believe, because the milk is stinted in making them, or poor, skimmed milk is used. Abundance of new milk should be employed, and more milk, or cream, should be added when they are taken. In Scottish households this matter is well understood, and a distinct pudding-plate, like a small soup-plate, is used for this course. The dry messes commonly served as milky puddings in England are exactly fitted to create disgust for what should be a most excellent and delicious part of a wholesome dinner for both children and adults."

On Tapping the Bladder from the Perinæum through the Hypertrophied Prostate.—Tapping the bladder is an operation which is not often necessary; I believe it may occasionally be resorted to even when a catheter can be passed. Assuming it to be required, how is it to be done? Tapping with the aspirator-needle above the pubes is a safe proceeding, and, for affording temporary relief, is to be recommended. A surgeon who finds himself in difficulties with a distended bladder, a large prostate, and false passages, is likely to do less harm with the needle than with the with the catheter, and is sure to give relief. Taking off the tension by withdrawing the urine generally permits the instrument to pass on the next trial. This method, however, can only be used for temporary purposes.

Tapping the bladder above the pubes with a trocar, for the purpose of establishing a more or less permanent drain, is very much like opening an abscess at its least dependent spot. Urine ascends the canula against gravity, and the products of inflammation of the bladder, usually present in some degree, remain behind in the pouch, undischarged. Tapping through the rectum requires the retention of the canula in the intestine, and is thus an obstacle to defæcation. Forcing the end of the catheter through the enlarged prostate is an unsurgical proceeding, not to be entertained. Tapping the membranous urethra leaves us in the position of having the obstructing prostate behind the opening. There is a point in the wall of the bladder, unconnected with peritoneum, through which a trocar and canula may safely be passed: I refer to the prostate gland, which in old men, where paracentesis is more frequently required, often affords a considerable area for the operation. I will illustrate this method by the following case, only premising that over twelve months ago I recognised its propriety, and tested it on the dead subject. I then had the instrument made for the purpose; but, though having considerable opportunity for dealing with retention of urine under all circumstances, it was not till quite recently that a case in point presented itself. I mention this as explaining how I came to be prepared, instrumentally, for doing that which I will briefly describe:—

N. D., aged 84, was admitted into the Liverpool Royal Infirmary at 2 A.M. on Nov. 4th, 1881. My house-surgeon, Mr. Laimbeer, found him bleeding from attempted catheterism, with a large prostate, and a distended bladder. Recognizing the urgency of the case, and finding catheterism impracticable, he emptied the bladder with the aspirator above the pubes. I saw the patient a few hours afterwards, and found that he had not passed urine since, and that no catheter could be introduced. His tongue was brown and he was much exhausted. Later on,

I again visited him, when the bladder had become fully distended. I then had him placed under ether, and succeeding in passing a gum-elastic prostatic catheter. Beyond demonstrating that the difficulty had been overcome, I declined letting any more urine be drawn off, for a reason arising out of recognizing that either the catheter must be retained, or reintroduced when required; neither of which proceeding I was disposed to recommend.

Retaining a catheter in the bladder of an old man, somewhat childish and disposed to remove any appliance if not closely watched, is not easy; and when it is done, it often ends with death from cystitis, pyelitis, and exhaustion. This was a case where, in my judgment, it was wisest to establish a permanent drain; and to do this in the manner on which I had determined required a tense, and not a flaccid, bladder. Taking a trocar which had been made for the purpose, with a silver canula, I introduced it in the median line of the perineum, three-quarters of an inch in front of the anus, and pushed it steadily through the prostate into the bladder, at the same time retaining my left index finger in the rectum for a guide. On withdrawing the trocar, a large quantity of ammoniacal urine escaped. The canula, being provided with a shield, was secured in its place by tapes much in the same way as a tracheotomy-tube. A piece of India-rubber tubing was attached to the portion of canula which projected beyond the shield, and conveyed the urine into a vessel placed at the side of the bed. Through this tubing urine continued to dribble. The patient was at once made comfortable by this arrangement, and in 48 hours he was up, sitting in an easy-chair—an important matter with old persons. To permit of this, the rubber tubing is shortened during the day-time, the end of it being tucked through a light abdominal belt, where it is compressed by a small pair of bulldog-forceps, which are removed when the patient desires to pass urine. He is quite as well as most men of 84 years of age are. He gets up daily, takes his food, and sleeps comfortably, either on his back or his side, without any narcotic, and is quite free from any urinary inconvenience other than wearing his tube. During the night, his sleep is not broken by calls to micturate or pass catheters, as his urine runs off by the tubing as it is excreted ; whilst in the day-time, when he is up and about, his act of micturition practically resolves itself into something equivalent to the turning of a tap. His urine, which had been fetid and ammoniacal, is now nearly normal, the bladder being readily washed out by applying a syringe to the canula twice a day. On two or three occasions the canula has accidentally slipped out whilst the tapes were being changed, but has been readily replaced by the nurse. The somewhat enthusiastic manner in which the patient compares his present with his past condition, cannot be passed by entirely unnoticed.

The operation was devised much on the same lines I endeavour to take in commencing my lithotomy incision—namely, the selecting of a point in the perineum which endangers no vessel of importance. My object in planning the operation was to obtain what I can best describe as a short low-level urethra, adapted to the altered relations of the bladder to the prostate when the latter becomes enlarged, for the purpose of securing the most complete drainage. I should add that since the tapping, as far as we are aware, the patient has only passed a few drops of urine by the urethra. —*Reginald Harrison in Brit. Med. Journal.*

A Modification of Lister's Antiseptic Dressing.—In a paper on Lister's " Antiseptic Method of Treating Surgical Injuries," which appeared in the " American Clinical Lectures " for 1878, I called the attention of the profession to a modification of this procedure, which I was then using in the treatment of small wounds, especially those of the hand and fingers. I have since continued its use, and have found its results, in a large number of cases, so satisfactory that I have deemed it of sufficient interest and importance to justify my calling your attention to it in a short paper this evening. Although having full confidence in Mr. Lister's antiseptic method, I, like many others, have long recognized the great difficutty that must needs be experienced by the general practitioner in attempting to carry out the minute details of the dressing, and have for a long time been hoping that a more simple method, equally efficacious, might be devised.

Dr. Markoe's " through drainage " was a decided step in

this direction—antiseptic in character, simple in detail, and successful in result. This method, however, is appropriate only where drainage is necessary, but, simple and efficient as it is, it requires a certain degree of attention, which, while easy for the hospital surgeon, is not sufficiently so to guarantee its extended use by the physician in charge of a large general practice. Aside from the difficulties incident to the application of Mr. Lister's dressing, it has been found that surgeons in country towns distant from large cities have great trouble, and often are unable to procure good antiseptic gauze at the time when it is needed. This would not be so embarrassing if, in the first place, the gauze was fresh when obtained from the dealers; and, in the second, if it could be kept for a reasonable time without spoiling. This, however, is not the case. The gauze sold in most of our stores is frequently not in an antiseptic condition. As to its keeping fresh, Dr. R. F. Weir has demonstrated conclusively that even when kept wrapped up in rubber cloth and in a box it will deteriorate in a few months. In assisting in surgical operations, I have in several instances found that the gauze used had no odor whatever of carbolic acid, although it had just been purchased from a responsible dealer in this city. In my own practice I have been obliged to depend for a reliable gauze on the kindness of the authorities of one of the hospitals with which I am connected. Furthermore, the materials necessary for fully applying Mr. Lister's dressing are somewhat expensive, a very important fact when we consider that the majority of accidents and operations that call for this procedure occur among those who are able to bear but little expense.

I have for several years been surgeon to a large factory in this city, in which three thousand hands are employed, and where injuries by machinery are quite frequent. These injuries consist chiefly of wounds of the hands and fingers, caused by their being caught in the cog-wheels and other parts of the machinery. In many cases the fingers are torn off, tendons are pulled from their sheaths, joints are opened, and the hands are often severely crushed and lacerated. In all of these cases I have, for the past six years, been using the following simple antiseptic dressing: Having put the parts in a condition for dressing, I wash the wound in a solution of carbolic acid of the strength of one to twenty; I then cover the parts with a thick layer of borated cotton, and then snugly and evenly apply a simple gauze bandage. At first I used bandages made of antiseptic gauze, but for the past three years have used those of plain uncarbolized cheese-cloth. These thin bandages distribute the pressure more evenly over the cotton, and are more easily saturated with the fluids than those made of unbleached muslin. The patient is instructed to keep the outside of the dressing wet with a solution of carbolic acid of the strength of one to one hundred. I frequently employ Squibb's solution of impure carbolic acid, which is of the strength of one to fifty, and which, when mixed with an equal bulk of water, gives a solution of the desired strength. The parts should be kept at rest, and the dressings may be left undisturbed for several days, unless there is pain, rise of temperature, or discharge through the dressings. These conditions are always to be considered indications for redressing. In many cases where rubber drainage tubes have been used they may be removed at the second dressing, and, if catgut has been used for sutures, this second dressing can be allowed to remain on for an indefinite period. In a number of cases of lacerated wounds I have allowed the first dressing to remain on until the wound has entirely healed. In these cases the external use of carbolic lotion was discontinued after the fifth or sixth day, and the dressings would become dry and hard, the wound healing, as it were, "under a scab." The patient should be instructed to loosen the bandage at once if any pain occurs. My experience with this dressing covers, as I have said, a period of about six years, during which time I have treated nearly three hundred cases of open wounds. Not one of this number has been followed by inflammatory symptoms. Extensive lacerated wounds have healed, and dead tissue has sloughed away, without giving rise to any of the so-called symptoms of inflammation. Neither pain, redness, heat, swelling, nor constitutional disturbance has resulted, In no case has there been reddening of the lymphatics or tenderness of the glands. No counter-openings have been necessary. Pain has been entirely absent, so that anodynes have not been needed, save in a single case, and that for one night only, to control slight restlessness. These results are the more remarkable from the fact that many of these patients were in an unhealthy condition, some suffering from anæmia, some from cardiac disease, phthisis, and the like.

Recently I used this modified dressing in St. Vincent's Hospital, in a case of amputation of the leg. The history of the case is as follows:

The patient, a boy nine years of age, was run over by a dummy engine, on September 28th. His left foot was crushed so that it was necessary to amputate the leg at the junction of the middle with the lower third. The operation was performed by Dr. John F. Luby, the House Surgeon, in my presence. The method of amputation was that by lateral skin flaps and circular incision through the muscles. All the details of Lister's method were employed except the spray. Catgut was used for ligatures and sutures. Short drainage tubes were placed in the anterior and posterior angles of the wound. After the wound was washed with a one-to-twenty solution of carbolic acid, it was dressed with several layers of dry borated cotton and a gauze bandage was applied. The outside of this dressing was kept constantly wet with a one-to-forty solution of the carbolic acid. The great and the second toe of the right foot were also crushed, so as to require amputation at the second joint of the great toe and at the metatarso-phalangeal articulation of the second toe. These wounds were dressed in the same manner.

October 2nd.—Four days after the operation. Patient has not complained of any pain. His highest temperature has been 99.8° F. Has slept well and has a good appetite. On removing the dressing, the cotton was found not to have been wet through by the carbolic acid lotion. The layer in direct contact with the wound was saturated with a watery discharge. The wound was in a perfect aseptic condition. The drainage tubes were removed and fresh borated cotton was applied.

October 7th.—The boy has been perfectly comfortable during the past five days. On removing the dressings very little discharge was found on the cotton. The wound was entirely healed, except at the points where the drainage tubes were inserted. The external application of the carbolic lotion was discontinued.

October 15*th*.—Dressings removed, and the wound found to be entirely healed, except at a point in the lower angle. The wounds of the right foot were dressed simultaneously with that of the stump. Although a small portion of the integument sloughed, there was no trace of inflammatory action. Granulations sprang up and the wound rapidly closed, so that on October 17th the cotton dressing was discontinued and unguentum resina was applied.

This case did as well as any case could have done under the most rigid Lister dressing. The value of cotton-wool as an antiseptic dressing is, I think, not fully appreciated by the profession. M. Guerin, of Paris, in 1872, and since then Mr. Gamgee, of Birmingham, England, have called attention to its great value. Used in the way I have indicated, it seems to me to be as perfect an antiseptic dressing as the gauze and other materials recommended by Mr. Lister, while at the same time it is free from all objections that pertain to the latter, and which materially hinder their use by the general practitioner. If applied in sufficient quantities around an open wound, it protects it thoroughly from the "floating matter of the air" which is supposed to be the real inciter of suppuration. It is the best germ filter known to us. Tyndall, whose experiments were very carefully made, found that while filtering the air, and endeavoring to get it perfectly pure, atmospheric dust, which would readily pass through sulphuric acid and a strong solution of caustic potash, was completely stopped by ordinary cotton-wool. I have used the very excellent borated cotton made by Mr. am Ende, of Hoboken, containing 15 per cent. of boracic acid* Keeping it wet externally with the solution of carbolic

* A great deal of the so-called borated cotton sold by dealers is made with a solution of borax, instead of boracic acid, which can always be ascertained by burning a piece of the cotton; if the cotton has been properly prepared with boracic acid, the flame is of a bright green color, but, if, as is generally the case, borax has been used, the flame will show very little of the green tint.

acid, in the manner already described, renders it more surely antiseptic. To insure success in the cases where the dressing is used, full precautions as to rendering the instruments, sponges, and the hands of the surgeon aseptic, and the use of drainage tubes if necessary, should not be neglected. Catgut or torsion should be used to arrest hemorrhage. The spray may be resorted to, if thought necessary, at the second dressing. I now usually apply carbolized oil, of the strength of one to twelve, to the wound to facilitate the removal of the cotton, which is otherwise apt to adhere after the first dressing.

I would state in conclusion, that my experience thus far seems to show that this simple dressing, so easy of application, is as thoroughly antiseptic as Mr. Lister's appliances, and that it has the very decided advantage of doing away with the necessity for using costly "protective oil-silk," "Mackintosh cloth," "carbolized gauze," etc., and gives us a dressing that can be used by any one under any circumstances, be it in the city or in the country. The borated cotton is easily kept for months unchanged. The fact that the dressing need not be done oftener than once in several days will especially commend it to the country physician. The success of this procedure in the treatment of large wounds after accident or amputation will increase its importance, and materially extend its field of usefulness.—*Dr. James L. Little in N. Y. Med Journal.*

Meat-Bread.—M. Scheurer-Kestner has discovered the remarkable fact that the fermentation of bread causes the complete digestion of meat. He found that a beefsteak cut into four pieces and mixed with flour and yeast, disappeared entirely during the process of fermentation, its nutritive principles becoming incorporated with the bread. The meat would also appear capable of preservation for an indefinite period in its new state; for loaves of meat-bread made in 1873 have been submitted to the French Academy of Sciences, where not a trace of worms or mouldness was observable. At the beginning of his experiments, M. Scheurer-Kestner used raw meat, three parts of which, finely minced, he mixed with five parts of flour and the same quantity of yeast. Sufficient water was added to make the dough, which in due time began to ferment. After two or three hours the meat had disappeared, and the bread was baked in the ordinary manner. Thus prepared, the meat-bread had a disagreeable, sour taste, which was avoided by cooking the meat for an hour with sufficient water to afterwards moisten the flour. The meat must be carefully deprived of fat, and only have sufficient salt to bring out the flavor, as salt, by absorbing moisture from the air, would tend to spoil the bread. A part of the beef may be replaced with advantage by salt lard, which is found to improve the flavour. The proportion of meat to flour should not exceed one-half, so as to insure complete digestion. Bread made with a suitable proportion of veal is said to furnish excellent soup for the sick and wounded.—*Sanitarian* —*Canadian Pharmaceutical Journal.*

Bicarbonate of Soda in Tonsilitis.— Dr. Giné, Professor of Clinical Surgery at Madrid, states that bicarbonate of soda, applied topically and repeatedly to the tonsils, is of incontestable efficacy in quinsy. The remedy may be employed by insufflation through a paper tube, or may be applied by the finger, even by the patient himself. Dr. Giné has rapidly cured dozens of cases by this procedure. In no single case was the application entirely without effect; most commonly a cure was obtained in 24 hours. Alleviation took place, ordinarily, at once. In none of his cases was it necessary to wait long for relief. But he especially recommends this remedy in the prodromic period to abort the disease. Dr. Giné considers tonsilotomy for enlarged tonsils as an entirely useless operation, for this affection is always overcome in a relatively short time by the frequent application of bicarbonate of soda.— *La Presse Méd. Belge*, July 17, 1881.

Small-pox and Anti-vaccinators.– The wickedness of encouraging the anti-vaccination agitation could not, it is opportunely pointed out by the *Globe*, be more strikingly proved than by an account it printed of the origin of an outbreak of small-pox in Rotherhithe. "A leading anti-vaccinator," Escott by name, who had none of his children vaccinated, had lost his wife and two children by small-pox, and four others have had the disease. Escott borrowed a suit of mourning from a friend named Angus to attend his wife's funeral, and returned the clothes without disinfection, with the result that the lender caught small-pox and died. Since then nearly every house in the neighborhood has been attacked, and sixteen patients have been romoved to the hospital.—*British Medical Journal.*

Lactic Acid in Phthisis.—A. D. Macdonald, M.B., C.M., writes as follows to the *British Medical Journal:*

"I have been struck by the observation that in some cases where there was a strong hereditary predisposition to phthisis, acute rheumatism had supervened early in life, and by middle age phthisis had not yet appeared. Besides, I understand that in Madras, for example, there is a large proportion of rheumatism to a comparatively smaller proportion of phthisis. May there not then exist some degree of antagonism between these diseases, and is there not in the latter a deficiency of the lactic acid poison of the former? On the 5th of June last I administered 10 minims of lactic acid thrice a day to a patient who had a vomica in the apex of the right lung, and the left apex had a deposit of tubercle. On the 11th the patient expressed herself as feeling better, but she complained of rheumatic pains in her joints for about two hours after each dose, and this in the absence of being informed as to any effect to be produced. Another patient to whom I gave the acid stated that it relieved her cough more than anything else she had taken. Both thought the acid very agreeable as a thirst-quencher."—*Med. Record.*

Capsicum in Uterine Hemorrhages.—Dr. J. Chenon (*Le Progrés Médicale*) says: From a large number of physiological experiments, I concluded that capsicum is a vascular remedy, acting especially on organs whose circulation is singularly active, such as the utero-ovarian, respiratory, and encephalic. Cayenne pepper acts like ergot of rye on the smooth fibre of the vascular coats, either directly or through the vaso-motors. But it presents a great advantage over ergot, in that it is well borne by the stomach, whose functions it simply stimulates. I have used it for several years in uterine hemorrhages with the best success, whether these hemorrhages were due to fibroid tumours, fungous endometritis, or even to epithelioma. The formulæ at which I have arrived are as follows:

℞ Powdered capsicum, 5 grammes. Make thirty pills. One before each meal, increasing to six pills a day.

℞ Aqueous extract of capsicum, 5 grammes. Make thirty pills. To be given in the same dose as No. 1.

℞ Tincture of capsicum, 5 grammes; rum, 30 grammes; gum julep, 120 grammes. Take by spoonfuls every two hours.

I have also successfully used capsicum in congestive headaches so common in the gouty, and in the hæmoptysis of tuberculous patients.

Pericardial Drainage.—Rosenstein, of Leyden (*Lancet*), reports the case of a child ten years old who had pericardial effusion, for which the pericardium was aspirated. A second aspiration was soon again required. A relapse occurred, whereupon an opening an inch and a half long was made in the fourth intercostal space. The soft parts were divided under antiseptic treatment, and two drainage tubes inserted. After four months of treatment the patient left the hospital in good general condition. An incision into the pleura was also required. The effusion was purulent.—*Chicago Med. Review.*

Epigastric Pressure in Obstinate Hiccough.—The *Journal des Sciences Médicales de Louvain* relates that M. Deghilage, of Mons, was called to a young lady suffering from very violent hiccough, with spasm of the glottis. The patient had been over an hour in this state, and was unable to articulate a syllable. There was no fever—no sign of heart trouble. The only cause that could be assigned was that the patient had the lower limb chilled a few days previously during her menstrual period. Inhalation of vinegar and Hoffman's anodyne and the application of sinapisms had been tried, without effect. Recalling Rostan's precept for such cases, M. Deghilage applied the palm of the hand to the epigastrium and exercised strong pressure. There was slight amelioration, the movements were less convulsive, and the dyspnœa less intense. A large pad of linen was then applied over the epigastric region and pressed strongly inward by means of a bandage passed around the body. In a very short time complete relief was obtained. The pad was left several hours in position, and when it was removed the symptoms did not return.—*Med. & Surg. Reporter.*

Benzoate of Soda in Whooping Cough.—Dr. Tordeus of Brussels writes that he has prescribed the benzoate of soda in a number of cases of whooping-cough, and that in all the cases the parents reported that the coughing fits began to diminish in force and frequency after one or two days of treatment. He gives four grains of the salt every hour to a child of two or three years. The drug seems not alone to diminish the force and frequency of the paroxysms, but also to exert a favourable influence on the mucous membrane of the respiratory tract, and to prevent the development of serious pulmonary complications.—*Journal de Med., etc., de Bruxelles.*

Salicylic Acid in Diphtheria.—Dr. Weise recommends very highly a two per cent. solution of salicylic acid in diphtheria. This is a strongly antiseptic solution, but not a dangerous one. He employs the following formula :—

℞ Acid salicyl., 1.09 ; sp. vini rectif., glycerine, āā 25.00. At the same time he uses benzoate of soda internally.

Neuralgic Headache with Constipation.—℞

Quiniæ disulph.,	- - - -	gr. xij
Acid. sulph. dil.,	- - - -	ʒ ss
Tinct. ferri perchlor.,	- - -	ʒ ij
Spt. chloroformi,	- - - -	ʒ ij
Magnes. sulph.,	- - - -	℥ jss
Syr. Zingiberis,	- - - -	℥ j
Aquæ	- - - - - - - - ad	℥ xij

M. Sig. Two tablespoonfuls three times a day.

CANADA

Medical and Surgical Journal.

MONTREAL, JANUARY, 1882.

THE BILLS FOR MEDICAL SERVICES.

If from feelings of personal delicacy, or from other equally unreasonable considerations, the physician has deferred sending his bill for services rendered to his patients, the time has arrived when the accounts for the year must be settled in some way or other. He knows full well that the general sentiment of the people whom he has attended is adverse to the prompt settlement of medical bills, and that too generally the latter are paid eventually under protest. While, according to the general law of domestic economy, the physician must live as well as the butcher and baker, each debtor to the doctor would much prefer to change places with any others who were free from such obligations. Thus, the medical man is often impliedly placed in the position of one who is tolerated rather than encouraged, who is supposed to belong to the class of individuals whose pay, in great part, should be taken in the mere consciousness of doing good to his suffering fellows. These are privileges denied to many, but in order to be properly appreciated by the physician he should be a trifle beyond want himself. These are our higher humanities, which can never attain their full function with an empty stomach. The smell of the lily may be a reasonable dessert after a hearty meal, but it is not specially tempting to the man who is forced to descend to the prose of an ordinary bread-and-butter struggle.

Physicians, as a class, are too often tempted to look on the soft side of charity, and suffer in consequence. Hence the practical business man makes allowance for him, and is ever ready in a patronizingly considerate way to take advantage of him. Of course this is the fault of the doctor as well as of his debtor. The readiness with which deductions are made from medical bills proves this. There is no doubting the fact that the prevalence of the practice has helped to create the too-widely entertained impression that medical services have no positive value, and that they should be paid for only after a heavy discount has been allowed. All these general considerations must have their bearing upon the medical men who are now making out their bills, and should help them to determine the amount of charges in given cases. It is well to recollect, while due allowance should be made for those who can pay little or nothing, that the maximum charges should be reasonably high. Physicians, as a rule, do not place enough pecuniary value on their services. Generally they are considered by their patrons worth no more than the small sum usually asked for them. The rich, as a rule, are of this opinion, and are usually disappointed in their estimate of the real value of the services of a doctor if a really small bill is presented. High charges are generally the only means by which the value of services rendered can be proven to such as are able to pay for them. There is far less likelihood of charging these persons too little than too much. An opportunity for practically testing this point is doubtless presenting itself to many of our readers engaged in bill-rendering. Another matter worth considering in connection with the squaring of accounts for the year, is how few patients shall be placed on the free list. Every physician who has a greater or less number of patrons whom he is not in the habit of charging, who occupy toward him the anomalous position of being his friends so long as they can use him to their advantage, or who, possibly, in consideration of some slight service rendered by them, give them a claim upon his good will and good deeds. It goes without the saying that these patients are the most troublesome and least profitable of the entire clientele of the physician. The best friends of the practitioner are those who pay him for what he does for them, and the sooner all services—no matter to whom rendered—can be placed on a cash basis, the better. It is quite easy to anticipate what may be the effect of cutting off worthless hangers-on by a formal bill. If they discharge their doctor in consequence of the insult of receiving his bill, they are the only ones that can possibly suffer by the change. At least the physician is relieved from the obligation of spending his time and his energies for naught.—*N. Y. Medical Record.*

Obituary.

Dr. Draper.—This eminent scientific man died on the 4th inst., at his residence, Hastings-on-Hudson, N. Y. Born near Liverpool in 1811, and partially educated at University College, London, he came to America in 1833, and in 1836 was graduated in Medicine at the University of Pennsylvania. Shortly after he was called to the Chair of Natural Sciences at Hampden-Sidney College, Va., and in 1839 to the University of New York, with which he remained connected until his death. He took an active part in the establishment of the Medical Faculty, and was the last of the six original founders. He lectured on Chemistry and Physiology for many years, and was an exceedingly popular teacher. His experimental investigations constitute some of the most important contributions to science made in the United States. He was one of the early workers at photography, and was the first to photograph the human face. Researches on light and the spectrum gave him a world-wide reputation, and he carried on at the same time many investigations into the mode of growth of plants and animals. In 1856 he published a Text-book of Physiology, which for many years was deservedly popular. He is best known to the public by his many purely literary works: "History of the Intellectual Development of Europe" (1862), "Thoughts on the Future Civil Policy of America" (1865), "The History of the American Civil War" (1867-70), and "The Conflict between Religion and Science" (1877). His death, we believe, was from kidney disease. Three sons survive him, all in the ranks of science; one, John C., is the Professor of Chemistry in the University of New York.

Medical Items.

TALL OAKS FROM LITTLE ACORNS.—Since the report that the child of the mother who, during gestation, carried a copy of Moore's Melodies, became a poet, "pre-natal culture" has become a study and the American Institute of Heredity is the result; most of its members are old maids.

HOW TO GIVE A SAVAGE DYSPEPSIA.—When a medical friend who could never resist disputing every pet theory of Sydney Smith, and always disagreed with him, accepted a professional call to Australia in the days of its savage condition, the clerical wit accompanied his friend to the ship, and, taking leave of him, remarked, "Good-bye, doctor; you have never failed to disagree with me, and I believe you will disagree with the savage who eats you."

TELEPHONIC TROUBLES.—Mistakes may happen even in the best regulated families. Here is an example. Chicago is blessed with a druggist of great experience and staid, modest habits of demeanour. It is his custom to replenish his stock when necessary, by ordering by telephone from other houses in the same line of business. With this purpose in view he called up such a house, and supposed he had it, when in fact he was still speaking to the telephone office. He was overwhelmed with chagrin and shame when, in reply to his question "Have you large black nipples?" only a hearty soprano cacchination was returned from the female operator in the office. For a number of days thereafter he was compelled to repeat his blushes as he caught the lady's laughter whenever she heard the tones of his voice on the wire.—*Chicago Med. Review.*

CHINESE REWARDS FOR MEDICAL SERVICE.—A correspondent of the *Globe* adds that this same decree throws some curious light upon the position which practitioners of the healing art hold in China. When the empress's illness became serious, several of the leading provincial governors were directed to seek out the most skilful doctors in their respective jurisdictions and send them on to the capital to consult with the medical college there as to the course of treatment to be pursued. About half-a-dozen were forwarded, and as the result has been so eminently successful, they are now all to get substantial government appointments. One is to be made a taotai, or intendant of circuit, upon the first vacancy; another a prefect; another a district magistrate, and so on. Suppose, after the recovery of the Prince of Wales, Sir William Jenner had been made a county court judge, and Sir William Gull a stipendiary magistrate, we should have a somewhat analogous case in England.—*Brit. Med. Journal.*

ÆSTHETICS AND CATHARTICS.—Bunthorne, the "fleshly poet," in the new opera, "Patience," gives the following as a "wild, weird, fleshly thing, yet very yearning, very precious. To understand it, cling passionately to one another and think of faint lilies":—

What time the poet hath hymned
The writhing maid, lithe limbed,
  Quivering on amaranthine asphodel,
How can he paint her woes,
Knowing, as well he knows,
  That all can be set right with calomel?

When from the poet's plinth
The amorous colocynth
  Yearns for the aloe, faint with rapturous thrills,
How can he hymn their throes,
Knowing, as well he knows,
  That they are only uncompounded pills?

It is, and can it be
Nature hath its decree.
  "Nothing poetic in the world shall dwell?"
Or that, in all her works
Something poetic lurks,
  Even in colocynth and calomel?
    I cannot tell.

—Heister, in his system of Surgery, whilst describing imperforate vagina, tells the following amusing story: "We have a merry recollection of a girl that was imperforated after this manner, who, when she became sensible that she could not be debauched by any one, enlisted a great many to her service, particularly some stout soldiers, who, upon trial, were all disappointed in their expectations, bilked of their money, and derided by the girl, who remained as much a maid as ever. Sometime afterwards this girl committed herself to the care of a surgeon, in order to be freed from the impediment; the case succeeded so well, that in a little time afterwards he got her with child, and she brought him twins into the world, as a testimony of his skill and a reward for his trouble.

PHYSICIANS.—Zimmerman says, if you need a physician, employ these three: A cheerful mind, rest, and a temperate diet. Pope declares that

> "A wise physician, skill'd our wounds to heal,
> Is more than armies to the public weal."

Butler says:

> "For men are brought to worse distresses
> By taking physic, than diseases,
> And therefore commonly recover
> As soon as doctors give them over."

—*Medical Bi-Weekly.*

—"What acid do we get from iodine?" asked the medical professor. "We get—a-n—usually get idiotic acid," yawned the student. "Have you been taking some?" quietly asked the professor.

VASELINE.—The attention of our readers is called to this valuable product obtained from petroleum. As a base for ointments, it is to be preferred to lard, as it never becomes rancid. There are also many valuable toilet preparations now manufactured from this base, amongst others being the *Vaseline Cold Cream*, one of the most soothing and elegant preparations obtainable at this season of the year.

—A new Pepsin, called *Pepsina Prorsa*, is being introduced to the notice of the profession by Kenneth Campbell & Co. The makers claim it to be an absolute Pepsin, without the addition of sugar of milk, starch or other dilutant. We have seen a sample that has been proved to us to answer the test given by the makers—one grain being capable of dissolving 220 grains of coagulated albumen.

Fig. 1.

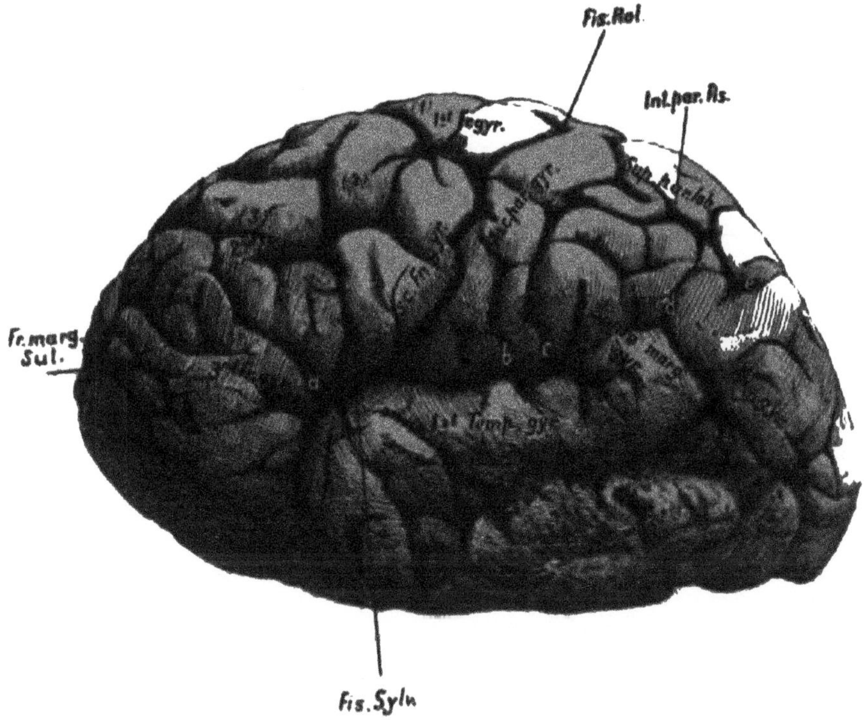
Fis. Rol.
Int. par. fis.
Fr. marg. Sul.
1st Temp. gyr.
Fis. Syl'n

Fig. 2.

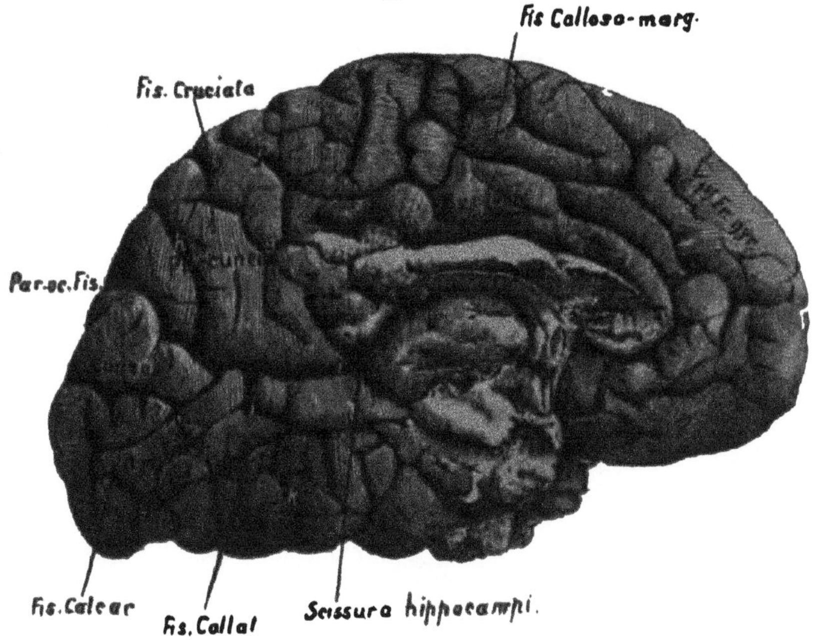
Fis Calloso-marg.
Fis. Cruciata
Par. oc. Fis.
Fis. Calcar
Fis. Collat
Scissura hippocampi.

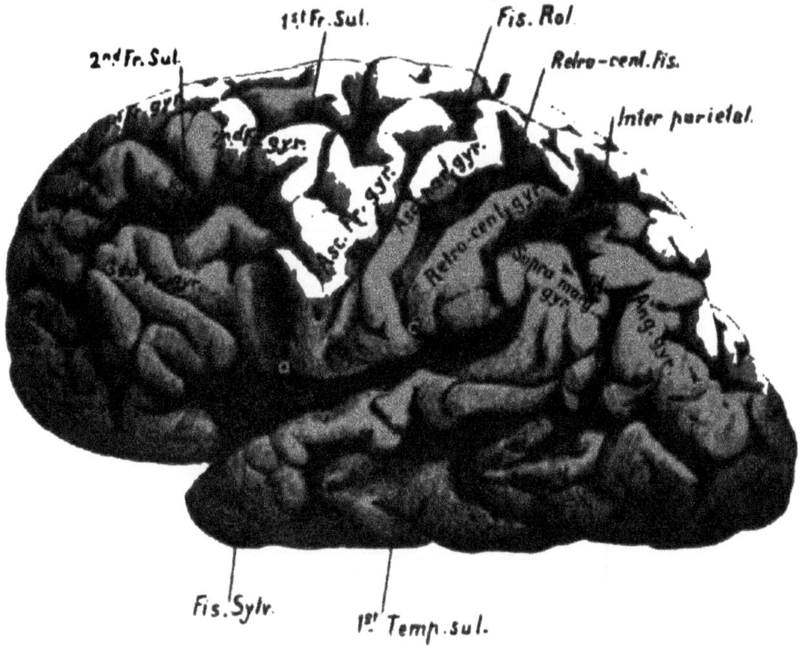
1st Fr. Sul.
Fis. Rol.
2nd Fr. Sul.
Retro-cent. Fis.
Inter parietal.
2nd Fr. gyr.
Asc. Fr. gyr.
Retro-cent. gyr.
Supra marg. gyr.
Ang. gyr.
Fis. Sylv.
1st Temp. sul.

Fig 4

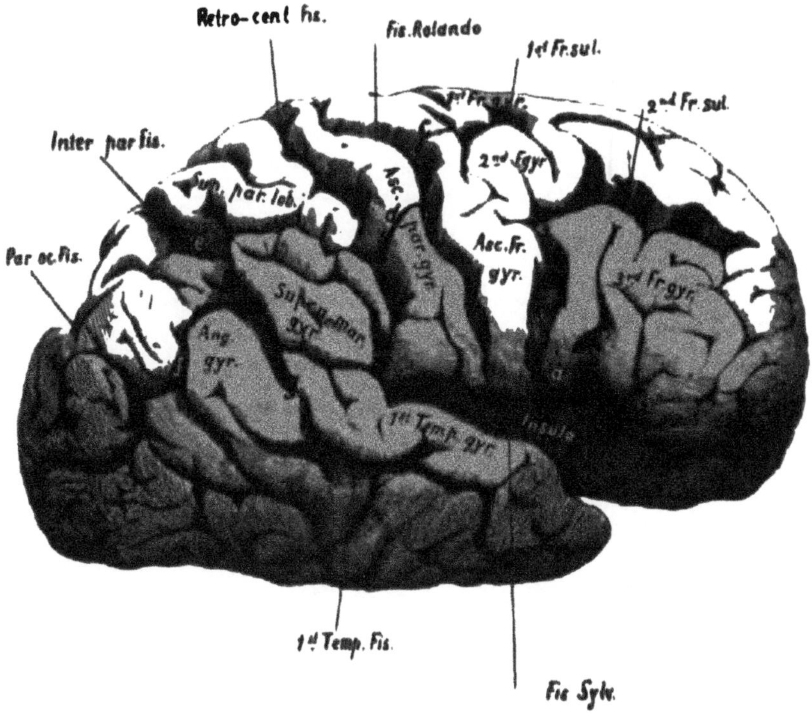
Retro-cent. fis.
Fis. Rolando
1st Fr. sul.
2nd Fr. sul.
Inter par fis.
Sup. par. lob.
2nd Fr. gyr.
Asc. par. gyr.
Asc. Fr. gyr.
3rd Fr. gyr.
Par oc. Fis.
Supra marg. gyr.
Ang. gyr.
1st Temp. gyr.
Insula
1st Temp. Fis.
Fis Sylv.

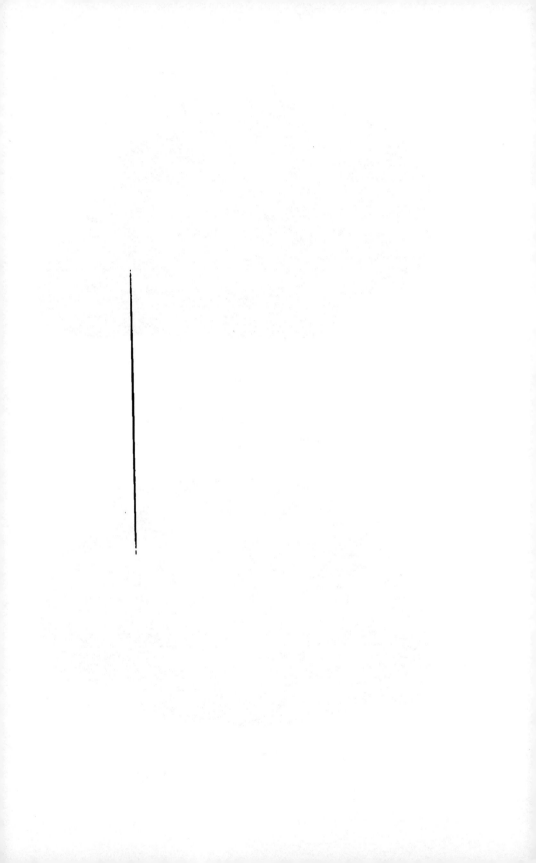

CANADA

MEDICAL & SURGICAL JOURNAL

FEBRUARY, 1882.

Original Communications.

ON THE BRAINS OF CRIMINALS.

WITH A DESCRIPTION OF THE BRAINS OF TWO MURDERERS.

(PLATES I. AND II.)

BY WILLIAM OSLER, M.D., M.R.C.P., LOND.

Professor of the Institutes of Medicine in McGill University, and Physician to the Montreal General Hospital.

[*Read before the Medico-Chirurgical Society of Montreal.*]

Mentally and bodily, we are largely the result of an hereditary organization, and the environment in which we have been reared. The child of a bushman nurtured in the family of a philosopher will not be able, with favourable surroundings, to rise much above his race level; the child of a philosopher, reared among the bushmen, will not reach his paternal standard, but the grossness of the savage natures around him will have weight to pull him down, and what is fine will learn to sympathize with the clay. In the former case, the individual cannot transcend his organization; and in the latter, he cannot burst the iron bars of his environment. That the mental and moral status of a man is determined by the conformation and development of his brain is an axiom with the school of physiological psychologists. The conformation is a matter of inheritance; the development, of education (in its widest sense). The different mental conditions of individuals are the expression of subtle differences in cerebral structure, just as the diversity in the features of men is the result of minute variations in the arrangement of the tissues of the face. That a faulty physical basis can have no other sequence than a faulty mental and moral constitution is acknowledged and acted upon by every one, so far as idiots and imbeciles are concerned, but that mental and moral obliquity is invariably the outcome of an ill-conformed or ill-developed brain is a doctrine novel and startling, though logical enough from the standpoint of modern physical fatalism. Endeavours have recently been made to put this theory on firm grounds by showing that in a large number of criminals the type of brain differs from that in tho law-abiding members of the community.

Anatomists and physiologists have of late paid much attention to the conformation of the brain surface, and the convolutions and fissures are now studied with care and minuteness. In a typical European brain, the cerebellum is completely covered by the cerebrum, and the general arrangement of the gyri and sulci is such that there is rarely any difficulty in mapping them out and assigning their proper names to each. Thus on the external surface of each hemisphere we recognize two fissures which are constant and invariable in position—the *fissures of Sylvius and of Rolando*, (*central sulcus.*) Other fissures constantly present, but less definite in their arrangement, are: the *inter-parietal*, which passes through the parietal lobe, the *parieto-occipital*; separating the parietal and occipital lobes, best seen from the median surface, the *superior* (1st), *inferior* (2nd), and *ascending* (3rd) frontal sulci and the 1*st* and 2*nd temporal.*

On the median surface, the *calloso-marginal*, the *parietal-occipital*, the *calcarine* and *collateral* are well marked and distinctive.

The convolutions or gyri separated by these fissures are remarkably uniform, and, though often intersected by subsidiary sulci, can usually be determined without difficulty. Of these, the only ones which need be now mentioned are the three frontal, 1st, 2nd and 3rd, the general direction of which is parallel to the longitudinal fissure and the two central gyri which bound the fissure of Rolando on either side.

In the typical brain the main fissures are unconnected with each other; thus the fissure of Rolando is isolated and does not unite with the Sylvian fissure below, or the ascending frontal or ascending parietal sulci on either side. The Sylvian fissure does not join with any of the sulci above or below it.

Prof. Benedikt of Vienna has made a special study of the brains of criminals,* and believes that he has met with peculiarities sufficiently marked to warrant the following proposition: "*The brains of criminals exhibit a deviation from the normal type, and criminals are to be viewed as an anthropological variety of their species, at least amongst the cultured races.*" The two peculiarities on which he lays stress are (1st) the confluence of many of the primary fissures and (2nd) the existence of four horizontal frontal gyri. He proposes to establish a confluent fissure type of brain, and he illustrates its most important characteristic by saying, "that if we imagine the fissures to be water-courses, it might be said that a body floating in any one of them could enter almost all the others." This, of course, means the absence of numerous bridges of nerve matter which normally separate the fissures—defects, marking an inferior development of the brain. Between the normal type with isolated fissures and the type with confluent fissures there will naturally be transitions, but he calls attention to the number and variety of the connections in his series of the brains of 22 criminals as supporting the truth of his proposition. He states that the brains of individuals in the lower grades of society approach nearer to the 2nd type, and it is probable, though, as yet, full data are wanting, that the brains of the inferior races of men also conform more closely to this than to the type with isolated fissures. Let us see now how far he has been able to establish the truth of this view. Of 38 hemispheres from the 22 criminals the following were some of the most interesting points:—

I. The *fissure of Rolando* communicated with:

(*a*) *fis. Syl.* completely in 18, incompletely in 6.

(*b*) with *3rd* or *ascending frontal*, complete in 11, incomplete in 2.

---

* On the Brains of Criminals, Vienna, 1879. Translated by Dr. Fowler. (Wood & Co., New York, 1881. *Cent. f. d. med. Wissenschaften*, 1876, and No. 46, 1880.

(c) with the 1*st* or *superior* *frontal sulcus*, complete in 9, incomplete in 1.

(*d*) with *inter-parietalis*, complete in 7, incomplete in 4.

Of the 19 brains there was not one in which the *fissure of Rolando* had not on one side a connection with some other fissure. Altogether there were 58 connections, 35 on the left and 23 on the right side.

II. The *Sylvian fissure* communicated with:

(*a*) *fis. R.* in 18 completely, in 6 incompletely.

(*b*) with *frontal sulci* in 18, incomplete in 7.

In 7 brains it existed on both sides; only absent on both sides in 3.

(*c*) with *fis. inter-parietalis* in 22, incomplete in 6.

(*d*) with 1*st temporal* in 18, incompletely in 4.

III. The *fis. inter-parietalis* communicated with:

(*a*) *fis. R.* complete in 7, incomplete 4.

(*b*) *fis. Sylv.* complete 22, incomplete 7.

(*c*) 1*st T.* complete 19, incomplete 6.

In the 38 hemispheres there were 51 complete and 16 shallow connections of the inter-parietalis.

IV. The *scissura hippocampi* communicated with: *parieto-occipital*, complete 17, incomplete 2.

V. The *calloso-marginal fissure*: with *parieto-occipital*, complete 8.

VI. The *parieto-occipital*: with *inter-parietalis* and *horizonal occipital*, complete 21, incomplete 6.

These were the most important connections; the others I shall not refer to.

The second peculiarity which Prof. Benedikt has noted in the brains of criminals is the existence of 4 horizontal gyri springing from the ascending frontal or anterior central convolution. This he regards as an animal similarity, and a reversion, so to speak, to the typical four primitive gyri of the brains of carnivora. The fourth gyrus is formed by the splitting, by a deep fissure, of either the 1st or 2nd convolution. In his latest communication on this point,* the results are given of the examination of 87 hemispheres (from 44 criminals), of which only 42 presented the normal type of frontal convolutions, and 27 showed four gyri. In these the additional gyrus resulted in 8 from the splitting of the superior; in 16 from the division of the middle convolution. In 13 there was an imperfect division into four gyri. In two hemispheres there were five frontal convolutions.

Through the courtesy of Dr. Desmarteau, Jail Surgeon, I was present at the autopsy, and secured the brain of the man Hayvern who was executed for the murder of a fellow-convict; and the Department of Justice permitted me to secure the brain of Moreau, who was executed at Rimouski.

I.—Hayvern, aged 28, was a medium-sized man, of no trade; Irish descent; parents living, and respectable; no insanity, inebriety or neurotic disease in the family. He had been a hard drinker, and as a child was stated to have had fits. There is no evidence of the recurrence of these in adult life. He was serving a term in the Penitentiary, having been sentenced for highway robbery in 1879. He had previously been in jail more than twenty times, and may be taken as a good representative of the criminal class. The details of the murder show deliberation, and there was no evidence to show that the act was performed during a paroxysm of epileptic mania.

The skull was somewhat ovoid in shape, dolicho-cephalic; the forehead rather low and retreating. The calvaria was of moderate thickness; no signs of injury, old or recent.

Brain, last organ examined. Pl. I.—Vessels were empty; drained of blood by the opening of the vessels of the neck, both in front and behind. Membranes were normal. Weight of organ, 1326 grammes (46½ ozs.) Cerebellum completely covered by cerebrum. I obtained the left hemisphere for special study, and the details of its structure are as follows:—

Antero-posterior diameter	16.5	cm.
Hemispheric arch	24.8	"
Anterior curve (tip of Fr. lobe to Fis Rol.)	14	"
Middle curve (from Fis. Rol. to Par.-occip. Fis.)	6.2	"
Posterior curve (from Par.-oc. to tip of Occip. lobe)	4.8	"

* *Centralb. f. d. med. Wissensch ft.*, No. 46, 1880.

Sylvian fissure (*Fig.* 1), in addition to the normal *ascending* and *horizonal* rami, presents a radial branch which passes into the *frontal gyri* (*a*), a short radial extension into the *asc. parietal* (*b*), and a shallow communication with *retro-central sulcus* (c).

The *fissure of Rolando* (F.R.) or *central sulcus* is separated from the F.S. by a very narrow bridge of brain substance. It has no other connections.

There are four well-marked *frontal gyri* [1, 2, 3 *and* 4]; the extra one (2) appears to be formed by the splitting of the *superior* or 1*st gyrus*, though its base, where it joins the *asc. front. gyrus*, is in the position of the *middle* or 2*nd. fr. gyr.* As can be seen in the plate, there are two radial sulci which pass from a point just behind *asc. ramus* of *fis. Sylv.* and ascend almost to the *long. fis.* They are deep, and the hinder one has a crucial extension in the position of the 2*nd fr. sul.*

The *sulcus inter-parietalis* presents a well-marked radial portion which passes up behind the ascending parietal convolution in its whole length (*asc. pariet.* or *retro-central* sulcus); the sagittal part passes back into the parietal lobe and divides into two branches, one of which (*d*) curves round the *supra-marginal gyrus* and unites with the 1*st temporal fis.*; the other (*e*) ascends to the median border, and is continuous with a sulcus which joins the *parieto-occipital*.

The *asc. par. gyrus* (retro-central) is well developed, as are also the *angularis* and *supra-marginal*.

The *horizonal* (or *sup.*) *occipital* sulcus is well developed; it does not join the *par. occip.*, but sends branches into the *gy. cuneus*. It appears to join the 2*nd temp. sulcus*, but the brain is lacerated at this point, and it is difficult to make out the connection.

The 1*st temporal sulcus* is strongly marked, passes up and joins the *inter-parietal*. The 2*nd temp.* cannot be well made out on account of the laceration.

On the median surface (*Fig.* 2), the *calloso-marginal sulcus* is strongly developed, presents numerous perpendicular branches, and terminates by two, one of which (*f*) ascends to the usual position behind the *retro-central gyrus*, the other (*g*) curves round and divides the *gyrus fornicatus* from the *pre-cuneus* (or quadrilateral), extending to within a short distance of the calcarine fissure, and uniting with the *fis. cruciata*.

The *gyrus fornicatus*, in the anterior half of its extent, presents a well-marked sulcus running along its centre.

The *parieto-occipital* is deep and well marked; it has a branch (*h*) which curves over the border and unites with the *inter-parietal*. The *calcarine* fissure unites with the *par. occip.*, and the conjoined sulcus communicates with the *scissura hippocampi* by a wide groove (*i*).

The *sulcus collateralis* joins the *calcarine* by a large fissure (*j*), which ends just at the handle of the fork of the *par.-occip.* and *calcarine*. Another sulcus (*k*) passes from it round the under surface of the occipital lobe, dividing the *temporal gyri* from the *occipital*.

The *orbital gyri* are separated from the frontal anteriorly, by a well-marked fissure (fronto-marginal of Wernicke).

The convolutions of the *insula*, normal.

According to Benedikt's views, this hemisphere is a-typical in the following particulars:—

(*a*) The union of the *Sylvian* with the 1*st frontal sulcus*.

(*b*) The junction of the *inter-parietal* with the *parieto-occipital* and with the 1*st temporal*.

(*c*) The extension of the *calcarine* fissure into the *scissura hippocampi*.

(*d*) The extension of the *calloso-marginal* fissure between the *gyrus fornicatus* and the *pre-cuneus*.

(*e*) The union of the *collateral* and *calcarine* fissures.

(*f*) The fission of the 1st frontal convolution into two parts, so that there appear to be four frontal gyri—a condition which Benedikt lays great stress upon as a marked *animal similarity* in the human brain.

II.—Moreau, a small farmer in the county of Rimouski, aged 40, French-Canadian, murdered his wife last summer, and was executed on the 13th of January. He was a short, very powerfully-built man, uneducated, and of a morose disposition; was temperate, and had never before been convicted of any crime.

He had not lived happily with his wife, and quarrels had been frequent; one day, when in the woods together, he cut her head open with an axe. The deed was apparently premeditated, as it came out in evidence that he had offered money to a man to do it for him. After the act and during the trial he maintained his usual stolidity, and did not appear to take a very deep interest in the proceedings. Indeed, it is stated that he was unaware, until some time after the sentence, that he was to be hanged. The autopsy was performed, about an hour after his death, by Dr. Belleau, and the brain was secured by H. V. Ogden, B.A., and brought to me in excellent condition for examination.

Organ large, weighed about 1587 grms. (56 ozs). [*Pl. II.*] The hemispheres, though large, did not completely cover the cerebellum. Membranes were normal; vessels of the pia mater and the subjacent grey matter deeply engorged.

Left hemisphere (*Pl. II., fig.* 3).—*Fis. Sylv.* is separated from ascending *parietal* by a very narrow and grooved gyrus, and joins the *inf. front.* by a shallow sulcus (*a*).

Fis. Rolando sends a deep fissure (*b*) across the upper end of *asc. par. gyr.*, which curves round the margin and unites with *fis. cruciata* of the *pre-cuneus.* There is not a well-marked *asc.* or 3*rd front. sul.* The 1*st fr. sul.* has a short vertical branch, and only extends for 2.5 cm. from *asc. front. gyr.*, when the 1st and 2nd convolutions fuse, but beyond this it is again apparent. 2*nd front. sul.* has a short vertical branch, and joins the fis. Sylv. by a narrow groove. Its anterior extension is well developed. The 3*rd front. gyr.* is large in comparison with the 1st and 2nd. The *asc. front. gyr.* is large.

The *asc. par. sul.* (retro-central), which is usually united with the inter-parietal, and called its radial portion, is isolated, and only joins the fis. Sylv. by a shallow furrow (c). The *asc. par. gyr.* is narrow.

The *inter-parietal fis.* runs almost parallel to the *asc. par.* and *fis. Rol.*, being separated from the former by a narrow convolution which joins the *sup. parietal lobule.* Below it joins the 1*st temp. sul.* (*d*); above it does not extend to the margin. Gyri of parietal lobe well developed.

The 1*st temp. sul.* is crossed in two places by bridging gyri uniting the 1*st* and 2*nd convolutions*. Posteriorly this sulcus has two branches—one which joins the *i. par.*, the other the *inf. occip*. The 2*nd temp. sul.* is not well marked.

The *sup. occip. sul.* joins the *par. occip.*; the *inf. occip. sul.* the 1*st temp.*

On median surface, *par. occip. fis.* unites with *sup. occip.*, and by a shallow sulcus with *fis. cruciata* of *pre-cuneus*.

Calcarine fis. normal; *cuneus* small.

Fis. collateralis long, and sends numerous fissures into *gyri lingualis* and *fusiformis*.

Sul. calloso-marg. has many fissures entering the 1*st front. gyr. Gyr. fornicatus* is fissured longitudinally. *Orbital gyri* normal; well marked *frontal marginal sul.* No external orbital fissure. *Insula* well developed, and has 9 gyri.

Right hemisphere (*Pl. II., fig.* 4).—*Fis. Sylv.* joins 3*rd* or *asc. front. sul.* (*a*), and the *asc. par.* (*b*) (retro-central) by shallow furrows. *Fis. Rol.* unites with 1*st front.* (*c*) and *asc. par.* (*d*) *sulci* by narrow grooves.

The *asc. front. sul.* arises by a shallow fissure from the *fis. Sylv.*, and then at the base of the 2*nd front. gyr.* joins the 2*nd front. sul.* 1*st*, 2*nd* and 3*rd frontal gyri* are well developed and distinct posteriorly. Anteriorly they are fused and crossed by many secondary sulci. *Asc. frontal gyr.* is very narrow in its centre.

Inter-parietal fis. has a well marked radial portion (the asc. par. or retro-central). The sagittal part passes back and presents three divisions—one (*e*) enters the *sup. par. lobule*, a second (*f*) passes directly back and joins a fissure in the position of *inf. occip.*, which reaches to the tip of occip. lobe, and the third (*g*) part passes vertically down and unites with 1*st temp. sul.* and has a branch which crosses the 2*nd temp. gyr.*

Asc.-par. convolution is large below, narrow above. The *angular*, *supra-marginal* and *sup. par. lobule* are much fissured.

1*st temp. sul.* joins *i.-par.*; the 2nd is not marked. Several oblique sulci cross the 2nd and 3rd temp. gyr. *Sup occip. sul.* joins *par. occip.*

On the median surface, *par. occip. fis.* joins *sup. occip.*; the *calcarine* enters *scissura hippocampi* and joins the *fis. collateralis* by a shallow groove. *Fis. collateralis* large and deep.

The *cuneus* is small; *pre-cuneus* (lob. quad.) is large and its anterior boundary ill-defined.

Calloso-marginal fis. extends to level of base of 1st frontal, and then curves up to the margin of the hemisphere, being interrupted by a broad annectant uniting the *gyr. fornicat.* with 1*st front.* Beyond this there is a short extension which joins a complex series of sulci in the *pre-cuneus.*

Orbital gyri normal. There is a narrow *fronto-marginal sul.* There is a well-marked *external orbital fissure.*

The chief points to be noted are:—

1. The absence of complete covering of cerebellum by cerebrum.

2. On both sides the *pre* and *retro-central fissures* were separated from *fis. of Sylvius* by very narrow and grooved gyri.

3. The left *fis. Rolando* joins *fis. cruciata* of *pre-cuneus*, and on the right side it is imperfectly separated from 1*st front*, and *asc. par. sulci.*

4. The *inter-parietal*, on both sides, joins the 1*st temp. sul.*, and on the right side is much more developed and joins the *occipital.*

5. On the median surface the *calcarine* on the right side enters the *scissura hippocampi.*

There remain two questions for consideration: first, to what extent does Professor Benedikt's confluent fissure type of brain prevail among ordinary members of the community, and how far is it reliable as an indication of defective development?

With a view of ascertaining how far the confluent fissure type of brain exists among the lower classes in this community, I have examined carefully 63 hemispheres from 34 individuals, all of whom were patients in, and died at, the General Hospital. Most of these were preserved by Giacomini's method, and as no special note exists as to the social standing or character of any of the individuals from whom they were obtained, the results are of value only so far as they show to what extent confluence of fissure occurs in that class from which the Hospital wards are recruited.

1. The Fissure of Rolando communicated with—
   a. *Fissure of Sylvius*, in 3 completely, in 7 incompletely.
   b. *Frontal sulci*, complete in 12; incomplete, 9.
   c. *Inter-parietal sulci*, complete in 7; incomplete, 9.
2. The Fissure of Sylvius joined—
   a. The *F. R.* [see above.]
   b. The *frontal* in 20.
   c. The *inter-parietal*, complete in 26; incomplete, 8.
   d. The 1st *temporal*, in 15.
3. The Inter-parietal united with—
   a. The *F. R.* [see above].
   b. The *F. S.* [see above].
   c. The *parieto-occipital* in 18.
   d. The *horizonal* or *sup. occipital* in 14.
   e. The 1st *temporal* in 19.
4. The *Calcarine* entered the *scissura hippocampi* in 25.
5. The *calloso-marginal* joined the *par.-occipital* in 1.
6. The *parieto-occipital* joined—
   a. The *inter-parietal in* 18.
   b. The *horizonal occipital* in 3.

From these limited observations we may conclude—

1. That a considerable proportion of the brains of Hospital cases are of the confluent fissure type.

2. The chief difference to be noted between Prof. Benedikt's series of criminals' brains and those which I have just gone over is the somewhat greater number of unions between typical fissures, more particularly between the *fis. Rol.* and contiguous ones. Thus in his set this fissure connected, completely or incompletely, with the *fis. Syl.* in 24 instances; in my series in only 10. In the other fissures the disproportion is not nearly so great.

3. Considering the number of brains of ordinary Hospital patients which present in some degree the confluent fissure type, it would seem more reasonable not to assign as yet any special significance to it until we have fuller information about the arrangement of the convolutions in the various races, and until a much larger number of the brains of criminals of all countries have been examined.

Professor Benedikt's cases were nearly all Slavonians or Hungarians, and though Betz of Kieff, a leading authority, acknowledged the atypy of his specimens, it would have been more satisfactory to have had a comparison between these specimens and an equal number taken from law-abiding members of the same races. It may be urged that in Hospital patients the brains should conform in considerable numbers to this 2nd or confluent fissure type, as many of them are individuals in the lower ranks of life, and not a few belong to the criminal class. This applies, however, much more forcibly to dissecting-room material, which, as Dr. Benedikt says, " consists of the remains of those who have suffered complete shipwreck in life through low grade of intelligence, imperfect motor development, or through crimes and vice." In the series of brains which I examined, there were no dissecting-room specimens, and it did not include the brain of any notorious criminal so far as I am aware.

As to how far confluence of fissures is indicative of a low type of cerebral organization we also want fuller information. When existing in high degree, there is certainly an absence of many important annectants or bridging areas of brain substance, but when we consider the variable size of convolutions bounding the typical fissures, it is easy to see that defect in one part might be more than compensated for by excess in another part, and even a neighbouring part. In several of the brains which I examined, notably No. 10, the confluent fissure type existed in an organ with a rich convolution system. In the brain of Moreau, the retro-central fissure on the left side was separated from the inter-parietal by a distinct gyrus, which might as well be regarded as an excess, as absence of an annectant and confluence of two fissures might be considered a defect.

With reference to the type of four frontal convolutions which Prof. Benedikt has found in such a large number of his specimens, I will only say that in 10 of the hemispheres examined it was observed in a greater or less degree of development. Nowhere was it better seen than in the brain of Hayvern. To enter upon the anatomical significance of this would be beside the question on this occasion.

Professor Benedikt's conclusions are those of a thorough-going somatist, who would bring all human conduct within the range of organic action. "The constitutional criminal," he says, "is a burdened individual, and has the same relation to crime as his next of blood kin, the epileptic, and his cousin, the idiot, have to their encephalopathic conditions." And again, "the essential ground of abnormal action of the brain" (*i.e.*, I take it, bad conduct,) "is abnormal brain structure. His 44 criminals were what they were because of defects in the organization of their hemispheres: they belonged to the *criminal variety* of the *genus homo.* No wonder he says "that this proposition is likely to create a veritable revolution in ethics, psychology, jurisprudence and criminalities." He wisely adds that it should not yet serve as a premise, and should not, for the present, leave the hands of the anatomists, since it must be repeatedly proven before it can finally rank as an undoubted addition to human science.

Crime is commonly regarded as the result of yielding to an evil impulse which could have been controlled; and this element of *possible control* is what, in the eyes of the law, separates the responsible criminal from the irresponsible lunatic. The belief in a criminal *psychosis* is spreading, and is the outcome of sounder views of the relation of mind to brain; and these investigations of Prof. Benedikt, to which I have so frequently referred, may serve as a foundation to a natural history of crime. But if this *is* the case, how are we to regard our criminals? What degree of responsibility can be attached to the actions of a man with a defective cerebral organization? Where is there scope to eschew the evil and to do the good, when men are "villains by necessity, fools by heavenly compulsion, knaves, thieves and treachers by spherical predominance." Any one who believes that with all our mental and moral processes there is an unbroken material succession, must consistently be a *determinist*, and hold, with Spinoza, that "in the mind there is no such thing as absolate or free will, but the mind is determined to will this or that by a cause which is determined by another cause, this by yet another, and so on to infinity." For a long time to come, however, the majority of individuals—including some who are inconsistent in so doing—will continue to hold the *intuitionist* view, nowhere better expressed than by Shakespeare, when he puts into the mouth of that arch-criminal, Iago, the words: "'Tis in ourselves that we are thus and thus. Our bodies are our gardens to the which our wills are gardeners; so that if we will plant nettles or sow lettuce, set hyssop and weed up thyme, supply it with one gender of herbs or distract it with many, either to have it sterile with idleness or manured with industry, why, the power and corrigible authority of this lies in our will."

"Theft and murder," as Huxley well says, "would be none the less objectionable were it possible to prove that they were the result of the activity of special theft and murder cells in the grey pulp." One thing is certain, that, as society is at present constituted, it cannot afford to have a class of *criminal automata*, and to have every rascal pleading faulty grey matter in extenuation of some crime. The law should continue to be a "terror to evil-doers," and to let this anthropological variety (as Benedikt calls criminals) know positively that punishment will follow the commission of certain acts, should prove an effectual deterrent in many cases, just as with our dogs, the fear of the whip exercises a restraining influence—immediate as well as prospective—on the commission of canine crimes.

REMARKS ON THE CAUSES OF DEATH IN DIPHTHERIA AND THE TREATMENT.

BY FRANCIS E. SHERRIFF, M.D., L.R.C.S.E., HUNTINGDON, P.Q.

Notwithstanding the continued and general prevalence of diphtheria, much diversity of opinion still prevails regarding its nature and treatment. Many believe that it is only a disease of the throat, while more, I think, contend that it is a disease of the system and governed by fixed laws like scarlatina and other zymotic diseases. I am of opinion that like other similar affections, an individual who has been ill of the disease is not liable to take it again, or at least for a long period. During the past four years I have followed one course of treatment with very gratifying success. My system was published in the CANADA MEDICAL AND SURGICAL JOURNAL in February, 1878. There are four causes of death which have to be guarded against. The first is a rapid and often sudden sinking, like syncope, which is apt to occur on the third, fourth and fifth days. The second cause arises from putrefaction of the false membrane causing septicæmia and hæmorrhage. The third is a diphtheritic croup, and the fourth is paralysis, sometimes taking place five or six weeks after apparent recovery. During the first two days of the attack the temperature often reaches 105°, although more frequently it is less. This can be speedily reduced by the free use of the salicylate and acetate of ammonia combined, also by the application of cold water to the throat under the chin and sponging with tepid water. As soon as the membrane is formed antiseptics must be applied either by a soft brush, atomizer or syringe. I do not believe it makes much difference what antiseptic is used as they are all good, such as brine, alcohol, iodine, sulphurous, salicylic, boracic or benzoic acids. The swabbing mixture I have always used is composed of Acid Carbolic, Tinct. Ferri Mur. Chlorat. Potass. Glycerine and Sulphurous acid. It has been my practice in severe cases to swab the throat every three hours, but lately I have learned that so frequent swabbing is unnecessary, and I am glad such is the case, as the operation causes a good deal of trouble both to the operator and patient. Three or four times a day is often enough. After the fever has been reduced I give every two hours a mixture composed of Chlorat. Potass., Tinc. Mur. Ferri, Sulphurous acid, Glycerine and water. This mixture acts as a powerful antiseptic and ought to be continued for two weeks after recovery, but only three times a day. If symptoms of sinking come on I give aromatic spirits of ammonia. The cold water application to the neck ought to be continued until all swelling of the throat internally or externally are dispersed. By attending carefully to these directions putrefaction of the membrane is almost certain to be prevented and thus obviating the second cause of death. It is doubtful if anything can be done to prevent croupal symptoms than by carefully attending to the first stage of the disease. Paralysis, I think, may be prevented by making the patient take medicine for at least two weeks after apparent recovery. This practice I have tried to pursue with all my patients, whether slight or severe, and I have seen only one fatal case of paralysis. As soon as the membrane has nearly disappeared I use a solution of salicylic acid, and borax and glycerine, both internally and by injection of the nostrils. Many writers insist on the necessity of supporting the strength by stimulants and nourishing food. This practice I have never followed, and only give such nourishment as the patient will take without much coaxing. Pure milk is probably the best.

THE USE AND ABUSE OF ALCOHOLIC DRINKS.

To the Editor of the CANADA MEDICAL & SURGICAL JOURNAL.

SIR,—In the Canada *Medical Record* for December I find a paper on the "*Use of Alcohol in Health*," by Professor Casey A. Wood, of Bishop's College, in which he criticises at length an address given by me to the medical society in this city, on the "*Use and Abuse of Alcoholic Drinks*," and subsequently published in the CANADA MEDICAL AND SURGICAL JOURNAL.

All must acknowledge the ability and ingenuity exhibited in Dr. Wood's paper; from his "standpoint," he has left little to be added. While I feel flattered and pleased at the notice taken of my address, for discussion often exposes the weak points on both sides of the question, Dr. Wood must pardon me if I feel that he has been hypercritical. I will not say that his arguments are "absurd." The word so often used by him not being an elegant one, should be expunged from discussions of this kind. though I fail to see the force of many of them. And making due allowance for the exuberant zeal so often displayed by speakers and writers upon this subject, I fear Dr. Wood perused my paper with a prejudiced eye when he classed me as an "*advocate*" of the uso of alcoholic drinks.

Every well-wisher of his race should hold up both hands in favor of any means that would lessen the shocking evil of intemperance, and I have no doubt Dr. Wood is one of them, consequently we are in accord upon that point, both wishing to arrive at the same goal. The issue between us lies in the fact that he takes one road I another, mine, I freely grant, possessing many obstructions, his—as acknowledged by himself—being impassable. Knowing that restrictions and prohibitory laws have effeeted little or nothing towards lessening the gigantic evil of intemperance, I was induced to write an address urging upon my professional brethren the propriety of exercising the influence they possess towards educating the "masses" upon the "*use and the abuse of alcoholic liquors*." In it I portrayed in as strong language as I could command the disastrous consequences of the *abuse* of them; that the great majority of persons are better without them; that they are not necessary aids in promoting health and vigor of body and mind; that, unlike other articles of diet, a dangerous craving is created by the continued and unseasonable use of them, and that the evils consequent upon the *abuse* preponderate over the benefits derived from them. I also cautioned my professional brethren when prescribing them medicinally to be particularly careful and avoid bringing the system into a habit of dependence upon the stimulus. I further stated that "the exhilarating effect of alcoholic beverages is so universally felt that the *use* of them has become a 'social habit,' and one so engrafted upon the human mind that no amount of persuasion or exertion can eradicate it." As well might we attempt to prevent the tide from rising as to prevent the production and consumption of them; therefore the efforts of the philanthropist should be directed towards the *possible*, not the *impossible*. I also stated that the "social use" often leads to abuse. "But if we are unable to combat the *use*, let us attack the *abuse*; let us teach those who use them how to do so with comparative safety, and how to avoid the danger." This, in the eye of Dr. Wood, is the language of an "*advocate*" of moderate drinking. As well might I be accused of wishing a patient to die because I said that his symptoms were such as to make his case hopeless.

The mind must be weak indeed that believes the word "abstain" possesses such magic power as to induce the millions of human beings who till the millions of acres in the cultivation of the grape in various parts of the world to abandon their occupation, or could this be accomplished, that alcoholic stimulants would not be produced from other substances in the vegetable kingdom *so long as the appetite for the stimulus exists.* Dr. Wood does not possess this belief, for he distinctly tells us (I quote his words), that " no amount of prohibition will prevent *in toto* the sale of liquor, that we are certain to have drunkards in spite of all coercive measures." Again he says, "I have no hope that our children's children will see drinking habits done away with, though all moderate drinkers were to join the ranks of teetotalism, nor even if the education and general amelioration of the condition of the masses (the real effective combatants of vice) were to be brought about; but drunkenness will always reign while the way is paved to it by the 'good intentions' of the so-called *use* of alcohol as a drink." A grave responsibility placed upon the shoulders of the men with "good intentions" by Dr. Wood; but he forgets that should all moderate drinkers join the ranks of teetotalism, there would be little need for his prohibitory laws. He also says, " yet *agitation for prohibitory laws* is the necessary outcome of the truth that alcoholic drinking is an injurious nuisance." It may be the necessary outcome. But Dr. Wood has rightly told us that "we will have drunkards in spite of all coercive measures." Then why agitate for laws which, if passed, will not produce the desired effect, and which must leave a large minority disapproving of them, whose ingenuity will be stimulated to evade them by every possible means, thus engendering deception, disregard for the sanctity of an oath, and moral degradation? And it may be asked why not agitate for something more practical and capable of being accomplished? For while all praise is due to "abstainers," who, by practice and precept, have doubtless saved many an individual from the horrors of intemperance, still it must be acknowledged that notwithstanding their efforts the drinking habit has increased with the increase of population, particularly in northern districts. If such is the case, and I think it will not be denied, then why find fault with a proposal to appeal to the understanding and the fears of the masses in favour of temperance? It is better to look facts in the face than to theorize about the abuse of over-eating, excessive bathing, swallowing too much camphor, &c. Every school boy should know that if he takes too much pudding it may make him sick. An individual eats a moderate dinner and feels well after it; he takes a glass of wine, and feels better, or thinks he does; but let him take too much of either, he pays the penalty. Hence, the necessity for exercising that self-control which is implanted in every individual, and which should be fostered and encouraged by all means, ennobling as it does the man who brings it to bear upon his acts and degrading him who declines to be governed by it.

Dr. Wood has taken exception to my remark that "every nation has its stimulant of some kind, that kind Providence has permitted the use of them, and that if they are abused evil consequences follow," and he enters into a lengthy argument to prove that the Mahommedans did not make use of a stimulant that will compare with alcohol. I did not say that all nations did, yet the Doctor acknowledges that the Mahommedans got drunk sometimes "on the forbidden juice of the grape." He concludes with the remark that "if it be stated that Providence really does approve of and sanction the employment of alcohol in health, I should neither agree nor disagree with the statement, for I do not know anything about it; but if He does approve of its use, there can be no shadow of a doubt but that He sanctions (on Dr. Bayard's own shewing) the employment of a very bad thing, and that the sooner He puts His veto on it, the sooner will He deserve the adjective with which Dr. Bayard qualifies His name." This argument is as pointless as it is blasphemous. I did not say that the Almighty *approved* of or sanctioned the use of alcohol. I said that he *permitted* its use. He permits sin. Possibly Dr. Wood may construe His permission to mean approval and sanction. Dr. Wood endeavours to prove upon hygienic and physiological grounds that the taking of "one drop" of alcohol is an *abuse*. So it would be if it could be proved that the drop produced intoxication and was injurions to health. He says that alcohol having "no *locus standi* in the human economy, it is no excuse whatever for drinking a daily glass of beer or wine to say that a dozen glasses of gin per diem will probably sooner or later produce cirrhosis of the liver." What does this mean? Who said that it did afford an excuse? Dr. Wood further says that "if it be illegal to explode fire-crackers within the city limits, surely the illegality begins with the explosion of the first cracker, not after the firing of the third." Certainly the illegality commences with the first act contrary to law. But is Dr. Wood credulous enough to believe that a law could be enacted to prohibit the use of "one drop" of alcohol, or that such a law could be enforced? I shall next expect him to urge that Lucifer matches should not be used, because by improper use of them they might set fire to a house.

Dr. Wood charges me with admitting that a goodly number of moderate drinkers must of necessity be kept on the tenter-hooks of eternal watchfulness. I acknowledge the correctness of the charge, believing that in spite of all coercive and prohibitory laws that can or ever will be enacted or enforced, there must and will be a "goodly number of moderate drinkers." I accept the inevitable rather than follow a shadow, and would have every individual kept on the "tenter-hooks of eternal watchfulness." As they would pray for forgiveness of sin, so let them guard themselves and exercise all the self-control they can command against the fascination of over-indulgence in the use of alcoholic liquors. And to aid this precept I would teach all who *will* make use of them how to do so with comparative safety and how to avoid the danger. And I would have my professional brethren aid in this work. Dr. Wood acknowledges that education is one of the effective combatants against vice. And so it is. The drinking habit is a vice, therefore let us educate upon it; let us instill into the minds of the "masses" the injurious consequences following the use of stimulants at *improper times*, in *improper quantities* and *without food.*

In conclusion, let me say to Dr. Wood that, while all praise is due to him and his co-workers in a good cause, still if he exercised the ability he evidently possesses towards educating the "masses" upon this point and towards urging upon philanthropists the necessity for comfortable and cheerful homes for the destitute, he would accomplish more good for his cause than by denouncing those who differ from him as encouraging drunkenness.

W. BAYARD, M.D.

St. John, N.B., January 26, 1882.

Hospital Reports.

MEDICAL AND SURGICAL CASES OCCURRING IN THE PRACTICE OF THE MONTREAL GENERAL HOSPITAL.

Two Cases of Cancer of the Stomach.—(Reported by Dr. J. A. MACDONALD, House Physician.)

CASE NO. I. UNDER THE CARE OF DR. GEORGE ROSS.

CASE I.—S. M., female, aged 73; admitted into Hospital Dec. 14th, 1881, to be treated for pain behind lower part of sternum and vomiting. No family history of cancer. Married at 20; husband only lived 10 months; no children. Has been a very hard drinker, especially last ten years; was a healthy woman till present trouble began. No history of any pain or vomiting previously. Eighteen months ago began to suffer from pain behind the lower part of sternum after eating; pain was not very severe, and after an hour or so would disappear. Two months ago she says she began to vomit; pain generally relieved by vomiting; has been losing flesh all this time: at present, patient is greatly emaciated, and is very feeble; requires help to get out of bed. The pain complained of is just behind ensiform cartilage, is of a burning character, and shoots through to the back. When food is taken she swallows without any forcing efforts, but experiences a sensation as if the food stopped just above cardiac end of stomach, and the pain begins at once. After a short interval, one to three minutes, the food begins to come up again; is simply regurgitated in mouthfuls; no effort at retching. After the food has been regurgitated the pain is usually relieved. This regurgitation was what she referred to when she spoke of vomiting before admission. At intervals between taking food spits up a quantity of glairy mucus. The abdomen is very empty, walls very lax; no tumour found on exploration of abdomen, epigastric region being specially examined. Liver extends two inches below ribs, and on its edge are two rounded irregularities; spleen not enlarged; heart and lungs normal; no albumen in urine.

Dec. 20th.—Since the patient has been under observation no marked change from the above symptoms observed. The amount of food kept down, if any, must be very small, as any taken is invariably regurgitated at once, always mixed with a quantity of mucus. The pain is not always relieved by the ejection of the food, especially towards night, but pain is never severe. Bowels are constipated; an enema caused a small movement of the bowels. An oesophageal bougie passed without diffiulty 17 inches, and met with a permanent obstruction.

Dec. 27th.—Bougie has been passed several times, but always meets an obstruction about 16 inches, evidently about cardiac end of stomach. Patient takes nothing but a little brandy and soda and small quantities of milk and lime water, but these are never retained. Is getting very feeble; speaks in a whisper. Pulse, 80; very weak.

Jan. 12th.—Enemeta of beef-tea and brandy tried several times, but were not retained, and patient absolutely refused to have anything more done for her. Is wasting slowly.

From this till date of death the symptoms remained about the same. Regurgitation of anything taken continued; towards the last would only take small quantities of soda water. For some days before death there was great dryness of skin, with blueish tinge of extremities, and a marked cadaveric odour. Death occurred Jan. 21st, 1882, about 19 months after first symptoms of pain, or three after vomiting set in.

Autopsy.—Body extremely emaciated. In abdomen, stomach very small and occupies the left hypochondriac region. Pharynx, œsophagus and stomach removed together. The gullet was dilated, fusiform; mucosa opaque; muscular coats thickened. Just above the cardia the walls were infiltrated and hard, but the mucous membrane was intact. In the stomach a flat cancerous ulcer, with smooth base, hard, sharp edges, occupied the cardia and the lesser curve, in an area about half the size of the palm. Great narrowing of the cardiac orifice was caused by the infiltrated state of the walls. Nothing special in the other organs, except the gall bladder, which was very large, contained about a dozen calculi, and attached to the upper wall was a large, flat, cancerous mass, confined entirely to the bladder, not involving the adjacent liver substance.

CASE NO. II. UNDER THE CARE OF DR. MOLSON.

CASE II.—L. F., aged 62, admitted into Hospital Jan. 17th, 1882, to be treated for indefinite pains in abdomen, constipation of bowels, and very rapid loss of flesh. Has been a healthy labouring man and a moderate drinker. No history of syphilis. No family history of cancer. Patient says he has suffered from a gnawing pain in abdomen for two months. The pain is not definitely located to any part; when asked where the pain is, he runs his hand over the abdomen without indicating any spot in particular. Pain has never been severe. Bowels very much constipated; says he frequently passes four or five days without going to stool, and then has to use purgatives. Loss of flesh is very rapid and marked. The pain, constipation and loss of flesh date back two months only. No vomiting or pain after eating. Is a pale, flabby man, decidedly cachectic. Arteries atheromatous. Last autumn weighed 168 lbs.; now weighs 128. Is able to walk about, but says he is getting feeble. Abdomen is very flaccid, so that a good examination is easily made. No tenderness; no tumour. Nothing found on examination of rectum; no albumen in urine. Liver extends slightly below ribs. Heart and lungs normal. Temperature normal; pulse 90, small and weak.

Jan. 20th.—Patient's bowels moved freely several times since admission by mild purgatives or enemata. Appetite is very poor. No pain or vomiting after eating. Nothing further made out. *23rd*—Patient had been doing about as usual till this morning, when he vomited for the first time; vomited matter decidedly stercoracious. Bowels moved daily; stools thin and very offensive. Pain is always present, but is slight, and not sufficient to prevent sleep at night. Is getting weaker. Refuses stimulants. *25th*—Bowels moved daily by teaspoonful doses of the compound liquorice powder. No further vomiting till this morning, when he vomited several times; vomited matter of same character as on previous occasions. Takes no nourishment but a little milk; is losing flesh very rapidly, and now makes no attempt to get out of bed. Temperature never goes above 98°F.; pulse 90, and very feeble.

From this time till his death, Jan. 31st, he vomited a little daily, never excessively; bowels moved naturally, but stools always thin and offensive. Death was slow, and resulted from pure exhaustion; patient much emaciated.

Autopsy.—Moderate emaciation; abdomen retracted. On inspection of intestines terminal part of duodenum is adherent to mesocolon and to the stomach, the parts being matted together and injected. Several greyish-white nodular masses in anterior wall of stomach. *Stomach.*—Opened along its anterior border. An enormous cancerous ulcer, with an irregular, sloughing base, occupies the mid-zone, almost encircling the organ. It measures 19 x 8 c. m. The edges are swollen and infiltrated; soft and greyish-white in color, evidently cancerous. The cardia and pylorus are not involved. At the base of the cancerous mass there are two large orifices of communication—one with the duodenum, which admits the index finger; the other with the colon, near the splenic flexure, admits the thumb, and has thickened edges. There are no secondary masses. Heart, lungs and other organs presented nothing of special note.

Correspondence.

To the Editor of THE CANADA MEDICAL & SURGICAL JOURNAL.

DEAR SIR,—The late tariff of medical fees in the Province of Quebec, is, I understand, to be revised during the coming session of Parliament. No mention of fees to be allowed in judicial cases was introduced into that tariff. It would be well to have this settled also whilst the tariff is being made. At present a physician appearing to give evidence is only allowed by an order in council a small fee over and above the amount payable to an ordinary witness as established by law, who has first to swear that he is poor and needy, having done which, he may be allowed the extra fee ordered in Council.

I hold that in all ordinary cases a physician attending a case is bound to give evidence as to what may come to his knowledge in that connection as any ordinary witness as to fact of any subject coming under his notice in the practice of his daily occupation; but when a medical man is called to give an opinion on the evidence as produced, or when he is called to give an opinion on some branch of the medical profession or scientific knowledge generally, he should be paid accordingly as an expert of these branches. He is called because his opinion is valued, and should be paid a fee commensurate with his position and experience. The use of the microscope and chemistry are the most frequently called into use, but anatomy or any other branch may be occasionally required, and a tariff should embrace these fees, both in the town and at a distance from home, and the fee for the examination separate, and according to time occupied.

I think that a representation made by the different medical societies to the College of Physicians and Surgeons of Quebec to secure their action in concert with the Government would be advisable.

Yours very truly, G. P. GIRDWOOD.

Reviews and Notices of Books.

A Manual of Ophthalmic Practice.—By HENRY S. SCHELL, M.D., Surgeon to Wills Eye Hospital, and Aural Surgeon to the Children's Hospital. With fifty-three illustrations. Philadelphia: D. G. Brinton.

This is a manual of handy dimensions, and appears to have been very carefully compiled. It contains a brief description of the anatomy and physiology of the eye, followed by chapters in systematic order upon the diseases of the various portions of the ocular apparatus. Special sections are devoted to the ophthalmoscope, and minute directions for its proper employment and the results which can be obtained with it. The anomalies of refraction and accommodation also receive the attention which their importance demands. The book is one intended specially for the assistance and guidance of the student of ophthalmology from the very commencement of his studies. It is well and clearly written, and seems to be thoroughly reliable. It can be strongly recommended to practitioners and to those following courses of instruction in this special branch in our hospitals.

Epilepsy and other Chronic Convulsive Diseases: their causes, symptoms and treatment.—By W. R. Gowers, M.D., F.R.C.P., Assistant Professor of Clinical Medicine in University College, Senior Assistant Physician to University College Hospital, Physician to the National Hospital for the Paralysed and Epileptic. London: J. & A. Churchill.

This last work of Dr. Gowers is a complete monograph upon this common and dreaded disease. It is based entirely upon his own original investigations, carried on with reference to a very large number of patients at the well-known National Hospital of Queen's Square. The etiology, symptoms, pathology and treatment of epilepsy are all exhaustively treated of and amply illustrated by the relation of numerous cases. Epilepsy is one of those affections which require for its successful management an accurate knowledge of the physiology of the nervous system and an extensive acquaintance with pathological facts which have a bearing upon it. A perusal of this treatise will furnish the reader with all the latest developments and the best founded theories of the disease, and the means which have proved most successful in arresting it, or, at any rate, lessening the violence and frequency of the attacks. The treatment by bromide of course receives considerable attention. Dr. Gowers' plan is somewhat different from that usually adopted. It is what he calls the method of *maximum dose treatment.* "The object is to give the nervous system, as it were, a series of blows with bromide in order to facilitate the occurrence of the condition which bromide produces in patients who are cured of epilepsy by its use. The method I usually adopt is to begin with doses of two or three drachms of bromide every second or third morning, and increase the dose to four drachms every fourth morning, and six drachms or an ounce every fifth morning." "It is only suitable in cases in which the attacks are influenced in a marked degree by bromide." "It has seemed to me to be of distinct value."

In addition to Epilepsy proper, Hysteroid-convulsions and Hystero-Epilepsy are also considered, with especial reference to their alliance with the former disease.

From the high reputation already enjoyed by Dr. Gowers as a writer upon nervous diseases, we need hardly say that this work is characterized by the scientific accuracy, the profound research, close reasoning and lucid exposition of every point, which we are led to look for in the products of his pen. It forms the most valuable original treatise on this obscure complaint which has appeared of recent years, and we cordially recommend it to the notice of the Canadian profession.

The Opium-habit and Alcoholism.—A treatise on the habits of Opium and its Compounds—Alcohol, Chloral Hydrate, Chloroform, Bromide Potassium, and Cannabis Indiea,—including their therapeutical indications. With suggestions for treating various painful complications. By Dr. FRED. HEMAN HUBBARD. New York: A. S. Barnes & Co.

This book treats of some very important subjects—subjects which are very frequently brought to the notice of the family physician—viz., the inordinate use (or rather the abuse) of certain stimulating and narcotic drugs. The opium-habit is specially dilated upon, and the details are given of a large number of cases treated by the author with more or less success. Many useful points are brought out with reference to the management of these very troublesome cases, but we do not find anything essentially different from the general rules which have been laid down by various previous writers. The treatise would have been more valuable to scientific physicians if these reports of cases had been put into more technical form, with definite descriptions of the exact nervous and other symptoms presented by the patients, for they are decidedly sketchy and rather popularly written. We must, moreover, take exception to several statements which we think are devoid of the scientific accuracy we should rightly expect. For instance, it is stated that the practice of using chloroform in accouchements is the cause of many persons acquiring the habit of the persistent use of the drug by inhalation, and then the cure recommended is the addition of turpentine and nitrite of amyl to the chloroform. It is said to have been *demonstrated* that the turpentine protects from the dangers of collapse or syncope. We would be glad to think that this had been demonstrated; on the contrary, a death from this very mixture was reported in this country last year. The writer condemns the use of chloroform in midwifery. He declares that it is quite possible to so mitigate the pains of labor that it will not be required. His panacea for this purpose is diet. He proposes to put the mothers upon a non-calcareous diet, so that "the framework of the fœtus may be yielding and pliable," thus "enabling it to glide through the pelvis easily." After these rather cartilaginous infants are born, the mothers are to have plenty of phosphates and harden their bones for them. It is also stated that by adopting this dietary, "puerperal fever and phlegmasia are entirely avoided, as the diet has facilitated the free elimination of those humors that excite inflammatory action during the puerperal state." We don't like the pathology, and cannot recommend the therapeusis based upon it.

The treatment recommended for alcoholism is the persistent impregnation during several days of every article of food by a mixture composed of nearly all the known varieties of alcoholic drinks. Great results are promised from the disgust thus excited in the patient's mind. We cannot feel the confidence here expressed in this plan. A singular admission is made with reference to the drinking habits of our grandfathers. Drinking in the mornings, in the degenerate people of the present day, is specially condemned, but in our ancestors it is said to have "had a salutary effect and to have been conducive to longevity." We know not what proof there is of this strange assertion, and cannot but think that, if the truth were known, topers in the old days produced diseases of their livers and kidneys just as they do in our own times.

We cannot recommend the adoption of all the author's suggestions, but, at the same time, we must say that any one interested in this subject will find in his cases much that will illustrate the many phases of the disorders induced in these victims to narcotics, and that will repay perusal.

On Spermatorrhœa : its Pathology, Results and Complications. —By J. L. Milton, Senior Surgeon to St. John's Hospital for Diseases of the Skin. Eleventh edition. London: H. Renshaw. 1881.

The fact that this work is now in its eleventh edition is a proof that it has been distributed widely, if not read widely. The book has been ostensibly written for medical men, but we certainly think it has not been bought by them to the extent of eleven editions. That large class of the youthful community known as "sexual hypochondriacs" have no doubt greatly aided in swelling the number of editions. The first chapter opens with a brief history of the disease, tracing it back as far as the period where men became transformed from hunters and shepherds to citizens. Why the history did not extend back to the *monkey* period of mankind it is difficult to say, especially as it is well known that monkeys, of all beings, are most addicted to the practices which lead to the disease treated of in the book before us. Hercules is made to contribute his quota to the history, and his name mingles familiarly with the names of Moses, Hippocrates, Celsus, and Horace. A long interval, in which history is silent about this disease, is passed over, and then the genius of the great John Hunter is invoked to grapple with the hydra-headed monster. In this connection Sir E. Home is quite unnecessarily, and without the least proof, accused of stealing his nitrate of silver treatment from Hunter. Mr. Milton then places on the roll of glory the names of Lallemand, Curling and Phillips for having "first elevated spermatorrhœa to its true position of a special and independent disorder." After a few remarks on the present state of professional opinion on the subject, he calls on the leaders of the profession "openly to recognize the disease and to devote more attention to its pathology and treatment," and relates how it reduces "hundreds, if not thousands, to impotence, weariness of life, insanity, &c."

In the second chapter the author treats of the pathology, results and complications of spermatorrhœa, and defines it as "all discharges which result from morbid states of testicles and excretory passages, producing greater expulsion of semen than is compatible with a healthy condition of the genital organs." Mr. Milton classes under this head every case of involuntary emission. If such symptoms constitute spermatorrhœa, how many men arrive at the age of twenty-five without having had an attack! Not many. Mr. Milton tells us that he has been abused for giving an overdrawn statement of the effects of spermatorrhœa, but he points the finger of scorn at his revilers and says, "I have not compiled my statements, but have taken them directly from the statements of patients." Now of all patients, with the exception of hysterical ones, those suffering from sexual hypochondriasis are most apt to exaggerate, and if the practitioner takes all that is told him, without the grain of salt, he will, indeed, make mountains out of mole-hills. It seems to us that true spermatorrhœa is one of the rarest of diseases. We do not recollect ever having met with but one genuine case; but young men who suffer from nocturnal emissions are common enough. Their fears are, as a rule, allayed by judicious counsel, together with advice as to diet, hygiene, &c. The only cases difficult to treat are those who have not entirely given up the vile habit of masturbation, and those whose disease is more mental than sexual. Full occupation is a great help in treatment, taking up certain hobbies, &c. Sir James Paget says that as men grow older they often get over this hypochondriacal state, because they have something more important to think of than their sexual organs. Mr. Milton, in support of his assertion as to the reality of spermatorrhœa, asserts that it is very common in members of our own profession, many of whom he has treated, and who always prefer therapeutic measures to moral instruction and advice. Well, medical men are constituted, mentally, much as other men, have quite as irritable spinal cords, and are not any more free from emotional conditions. Sexual hypochondriasis is the hysteria of males, and in the majority of cases the condition of the genital organs has about as much to do with the one as the uterus has to do with the other.

Mr. Milton, after all that he has said about the pathology of the disease, and after all his urgent appeals to the leaders of the profession to investigate, concludes that spermatorrhœa is "due to an irritable state of testicles, vasa deferentia, and common seminal and ejaculatory ducts." Very simple pathology, truly. The most fearful result of spermatorrhœa is impotence, and a chapter is devoted to *its* pathology. All attention is directed to the conditions of the sexual organs themselves as a cause for (so-called) spermatorrhœa and impotence, but nothing is said of the state of the nervous system, the irritability of the cord, or the emotional temperament of the individuals. Numbers of cases are given, all of which, of course, were cured; in some, the patients were startled by the author telling them that in another year they would have been *impotent*, but he, of course, was able to snatch them from that valley of the shadow of death.

The first 73 pages are devoted to the pathology of the disease, and the last 100 pages to its treatment. One thing may be said of the treatment, viz., that there is plenty of it. The patients are well "worked over," and get the worth of their money. The variety of treatment vies with that of many other specialties, as, for example, that devoted to the cure of the various flexions and curves of the uterus. Of course, the usual tonics are prescribed, as quinine, iron, strychnia, &c., also bromide of potassium, digitalis, lupulin, ergot of rye, &c. Seven pages are devoted to extolling the merits of the tincture of the sesquichloride of iron, given in heroic doses of a drachm to a drachm and a-half three times a day. Cold bathing and "sleeping cool" is advised; also discarding clothing, "especially in the shape of that rubbish which is known by the inappropriate name of underclothing." Blistering, cauterization of the urethra, injections, galvanism, diet, &c., are among the remedies recommended.

Some marvellous instruments are figured to prevent nocturnal emissions, as, for example, several instruments of torture called urethral rings, which look like spiked dog collars, with the spikes worn inside. There is one specially novel instrument which is worthy of this progressive and inventive age. It is called the *Electric Alarum*, and is made somewhat on the principle of the burglar's alarm, and, after the connections are made, is placed under the patient's pillow. A wire cage with a padlock is recommended for those who practice masturbation when half awake and half asleep. Mr. Milton recognizes, in common with other specialists, the production of stricture due to the irritation set up by omissions. We have never happened to meet with such strictures, but Dr. Gross, jr., of Philadelphia, says they can be detected with a No. 22 sound, and Mr. Milton informs us that they occur. According to Mr. M., they are easily amenable to treatment, especially after cauterization with nitrate of silver and the use of his screw dilator. The nature of the stricture is not mentioned ; if it does exist, it is probably spasmodic.

In conclusion, we may say that the book recommends itself in one particular, viz., it is quite free from the disgusting details so often seen in works on this subject. The letterpress is good and typographical errors are few, if we except the leaving out of the capital in such words as Italian, English, &c. Appropriate quotations are interspersed, both from the ancient and modern classics, which, doubtless, will prove attractive to lay readers. We are of opinion that the book under consideration might be compressed into a much smaller compass by leaving out long quotations from other medical authors, and by the author himself being less prolix ; the book would be quite as valuable and take less time to read. We are also of opinion that both lay and medical readers would be much more benefitted by the perusal of Sir James Paget's classical essay on Sexual Hypochondriasis.

Antiseptic Surgery : The Principles, Modes of Application, and Results of the Lister Dressing.—By Dr. JUST LUCAS-CHAMPIONNIÈRE. Translated from the second and completely revised French edition, and edited by FREDERICK HENRY GERRISH, A.M., M.D. 8vo., pp. 239. Portland: Loring, Short & Harmon.

This book supplies a want long felt by the English-speaking portion of the profession everywhere. Hitherto it has been necessary for those who attempted to practice Listerism to obtain the information desired from scattered articles on the subject in the various medical journals of the day, and these were often found to be indifferent guides. Dr. Gerrish deserves, then, the thanks of English and American surgeons for having put this important subject so neatly and concisely before them.

Dr. Championnière is undoubtedly the pioneer of antiseptic surgery in France. He has been a close follower of Lister since 1867, and kept the system constantly before his colleagues until he succeeded in convincing such men as Guyon and Vermeuil of its immense value. In 1875 he spent some months with Lister in Edinburgh, and at the time of writing the second edition of his book, Championnière appears to have had a very extended and remarkable experience of the method. In his introduction he says, "Whatever I state, I have tried and observed. I have educated myself upon all points, and, confident of success, I have fearlessly performed operations which formerly one could scarcely have ventured on." To those who are faithful to the method he promises the following: "The disappearance of wound accidents even in the worst circumstances. A regularity of repair hitherto unknown. Surgery without suppuration; union by first intention habitually and without danger. Such rapidity of healing as to surpass all anticipation. The possibility and safety of operations hitherto considered dangerous and even unjustifiable." All imitations or so-called modifications of Listerism are strongly condemned, and justly, too, as in this way much discredit has been brought upon the method. Doubtless the results of the surgery of all these imitators are vastly improved, but they must be still very uncertain and unsatisfactory. However, even they cannot afford to be without this book, because it is well known that, in order to produce a good counterfeit, the imitator must have some knowledge of the chief characteristics of the genuine article.

The two first chapters are devoted to the history of antisepsis and to the theoretical views on which the practice is based. The author is, of course, as indeed are all the true antiseptic surgeons, a disciple of his clever countryman, Pasteur. He tells how Lister had struggled ceaselessly and in every possible way with the insalubrity of the Glasgow Infirmary, and was constantly vanquished by its fatal influences; how, in 1865, he became a convert to the doctrines of the eminent French chemist, and made for himself numerous experiments which demonstrated the presence of germs in the atmosphere and their influence upon fermentation and putrefaction, and how he then proposed to enter into a struggle with these disturbing elements.

The subsequent chapters are devoted to an exhaustive and very truthful description of the antiseptic apparatus generally, with the influence of the method on the phenomena of repair, &c. Particular operations and dressings are also fully described, and one chapter is devoted to "objections to the antiseptic method." These are all well answered, but especially so is that frequently raised objection—the cost of material. On this point the author says: "I am prepared to assert that this is a remarkable exaggeration, and I have good reason for knowing, as during the first six months I dressed at my own expense all the patients on whom I operated. I privately imported from Edinburgh all the materials, when, too, they were very high-priced. I found the expense of the pieces necessary for the seven dressings, after an amputation of the leg at the upper third, to be about two dollars and forty cents. This patient was healed in twenty-four days, and was able to leave the hospital on the thirtieth. In Nussbaum's excellent work I find an estimate of the pieces of dressing which he considers necessary in a thigh amputation, and reckoning on the same basis, fifteen dressings would cost about five dollars."

A portion of Chapter XX. is devoted to "Listerian Midwifery." In the author's service at the Cochin Hospital, where antiseptic precautions are taken in all obstetrical cases, the statistics have been admirable: In 1878 there were 778 deliveries, serious operations being performed in a good number of them, and only two deaths are recorded from puerperal disease. In a series of 1,455 cases there were only six deaths from all causes, showing a mortality of about 0.41 per cent.

It is to be regretted that the work is not more fully illustrated. It is, however, elegantly printed, and for the convenience of those not familiar with the metric system, the translator has appended a table of equivalents.

Society Proceedings.

MEDICO-CHIRURGICAL SOCIETY OF MONTREAL.

Stated Meeting, December 23rd, 1881.

GEORGE ROSS, M.D., PRESIDENT, IN THE CHAIR.

Acute Tuberculosis.—Dr. McConnell read a paper on "A case of Acute Tuberculosis in an Infant."

The discussion following was confined principally to the subject of tubercular meningitis as to recovery.

Dr. Mills, who had made the *post-mortem* in this case, said he looked specially for tuberculosis in the dura mater, but in this, as in eight other cases he had examined, tubercles there are rare. Enlarged glands pressing on the bronchus would occasion the pneumonia found in the left lung.

Dr. Geo. Ross said that as regarded the attacks of distinctly asthmatic respiration, these, in his experience, were rather suggestive of obstruction by pressure upon a bronchus rather than pressure upon the recurrent nerve, which will cause suffocative attacks from spasm of the glottis. He had recently been observing three cases, in all of which there was respiratory disturbance from pressure on the main tubes; in two of these the trouble arose from secondary cancerous nodules, and in the third from aneurism. In one of the former the attacks of asthma were exactly similar to those of the ordinary spasmodic disorder arising without any local organic change. Had recently had two cases of tubercular meningitis in adults. (These have since been published amongst the Hospital reports in this journal for 15th January.) In the first there had existed an old pleuritic disorder, from which the system became contaminated; in the other there was suppurating disease of the kidney, from which the acute brain trouble was developed.

Dr. Mills asked the opinion of members for prognosis in these cases of tubercular meningitis. He found that Drs. Stephen McKenzie, Sutton and Hughlings-Jackson had a case in which all agreed it to be tubercular meningitis, and this case recovered with the treatment of pot. iod. Cases seen in London were treated with pot. iod. and mercury.

Dr. F. W. Campbell, some years ago, had a case of tubercular meningitis in a boy aged 15; was comatose for from 3 to 5 days; was seen in consultation with Dr. Godfrey, and both concluded that patient would die, but he rallied and lived for two years, and died of phthisis. Treatment was large doses of pot. iod.

Dr. Cameron said some five years ago he saw a case which he thought to be tubercular meningitis in a child aged 4, who died. Two years later, a younger sister, when arriving at the same age, developed similar symptoms; was seen in consultation with Dr. Roddick, and unfavorable prognosis given, but under pot. iod. and brom. and a little calomel, the child recovered. A third child, when arriving at the same age, evinced similar symptoms, and under treatment recovered. The family history was markedly phthisical.

Dr. Wood said he saw a case lately in which tubercular meningitis was diagnosed, and the child recovered.

Dr. Mills related a case of recovery in a girl aged 19, brought into the hospital at Hamilton, with all the symptoms of meningitis. She continued unconscious for four weeks, and then became convalescent in six weeks. During that time the syphon tubing with ice-cold water was used, and whenever the tubing was removed, the temperature rose.

Dr F. W. Campbell mentioned a case of a patient, mother of a large family, who, 10 years ago, had all the symptoms of phthisis, and was attended by her father and another physician. Two years ago extensive disease in the left lung was found, and her appearance indicated fatal issue, but she recovered. Lately the right lung showed decided pneumonic symptoms, and now the left lung appears sound. There is no phthisical history. Treatment last spring was 10 grs. doses of quinine at bed-time and Hydroleine, and subsequently Trommer's Ext. of Malt; now taking 1-120th gr. of atropia in pill and oxymel scillæ to relieve cough.

Stated Meeting, January 6th, 1882.

GEORGE ROSS, M.D., PRESIDENT, IN THE CHAIR.

Pneumonia, Diphtheritic Gastritis.—Dr. Osler exhibited the specimens, which were taken from a man aged 66, who was admitted to the General Hospital with great shortness of breath and prostration, and died in six hours. He was sent in from the House of Refuge, and the surgeon in charge, Dr. Burland, stated that he had noticed the man two days before walking about looking very blue and short of breath. He sent him to bed, and on examination the next day the signs of pneumonia were evident, and he sent him to the Hospital. At the autopsy the stomach and duodenum were enormously distended with gas, the diaphragm on the left side was pushed up in front to a level with the second intercostal space. In the thorax the heart was displaced upwards and to the right, the apex being under the sternum. The right lung was universally adherent; the left was free, but pushed up and compressed by the distended stomach. The right lung was in a state of grey hepatization; the only crepitant parts were a small area at the apex and part of the lower lobe. The left lung was small, compressed, but feebly crepitant. The stomach presented an area of diphtheritic inflammation 12 + 10 cm., just to the left of the cardiac orifice. The mucosa of this region was deeply injected and covered with a closely-adherent greyish-white false membrane, from 1 to 2 mm. in thickness. When stripped off, the membrane beneath was deeply congested and rough. In the centre of the patch was a spot from which it had been removed. In the vicinity of the large area were other small bits of false membrane on congested bases. Œsophagus and duodenum normal. Dr. Bristowe, of St. Thomas's Hospital, was the first to describe diphtheritic inflammation of the alimentary canal in pneumonia; he met with it in the colon in 2 out of 30 secondary, and in 4 out of 16 primary, pneumonias. Dr. Osler, in about 50 autopsies in primary pneumonia, had met with five instances of croupous or diphtheritic colitis. This was the first specimen in which the stomach was affected. In connection with this, he called attention to the frequency of the so-called diphtheritic endocarditis in pneumonia; thirty-eight per cent. of the cases which he had analyzed occurred with inflammation of the lungs. The extreme distention of the stomach has probably taken place during life and in connection with the gastritis; it doubtless assisted in bringing about the fatal termination by embarrassing the heart and compressing the healthy lung.

The President remarked on the latency of pneumonia in old men, and on the special liability of these cases to sudden death from heart failure.

Mitral and Tricuspid Stenosis.—Dr. Molson related the case—a woman aged 39, who died in the Hospital after a residence of four days. She had had rheumatic fever when nine years of age, and ever since had been troubled with short breath and cough on exertion. The chief symptoms on admission were dyspnœa, extreme rapidity and irregularity of the heart, scanty urine, albuminous, and with granular casts. There was no dropsy. Nothing positive could be determined as to the character of the murmurs; under an aggravation of the symptoms, the woman sank on the fourth day. Dr. Osler presented the specimens. The heart showed extreme mitral stenosis, with great thickening of the fused segments; left ventricle small, walls of average thickness; left auricle dilated and hypertrophied. The tricuspid orifice admitted the index-finger, the segments of the valves had united, and the edges were thickened. The right ventricle was dilated and hypertrophied; the right auricle much dilated. The lungs were universally adherent: pleura at left apex very thick, and for an inch or more the lung tissue beneath it was cirrhosed, and had dilated bronchi and fibrous bands passing through it. The lungs were in a state of brown induration, but not congested. The kidneys were slightly reduced in size, granular and rough on the surface, and in a state of tolerably advanced cirrhosis. Dr. Osler, in reply to a question by Dr. T. W. Mills, stated that he thought the condition of the kidneys might have been the outcome of the chronic valve disease, and represented a later stage of the large indurated organs commonly met with. There was not extensive arterial disease or hypertrophy of the left ventricle.

The Brains of Criminals.—Dr. Osler read a paper on this subject, and recorded the results of an examination of the brain of the murderer Hayvern, who was executed at Montreal on 11th Dec., 1881. (*See page* 385.) He first referred to the observations of Benedikt of Vienna, who, in 87 hemispheres from 44 criminals, has found certain peculiarities which he regards as indicative of a lower type of cerebral organization. The points upon which he most dwells are the confluence of many of the principal fissures, and the existence in a considerable proportion (27 of the 87) of four frontal gyri, the fourth being formed by the splitting of the first or second gyrus. This is regarded as an animal similarity. Hayvern was a low, dissolute fellow, addicted to drink, with no special neurosis in his family, who, on June 29, stabbed a fellow-convict. The brain weighed 46½ ozs., and was fairly well formed; the cerebellum was completely covered by the cerebrum. On examination it was found to conform in many respects to Benedikt's cases, and was atypical, according to his views, in the following particulars: The union of the Sylvian fissure with the first frontal gyrus; the junction of the inter-parietal with the parieto-occipital and first temporal fissures; the extension of the calcarine fissure into the scissura hippocampi; the union of the collateral and calcarine sulci, and in the fusion of the first frontal gyrus, so that there appeared to be four frontal convolutions arising from the ascending frontal or anterior central gyrus. To ascertain how far these peculiarities existed in the brains of hospital patients, Dr. Osler examined 43 hemispheres from 24 individuals, and found that a very considerable proportion were of the confluent fissure type. Thus, the Sylvian fissure joined the fissure of Rolando in 8 hemispheres, the frontal sulci in 18, the interparietal in 19, and the first temporal in 12. The chief difference between Benedikt's series of brains of criminals and those examined was a greater number of unions between the typical fissures, more particularly the fissure of Rolando, which in the former joined contiguous sulci in 24 instances. In 9 of the 43 hemispheres there were four more or less distinct frontal gyri. He thought that much fuller information was needed about the arrangement of the sulci in the different races, and many more criminals would have to be examined before any positive result was arrived at as to the constant atypical character of the brain in members of this class. Speaking of Benedikt's conclusions, he questioned whether it was wise to speak of criminals as an anthropological variety of their species. On his views there is no place left for responsibility; but society cannot afford to have a class of criminal automata, and every rascal pleading faulty gray matter in extenuation of his crimes.

Dr. Henry Howard (Med. Supt. Longue Pointe Asylum) asked if it were known how many of the brains of the series of hospital cases were from criminals, and whether a larger proportion presented abnormalities than could be reasonably thought to belong to this class. He believed in a criminal class as distinct as a mercantile class, and regarded the mental and moral condition of the individuals belonging to it as dependent absolutely on their physical organization. Hayvern was not responsible for his act; it was not premeditated, but performed under the influence of an uncontrollable impulse; and he thought that there was evidence to show that it may have been connected with the epileptic neurosis.

Dr. Hingston wanted to know how it was, if viciousness and crime were the product of defective cerebral organization, that some notoriously wicked men had reformed and lived sober and honourable lives? Was it probable that with such a change there was any alteration in the structure of the brain?

Dr. Cameron thought that, for Benedikt's conclusions to have any value, it must be shown that criminals have invariably atypical brains and all other people normal ones. Most criminals have some degree of control over their actions, and the law is an effectual deterrant in many instances, particularly where the penalty enacted touches the person. He illustrated the rapid abolition of garroting by the introduction of the lash, and quoted facts to show the good effects of capital punishment.

Dr. Shepherd remarked that it was somewhat difficult to say what was the typical brain. The majority of observations were upon the lower classes; we lacked data as to the arrangement of the fissures and convolutions in a large number of the intellectual members of society. He had frequently seen brains of the confluent fissure type in the dissecting-room.

Dr. Mills said that, with reference to the series of brains from hospital patients examined by Dr. Osler, the question arises as to how far such patients belong to the criminal class. In about one thousand patients that he had observed closely, he did not think that many of them ranked in this class.

Dr. Osler, in reply to Dr. Howard's question, stated that the series of brains which he had examined were nearly all preserved by Giacomini's method, and no data existed from which the social status of the individuals could be ascertained. In the 43 hemispheres (19 perfect brains and 5 halves), 19 presented one or more atypical features.

Dr. Hingston then showed an instrument, lately made by Tiemann, for facilitating the finding of the urethral canal when a number of false passages existed.

Foreign Bodies in the Windpipe.—Dr. Hingston narrated two cases. *False tooth in the trachea for over three months, tracheotomy, removal.* The patient, an elderly lady, who had worn a false incisor tooth for over 40 years, and had never been in the habit of removing it at night, noticed one morning that she could not find it. After searching in vain for some time, her attention was directed to a suspicious cough, and she began to think she might have swallowed it; though she had not been disturbed during the night, and had no remembrance of its dropping into the throat. When she consulted the doctor there was very little inconvenience, no difficulty of breathing; but while in his house a violent paroxysm of coughing came on, and she appeared to be choking. Brunelle's method of inversion was at once practised, and she was relieved. An operation was urged and consented to, but the following day she felt so well that she refused to submit. Dr. H. heard nothing more of her for several weeks, when she came again, the cough having become troublesome. She again refused operative measures. After consulting several other medical men, all of whom assured her that the tooth was in the windpipe and must be removed, she returned to Dr. H., and finally decided to have the operation performed. On November 1st the trachea was opened, and with a pair of slightly curved laryngeal forceps the offending tooth was readily grasped, being situated in the neighbourhood of the orifice of the right bronchus. It was a small incisor, with a flat gold plate and two lateral extensions to fasten it to the contiguous teeth. It was coated with dark mucous. In the operation, he adopted a device which answered admirably. After a long incision through the skin and superficial fascia, he made a transverse incision just below the cricoid, inserted the director upon the trachea and tore down, with the greatest ease and without any bleeding, the tissues covering the first five or six rings. The remarkable feature about the case was the length of time the foreign body existed without producing very serious inconvenience. Dr. H. stated, in response to a question from the President, that he thought there was some little difficulty to the entrance of air into the right lung. The second case was that of a young boy, son of a farmer in New York State, who had had *a pin in the windpipe for eleven months.* A day or so after swallowing it, the child was brought to Dr. H., but, as there were no special symptoms, an operation was not deemed advisable. The child subsequently suffered a great deal from cough, fever and expectoration. He would be better at times, and then severe fits of coughing would come on. One day, after riding on a comrade's neck, he had an unusually hard coughing spell, and ran to his mother, who put him across her knees and struck his back forcibly. Shortly after he went out to the doorstep, and, while coughing, put his finger down the throat and drew out the pin. He has since been quite well.

Chloral Poisoning.—Dr. Cameron reported a case of a lady who took 160 grains of chloral hydrate at a single dose, for suicidal purposes. When seen three hours after, the pulse was 18, pupils contracted, and features pale. Believing that the chief indication was to support the failing heart, sulphuric ether, ♏ xxx, was injected subcutaneously every half-hour for four doses, with marked improvement of the pulse and general symptoms. Emetics were employed, but very little came up in the vomiting. The patient made a good recovery.

Dr. Proudfoot mentioned that in Boston, when chloral first came into use, he gave sixty grains an hour, for six hours, to a man with *delirium tremens.* No dangerous symptoms followed; so far as he knew, the drug was good, having been imported from Germany.

Extracts from British and Foreign Journals.

Unless otherwise stated the translations are made specially for this Journal.

Chyluria.—The members of the London Pathological Society a few days since enjoyed the rare opportunity of seeing the *filaria sanguinis hominis* in the living state from a patient in the London Hospital, suffering from bemato-chyluria, under the care of Dr. Stephen Mackenzie. Briefly, the facts known about the blood-worm and their bearing on the pathology of obscure lymphatic disease are as follows: The parasite presents an example of the alternation of generations, requiring two hosts for its complete development. The minute, almost structureless worms found in the blood of the human subject in such vast numbers are the embryonic forms of the filaria, which requires the musquito in which to develop into the sexually-mature worm. The musquito, feeding on the blood at night, when the filaria are generally alone to be found, becomes gorged with them. Their growth in the musquito has been traced by Lewis and Manson, and it is presumed that they are only liberated from the body of their host by its death in the water, to which it always finally resorts. The hematoid is thus set free, and probably undergoes further development; for the mature worm measures some three inches in length. Its passage into the human body is easily explained, and the analogy in this respect with the guinea-worm is one which Dr. Vandyke Carter ably illustrated. Once within the human body, the worm lodges in the tissues; but as to its migrations, and, indeed, its ultimate resting-place, but little is known. It seems, however, to have a peculiar aptitude for selecting the lymph-channels for its habitat—a selective power not more remarkable than that which urges the trichina to select the muscular tissues. This is further borne out by the fact that its embryos—the filaria sanguinis hominis—are met with in the blood and urine of the subjects of chyluria and nevoid (or lymphatic) elephantiasis. The precise mechanism of chyluria still requires to be explained, and until it is elucidated an important part of the subject will remain obscure. Dr. Mackenzie hardly touched upon the pathology, limiting himself to the statement of the facts observed in his case, the most important in connection with the urine being that besides having all the chylous properties, it invariably contained more or less blood, that passed by day containing more blood and filaria, that passed by night being more milky; and that filaria were found in it, especially in connection with blood-coagula. The most remarkable feature of the whole case lay in the periodicity shown by the filaria in the time cf their appearance in the blood. During the whole period of the man's stay in hospital his blood had been examined regularly every three hours, with the constant result that by night the filaria abounded, by day were entirely absent. It is certainly singular that the time selected by the musquito should correspond with the presence of the parasite in the blood-stream, and the connection of these two facts is not the least wonderful in the life-history of the parasite. Dr. Mackenzie found that the ingestion of food bears no relation to the presence of the parasite in the blood, but that the time of rest and sleep does; for when the patient was up all night and slept during the day, the period of filarial migration was similarly inverted. Dr. Mackenzie did not venture to speculate on these curious points; he wisely contented himself with laying the facts he had observed before the Pathological Society; and we may congratulate the Society upon having had the advantage of this valuable demonstration upon a class of diseases seldom met with in England, it is true, but the study of which may throw light on other obscure affections, and enlarge our conceptions not only of the manner in which parasites may infest the human organism, but of the remote effects their presence is capable of producing.—*American Practitioner.*

Tobacco Poisoning.—Dr. J. M. Bigelow reports the case of a young man who had been suddenly seized, on the street, with a convulsion, of which there was no premonition. Found him pallid; countenance pinched and contorted; pulse variable, being for a few seconds 136 to the minute, then 38, and intermittent. Heart action was very irregular, the sounds muffled and running into each other. Temperature was normal.

Eyes were staring, pupils dilated. He had severe pain and distress in the left side, especially over the heart. Dyspnœa was marked ; respiration sighing ; hiccough ; cold perspiration and great prostration. Convulsions rapidly succeeded, with great agitation of the extremities, without loss of consciousness, and at their termination, anæsthesia, especially of the left side, with uncontrollable nervous tremor. After the transit of the convulsions a cataleptic condition was observed. This passed off, and was succeeded directly by hysterical tremors, convulsive twitching of the flexor muscles of the whole body, with agonized apprehension of approaching catastrophe and death. He would clutch the arm of a by-stander and beseech him to save his life, to relieve him of the great precordial distress and threatening suffocation. Conversation or any violent motion of the attendants provoked these spasmodic attacks. It was learned that this was his third attack within a year. He was an excessive tobacco smoker, sometimes consuming ten cigars a day ; he had begun its use at the age of twelve. He had little appetite most of the time, was pale and cadaverous, enfeebled, restless, starting in his sleep, and his disposition had become irritable. There was no family history of nervous disease ; his own health, aside from this, had been good. Morphia was given hypodermically and bromide of potassium and carbonate of ammonium internally, and in a few days iron, quinine and strychnia : tobacco was interdicted. The latter injunction was disregarded, and four days later he had another even more violent convulsion ; he then gave up tobacco, and has since been in good health.—*Med. Annals*, Nov., 1881.

In the *Revue Scientifique* for Nov. 19, 1881, there is a paper by M. Thorens on this subject, in which attention is particularly directed to tobacco poisoning as productive of symptoms closely allied to those of angina-pectoris, particularly when the tobacco smoke is inhaled.

A New Method of Detecting Small Stones in the Bladder.—Dr. S. Cuthbertson Duncan has used for about three years the following method of detecting stone when small or in fragments. He takes a nickel-plated sound, such as is commonly used for that purpose, and holds it over the flame of an ordinary lamp or candle until the point is covered with a thin black film. After it has become quite cool, it is dipped in a solution of collodion and allowed to dry. He then oils it with castor-oil, and introduces it a short distance in the urethra and withdraws it, to see if it be injured. If not, he proceeds to explore the floor of the bladder with a sweeping lateral movement. If there be a stone or any fragments left after lithotrity, its black covering will be removed in patches, and the bright metal will show through. The author thinks this more delicate than Mr. Napier's indicator, the point of which is made of lead, blackened by chemical agents; and this very method does not impair the conducting power of the sound in any degree. A short beaked solid steel sound is preferred, with a round handle, which has a flat disk about two inches from the end, at right angles to the curve of the beak, to serve as a guide for the direction of the point. The round handle allows it to be rotated between the index-finger and thumb, the most sensitive part of the hand—two things necessary for rapid and delicate manipulation.—*Brit. Med. Jour.*, Nov. 12, 1881.

Milk Indigestion in Young Children.—Dr. Eustace Smith (*Brit. Med. Jour.*) says that when indigestion is due to catarrh of the stomach it is readily amenable to treatment. All that is necessary is to put a stop to the milk for a day or two, and to clear away the curd by a full dose of castor-oil. If, however, the fault be in the milk, and not in the digestive organs of the child, some change in the method of feeding is indispensable. In one case, where curding took place, with resultant griping and indigestion, and where various remedies had failed, Dr. Smith at last adopted the plan of giving the child barley-water from a bottle immediately before he took the breast, in the hope that by this means the milk might be diluted directly it reached the stomach. This method succeeded perfectly, and the child had no further unpleasant symptoms. In cases of gastric catarrh, when the complaint is acute and severe, vomiting is usually the most prominent symptom. Under such circumstances milk becomes a positive poison, and no hope of alleviating the symptoms can be entertained while this diet is persisted in. In the case of an infant two months old, brought up by hand, and fed upon milk and barley-water, uncontrollable vomiting and diarrhœa had reduced it to the last extremity. Dr. Smith directed a weak mustard poultice to the epigastrium. The milk was stopped, and the child fed with weak veal broth and thin barley-water, mixed together in equal proportions, and given cold at intervals with a teaspoon. A few drops of brandy were given occasionally, as seemed desirable. As a result of this treatment, the vomiting stopped at once, and the child, when seen three days afterwards, was found to be much improved, and was cured by the end of a few days' further treatment. The most important part of the treatment in this case was the substitution of veal broth for milk. Directly the supply of fermentable matter was stopped, fermentation ceased, acid was no longer formed, and the digestive organs returned to a healthy condition. Here the derangement was acute.

Psoriasis from Borax.—Among the cutaneous eruptions which may result from the administration of drugs, psoriasis has not, according to Dr. W. R. Gowers (*London Lancet*), been hitherto included. The following facts which he narrates show that an eruption of characteristic psoriasis may result from an internal administration of borax. The facts have been met with in the use of borax in the treatment of obstinate cases of epilepsy in which bromide fails. The first instance was in the case of a man who had taken borax for nearly two years in doses of first fifteen grains and then a scruple three times daily. An eruption of psoriasis made its appearance on his limbs and trunk, developing to a considerable extent in the course of a few weeks. Five minims of arsenical solution were added to each dose of borax, and the eruption rapidly disappeared. Shortly afterward Dr. Spencer, of Clifton, in mentioning to me a case of epilepsy in which he had given borax with advantage, inquired if I had met with any inconvenience from its use. I told him of this case, in which I thought it possible that the psoriasis was produced by the borax, and he informed me that in his patient the same eruption had just appeared. In this case also the rash rapidly cleared away under the influence of arsenic, and a few weeks later Dr. Spencer wrote to me, " I have not the slightest doubt that the borax caused the psoriasis or that the arsenic cured it." A third instance has lately come under my notice. The patient was a young mon who had suffered from epilepsy since infancy, and who was always rendered worse by bromide, so that he was brought to me with the request that bromide might on no account be given. He took borax, first fifteen grains and then a scruple three times a day, with greater benefit than had resulted from any previous treatment, and after eight months an eruption of psoriasis appeared. Arsenic was added, but the result of treatment has not yet been ascertained. The eruption in these cases occurred on the trunk, arms and legs, but more on the arms than elsewhere. The face was free. It was located on both the flexor and extensor aspects. The patches varied in size, up to an inch and a half in diameter. Their appearance is quite characteristic, but the scales were not quite so thick as they sometimes are in ordinary psoriasis. In no case was there a history of syphilis, and in Dr. Spencer's patient syphilis could with certainty be excluded.

Extractum Carnis and Urine as Medicinal Agents.—Mr. G. F. Masterman has already by several analyses shown that the ordinary Liebig's extract has very much the composition of urine, except that it contains less urea and uric acid. Beef-tea, as ordinarily made, does not contain, including alkaline salts, more than from 1.5 to 2.25 per cent. of solid matters. These solids are chiefly urea, creatine, creatinine, isoline, and decomposed hæmatin—exactly the animal constituents of urine, except that there is but a trace of urea. Dr. Richard Neale, in the *Practitioner*, comments upon the above facts, and says that the real value of beef-tea as a nutriment is still not appreciated, especially among the laity. Even some physicians are apt to class it as of almost equal value to milk. Dr. Francis Sibson has shown how detrimental beef-tea may be to persons who are suffering from Bright's disease, where the kidneys are already taxed to their utmost to throw off metamorphosed matters. The addition of the nitrogenous metabolites of the cow cannot but be dangerous. Frequently, says Dr. Neale, beef-tea is recommended by practical physicians in diarrhœa, dysentery, and during diarrhœa of typhoid fever. This he considers a very dangerous practice, and looks upon beef-tea in such cases as little better than a poison. Dr. Lauder Brunton is also quoted as raising the question whether beef-tea is not actually injurious. After thus emphasizing the fact of the non-nutritive, but stimulating properties of beef-tea, Dr. Neale states that similar properties have long been known as pertaining to urine. In South America urine is a common vehicle for medicine, and the urine of little boys is spoken highly of as a stimulant in malignant small-pox. Among the Chinese and Malays of Batavia, urine is freely used. One of the worst cases of epistaxis ceased after a pint of fresh urine was drunk, although it had for thirty-six hours or more resisted every form of European medicine. This was by no means an unusual result of the use of urine, as Dr. Neale was informed by the natives As a stimulant and general pick-up, he had frequently seen a glass of a child's or young girl's urine tossed off with great gusto and apparent benefit. In some parts of England the use of urine as a medicinal agent is not unknown. In 1852 Bauer recommended the external use of urate of ammonia in lepra, morphœa, and other obstinate skin diseases. In 1862 Dr. Hastings made a report on the value of the excreta of reptiles in the treatment of phthisis.

The Pre-Cancerous Stage of Cancer, and the importance of Early Operations. —GENTLEMEN: The patient who has just left the theatre is the subject of cancer of the tongue in an advanced stage. As I demonstrated to you, the lymphatic glands are already enlarged. It is hopeless to think of an operation, and there is nothing before him but death, preceded and produced by a few months of great and continuous suffering. His case, I am sorry to say, is but an example of what is very common. Not a month passes but a case of cancer of the tongue presents itself in this condition. The cases which come whilst the disease is still restricted to the tongue itself are comparatively few; nor does this remark apply only to the tongue. "Too late! Too late!" is the sentence written but too legibly on three-fourths of the cases of external cancer concerning which the operating surgeon is consulted. It is a most lamentable pity that it should be so; and the bitterest reflection of all is, that usually a considerable part of the precious time which has been wasted has been passed under professional observation and illusory treatment. In the present instance, the poor fellow has been three months in a large hospital and a month under private care. I feel free, gentlemen, to speak openly on this matter, because my conscience is clear that I have never failed when opportunity offered, both here and elsewhere, to enforce the doctrine of the local origin of most forms of external or surgical cancer, and the paramount importance of early operation. I have tried every form of phraseology that I could devise, as likely to impress this lesson. Nearly twenty years ago, I spoke to your predecessors in this theatre concerning the "successful cultivation of cancer"; telling them how, if they wished their patients to die miserably of this disease, they could easily bring it about. The suggestion was, that all suspicious sores should be considered to be syphilitic, and treated internally by iodide of potassium, and locally by caustics, until the diagnosis became clear. More recently, I have often explained and enforced the doctrine of a pre-cancerous stage of cancer, in the hope that, by its aid, a better comprehension of the importance of adequate and early treatment might be obtained. According to this doctrine, in most cases of cancer of the penis, lip, tongue, skin, etc., there is a stage—often a long one—during which a condition of chronic inflammation only is present, and upon this the cancerous process becomes engrafted. I feel quite sure that the fact is so. Phimosis and the consequent balanitis lead to cancer of the penis; the soot-wart becomes cancer of the scrotum; the pipe-sore passes into cancer of the lip; and the syphilitic leucoma of the tongue, which has existed in a quiet state for years, at length, in more advanced life, takes on cancerous growth. The frequency with which old syphilitic sores become cancerous is very remarkable; on the tongue, in particular, cancer is almost always preceded by syphilis, and hence one of the commonest causes of error in diagnosis and procrastination in treatment. The surgeon diagnoses syphilis, the patient admits the charge, and iodide of potassium seems to do good; and thus months are allowed to slip by in a state of fool's paradise. The diagnosis, which was right at first, becomes in the end a fatal blunder, for the disease which was its subject has changed its nature. I repeat that it is not possible to exaggerate the clinical and social importance of this doctrine. A general acceptance of the belief that cancer usually has a pre-cancerous stage, and that this stage is the one in which operations ought to be performed, would save many hundreds of lives every year. It would lead to the excision of all portions of epithelial or epidermic structure which have passed into a suspicious condition. Instead of looking on whilst the fire smouldered, and waiting till it blazed up, we should stamp it out on the first suspicion. What is a man the worse if you have cut away a warty sore on his lip, and, when you come to put sections under the microscope, you find no nested cells? If you have removed a painful, hard-based ulcer of the tongue, and with it perhaps an eighth part of the organ; and, when all is done, and the sore healed, a zealous pathological friend demonstrates to you that the ulcer is not cancerous, need your conscience be troubled? You have operated in the pre-cancerous stage, and you have probably effected a permanent cure of what would soon have become an incurable disease. I do not wish to offer any apology for carelessness, but I have not in this matter any fear of it.—JONATHAN HUTCHINSON *in Brit. Med. Jour.*

Darwin on Worms.—The habits of worms and the purpose they fulfil in the economy of nature do not at first sight appear to be very promising subjects of inquiry, nor likely to lead to interesting results; yet the work which has just been published by Mr. Darwin, "On the Formation of Vegetable Mould through the Action of Worms," shows how the facts accumulated by a careful and accomplished observer may render an uninviting subject extremely interesting, and serve as a basis on which theories having an important relation to geology may rest. It is remarkable, that, notwithstanding their common occurrence, no monograph of the British species has been written. It is probable, however, that there are about eight species. All of them are probably terrestrial, though they resemble other annelids in being able to live for a considerable period under water. Salt or brackish water proves rapidly fatal to them, as was demonstrated not long ago on the occasion of a high tide overflowing the banks of the Medway at Rochester, when many thousands of worms might be seen lying dead on the surface. Worms are nocturnal in their habits, and only exceptionally leave their burrows by day; those that are found wandering on the surface are, Mr. Darwin thinks, sick individuals affected by the parasitic larvæ of a fly. They do not, however, bury themselves deeply except in very hot or very cold weather, but lie with their heads near the surface, partly perhaps for warmth, but more probably for respiratory purposes. The senses of worms, with the exception of that of touch, appear to be very feebly developed. Their sensitiveness to light varies remarkably, the sudden admission and shutting off of a bright light concentrated on the head sometimes producing no effect, whilst at others it induces a rapid retreat of the animal into its burrow. Both Mr. Darwin and Hofmeister agree in thinking that light affects worms by its duration as well as its intensity, the light of a candle even causing them to withdraw or preventing them from issuing from their holes at night. They do not appear to possess any sense of hearing, remaining quiet both when a shrill metal whistle and a bassoon were sounded near them. The faculty of smell, again, seems to be only developed so far as to enable them to distinguish the proximity of the favorite objects of food, for they remained unexcited by many odors, though they soon discovered and carried off fragments of onion and cabbage. Their sensitiveness to contact, on the other hand, is very acute, and the slightest vibration, or even the impression produced by a feeble puff of air, is sufficient to induce rapid movement. They are omnivorous; they like particles of meat and fat, and do not refuse the dead body of another worm. Their digestive fluids are found to resemble the pancreatic juice, and to digest albumen, fats and starch. Everyone must have been struck with the leaves and petioles of leaves, that are so frequently found standing nearly vertically in the soil. These are probably often thought to be merely accidentally imbedded, but it is well known that they are objects seized by worms and dragged into their burrows, partly for food and partly to close the orifice; the latter object being demonstrated by the fact that small stones are gathered together and similarly placed. Mr. Darwin's observations on this point are very interesting. He describes the mode in which they seize such objects, showing that it is partly by the lips and partly by suction, and that they evince a certain amount of intelligence in the mode in which they, if the expression may be allowed, manipulate them, so that they are always dragged to their holes with the least expenditure of force. The mode in which worms form their burrows has engaged Mr. Darwin's attention, and he thinks it partly effected by a wedge-like cleaving process, and partly by swallowing the earth immediately in front of them. They penetrate sometimes to a depth of five or six feet, and there form chambers, where many hibernate, rolled together in a ball. He does not think Hensen's estimate of 53,767 worms to an acre too high an estimate, and this number would weigh 356 lbs., whilst their castings reached the surprising amount in one instance of 7.56 tons per acre, and in another of 16.1 tons per acre—an amount that, considering all this had passed through the bodies of the worms, is sufficient to show how important a part these animals play in the economy of Nature.—*Lancet.*

Communication of Syphilis by Skin-grafting.—At a recent meeting of the Société Médicale Hôpitaux de Paris, M. Féréol related the following curious instance of the above:—A man, aged 49, suffered from gangrenons erysipelas of the upper third of the left thigh, which left a large obstinate ulcerating surface. On March 7th, M.

Doubel, the surgeon in charge, applied forty-five pieces of skin taken from five different persons to the outer part of the sore. Thirty-three of the grafts adhered. On March 18th, twenty-eight grafts taken from the buccal mucous membrane of a rabbit were applied, but all failed. On March 23rd forty grafts supplied by seven persons were placed on the internal portion of the ulcerated surface. Thirty of these were successful, and cicatrisation was proceeding rapidly, when, on April 5th, a greyish ulcer appeared at the site of the first grafting; other similar ulcers quickly followed, and in three days involved the whole of the cicatrix. About ten weeks after the first series of grafts had been applied (May 19th), a copious roseolar rash appeared, and was soon followed by crusts on the hairy scalp and mucous patches in the mouth. About this time the son of the patient, who had furnished part of the grafts on both occasions, consulted M. Doubel, who subsequently discovered that the young man had had a chancre eighteen months before, which had not been attended to.—*Med. News.*

Hysterical Affections of the Larynx.—Some observations of Dr. Thaon have been translated for the *Edinburgh Medical Journal* as follows:—

Hysterical Aphonia is caused by paralysis of the muscles of the larynx. The muscles most commonly seized are the vocal muscles. Nevertheless, paralysis of the posterior crico-arytenoids is not absolutely rare, and we have known a case of this kind in which a hysterical female has been twice tracheotomized. A primary symptom of hysterical paralysis is that it is frequently bilateral, or else the paralysis is one-sided, but complicated with paresis or contraction of tho opposite muscle. Thus hysterical aphonia is often complete. It is, besides, a common enough occurrence, this diffusion of hysteria in organs which are impaired, and which are not symmetrical, as the ovaries. A second symptom of hysterical aphonia is that it frequently gives a laryngoscopic image differing the one day from the other. A third characteristic is to leave the cough intact, which even gains in intensity and breaks forth into roaring. We have even seen some cases of hysterical aphonia where the patient could sing, and some who could speak in their dreams.

Spasm of the Larynx.—The hysterical laryngeal spasm has its characteristics which distinguish it from the spasm of infancy, from the spasm from an irritation of the vagus nerve or of the recurrent, and from the spasm from the introduction of a foreign body into the larynx, This spasm is expiratory or inspiratory. The expiratory spasm is nothing else than the whimsical cough of the hysterical, a symptom common to nearly every hysteric, but one the most painful. In a boy 14 years of age we have counted as many as twenty-five coughs per minute during weeks. This child was cured by a heavy rain which overtook him during a walk, and to which he was exposed for two hours. At other times the hysterical cough is cured by the intercurrent affection which has been its primary cause. We know the fortunate consequences of the cure of uterine maladies from the hysterical cough. This hysteric cough was the cause of many errors being made before the laryngoscope had unveiled the exact state of the larynx. When it is met with in young girls associated with supplementary hemoptysis, it gives rise to a prognosis of which the gravity is only apparent.

Laryngeal Hyperesthesia.—Hysterical laryngeal hyperesthesia is very common. It is perhaps the most frequent mani. festation of hysteria in the larynx. It is sometimes diffuse, and manifests itself by various sensations—sensations of burning, tearing, pulling, going from the throat to the sternum, sensations of a foreign body. Who does not remember being called out in great haste to see a woman who had swallowed a pin, a fish-bone, etc., and who was in the greatest agony. After a conscientious examination, we find that the patient has been mistaken by a false sensation, and that we ourselves have been the victim of a false alarm. But it is not always easy to convince these same subjects that it is not a rare thing to find among them veritable cases of laryngeal hypochondriasis.

Laryngeal Anesthesia.—The result of our inquiry on this subject is that only in one-sixth of hysteric patients we have met with more or lèss complete anesthesia of the epiglottis. It is the epiglottis which is frequently attacked by anesthesia, and frequently to the exclusion of every other part. Anesthesia may have completely mastered the whole of the larynx, and be absolute. Generally it is bilateral, and is not limited to any well-defined nervous territory. This characteristic sometimes sufficiently distinguishes it from other anesthesias, which are as extensive as one of the areas of one of the superior laryngeal nerves, such as diphtheritic anesthesia. Another important and special characteristic of this anesthesia is that it is frequently associated with a cutaneous patch of anesthesia on the front of the neck, a peculiarity already noticed with reference to hysteric aphonia. The simple introduction of the mirror is sufficient to cause many of these anesthesias to disappear.

Treatment of Hydrocele and Serous Cysts in general by the Injection of Carbolic Acid.—Dr. Levis states that he has been experimenting with a view of determining what substance may best secure the obliteration of the secreting surface and the adhesion of the walls of the cyst with the most certainty and the greatest freedom from suffering and danger. Having selected carbolic acid as an agent which would provoke simply a plastic inflammation, he injected one drachm of the deliquesced crystals into the sac of a large hydrocele. The new procedure was entirely painless. A sense of numbness alone was experienced, and no inconvenience was felt until, on the next day, the desired inflammatory process developed. A nine years' hospital and private experience leads the author to believe that this method is the most satisfactory for the object. For the purpose of injection, crystallized carbolic acid is maintained in a liquified state by a five to ten per cent. solution of either water or glycerine ; the crystals are to be reduced to the fluid state with no more dilution than may be necessary for this. After the usual tapping, he injects the liquified crystals with a syringe having a nozzle sufficiently slender and long enough to reach entirely through the canula. He has never been able to detect any general toxic effects upon the system, but believes that the action of strong carbolic acid on surfaces secreting albuminous fluids is to seal them, to shut them off from the system in such a manner that absorption cannot readily take place. The occluding influence of strong carbolic acid he regards as an important surgical resource in certain cases of compound fracture, destructively lacerated wounds, and ulcerating surfaces, where septic infection is inevitable. All forms of serous cysts which are usually subjected to any form of operative treatment, on the principle of producing plastic adhesion of their walls, may be deemed amenable to the treatment indicated.—*Medical Record.*

Oil of Wintergreen as an Effective Salicylate in Rheumatism.—An able chemist, namely, Mr. P. Casamajor, of Brooklyn, informs the writer of this paragraph, that, arguing from a purely chemical position, he expected to obtain better results in acute or subacute rheumatism, and perhaps in chronic rheumatism also, from the use of Oil of Gaultheria, or Wintergreen. This oil is mainly Methyl Salicylate, and was among the earliest sources of Salicylic Acid. Mr. Casamajor supposes that this salt of Salicylic Acid would be easily appropriated in the economy, and would prove more effective than other salicylates of more fixed character. Carrying out his ideas, he had treated himself and several friends who had been subjected to rather sharp attacks of rheumatism with Oil of Wintergreen, and with somewhat marked benefit in every case tried. He takes and gives the oil in doses of ten drops dropped on sugar, and the sugar then mixed with a little water and swallowed about every two hours until the pain is relieved. This simple procedure is well worthy of extended trial and closer observation.—*Ephemeris of Mat. Medica.*

Billious Headache with Flatulence.—

℞ Magnes. sulphate - - - ʒ vj
Magnes. carbonat. - - - ʒ j
Tinct. lavand. co. - - - ℥ iij
Aquæ menth. pip. - - ad ℥ viij

M. Sig. A six part to be taken early in the morning, and repeated as may be necessary.

CANADA

Medical and Surgical Journal.

MONTREAL, FEBRUARY, 1882.

PROVINCIAL HEALTH BILL.

At the meeting of the Canada Medical Association, held in August last at Halifax, the Hon. Dr. Parker, in introducing the report of the committee on Public Health, said:—"Law-making on sanitary matters should begin with the separate provinces, each for itself, and the whole should be consolidated under some Act governing the entire Dominion, and passed by the House of Commons. Sir John Macdonald used formerly to say that all matters connected with statistics belonged to the Provincial Legislatures, but he has seen reason to change this opinion, and would be ready to admit the control of the general Government over statistics and such like matters which are necessarily intimately connected with sanitary legislation." The opinion that the initiative should be taken by separative provinces, and that consolidation under a Central Board should remain a matter for future consideration, was very generally entertained. The plan is entirely feasible, and it is encouraging to find indications that the profession are alive to the importance of lending their assistance for the immediate prosecution of this important work. Exertions are already being made in Ontario for developing suitable legislation on public health, and the Province of Nova Scotia has also been moving in the matter. We in Quebec have not been idle. For several months past Dr. Larocque (the Health Officer of Montreal), with the assistance of the City Attorney and other civic officials of experience, has been preparing a Bill to be submitted to the Provincial Legislature during the coming session. The provisions of the Bill have received much careful thought at their hands, and is based upon a consideration and comparison of the laws in existence in Great Britain and in many of the United States. When sufficient progress had been made, and a draft of the clauses had been printed, the matter was brought to the notice of the Medical Societies of this city, and committees were appointed therefrom to confer with the Health Officer and make suggestions. These committees had several meetings, and went over the separate clauses with care. This done, a joint meeting was held of the Board of Health and the Medical Committees. A further careful revision was had, and many important alterations made. The attendance at these meetings was large, and much interest was taken in the proceedings. The Bill is now in the hands of the City Attorney for final preparation. The Attorney-General of the Province, Hon. Mr. Loranger, has expressed his entire approval of the proceedings thus far, and has promised that if, on examination, he is satisfied with the provisions asked for, he will have the matter taken up and introduced as a Government measure. There is, therefore, a reasonable expectation that before another year a regular scheme for the supervision of the public health of the Province will be in operation. The principal features of the Bill as at present drafted are as follows:—A Provincial Board of Health is to be organized, composed of certain members of the Ministry *ex officio*, medical men of experience and standing, and lay members; these to be selected by the Lieutenant-Governor in Council. In all matters affecting the sanitary condition of all districts of the Province this Board shall be supreme. It shall institute enquiries and investigations into the prevalence, mortality and causes, of all epidemic and infectious diseases. It will also have the supervision of the Provincial system of registration of births, marriages and deaths, and also of the registration of infectious diseases. It will have power to examine into and abate nuisances not attended to by the local Boards. It will advise and direct all local Boards, and see to uniformity of action amongst them. If a municipality neglect to organize a local Health Board, the Provincial Board will have power to appoint suitable persons to act in that capacity.

The second portion of the Bill provides for the establishment of local or municipal Boards of Health throughout the Province. Thus the Mayor and Aldermen in each locality, assisted by physicians, are empowered to assume the functions of a local Board, and each such Board is to appoint a local Health Officer, who will have the usual executive powers of such an official, and will report annually to the Provincial Board. The provisions which occupy the following clauses give the necessary authority to these Boards to regulate sanitary matters in their own districts. These need not be particularized. They resemble closely those under which the Board of Health of this city has been acting, giving them, however, even more ample powers with reference to the compulsory isolation and quarantining of persons afflicted with infectious diseases. It is made the duty of householders to report cases of infectious disease to the Board. The third and last division of the Bill is that to provide for "the collection of vital statistics in the Province of Quebec by means of the registers now being kept, or by civil registration." The scheme here proposed is that the statistics shall be obtained in the first place from all "persons authorized to keep a register of the Acts of the Civil Status," and in the second place by compulsory legislation in all cases unprovided for as above. It is also proposed to make stringent regulations concerning death certificates. In the absence of the regular certificate from the attending physician of a deceased person, the Coroner must be notified, and it must then rest with him to say whether any further investigation is requisite. Such is the general scheme of the proposed Bill. It appears well suited to our wants. We shall watch with interest for its appearance at Quebec, and trust that before long it may, with any suitable amendments, become law.

A MEDICAL MAYOR.

It is publicly announced that Dr. J. L. Leprohon has consented to become a candidate for the Mayoralty of the city of Montreal. We cannot but congratulate Dr. Leprohon upon this mark of the esteem and respect entertained for him by his fellow-citizens. A better selection could not have been made. The Doctor possesses the courtesy, dignity, tact and experience of public matters, which are requisite to a proper fulfilment of the important duties of this office. He has for many years past devoted much attention to the subject of sanitary science, and will thus become a valuable practical member of the Board of Health. He bears the highest character as a professional man, and will therefore be a most proper person to do the honors of our city to the delegations of scientists who will next summer attend the meeting of the American Association for the Advancement of Science. We have no doubt that Dr. Leprohon will receive the unanimous support of his *confrères* during the election, and we hope to have the pleasure, on a future occasion, of announcing that he has been successfully returned.

THE HAYVERN CASE.

The evidence in this now celebrated case is reviewed at length in the last number of the *Journal of Mental Science* (January, 1882.) Our readers are well aware, through the general press and through the controversy carried on in the columns of some of our medical contemporaries, of the wide divergence between the opinions held by the medical experts for the prosecution and defence respectively. They know that Dr. Henry Howard took very strong ground in asserting Hayvern's insanity, and that his evidence was entirely overborne by the conjoint statements to the contrary of several others who have given the subject of mental disease some attention, and the man was executed. It will, therefore, interest them to hear the result arrived at by the *Journal of Mental Science*, after a review of the whole case. It says :—

" Legal opinion in regard to the test of insanity does not appear to have made so much progress in Canada as in some of the States of America, where the test of knowledge of right and wrong has been departed from in a marked manner. Dr. Howard, who has had long experience of the insane, has done good service by ventilating more advanced views on the subject. We hesitate to express a decided opinion on the irresponsibility of this particular prisoner, seeing that several physicians on the spot differed from the conclusion arrived at by Dr. Howard, that he was insane and unaccountable. At the same time the history of the ease strongly suggests epilepsy, and the intemperate habits were probably symptoms rather than causes of the low mental condition present. The absence of motive for the crime is a striking feature of the case, as well as the prisoner's indifference to the verdict pronounced upon him."

THE *Illustrated Quarterly of Medicine and Surgery.*—We have just received the announcement and the first number of the journal bearing the above title. It is edited by Geo. Henry Fox and Fred. R. Sturgis, and is intended to contain articles upon all the departments of medicine and surgery. The great feature of the work will be the illustrations. These are of large size, and executed in the very best artistic style. Of these there are no less than twenty in the first number. We shall pay this excellent new work some attention in our next issue.

Obituary.

DR. KENNETH REID.—Few of our readers who were acquainted with the deceased could have read without painful emotion the announcement of the sudden death of Dr. Kenneth Reid, of New York. It is eighteen years since Dr. Reid left Montreal for a wider sphere of action, and his career in the commercial metropolis has always been watched with interest by his Canadian friends. Dr. Reid was but 42 years of age at the time of his death. He was born at Huntingdon in 1840 ; received his education at the Academy there, became an articled pupil of Dr. Hingston, and graduated at McGill University in 1864 with distinction. He then went to Europe, where he spent two years, devoting his time chiefly to diseases of the eye. On his return he had charge of an emigrant vessel, and his report on the health of the passengers was of a nature to attract the notice of the officer of quarantine, Dr. Swinburne, who at once offered him a position on the staff, which, with some hesitation, he accepted. He continued in that office during the remainder of Dr. Swinburne's term of office, and until that of Dr. Carnochan, was brought to an abrupt termination. He then commenced practice in New York, and while brilliant success was not his, he was, in the opinion of those most competent to judge, laying the foundation of a solid and permanent reputation. Dr. Reid's zeal was untiring, with great capacity for labour. His memory was most retentive, rarely forgetting anything he had ever read. But what most endeared him to those around him was a modest demeanour, a mild and gentle manner, and a delicate appreciation and practice of what was right and honorable. A widow and one child survive him.

Medical Items.

PERSONAL.—W. R. Sutherland, M.D., has been appointed curator of the museum of the Medical Faculty McGill University.

—A vigorous effort is being made by Oliver Wendell Holmes and others to secure an endowment for Harvard Medical School. $500,000 is the amount named. The effort will doubtless be successful. The regular course of four years will then be made obligatory upon all its graduates.

A WAIST LARGER THAN LIFE:

" Still she strains the aching clasp,
  That binds her virgin zone;
I know it hurts her, though she looks
  As cheerful as she can—
Her waist is larger than her life,
  For life is but a span."

—*Dr. O. W. Holmes.*

—An Evangelical of Hobart, Australia, it is said, refused to permit his child to be vaccinated, because the virus came from a member of the family of a Ritualist. He indignantly declared that his child should not be inoculated with Ritualism. "On the vaccination theory," says the *Independent*, "he did not act wisely. If the child had been inoculated, he could have only a very mild attack of Ritualism, a sort of religious varioloid."

CONVERSATION FOR A HOSPITAL.

Why has the powder which I have just taken such an exceedingly pungent and bitter taste?

Now that I examine the paper containing the powder, I find a card attached to it, stating it to be "Poison." Is this the usual designation for Quinine?

If there is no special place set apart for medicines, I should be obliged if you would kindly *not* mix mine with the morphia, aconite, laudanum, and oxalic acid powders in the basket now lying on the table.

If neither the Sister, the Nurse, the House Physician, or the Dispenser are responsible for the proper medicines being administered to me, would you have me removed at once to my own house for further treatment?

Why does the Hospital Dispenser put his Poisons and his Medicines in precisely similar Wrappings?

The Doctor and the pretty Sister seem to be discussing my symptoms at considerable length.

I wonder if the Nurse is doing right in bandaging the artisan's broken head with brown paper soaked in solution of turpentine, without consulting the doctor?

Supposing I am killed in this Hospital, will a Jury bring in a verdict of Manslaughter against anybody?

Now that I have swallowed five grains of Prussic Acid, given to me by mistake for Quinine Powder, perhaps you will kindly have my Executors communicated with, and tell me the name of a good Undertaker in this neighbourhood.—*Punch.*

MALTINE AS A CONSTRUCTIVE—BY L. P. YANDELL, M.D.—"Maltine in its different forms is the only malt preparation I now employ, being so palatable, digestible, and easily assimilated. Of its efficiency in appropriate cases there is no more doubt in my mind than there is of the curative power of quinine, cod liver oil, the bromides and the iodides. It deserves to stand in the front rank of constructives; and the constructives, by their preventive, corrective and curative power, are probably the most widely useful therapeutical agents that we possess."—*Louisville Medical News.*

CANADA

MEDICAL & SURGICAL JOURNAL

MARCH, 1882.

Original Communications.

A CASE OF AMMONIA POISONING.

BY A. A. BROWNE, M.A., M.D., MONTREAL.

R. W., aged 54 years, had been drinking heavily for two weeks, and on Sunday evening, Feb. 5th, 1882, he took, by mistake, a draught of strong liquor ammoniæ. He had left the tea-table and gone up-stairs, when, in a few minutes, he returned very much agitated, and stated to his brother that he had, by mistake, swallowed strong liquor ammoniæ instead of a bromide of potassium mixture which he had been in the habit of taking. He had, in the dark, taken the wrong bottle, and, raising it to his lips, swallowed the ammonia before he was aware of the difference. The two bottles were similar in size and shape, and were standing side by side on a shelf. The liquor ammoniæ had been put into an ordinary medicine bottle, on which the original label still remained, and there were no marks on the bottle by which it could be distinguished from any other ordinary medicine bottle. When he returned to the dining-room and told his brother that he had taken ammonia, he fell insensible on the floor. His brother hastened to help him, and managed to make him swallow some milk with considerable difficulty. Previous to the accident, R. W. had taken two plates of strong soup.

Drs. Ross and Proulx were summoned, and after free emesis he appeared rather better. The vomited matter smelt very strongly of ammonia, and contained some blood. The voice was husky, but there was no dyspnœa. I saw him at 10 P.M., about three hours after the accident. He was then very weak; pulse

130, and weak. He vomited about every 15 or 20 minutes, and the vomited matter was almost pure blood. The blood was partly in clots and partly fluid. The pain of which he complained at the epigastrium was relieved for a few minutes by vomiting, but it soon returned. The features were pinched and the surface generally cool, and covered by a clammy sweat. Urine not suppressed. He constantly hawked and endeavoured to clear his throat, but the voice, though husky, was not lost. Respiration not impeded. He remained in this condition until about 7 A.M., Feb. 6th, when the hemorrhage ceased, and the vomiting became less frequent. During the day he remained in much the same condition, constantly hawking and unable to retain fluids, the smallest mouthful of water bringing on vomiting almost immediately. He complained of pain on the right side of the chest, and constantly struck his right breast with his hand. Pulse very weak and rapid. Towards evening he became delirious, and was so all night. On the 7th, his condition remained much the same. Some delirium, but less noisy. Had morphia, gr. ss., and liquor atropiæ, ℳ ii, hypodermically, which gave him a good night's rest, comparatively: that is to say, the pain was very much relieved, and he dozed almost all night, only speaking at intervals, Next morning (Wednesday, Feb. 8th) he seemed easier and more comfortable. Pulse still very weak; it has never been less than 130 since Sunday evening. Is quite rational. He cannot keep anything on his stomach; hawks and spits a great deal, and occasionally, but rarely, vomits. In the evening, Dr. Ross saw him with me for the third time since his illness. He was then much weaker, but sensible, and spoke intelligently of his case, expressing the conviction that he should not recover, and that the mucous membrane of his œsophagus and stomach were sloughing. His opinion seemed to be justified by the odour of what he hawked up, which was exceedingly offensive. The abdomen was very much swollen and tympanitic, but there was not much tenderness, if any. Bowels move involuntarily. His condition remained much the same until he died of exhaustion at 4.30 P.M. on Thursday, Feb. 9th, about 94 hours after taking his fatal dose. He was quite sensible until about a quarter of an hour before his death.

QUARTERLY REPORT ON THERAPEUTICS AND PHARMACOLOGY.

By JAS. STEWART, M.D., L R.C.P. & S., Ed., Brucefield, Ont.

Carbolic Acid and its Substitutes.

For many years carbolic acid has been almost the sole antiseptic used for surgical purposes. Lately, however, there has been accumulating a mass of evidence which has had the effect of throwing doubt, not on its antiseptic properties, which are still recognized as second to none, but on its harmlessness. There are several authentic cases now on record where carbolic acid, used in the form of spray or gauze dressing, has been the direct means of causing death.

There are two distinct forms of carbolic acid poisoning—one, where the symptoms set in with a very extraordinary rapidity; the other, where its injurious effects are later (a few hours) in manifesting themselves. Cases of the very acute form of poisoning have not, as yet, been described as resulting from the practice of Listerism, but have followed the injection of the acid into the rectum and the local application of the pure acid or highly concentrated solutions of it to the skin. The prominent symptoms of this form of poisoning are vertigo, weakness, condition resembling intoxication, then loss of consciousness, small, weak pulse, frequently cyanosis, and contracted pupils. Müller reports the case of a man who applied the pure acid to two-thirds of his shaven scalp. Immediately he complained of pain in the head, and vertigo. In a few minutes he was unconscious and cyanotic, and died shortly afterwards. Müller also reports the case of a woman troubled with diarrhœa who received an injection per rectum of not more than six ounces of a half per cent. solution. Almost immediately she complained of vertigo, noises in the ears, great weakness and faintness. She recovered. A three-year-old child, for the treatment of thread-worms, received an injection of a half per cent. solution; scarcely the half of a medium-sized syringe was injected when the child became pale, limpid and insensible. It was fifty minutes before the child was considered out of danger.

It appears that the rectum, especially its lower part, is more sensitive than even the stomach to the action of the acid. The male urethra can withstand injections of from ½ to ¾ per cent. solutions with apparent impunity. The writer has had considerable experience with Ultzmann's method of treating spermatorrhœa by carrying injections of the above strength down to the prostatic portion of the urethra, and has never seen any alarming symptoms set in either during or after the procedure. According to Müller, no cases of poisoning have as yet been recorded from the hypodermic use of carbolic acid, although solutions of the strength of 5 per cent. have been used in this way, neither has any dangerous symptoms arisen from the inhalation of the acid.

All animals, except mice and rats, can live for an indefinite time in an atmosphere of carbolic acid.

There are several cases now recorded where death has followed and was clearly due to carbolic acid used in the form of spray and gauze dressing. Mr. Pearce Gould reported a case of antiseptic osteotomy of the tibia to the Clinical Society during the last year where death was clearly attributable to the acid. A fatal case has also been reported by the late Prof. Busch of Bonn, in a child of five years of age who had undergone a knee resection. Several cases of ovariotomy have been said to have ended fatally from the use of carbolic acid. Nearly all the fatal cases, and those where dangerous symptoms have arisen, have been in bone operations and abdominal incisions. Puky, of Buda-Pesth ascribes two cases of sudden death occurring soon after severe operations to carbolic acid poisoning, but where, according to Muller, the chloroform was the real agent in bringing about the fatal event. A case reported by Lawson Tait is better explained in this way also. The symptoms of carbolic poisoning induced in this way are different from those attending the terribly acute form already described. The most prominent symptom is a very low temperature; the general state being very like that attending a diffuse peritonitis. The mind remains clear until about the end. It is not the intention to refer here to those cases of subacute or chronic intoxication by carbolic acid, as they never assume an alarming character; at least, their appearance is so gradual, that the surgeon is well aware of their nature before they can possibly take on a serious aspect.

Many substitutes have been proposed for carbolic acid, prominent among which are Iodoform, Eucalyptus, Resorcin, Chinolin, etc.

Iodoform.

The following is a summary of the actions of this drug, as determined by Högyes from a series of very complete experimental investigations :—

1. Iodoform, in suitable doses for dogs, cats and rabbits, is a poison, and causes, in a few days, emaciation, with slow death, without convulsions. It is both a heart and respiratory poison.

2. Fatty degeneration of the liver, kidneys, heart and voluntary muscles is found after death.

3. In cats and dogs it induces sleep, but not in rabbits ; reflex action is not diminished during the deepest narcosis.

4. If applied in an undissolved condition to the skin, or under it, in the intestinal canal or to serous membranes, it dissolves in the fats of the part and free iodine is liberated, which unites with the albumen, and as such it is absorbed.

6. A similar formation of the albuminate of iodine takes place when iodoform is injected as an oil solution under the skin or into the serous cavities.

Iodoform has a very powerful effect on the heart, its influence in this way being much stronger than chloroform. Ringer has shown that one-fifth of a grain is quite sufficient to arrest the ventricle of the frog's heart, while it takes from 1 to 2 minims of chloroform to bring about a like result. For a number of years iodoform has been extensively used in the treatment of ulcers, chancres, &c., but it is only lately that its use has been extended so as to include the treatment of all forms of wounds. It is now the fashion among some German surgeons to treat both recent and old wounds with it. Mikulicz publishes an account of 18 cases of major operations on bone and joints where the use of iodoform gauze was attended by complete antiseptic results ; five cases of extirpation of the thyroid, four of them taking antiseptic courses, the fifth case becoming septic from the proximity of a tracheotomy wound. In all, he reports 53 major operations treated by iodoform. In 49 of these the wound was antiseptic throughout ; in the remaining four cases, the wound became septic in two from erysipelas, and in two from local conditions. Mikulicz believes that (1) iodoform gauze is much preferable to carbolic acid gauze; (2) that in already infected wounds or ulcers, iodoform acts quicker than any other antiseptic, and is free from any irritating qualities; (3) that it has a special action on syphilitic, tuberculous, scrofulous and lupoid infiltrations. Leisrink, Mosetig-Morrhaf and many others have published results very favourable to iodoform as an antiseptic.

There have already been reported several deaths caused by the free application of iodoform to wounded surfaces. "In one instance, after an extended resection of the elbow on account of fungous synovitis, with intra-muscular abscesses, in a man 57 years of age, the cavity was packed with about 2,000 grains of iodoform. The patient died on the fifth evening in deep coma, with symptoms of pulmonary oedema. The only abnormalities of consequence revealed by the *post-mortem* were fatty degeneration of the heart, kidneys and liver. A second case died under similar circumstances, with the same symptoms and lesions."—(*Phila. Med. Times Editorial.*)

It is not surprising to see 2,000 grains kill a man, when the 1-10 thousandth part of it is sufficient to arrest a frog's ventricle. Whether there is any danger or not attending the use of iodoform in legitimate quantities remains to be seen. Judging from the present state of the subject this drug is not at all likely to fill the place of carbolic acid. There are some few cases reported where, when used even in small quantities, it brought about a temporary albuminuria and considerable increase in the body temperature.

Resorcin.

Although this agent has not as yet been extensively used, the little that is known about it tends to show that it possesses many desirable qualities both as an antiseptic and as an antipyretic. The following are the conclusions reached by Dujardin-Beaumetz and Hippocrate Callias from an extended experimental investigation into its action:—

1. Resorcin has the same properties as carbolic acid, salicylic acid, and the other substances of the aromatic series.

2. It possesses a toxic influence inferior to carbolic acid.

(*a*) 30 to 60 centigrammes per kilogramme of the weight of the animal produces trembling, clonic convulsions, acceleration of the pulse and respiration. All symptoms disappear within an hour. Sensibility and consciousness remained intact.

(*b*) Doses of 60 to 90 centigrammes per kilogramme causes intense vertigo and loss of consciousness. Sensibility is blunted. Clonic convulsions are violent and frequent, and are especially localized in the anterior extremities. The temperature is little influenced. The normal state is regained in from one to two hours.

(*c*) In doses of 90 centigrammes to 1 gramme per kilogramme, it causes death in about 30 minutes. The temperature rises gradually, and without exception, until it reaches about 41° (C.) at the moment of death.

Resorcin is therefore an excitant of the central nervous system.

3. Resorcin has no influence on the morphological state of the blood, except when it is brought into direct and prolonged contact with it.

4. It can be used both internally and externally for all those diseases due to contagious germs, or in those which favour their development. Its antirheumatic, febrifuge, and antithermic properties are not as yet well defined.

5. Owing to its extreme solubility, slight odour, and its feeble toxic and caustic properties, it should be experimented with for surgical purposes, for it does not possess any of the grave inconveniences of carbolic acid.

A one per cent. solution of resorcin arrests all forms of fermentation. Blood, urine and other substances which tend to rapidly putrefy can be kept for an indefinite length of time by the addition of a few grains of this new antiseptic. Even when decomposition has already set in, it is speedily arrested by resorcin. Dujardin-Beaumetz has administered it in a large number of cases of typhoid fever, in doses of from 30 to 45 grains. It appeared to have no favorable action on the course of the disease. The temperature, which was carefully noted, did not appear to be modified. This result is in contradiction to the results obtained in Germany. Lichtheim says that he has obtained a notable diminution in the temperature, often as much as 3° (C), especially in intermittent and typhoid fevers. The reduction of temperature does not last over an hour or two. Lichtheim says that in order to obtain the anti-febrile action of resorcin it is necessary to give it in large single doses (30 to 60 grains). These large doses are inconvenient to the patient on account of the irritant action of the drug. That resorcin is not destitute of toxic properties is proven by a case reported by Dr. Murrell. The patient was a young woman who suffered severely from asthma. Resorcin was given in gradually increasing doses until two drachms was reached. A dose of one drachm caused giddiness and drowsiness. The attacks of dyspnœa were relieved and in a quarter of an hour she was fast asleep. This was tried on four different occasions, and always with the same result. On increasing the dose to two drachms, decided effects were produced. The patient complained that it flew to her head, and she felt giddy, and had "pins and needles" all over. In a few minutes she became insensible, and was found on her side faintly moaning, her eyes closed, and her hands clenched. She was in a profuse perspiration from head to foot; there was complete loss of voluntary power and reflex action, the pulse at the radials was weak and thready, and the temperature in the axilla was only 94° Fah. The stomach pump and emetics were used, and she was made to inhale nitrite of amyl. She recovered in the course of a few hours. The urine first passed had an olive green colour. It is stated that the resorcin first used in this case was impure, being contaminated with carbolic acid; but the specimen from which the 2 drachm dose was taken had been specially prepared, and contained not more than two or three per cent. of impurity.

Dujardin-Beanmetz has treated six cases of acute rheumatism with resorcin. The average duration from the commencement of treatment until convalescence was nine days, and the average duration of the disease in the six cases was thirteen days. Andeer considers that it is of great value in affections of the stomach, and especially recommends its administration in gastric ulcer, from its peculiar action on mucous membranes, which heal without the formation of a cicatrix after cauterization with resorcin. For the disinfecting of large putrid abscess cavities, and for the treatment of common and syphilitic ulcers, he says there is no remedy equal to it. In the treatment of ulcers he recommends an ointment of resorcin, glycerine and vaseline. Incised and punctured wounds are said to heal always by first intention when treated with a one per cent. solution. As an inhalation, it is recommended in diphtheria and diphtheritic affections of the throat.

Resorcin is almost completely eliminated by the urine, and that elimination is excessively rapid. In about an hour after its introduction into the circulation, it is found that the urine is changed in colour to an olive green, and on the addition of the perchloride of iron it turns black. The average adult dose is from 15 to 30 grains. It may be taken dissolved in water and flavoured with a little glycerine and syrup of oranges.

CHINOLINE.

This is a transparent, colourless, oily fluid, having a penetrating odour resembling bitter almonds and a hot, pungent taste like peppermint. It is procured from cinchonin, and also from nitro-benzol; from the latter, a purer and cheaper article is obtained than from the former. It is a very powerful bacteria poison; a one-fifth per cent solution arrests fermentation in cultivating fluids. In the same proportion it prevents lactic acid fermentation and decomposition of urine. It is therefore a stronger antiseptic than salicylic acid, carbolic acid, boracic acid, quinine, sulphate of copper and alcohol. In a two-fifth per cent. solution, it completely prevents decomposition taking place in blood and retards the coagulation of milk. In a one per cent. solution, it prevents entirely the coagulation of the blood. Although superior to quinine in the above respects, it is inferior to it in its action on yeast cells, but this is practically due, as Binz says, to the yeast being exposed to a too favourable temperature.

Biach and Loimann have performed twelve experiments with it on rabbits, and found that it reduced the temperature in every case. The fall took place from its internal administration, as well as from its hypodermic use. The greatest fall noticed was 1.1° (C.), and the least 0·3° (C.) The temperature reached its lowest generally within an hour, and began gradually to ascend, often reaching a higher point than before the commencement of the experiment. It appears to have an influence in reducing the respiration, but this is not constant.

It possesses anti-periodic powers of the highest order, according to Donnetti and Salkowski. It has been used by the latter in typhus and malarial fevers with excellent results. Dr. Lowey records forty cases of intermittent fever successfully treated with it, besides many cases of neuralgia. The tartrate is the salt which is generally used; it occurs in small, colourless, acicular crystals. It can be given in doses of from 5 to 15 grains. It does not cause any unpleasant head symptoms, like quinine and salicyic acid.

Eucalyptus Globulus.

Of all the substitutes for carbolic acid in the treatment of wounds the above is likely to prove the most trustworthy. It is entirely free from toxic or locally irritant effects, while its antiseptic powers are undoubted. The oil of eucalyptus has, however, the disadvantage of being insoluble in water, and of evaporating very quickly from an oily solution. Prof. Lister has found that gum dammac holds it exceedingly well, and the mixture remains soft and strongly odorous of the oil even at the end of several weeks. He has had a gauze prepared with a mixture of one part of the oil, three of dammac, and three of paraffine. It is Lister's opinion that a gauze prepared in this manner can be thoroughly trusted as an antiseptic where carbolic acid was inadvisable.

In some of the Australian hospitals the eucalyptus tree is grown in large boxes in the wards and court-yards. It is claimed that these experiments have proven highly beneficial in rendering the wards free from malarial and other septic influences.

It is as yet too early to say to what extent eucalyptus will replace carbolic acid in the surgical treatment of wounds. That it will entirely supersede it is very unlikely. When we know more about so-called "idiosyncrasies" we will be in a better position to give a definite place to each of our different antiseptics.

The Action of Calomel on Fermentation Processes and the Life of Micro-organisms.

Wassilieff of St. Petersburg has quite recently performed a very valuable series of experiments in Hoppe-Seyler's laboratory on the action of calomel in artificial digestion and on its action in preventing the formation of low forms of life in fluids prone to undergo decomposition. Calomel has, from time almost immemorial, been used with alleged success in disorders of the stomach and alimentary canal, especially in children. Its use is also greatly commended in the early stages of typhoid fever (Liebermeister.) It has also an undoubted good influence in cholera, infantile cholera, etc. With the exception of a passing notice in one or two hand-books, there is no attempt to explain the method by which these results are produced.

Köbler, in his compendium, attributes the beneficial action of calomel in typhoid fever, cholera, dysentery, etc., to its power of destroying fermentation. Voit, in 1857, observed that the white of egg and blood mixed with calomel would remain for a day without putrefaction. Hoppe-Seyler, in his work, mentions the anti-putrefactive property of calomel, and explains in this way the appearance of green stools after its administration. The first set of experiments conducted by Wassilieff was to ascertain what, if any, influence was exerted on the artificial digestion of fibrine by the addition of calomel. The result was that this agent was found to possess no influence in either furthering or retarding the albuminoid gastric digestion. It was also found that calomel had no influence on albuminoid pancreatic digestion. Besides the formation of peptones, leucin and tyrosin, pancreatic digestion is attended by the formation of other substances, as Indol, Phenol, Scotol, Kresol, &c. These have been supposed to arise from putrefactive changes taking taking place in the albuminoids in the intestinal canal. In proof of this, we have it demonstrated by Wassilieff that calomel has the power of preventing their formation, while it exerts no influence on the manufacture of peptones, leucin, or tyrosin. It has been shown by

Hufner that not all gases which are found in the intestinal tract are the consequence of the unorganized ferments of the natural secretions on the food, but gases such as hydrogen and sulphuretted hydrogen, which are constantly present, are due rather to fermentation and putrefaction, brought about by active, low organisms. If artificial digestion of pancreas extract is carried on with the precaution of avoiding the introduction of organisms, with the exception of carbonic acid, no other gases are formed. In many experiments Wassilieff did not once find either hydrogen or sulphuretted hydrogen present in a digestive pancreatic mixture, to which calomel had been previously added, thus showing that calomel acts in the same manner as does the procedure which prevents the introduction of organisms. It was also noticed that carbonic acid appeared in much smaller quantities when calomel was added to the digestive mixture than in the control experiment.

The next problem that Wassilieff undertook to decide was the cause of the saponification of fat. Is this change owing to a special ferment in the pancreas, or is it due to the decomposition of the albuminoids? Wassilieff concludes that the pancreas possesses a special ferment for the saponification of fats, on account of the fat undergoing this change in the absence of putrefaction, as it does when calomel is added. From another series of experiments, it is concluded that calomel behaves itself in the same way towards the *amylolytic* ferment of the pancreas as it does towards the *albuminoid* and *fat* ferments of the glands. Calomel acts therefore in the same manner as does salicylic acid (Kulme) and arsenic (Scheffer and Böhm). In short, calomel in artificial digestion prevents the formation of those products which result from decomposition, and exercises no influence on the normal ferments. Calomel also possesses the power of preventing butyric acid fermentation. As regards the influence of calomel on micro-organisms, Wassilieff concludes (1) that it prevents the development of organisms in a cultivating fluid [Bucholtz-Wernich]; (2) the activity of already developed bacteria and micrococci is destroyed. According to Wernich's nomenclature, calomel is both antiseptic and aseptic.

LITERATURE.

Reichert—Carbolic Acid; a summary of fifty-six cases of poisoning. (Am. Tr. Med. Soc., Oct., 1881.)

Muller—Ueher die Acuteste Form der Carlbolsäure vergiftung. (Virchow's Archv. Band 85.)

Högyes—Iodoform. (Archv. fur Exp. Path. und Pharm., Band X, § 228.)

Ringer—Influence of Anæsthetics on the Frog's Heart. (Practitioner, July, 1881.)

Mikulicz—Weitere Erfahrungen uber die Verwendung des Iodoforms in der Chirurgie. (Berl. Klin. Woch., Nos. 49, 50, 1881.)

Beaumetz et Callias—De la Resorcine et de son emploi en Therapeutique. (Bull. Gen. de Therapeutique, Tome 101, 1 and 2 Liv.)

Murrell—Case of Poisoning by Resorcin. (Med. Times and Gasette.)

Andeer—I. Ueber die Ausscheidung von Resorcin und uber das Resorcinblau. II. Resorcin-catgut. (Cent. fur. Med. Wisseneh., No. 51, 1881.)

Donalth—Chinolinum Tartaricum, ein neues antipyreticum und antisepticum. (Transactions of Int. Med. Congress, Vol. I, p. 463.

Biach und Loiman—Versuche uber die Physiologische Wirkung des Chinolins. (Virchow's Archv. Bd. 86, s. 456.)

Wassilieff—Ueber die Wirkung des Calomel auf Gahrungs prozesse und das Leben von Mikroörganismen. (Zeitschrift fur Phy. Chemie., Band 6, Heft 2.)

QUARTERLY RETROSPECT OF SURGERY.

PREPARED BY FRANCIS J. SHEPHERD, M.D., C.M., M.R.C.S., ENG.

Demonstrator of Anatomy and Lecturer on Operative and Minor Surgery McGill University; Surgeon to the Out-Door Department of the Montreal General Hospital.

Recent Operations for the Cure of Club-foot.—In ordinary cases of this affection in children, tenotomy with proper after-treatment by apparatus or plaster of paris, &c., is nearly always found to be successful, if sufficient care is given by the surgeon to the after manipulation. When failure occurs it is usually because, after the tenotomy and the placing of the foot in proper position, the patient is not seen again, or if seen, at long intervals. There are some cases of club-foot, however, which are but little benefited by dividing the tendoms and replacing the foot in position. In these intractable and relapsing cases some surgeons, especially Mr. Davy, of Westminster Hospital, London, advocate excision of part of the tarsal arch. The general opinion is that this is rather too severe an operation to be resorted to in children. Mr. Davy thinks otherwise, and has operated successfully in these cases. In seventeen operations on fourteen patients he has lost one case, from septicæmia. All his cases were treated without antiseptics, and in fact without dressing of any kind. The majority recovered with bony union, but he states fibrous union would answer well. He has had no case of relapse. Mr. Davy commenced by excising the cuboid bone, but now removes a wedge-shaped block of the tarsal arch. He at first insisted strongly that the foot should be firmly fixed in a vice to render it sufficiently steady for the chiselling to be done during the operation. (Davy's Surgical Lectures.) Now he uses a fine saw, instead of the chisel, to remove the wedge-shaped piece of bone. (*Brit. Med. Jour.*, Oct. 31, 1881.) The position of the wedge-shaped piece of the tarsal arch to be removed depends on the kind of talipes to be operated on. For instance, in talipes equinus, a wedge, having its base upwards, is taken from the arch ; in talipes varus, the base of the wedge would be more inwards to overcome the deformity. A portion of the skin is first removed, then the soft parts are raised away from the dorsum by a blunt periosteal knife and a grooved director passed between the soft structures and the bone, a probe-pointed saw is then slid along the groove on the under surface of the director and an accurate wedge of bone sliced out. The wedge generally includes slices of the astragalus, os calcis, scaphoid, and cuboid bones. The gap is then approximated, and the foot is placed in proper position by means of a back splint, with a foot-piece, and the leg put up in gum and chalk bandages over a flannel roller. The wound is left open and swung, so that it is dependent.

Mr. Bennett exhibited a man, aged 47, at the Clinical Society in London on Dec. 9th last, who had been the subject of severe talipes equino-varus, and on whom he had performed excision of the tarsal arch. (*Lancet* Report, Dec. 17, 1881.) He had previously been treated by tenotomy with only partial success. The operation of excision was performed on June 30th, 1881, antiseptically, and drainage tube and antiseptic dressings applied. By July 8th the whole wound had healed except a small sinus. The antiseptic dressing had now to be discontinued on account of severe carbolic irritation of the skin, and a few days later erysipelas attacked the wound, which had to be opened up. The union of the bones all broke down. By Sept. 8th the wound had again healed, and by Nov. 8th he was allowed to walk with boot and iron support. When exhibited the union of the bones was firm but not bony. The patient had a useful loot.

It is plain that this is a most formidable operation, and should not be undertaken except for the most intractable cases which have not been benefited by other treatment. In Mr. Davy's cases the average duration of treatment was about two months. The short time taken in effecting a cure is an important consideration in patients of the poorer classes, especially when they are unable to purchase suitable apparatus. Mr. Davy has lost one case out of seventeen operations, and König, one out of three. Both patients died of septicæmia. It seems to be a more scientific and conservative operation than Chopart's, which is sometimes resorted to.

Dr. A. M. Phelps, of Chateaugay, N. Y., has lately introduced a new operation for club-foot. The number of cases operated on are too few to, as yet, pass a definite opinion upon it. The cases reported so far have been wonderfully successful, the patients being able to walk about at the end of six weeks to two months. As a detailed description has been given in the November number of this Journal of Dr. Phelps' method of operating, I shall only state that that operation is performed by making an incision across the sole of the foot and dividing all the resisting structures down to the bones. The foot is then brought into normal position on a special splint and the wound left open. By drawing a pointed stick of nitrate of silver through the bottom of the wound the granulations are prevented from springing up too rapidly, and the wound is induced to heal from the sides "by the skin gradually crawling downward into the wound." In making the incision the arteries and nerves should if possible be avoided. Esmarch's bandage should be used. Dr. Hingston, of this city, a short time ago exhibited to the Medico-Chirurgical Society a patient who had been operated on in this manner. The result seemed to be satisfactory, the patient having a useful foot and being able to walk on the sole.

Extirpation of the Lung.—The latest attempt to extend the domain of surgery, at any rate, as regards the lower animals, is the removal of the lung. Gluck appears to have first conceived the idea that so tremendous an operation might be endured, and after some experiments on dead bodies, he performed the operation on dogs, and found that it was fairly well borne, and that the animal might recover perfectly. When death occurred it was due to pericarditis or to pleurisy on the remaining side. He believes that in man diseases of the lungs are not so far removed from surgical interference as is commonly believed, and that the excision of a diseased lung or part of a lung, would, under certain circumstances, be a justifiable operation. Analogous experiments have been made by Schmid. On eight dogs operated on, five died from two to three days after the operation; three of the animals recovered. Schmid concludes that the lung can be operated on without special mechanical difficulties and without important hemorrhages. He has practised a similar operation on the human (dead) body, and found that after resection of two or three ribs there was no special difficulty. M. Marcus in France has been unsuccessful in his attempts to excise the whole lung in dogs, as the animals quickly died, but a rabbit survived the operation. These experiments may encourage the minor applications of surgery to the lung; but it may be doubted whether the excision of a part would ever be justifiable, since the diagnosis of malignant disease can rarely be made with such certainty and sufficiently early to permit its excision; and the applicability of the operation to the cases for which it is suggested by Schmid, tubercular disease of the apex, is manifestly absurd.—*London Lancet*, Dec. 24, 1881.

Treatment of Gonorrhœa.—There is perhaps no affection for which there is such a variety of treatment and such a number of specific cures. Its treatment is not confined to medical men; every druggist thinks he has a heaven-born genius for managing this disease, and the number of powerful caustic and astringent remedies patented for the cure of gonorrhœa and gleet exceeds the wonderful pills sold for the cure of all uterine diseases. Both internal and local remedies are in great variety, and fashion rules in this as in many other things. Every new remedy is, of course, highly recommended, and is better than any that has preceded it.

Zeissl, in *Wiener Med. Woch.*, advises for acute gonorrhœa three or four injections daily, feebly astringent, viz., 1 to 3 grs. of hypermanganate of potash in eight ounces of water. If the patient is no better in eight days the strength is increased. Later on gr. v. of sulphate of zinc in eight ounces of water are given. If this fails he advises solutions of subnitrate of bismuth or pure powdered kaolin, seventy-five grains in eight ounces of water, or sulphate of zinc and acetate of lead, each half a drahm to eight ounces of water. If the affection becomes chronic, he introduces bougies into the urethra, allowing them to remain five to ten minutes. He is opposed to strong injections at the commencement of the disease, and even later he says they should only be employed with great prudence. In regard to internal treatment, he uses matico, cubebs, copaiba and perchloride of iron. Prof. Zeissl insists on the known fact of the co-existence of prostatic hypertrophy and chronic urethritis.—(*St. Louis Med. and Surg. Jour.*)

In gleet, Mr. Reginald Harrison advises frequent irrigation of the deeper portions of urethra by means of a soft catheter and slightly astringent solutions. By thus washing away the discharge which collects in the bulbous portion of the urethra the liability to stricture is lessened.

Dr. Wilson (*London Lancet*, 1881), has treated sixteen cases of gonorrhœa with the greatest success, his patients being at work in an average of six days. His method is placing the patient on low diet and administering injections of sulphurous acid diluted in water (one to fifteen) three times a day. The injections to be effectual should be kept in the urethra three to five minutes. At the end of three days the purulent discharge will be replaced by a gleety one, and then only one injection should be used daily. The first injection often causes pain, which is not complained of afterwards.

Dr. R. Park, in an article on "Therapeutics of Ol. Sant. Flav." in *London Practitioner*, of December, 1881, says oil of sandalwood has been employed largely for the last twenty years in the treatment of gonorrhœa and urethral and vaginal discharge generally. He says there is no use prescribing it for the purpose of *curing* a gonorrhœa, if by that term is meant urethritis or other pathological condition causing discharges. For the discharge, however, he asserts the Ol. Sant. Flav. is distinctly the most specific drug he is acquainted with. It restrains the "running" at once, very frequently stopping it in forty-eight hours; but it requires to be continued *quite a fortnight after entire cessation of discharge* to make sure the latter does not return. It produces these effects in the most acute and the most chronic cases alike. He gives fifteen to twenty drop doses three times a day. The average duration of cases treated by this method, he says, may be broadly stated to be three weeks. Twenty drops is a full dose, and this quantity invariably produces griping of the bowels and dull, lumbar aching. He also uses in some cases a large bougie smeared with a liniment of vaseline and Ol. Sant. Flav. The *modus operandi* of this drug he believes to be (1) (Neuræsthetic ?) upon the pelvic and genital nervous system; (2) Antiseptic, or rather *contra purulent*. It also appears to be a special stimulant to unstriated muscular fibres, and in this way constringent. It has a drying effect on all mucous surfaces, when healthy or diseased.

Nerve Stretching.—The operation of nerve stretching is coming more and more into favour for the purpose of curing or relieving certain affections of the nervous system, as locomotor ataxy, spasmodic tic, neuralgia, &c. Dr. Langenbuch, of Berlin, introduced a discussion on the subject in the late International Congress in London. With regard to the *modus operandi* of nerve stretching, we are as yet much in the dark, and much has still to be found out about the class of cases to which this operation is most applicable. The German surgeons publish more favourable results than those obtained by others, but even in their cases results differ very widely in different cases.

Dr. Davidson has recorded two cases in the *Liverpool Medico-Chirurgical Journal* of stretching the sciatic nerves for locomotor ataxy. In one case, after three weeks, there was improvement as to co-ordination, and the lightning pains had ceased. At the end of two months the patient could walk fairly well, and the patellar reflex was very evident. The degree of stretching was 40 pounds, or half the breaking weight of the sciatic nerve. In the other case the ataxia was not improved, though the pains were much less. The disease in this case was much more advanced than in the first case.—*Lancet.*

Mr. F. A. Southam, in an article on "Nerve Stretching," with particulars of three cases (*London Lancet*, Aug. 27, 1881), says:—"Since the nerves of the brachial plexus were stretched by Prof. Nussbaum in 1872, for spasm of the arm, numerous are the affections in which this method of treatment has been adopted. For a time it was restricted to neuralgia and other painful or spasmodic affections of a simple localized nature, but more recently it has been adopted in diseases of a more general character, as for example, tetanus and locomotor ataxy; and during the last few months, cases of anæsthetic leprosy have, in India, been successfully treated by this plan."

Mr. Southam's three cases were all cases of clonic spasm.

In Case I., of clonic torticollis, he first stretched the spinal accessory nerve, and though temporarily relieved, no permanent benefit following, he afterwards excised a portion of the nerve, also without good result, owing to the fact, he thinks, of his not getting above the point where the spinal accessory gives off some muscular branches to the sterno-mastoid muscle.

Case II. was also a case of clonic torticollis. In this case he stretched the spinal accessory. The muscular spasms came on in paroxysms, separated by brief intervals of complete rest. In addition, the deep muscles of the neck, back, and also both arms, were affected with clonic spasm. Locomotion was somewhat impaired—both legs—but more especially the left, dragging slightly; spasms much increased by emotional disturbance. Eating was performed with the greatest difficulty, and it was with the greatest effort he could bring his hand to his mouth. The operation was followed by great relief for about six weeks, when a relapse set in, but this passed off. At the time of writing a decided improvement had taken place in the patient's condition, the spasm only coming on at long intervals, especially when his attention is directed to it.

The operation is simple. An incision two inches long is made along the posterior border of the sterno-mastoid, its centre being on a level with the upper border of the thyroid cartilage. After cutting through the deep cervical fascia the spinal accessory nerve will be readily found running obliquely along the floor of the posterior triangle.

Case III. was one of clonic spaasm of the muscles of the face, and the facial nerve was stretched, with the result of completely relieving the spasm. The facial paralysis caused by the stretching was disappearing five weeks after the operation.

Mr. Southam states that previous to his case only five cases are recorded of this operation having been performed; once in England by Mr. Godlee, of University College Hospital; three times in Germany, by Baum, Schussler and Eulenberg; and once in America, by Dr. James J. Putnam. The operation is performed by making an incision behind the ear, from the level of the external meatus to near the angle of the jaw; the sterno-mastoid and parotid gland are then pulled in opposite directions, exposing the upper border of the digastric, close to which the nerve is found as it emerges from the stylo-mastoid foramen. Since writing his paper Mr. Southam has adopted nerve stretching as a means of relief in three cases.—(*Lancet*, October 8th, 1881.) The first was a case of idiopathic lateral sclerosis in a man, aged 36, under the care of Dr. Morgan, at the Manchester Royal Infirmary. At Dr. Morgan's suggestion, Mr. Southam stretched the sciatic nerve; on the second day after the operation the shooting pains ceased, and in the course of a fortnight ankle clonus and patellar reflex began gradually to reappear. Six weeks later there had been no return of the pain. In the second case, under the care of Dr. Dreschfeld, the left sciatic nerve was stretched by Mr. Southam for locomotor ataxy in a man aged 51, at Dr. Dreschfeld's suggestion. The operation was not at first attended by any apparent result. After about ten days, the shooting pains, in both legs, began gradually to disappear, and he left the Hospital greatly relieved in this respect, but with the other symptoms in no way affected by the operation.

The third case was one of clonic spasm of the muscles of the face in a woman aged 32; duration 4 years. Four weeks after the operation there was no return of the spasms, and paralysis was only present to a slight extent.

At a meeting of the Surgical Society of Ireland, in December last, Mr. Wheeler detailed the treatment of a case of acute tetanus, by nerve stretching, which was successful. The patient, a girl aged eight, last October received a lacerated wound of the hand, and when tetanic spasms came on the usual remedies were administered without effect. The median nerve of the forearm having been exposed, was stretched, and the patient progressed gradually towards recovery.—(*Lancet*, December 10th, 1881.)

H. E. Clark in July, 1879 (*Glasgow Medical Journal*), reports a successful case of nerve stretching in a case of acute tetanus.

R. M. Simon, in the *Brit. Med. Jour.*, Feb. 25th, 1882, reports a case of infantile paralysis affecting the right leg in a child five years of age, greatly benefited by stretching the sciatic nerve.

L'Union Medicale, of November 8th, 1881, states that at a meeting of the Societé de Chirurgie, November 2nd, M. Le Dentu presented a patient in whom he had successfully practised stretching the lingual nerve for neuralgia of the face with epileptiform convulsions. The pain was located in the temporal region, auricle, lower jaw, and the left side of the tongue; it had lasted for 5 years, but in the last few months it had so increased in severity as to be insupportable. M. Le Dentu reached the nerve through the mouth, held the tongue aside and gently raised the nerve above the mucous membrane with a small hook for a few moments. On the second day the patient was able to sleep. Thirteen days after the operation the pain had entirely ceased and the patient was able to eat and sleep well. M. Le Dentu said that he had previously in another case practised, with success, resection of the auriculo-temporal nerve for neuralgia. M. Polaillon said, that three months before, he had stretched the inferior dental nerve for violent neuralgia, and the patient had been free from pain ever since.—*Am. Journal Med. Science*, January, 1882.)

Dr. Drake of this city was the first, as far as I know, who practised nerve stretching in Canada. The case was one of acute tetanus in a Swede aged 28, produced by running a rusty nail into the foot.—(*Canada Med. and Surg. Journal*, Vol. V.)

The left sciatic nerve was cut down on the posterior border of the gluteus maximus muscle and stretched. There was amelioration of the spasms for a few hours, but they soon returned more violently than ever, and the man died 12 days after the operation from exhaustion. This operation was performed August 26th, 1876.

Dr. Norman McIntosh of Gunnison, Colorado, reports in the April number of *American Journal of Medical Science*, a case of sciatic neuralgia of sixteen years standing which had resisted all ordinary treatment. The paroxysms lasted from five to six weeks, during which time the patient could neither eat nor sleep. The sciatic nerve was stretched and complete relief followed, and four months after the operation there had been no return of the pain.

Billroth, of Vienna, recommends a subcutaneous nerve stretching in sciatic neuralgia, by extending the leg and flexing the thigh forcibly on the pelvis.

Dr. J. Cavafy of St. George's Hospital, London, in the *British Medical Journal* for December 10th and 17th, 1881, in an article on nerve stretching in locomotor ataxy, gives an account of 18 cases besides his own, where this method of treatment was employed for locomotor ataxy. The cases are derived chiefly from German and French sources. In four cases the ataxy was cured (three of Langenbuch's and one of Esmarch's).

In eight cases the ataxy was diminished; in four there was no improvement. In one case, patient died 15 days after from pulmonary embolism. In the greater number of the cases the pains were removed or at least greatly alleviated by one operation; but in three cases they subsided only in the territory of the operated nerve, while in one they disappeared from the part operated on, but increased elsewhere. The improvement seems to have been permanent in the majority. Dr. Cavafy comes to the conclusion that the operation is applicable, especially to early cases where pain is a prominent symptom; but he would not hesitate to employ it in later ones, especially as the operation has not been followed by injurious results beyond temporary paralysis, and this very rarely. The wound is often slow to heal, as in his own case, where it was unhealed after six weeks.

Dr. Julius Althaus (*Brit. Med. Jour.*, January 7th, 1882), referring to Dr. Cavafy's paper, says that it may not be out of place to mention that at least five fatal cases have been recorded, due to nerve stretching in locomotor ataxy—one by Socin (mentioned by Dr. Cavafy), another by Langenbuch, who originated the operation; a third by Billroth and Weiss; a fourth by Berger and a fifth by Benedict. In most of the cases the cause of death appears to be undue violence in stretching, whereby the medulla oblongata would appear to have received a shock. Dr. Althaus goes on to remark that the operation cannot be considered a slight one, and we must be careful not to conceal the risks attending it from the patient and friends; also that undue violence and stretching should be avoided, and where there is the least suspicion of an affection of the medulla, such as asthma and certain cardiac and respiratory diseases, the operation should not be resorted to.

Medullo-Arthritis.—Mr. J. Greig Smith, Surgeon to the Bristol Infirmary, in a lecture published in the *Lancet* of Dec. 24th and 31st, 1881, on Medullo-Arthritis, proposes to name the two forms of so-called white swelling of joints, which are commonly called strumous, as follows:—The one where the inflammation commences in the synovial membrane, *synovio-arthritis*; and the other, where it commences in the pink marrow of the cancellated ends of long bones, *medullo-arthritis*. He proceeds to remark that the pink marrow in the cancellated ends of long bones belongs to the lymph-glandular class of organs, and probably discharges most of the functions of lymphatic glands. In disease of bones in persons of a strumous habit, it is this pink marrow which is affected with a form of inflammatory disease, similar to that found in strumous diseases of lymphatic glands in connective tissue. The inflammatory products are of the same histological type, they show the same sluggishness, and have a like tendency to undergo caseous metamorphosis. There is this difference, however, a strumous gland has room to swell, and if it suppurates, its contents perforate the skin and so are discharged. But it is not so with bone glands. They are bound down by a bony shell, and the swelling results in compression and strangulation ; an outlet is forced where there is least resistance, and it is for this reason the inflammatory products in the ends of long bones take a most dangerous course—through the articular cartilage into the joint cavity. Suppurative synovitis is set up, which generally leads to complete destruction of the articulation and even to the loss of the patient's life.

After describing synovio-arthritis, he gives the symptoms of medullo-arthritis, and states that it may be distintinguished from the synovial form by the intense starting pains, by percussion round the joint causing pain, and by the great tenderness during any sharp movement. In the synovial variety the pain is not a prominent symptom ; the joint has a pale, smooth, sometimes glassy and lustrous skin, and large, blue veins course over it. In medullo-arthritis the skin is not pale, but a dingy red ; instead of being smooth, it is rough and mottled, and frequently covered with long hairs, &c. He believes if the pathological condition of medullo-arthritis is recognized sufficiently early the progress of the disease may be nipped in the bud ; and that if we can reach the inflammed marrow and remove it, we ought to cure the patient. Even after suppuration has taken place, the treatment he advises is better than excision. He relates two cases of advanced medullo-arthritis, both at the lower end of the femur, in young girls, where, after making an opening in the condyles and gouging out with a Volkmann's spoon the cancellated tissue of both condyles and inserting a drainage tube, the best results followed. In the first case, after several months, the cavity filled up, and the girl now walks about without the slightest lameness. In the second case, after first trying simple drainage of the joint, it was determined to remove the whole contents of the condyles. At the time of writing the child was progressing most favorably, but had not commenced to walk. In this case it is probable a permanent stiffness of the joint will remain. Both cases were treated antiseptically. Mr. Smith says that this operation will be most frequently performed in morbus coxæ, because the hip joint is most frequently affected with medullo-arthritis. In medullo-arthritis of the hip, he taps the great trochanter a little above and posterior to its anterior inferior angle. The opening is made with a gouge, keeping carefully in the centre of the neck of the femur. He drills through this, through the epiphysal cartilage, and taps the marrow inside the head of the bone; if the bone is soft here, it may be scooped out; if not, it ought to be left; the incision in the skin is closed, antiseptic dressings applied and left on for ten days, at which time complete union will probably have taken place. As the gouge approaches the epiphysal cartilages care must be taken to handle the gouge gently, as any roughness might break off the diaphysis and set it loose in the joint.

In *Lancet* of Dec. 10th, 1881, Mr. G. A. Wright, F.R.C.S., reports a *case of pulpy disease of the knee*, treated by erasion, on the lines already laid down by Prof. Lister. On Jan. 22nd, 1881, an incision was made as for excision of the joint, but not dividing the ligamentum patellæ. The synovial membrane, which was thick, pulpy and very vascular, was cut and scraped away, and some of the cartilage removed at the margins; a softened cavity in the outer tuberosity of the tibia was gouged out, and the articular surface of the patella was scraped. The whole of the diseased material was removed as far as possible. The wound was closed with silk ligatures and an India rubber drainage tube inserted. The limb was packed in a Gooch's splint. On February 5th the wound was healing without suppuration, and on February 16th the wound had quite healed; except on the second day, the temperature had never reached 100°. The knee was dressed seven times in all. On the 21st the splint was removed, and passive movement began. On the 28th the joint was fully flexed under chloroform, and one adhesion gave way; passive movement was kept up, and on March 9th the child was sent out with full range of movement of joint and free from pain. When last seen, May 27th, she could walk, run, kneel down on the bad leg, and flex it to its full extent without pain or difficulty. The patella was freely movable. The operation was performed antiseptically. This certainly seems too good to be true, and is a great improvement on the operation of excision.

New (?) Treatment of Varicocele.—Dr. R. J. Lewis, in the *Phila. Med. Times*, Nov. 5th, 1881, recommends the excision of the redundant scrotum as a radical cure for varicocele. The excision should embrace a portion of the anterior and inferior part of the scrotum; a clamp is used to fix the skin before cutting, and is also kept on whilst the metallic sutures are applied. Dr. Lewis has not seen hemorrhage follow the operation. The wound is then dressed with carbolized oil, and a perineal bandage is somewhat tightly applied. (*Amer. Jour. Med. Sc.*, Jan., 1882.)

This is merely a revival of Sir A. Cooper's operation, which is fully described in Guy's Hospital Reports (Vol. III) for 1838. Scissors were used to cut off the redundant scrotum, and the parts united by ordinary silk ligatures. Every case reported did well, and healed without a bad symptom. But this is by no means a radical cure, and is only advised where there is great pain. It relieves the pain, but does not cure the varicocele; in fact, it acts in much the same way as a well-fitting suspensory bandage.

Sponge-Grafting.—D. J. Hamilton, M.B., Pathologist to the Edinburgh Royal Infirmary, has contributed a valuable series of original observations on the above subject in the *Edinburgh Medical Journal* of November, 1881. In an article on the "Process of Healing," published in Vol. XIII *Journal Anat. and Phys.*, 1879, Mr. Hamilton endeavoured to show, experimentally and otherwise, that the vessels of a granulating surface are not newly formed, but are simply the superficial capillaries of the part which have become displaced. They have been thrown upwards as granulation loops by the propelling action of the heart, because the restraining influence of the skin has been removed. He goes on to remark that one of the great functions of the skin is to counteract the tendency which superficial vessels have to be pushed outwards, and a similar restraining action is conferred upon the deeper branches of the fasciæ which surround them. These hold the vessels in their proper places, and overcome the tendency to this peripheral displacement.

It was whilst getting the information for the paper above mentioned, and also when subsequently studying the subject of organization and healing still further, that Mr. Hamilton was struck with the similarity of the process of vascularization, as seen on a granulating surface, and that which occurs when a blood-clot or a fibrinous exudation is replaced by a vascular cicatricial tissue. The author states that blood-clot or fibrinous lymph plays merely a mechanical and passive part in any situation, and that vascularization is not due to the formation of new vessels, but rather to a displacement and pushing inwards of the blood-vessels of the surrounding tissues. Being convinced that the blood-clot or fibrinous lymph, before organization takes place, was just so much dead matter in a tissue, it occurred to Mr. Hamilton that if he could employ, instead of blood-clot or fibrinous lymph, some dead porous animal tissue, it also would, in the course of time, become vascularized and replaced by cicatricial tissue. He thought that sponge, if placed under proper conditions, would fulfil the object in view, for the following reasons: 1. It is a porous tissue, and would imitate the interstices of the fibrinous network in a blood-clot or in fibrinous lymph. 2. It is an animal tissue, and, like other animal tissues, such as catgut, would, if placed under favourable conditions, become absorbed in the course of time. 3. It is a pliable texture, and can be easily adjusted to any surface. If, therefore, the blood-clot or fibrinous exudation merely acts mechanically in the process of organization, there is no reason why sponge or other porous texture should not similarly become vascular and organized. The first experiment was performed on a female patient suffering from several ulcerated wounds in different parts of the body. The largest of these was situated on the outside of the left leg. It was circular in a shape, and five inches in diameter by from a half to three-quarters of an inch in depth; the edges were indurated, slightly raised, and in some places undermined. There was a cellular tissue slough at the deepest part of the wound, which gave to the whole ulcer a putrefactive odour. The rest of the floor was in a granulating condition.

The usual antiseptic dressings were first applied, but very little progress was made in its contraction, and on the 3rd of August, 1880, Mr. Hamilton filled the wound with one large piece and several small pieces of very fine sponge prepared by dissolving out the siliceous and calcareous salts by means of dilute nitro-hydrochloric acid, subsequently washing in liquor potassæ and finally steeping it for some time in a 1 to 20 solution of carbolic acid and water. The sponge in the central part of the wound rose a little higher than the edges, so that at its greatest thickness it must have measured from half to three-quarters of an inch by five inches in width. The sponge was made to fit the wound very accurately and was inserted beneath the undermined edges. A piece of green protective was placed on the surface and above this, lint soaked in a 1 to 20 solution of carbolic acid and glycerine, with a little tincture of lavender in it. The whole was covered by a pad of boracic lint. An ordinary bandage was applied. The patient was kept in bed, with the limb at absolute rest. Next day it was redressed. There was not any marked putrefaction odour. On the 5th of August there was a distinct putrefaction odour. It was dressed as formerly, but the wound was irrigated with 1 to 40 carbolic solution. This was continued throughout the progress of the experiment, and at one time when the putrefactive odour became great a 1 to 20 solution was employed. Oakum was now used as a top dressing over the glycerine and carbolic acid. The sponge at its shallowest part appeared to be slightly red in one or two points, and the undermined edge had extended for a short distance further over it. On the 6th of August the sponge was irrigated as before, and was gently squeezed so as to remove any waste materials which were contained in it. The edges of the sponge were now adhering to the granulating surface. Five days after the commencement of the experiment the wound seemed to have shrunk a little, there was very little putrefactive odour. The thin parts of the sponge felt firm and their interstices were evidently filling with organizing tissue. If the surface was pricked it bled freely. Healing seemed to be going on from the edges to the centre and upwards. The edges of the sponge seemed to be dissolving as it became infiltrated with the new tissue. Its surface was covered by a grayish colored pellicle, very much like that seen on the surface of wounds healing under antiseptics. From this time onward the sponge rapidly became filled with organizing tissue, until on the 29th of November there was only a small piece of it seen on the surface. As soon as it became vascular and filled with new tissue the epithelium spread over it.

Mr. Hamilton remarks that in the healing of this wound instead of the edges and surrounding skin being drawn downwards and towards the centre, the reparative material had in reality grown up and so filled the vacuity caused by the cellular tissue slough. The first experiment showed that if sponge be placed over a granulating surface its interstices will, in course of time, be filled with blood vessels and cicatricial tissue, just as in the case of a blood-clot, and that ultimately the whole sponge will disappear in the wound, leaving an organizing mass of new tissue in its place. It further showed that even where the wound continues in a putrescent condition organization will go on. In the case of blood-clot, putrefaction tends to destroy it; in that of the sponge, its texture being more resistent, it does not seem to make much difference.

Four other experiments were made of healing wounds by sponge grafting on the human subject, all of which were successful except the last, which was a case of old necrosis of the lower end of tibia communicating with a wound of considerable size. There was no granulating surface at any part, and no attachment of the sponge occurred after several weeks, for the simple reason that the part could not furnish sufficient embryonic tissue to pierce the sponge and organize it.

Other experiments on animals were carried out in Vienna for Mr. Hamilton, by Dr. Woodhead, in Prof. Stricker's laboratory, for the details of which I must refer the reader to Mr. Hamilton's article. A minute account, accompanied by beautiful plates, is next given of the microscopic appearances of the various stages of the organization of this new tissue. The first thing noticed, in all the experiments made, is the infiltration of the interstices of the sponge with a certain amount of fibrinous lymph. The canals do not become occluded by it, but fibrin with entangled leucocytes is found adhering to the sponge framework. The line of demarcation between the fibrinous and organizing layers was in all cases quite distinct, and in no instance was organization found to commence within the interior of the sponge among the primarily effused lymph. Without exception the cicatricial elements grew into the sponge in the form of a distinct layer springing from the tissue to which it had become attached, and from this attachment blood-vessels also arose.

The blood-vessels first become much distended and unduly tortuous. When the loops of blood-vessels reached the sponge framework, they were pushed into it, and always maintained the character of complete capillary loops. He was unable to detect anything like free, newly-formed and pointed offshoots. No evidence of sprouts from their sides could be detected after the most searching examinations. Mr. Hamilton noted a significant phenomenon supporting the theory that blood-vessels were pushed into the sponge as loops, viz., that when the convexity of a loop came in contact with the sponge framework, instead of one of its pores, a curvature formed on the vessel at the opposing point, and on each side of the obstacle there was pushed a secondary loop similar to that from which both had arisen. The blood-vessels which have been pushed outwards from the neighbouring parts bear with them great numbers of the actively proliferating connective tissue corpuscles derived from the neighbouring connective tissues. These, he affirms, and not the leucocytes, as described by Conheim and others, are the tissue-forming cells. Mr. Hamilton says that fibrinous lymph has no more power of forming *per se* a fibrous tissue than blood-clot or a piece of sponge has. The blood-vessels are the primary, and the connective tissue corpuscles the secondary factors in the organizing process. Mr. Hamilton thinks the method of sponge-grafting is excellently suited for growing new tissue where that is insufficient to cover a part or to allow of stretching, but whether it may not have a wider range of application remains for future experience to demonstrate. The only objection seems the somewhat long time needed to organize it. Instead of sponge, charcoal or calcined bone might be employed in certain cases, as, for instance, where the formation of new bone is needed. To prevent contraction of the newly formed tissue when it cicatrizes, such a solid framework would be useful.

When speaking of the displacing action of the heart upon the blood-vessels, Mr. Hamilton asks, "Why is it that in different individuals there is such a difference in stature?" and answers, "May it not be that the cause of it, in reality, is that the propelling action of the heart is specially vigorous in those of great stature, and the resistance of the tissues slight, while in those of small stature the reverse conditions are present." "Why is it that growth goes on to a certain age?" "May it not be that the heart is relatively more powerful than the delicate stretchable tissues of youth, but as adolescence is reached, the tissues become sufficiently rigid to counteract the heart's action, &c." He says much the same thing is seen in plants. When growth is most active, the plant is in a cellular, pliable condition, and as it becomes older, and more woody fibre is formed within it, a stable condition is reached.

For a further account of this most interesting subject, I must refer the reader to Mr. Hamilton's original article, which will well repay a thorough perusal.

BI-MONTHLY RETROSPECT OF OBSTETRICS AND GYNÆCOLOGY.

PREPARED BY WM. GARDNER, M.D.,

Prof. Medical Jurisprudence and Hygiene, McGill University; Attending Physician to the University Dispensary for Diseases of Women; Physician to the Out-Patient Department, Montreal General Hospital.

On Antiseptic Midwifery and Septicœmia in Midwifery, by Dr. Robert Barnes, of St. George's Hospital, London.—This is the title of a recent (*Am. Jour. Obstet.*, Jan., 1882,) and most pertinent paper to the present position of the burning question of the day in obstetrical circles. At the outset, Dr. Barnes makes a statement which contains an important and, we believe, often-forgotten truth, that antiseptic appliances can strictly only be regarded as subsidiary means in the carrying out of the great principle that lies at the bottom of all good obstetric practice, namely, to screen the lying-in woman from those poisons and other noxious influences which threaten her from within and without. "The foundation of puerperal disease is laid during gestation. With the completion of labour, the conditions predisposing to disease gather strength. During the puerperal state fresh elements of danger accumulate." The diseases of the pregnant woman differ from those of the puerperal woman. The diseases of the gravida are diseases of high nervous and vascular tension. Those of the puerpera are of low nervous and vascular tension. In the gravida, the balance of osmosis is centrifugal; in the puerpera it is centripetal. During pregnancy there is an active process of building going on. The moment this work is complete, the reverse process of demolition and carrying away of refuse is begun. Absorption and excretion are now the ruling energies. Active absorption, it is true, goes on during gestation, but it is a very different thing from the absorption of the refuse-stuff, which must now be cast out of the body. If not cast out of the body, this refuse may be as poisonous as the elements of the urine. For these reasons, thrombosis, phlegmasia dolens and septicæmia are rare during pregnancy, but common during the puerperal period.

Before discussing antiseptic midwifery, we ought to have a clear idea of what constitutes septicæmia in midwifery. When a lying-in woman is assailed by a fever-producing cause, her condition is complex. If by the word septicæmia, as used in obstetric discussions, we understand simply that a special poison has been taken into the blood of the puerpera, then we have a very imperfect idea of the case. We have not a correct picture in the mind of what is going on in the poisoned puerpera. If we continue to use the word, and it is very convenient, it must be used broadly. Dr. Barnes suggests that it be used to designate an empoisoned condition of the blood. We cannot as yet, physically or clinically, identify sepsin, nor can we clearly and certainly distinguish between pyæmia and septicæmia. For these reasons Dr. B. advocates the old word "toxæmia." It implies no theory.

It only expresses the fact that a poison has entered the blood. Dr. Barnes traces as follows the several factors which enter into the problem of a case of septicæmia:—

1. The modified blood condition of the gravida: excess of fibrin, diminished red blood-globules, increase of water and white blood globules. If there have been hemorrhage during or after labour, the blood has become more watery and more charged with fibrin. The excess of albuminoid or colloid materials increases centripetal osmosis. 2. There is a fall of nervous and vascular tension, involving a change in the dynamic state of the circulation. 3. There is a period of rest after labour, of preparation for the active processes of breaking up of the tissue used during pregnancy, now superfluous, and of casting out refuse-stuff. This lasts 48 hours. It is rare to see evidences of self-empoisonment before the third day. 4. At the end of this time the disintegration of the uterus and other organs has begun. There is a great revolution at hand. The proceeds of the disintegration of the uterus, &c., are rapidly taken up into the circulation, and ought to be as rapidly converted and excreted. Absorption revives. The lymphatic vessels and venules have come into active function. If the lymphatic system and liver fail to prepare this waste-stuff brought to them, so as to fit it to enter the circulating blood, then it (the waste-stuff) is noxious, poisonous. Hence one form of toxæmia. 5. But even if this waste-stuff enters the blood, and is properly prepared or digested for removal, if it be not removed *pari-passu*, there will be accumulation in the system. This is another form of toxæmia. Hence the necessity for easily-working excretory organs; sound lungs, kidneys, and skin. 6. Both evils may co-exist,—conversion of waste-stuff and excretion may both be defective. Hence a complex toxæmia, endogenetic, derived from no external force. 7. Other dangers exist,—the ruptures, lacerations, and violent bruisings of the parturient tract by the passage of the child, and the separation of the placenta. Barnes draws especial attention, in this connection, to the extravasation of blood and serum in the pelvic connective tissue, and the baring of the mucous membrane by removal of its epithelium. In these various ways traumatism obtains

in the puerperal woman. Absorbing surfaces are produced. If there be foul, decomposing, septic material about the wounded parts, it may be absorbed—another form of autogenetic toxæmia. But this may be combined with the other two forms or sources, and a complex case be produced. Simple septicæmia, as described and imagined, probably does not, cannot exist. Whenever the blood is poisoned, be it with septic stuff or other, the natural processes of purification, of excretion of the waste-stuff, are obstructed, the balance between disintegration, absorption, and excretion is lost. 8. The puerpera is still open to poisoning from other sources. Poisons foreign to her may be brought in contact with the raw surfaces and absorbed. Cadaveric poison and others may be conveyed by the examining finger, tainted sponges or linen, may also carry such poisons Bacteria probably play an important part in some of these. 9. The lying-in woman, again, is peculiarly susceptible to the ingestion of zymotic poisons. Typhoid fever, variola, scarlatina, rubeola, and erysipelas act with special virulence in the blood of the puerpera. These poisons in the lying-in woman are in contact with blood loaded with refuse stuff which it cannot excrete, and are therefore most favourably circumstanced for the development of mischief. The patient may have had scarlatina before. She may have enjoyed immunity to the full extent till she became pregnant. If inhaled, the poison was quickly eliminated. But in puerperal blood, climination is arrested and the morbid train is fired. Under such circumstances we get a toxæmia very complex in nature. It is neither waste-stuff poison, septicæmia, pyæmia, nor scarlatina, but is a compound of all, the product of their interactions.

How is the lying-in woman to be protected from these various sources of danger? There are two main objects. First, keep all extraneous poisons out. Second, if any gain entry, counteract their ill effects. It is an essential condition to success to put the system in the best condition for defence. Secure efficiency of the organs of nutrition and excretion. The carrying out of this programme fully is antiseptic midwifery in the broad sense. The adaptation of the Listerian or conventional antiseptic precautions is antiseptic midwifery in the partial and narrow sense.

But we cannot always get a healthy puerperal subject. We must take her as we find her, perhaps with damaged kidneys or liver, deficient in nerve power and fibre, with skin and lungs unequal to the new task thrown on them. Pregnancy is the great test of the soundness of the subject. Under it many women break down; some abort, others go on a little longer, some fail in labour, others in childbed.

Dr. Barnes is sceptical as to the occurrence of anything like milk-fever, strictly speaking. It is not physiological; it is not constant. When the breasts are sound, there is no fever. If there be fever, it obstructs the due secretion of milk. If the breast be not in a condition to secrete, fever is excited. The truth is that the third day is the epoch for the establishment of the absoption process. The two days immediately following labour are a period of rest. Blood or other matter in the uterus has not had time to decompose. But both begin at the third day. Active absorption finds material ready to work upon. This is the cause of febrility on the third day. The mammary glands labour under the disturbance thus induced. Their healthy action is impeded, and as they are under easy observation, their struggle against the fever is interpreted as the cause of the fever.

Antiseptic treatment of our lying-in patients must be begun early. 1. It begins with the management of labour. The great point is to secure firm contraction of the uterus. The immediate object, of course, is to prevent hemorrhage. To prevent hemorrhage is to oppose septicæmia. Dr. Barnes insists on the utility of the pad and binder to provoke contraction and counteract aspiration or the suction-force which tends to draw air, one of the factors of decomposition, into the uterus. The author further advocates the custom of giving an aperient the day after labour. In the effort of defecation the uterus, compressed, often expels a clot and contracts more effectually. For many years he has given to every patient after labour a mixture of quinine, ergot, and digitalis, three times daily for two or three weeks, and asserts that it contracts the uterus remarkably. The patient often feels a contraction soon after each dose. This ought to be regarded as the foremost measure in antiseptic midwifery. It shuts the gate in the face of the enemy. 2. Wash out the uterus. Use a two per cent. solution of carbolic acid once or twice a day, from the second day onwards. It is best done by a gravitation or syphon tube. The good results on pulse, temperature and rigors is well known to be remarkable. In this connection the author points out that " Harvey the Immortal " thus cured a lady in imminent danger of death from septicæmia. Keep the uterus in position. Retroflexion or anteflexion favour retention of discharges. Keep the catheter and other appliances soaked in carbolic acid solution. Use no sponges, but soft tow soaked in the solution; it can then be thrown away. The napkins or diapers are a source of contamination, as they come from the wash which does not mean purification. The modern " ladies' towel " should be used. It consists of cotton or tow impregnated with carbolic acid. After use they are burned. Physician and nurse must wash in carbolic solution, and use carbolized vaseline for lubricating the hand. Dr. Barnes suggests that sulphurous acid will be found better than carbolic acid, which sometimes poisons. He has used it recently at St. George's Hospital. Dutrochet, in his investigations on osmosis, found that the slightest trace of it stopped osmosis. It may be used in a solution of one to forty of water. 3. While we take care to exclude foul stuff from the genital canal, it is also important to exclude foul air from the lungs. Supply pure air. Sometimes it is difficult. If the sun shines, open the window. At night, a fire will furnish good ventilation. Avoid a chill to the surface, or any check to the secreting action of lungs, skin, kidneys and alimentary canal. 4. Secure drainage of the uterus. Dr. Barnes is rather lukewarm in his advocacy of Goodell's plan of raising the patient at times to the sitting posture. In the weakly, those who have suffered from hemorrhage, syncope and sudden death have occasionally been the consequences. There is no objection to having the bed made so that the head and shoulders are kept at a higher level than the pelvis. 5. Supply healthy nutriment by the stomach. This is an effective barrier to absorption of noxious stuff from the parturient canal. The more the system is supplied in this way, the less will it absorb in other ways.

Although the diet ought to be generous in quantity it ought to be easily assimilable. Broths, beef-tea, milk toast, eggs, plain cr combined are enough for the first two days. After this more solid food ought gradually to be allowed.

Dr. Barnes summarizes Antiseptic Midwifery in the following rules :—

1. Keep the door shut against the enemy by maintaining contraction of the uterus.

2. Prevent the enemy from forming and collecting by irrigating the parturient canal with antiseptic fluids.

3. Eject the enemy as fast as he effects an entry; that is, keep the excretory organs in activity.

4. Guard the lying-in chamber against the approach of foreign poisons.

5. Fortify the patient against the attack of the enemy by keeping up due supplies of wholesome food.

The practitioner who adopts these principles for his guidance will rarely meet with septicæmia in women confined in their own homes. It is otherwise in hospital practice. Here in addition to most careful attention to purity of clothing, beds, linen, fingers of accoucheur and nurse, &c., he recommends the carbolic spray. These measures within the last few years have saved many lives in Maternity Hospitals. Dr. Fancourt Barnes' results at the British Lying-in Hospital are amongst those most recently published.

The Treatment of Puerperal Hemorrhage.—This ever-interesting subject to the obstetrician was discussed at the June (1881) meeting of the Medical Society of the County of Kings, Brooklyn, N. Y. Dr. T. G. Thomas, of New York, participated in an able address containing many practical and some original ideas. He said that many individual remedies had been brought forward of late, but he did not believe that we had advanced much from olden time. The influences than which there are no other which prevent post-partum hemorrhage are contraction of the uterus, which ligates the vessels, and coagulation—the formation of thrombi at their mouths. In ante-partum hemorrhage there is a direct influence, pressure of bleeding points directly against the body of the child. Post-partum hemorrhage is often due to hasty action on the part of the accoucher, effecting rapid delivery. It occurs much more frequently in cases managed by men who do not watch the uterus, who do not allow nature to deliver the child, who do not superintend the third stage of labor, and who do not fix in their mind the fact that the third stage of labor consists, not in the delivery of the placenta, but in *persistent uterine contraction.* As regards prognosis. he believed that this depends much more on the practitioner in charge than upon the case ; that a case of puerperal hemorrhage, ante or post-partum, if managed carefully and thoroughly in the beginning, will almost invariably get well. In hemorrhage at the beginning of labor, before the rupture of the membranes, (the child and liquor amnii are in the uterus) and the os uteri is not dilated, unless it be furious—the tampon is to be employed. Internal hemorrhage is, of course, possible in these cases, but only when there is not firm tonic contraction of the uterus, which latter condition must be secured. The practitioner must not, therefore, put in a tampon and leave his patient, for if the uterus relax she may die of internal hemorrhage. In speaking of the tampon, Dr. Thomas said:—"I do not mean that painful and inefficient measure known to our grandfathers, which consisted in stuffing a silk handkerchief into the vagina, or in using the kite-tail structure which accomplished nothing towards obtaining the desired result, but I mean the tamponing which is secured by placing the woman upon her left side, with one arm thrown behind her, and, with a Sims' speculum, or the two fingers of an assistant, lifting the perineum and depressing the anterior wall of the vagina, removing all blood from the vagina, and then taking balls of wet cotton, not containing any astringent whatever, and stuffing them all around the cervix so as to make a collar, and then thoroughly filling the entire vagina with this wet cotton." If in spite of such efforts well and persistently directed, hemorrhage goes on, the tampon is to be removed, the membranes ruptured by introducing the sound through the narrow cervix, and uterine action secured. If these fail, the uterus is to be emptied by rapid dilatation, begun by Barnes' bags and completed by introduction of the hand folded into a cone, and then opened so as to spread out the tissues till it can grasp and extract the child, placenta and clots. The same treatment identically is that which is to be adopted for hemorrhage from separation of the placenta, as by a blow or fall on the abdomen, as labor is progressing.

In placenta prævia, we cannot trust to the same principles. The mouths of the bleeding vessels cannot be permanently sealed with coagulated blood so as to arrest the hemorrhage, because by reason of contraction of the uterus no sooner is one set of vessels closed than another is freshly opened, and unless something more is done the woman may die in the first stage of labor. Neither can we depend upon pressure and counter pressure, for the head of the child is quite above the placenta and out of reach. As regards ligation of blood vessels by contraction of uterine fibres, this is not to be depended on,—the cervix contracts very badly at best; besides, nature wishes to have it open. For all these reasons hemorrhage with placenta prævia is the most difficult to treat. It is in the first stage that the dangers and difficulties chiefly exist. In this stage Dr. Thomas advocates a properly applied tampon, which he prepares and applies as follows:—" My plan, when I wish to tampon for placenta pravia, is to take an ordinary piece of linen, make a conical bag, stuff it with carbolized cotton till it is quite hard, and sew up the base. I then turn the woman on her side, introduce a Sims' speculum, remove all the blood I can, and then push the apex of that cone into the uterus as far as I can make it go. It can do no harm. I then tampon around it, fill the vagina, and put on a strong T bandage, which keeps the compress against the uterus constantly, and when the uterus contracts it is forced up on this cone, and gradually three things are accomplished: First, coagulation of blood is favoured; second, the cervix is dilated by the pressure of the elastic plug; and third, direct pressure is brought to bear upon the bleeding blood vessels." When the first stage is complete the greatest difficulty is overcome; the uterus can be emptied at once, and the case is at an end.

In post-partum hemorrhage, when ordinary measures to induce contraction of the uterus have failed, then hypodermics of ergot or ether, or both should be employed. If the hemorrhage is not severe enough, or if for other reasons we do not wish to pass the hand into the cavity of the uterus, excessive cold or heat may be applied to the fundus, the uterus is to be forced into firm contraction under the hand, and never let go till the bleeding stops. Dr. Thomas asks the question as to how long the uterus ought to be held? And replies: "I have repeatedly held it, under such circumstances, for 12 hours." But if these measures fail and hemorrhage continues, "then wash the hand and arm thoroughly with soap and water, use a nail brush thoroughly, dip the hand and arm in warm, strong, carbolized water and without wiping them, carry the hand up to the fundus uteri, sweep everything out, and keep the hand there until the uterus contracts. Pass the pulp of the fingers up and down the sides of the uterus in any direction, and at the same time make counter pressure from the outside." Dr. Thomas believes that in ninety-nine cases out of a hundred of post-partum hemorrhage seen before the woman's nervous system is entirely prostrated, if the hand is introduced and used in the manner described, the uterus will contract. He does not believe that hot water injections or the use of a sponge dipped in hot water and introduced into the interior of the uterus act otherwise than by mechanical irritation, and then the hand is more effectual. Injection of solutions of iron he rejects absolutely, except as a *dernier ressort* in the strictest possible sense.—(The proceedings of the Medical Society for the County of Kings, Brooklyn, N.Y., for July, 1881.)

A Case of Pyosalpinx bursting into the Abdominal Cavity.—Dr. H. Burnier reports a case of right-sided purulent salpingitis with the termination just mentioned. A woman, 69 years of age, suffering from prolapsus uteri, died soon after admission to the hospital. In the right side of the pelvis a pus-cavity was found communicating with the right fallopian tube. The portion of intestine attached was thinned at several points, and actually perforated at one. Burnier believed that the metritis and endometritis resulting from the prolapse had given rise to the purulent salpingitis. The free end of the tube was closed, and the consequent accumulation led to rupture. Eleven days before death the patient suffered from tolerably well marked symptoms of peritonitis. It was probably at this time that the rupture took place.—(*Zeitschrift f. Geb. & Gynak.*, Bd. vi., Hft. 2.)

Treatment of Incontinence of Urine in Women.—Dr. J. M. Chapman reports (*Edin. Med. Jour.*, June, 1881), a case of vesical catarrh, with inability to retain the urine for more than half an hour, which, after having cured the catarrh, he treated by gradual dilatation of the bladder with daily injections of a warm two-per cent. solution of carbolic acid in increasing quantity. At the beginning of the treatment the patient could retain the urine only one hour, and the bladder held one fluid ounce. After six weeks' treatment the capacity was sixteen ounces; during the night she micturated once or twice only, and during the day at normal intervals. We have had some very favourable experience of this method of treating this form of incontinence.

A New Method of Intra-Uterine Application of Perchloride of Iron.—Dr. Von Teutleben, of Berlin, has recently (*Centralblatt für Gynakologie*, 26th Nov., 1881), proposed to use perchloride of iron in the form of solid sticks. These are made of the pure salt, of suitable size, and are kept in stoppered bottles, as they are deliquescent when exposed to the air. They are introduced to the uterine cavity by means of a parti-caustique with as large a fenestra as possible. The instrument is to be moved about several times in various directions, and partially withdrawn and reintroduced to remove coagula, and so favor the escape of the melted salt. After a few minutes the instrument may be removed, and will be found empty, the perchloride being dissolved and remaining in the uterine cavity. The advantages claimed by Teutleben for this method are facility of application, as the parti-caustique is easily guided to the uterine cavity by the finger without the use of a speculum, which, in women with very narrow or sensitive vulva or vagina, is painful or disagreeable, and further, the absolute impossibility of any escape of the iron into the abdominal cavity. This plan certainly commends

[illegible]

[illegible] Leopold [illegible] [illegible] — Prof. Tergen [illegible] [illegible] [illegible] [illegible] [illegible] The method is [illegible] [illegible] [illegible] [illegible] [illegible] [illegible] [illegible] [illegible] [illegible] changes are necessary during the first [illegible] days, but [illegible] after this the [illegible] [illegible] [illegible] the discharges was found to be maintained [illegible] [illegible] [illegible] sufficiently often. This was proved by Prof. [illegible] [illegible] [illegible] Tergen's [illegible] [illegible] the discharges for four or five days and found no bacteria [illegible] [illegible] them.

[illegible] of Heidelberg, in the number of the [illegible] January, 1882, of the same periodical, [illegible] the use, in the cases, of a modification of Tergen's method. [illegible] [illegible] strands of cotton [illegible] [illegible] [illegible] lies between the edges of the wound, the free ends [illegible] in the abdominal cavity and outside the wound.

Reviews and Notices of Books.

Eczema and its Management [illegible] *based on the study of* [illegible] *cases of the disease.*—By L. Duncan Bulkley, A.M., M.D. [illegible] pp. 324. New York: G. P. Putnam's Sons. 1881.

Dr. Bulkley is so well known as a teacher of, and writer on, skin diseases (especially eczema), that anything coming from his [illegible] to be the result of matured experience. This book, [illegible] [illegible] represents the personal views of the author, and on that account is much more valuable as a contributien to the Science of Dermatology. Most of the matter has appeared from time to time in the various medical journals. The basis of the work being, however, an Essay on "The Management of Eczema," read before the American Medical Association in 1874. In the opening chapter we find a definition of the disease and also the author's valuable general classification of diseases of the skin. In Chapter II an interesting analysis of 2,500 cases of eczema is given, from which it appears that eczema occurs with greatest frequency between the ages of 20 and 40, and most often on the face and head, hands, thighs and legs. In about 8 p.c. of the private cases it occurs with other eruptions, these eruptions being psoriasis, boils and severe acne. The frequent occurrence of hordeoli or styes is considered by Dr. Bulkley to be significant of an eczematous diathesis. He has little belief in the heredity of the disease and gives, in proof, a table, where out of 2,153 relatives of 500 eczema patients only 422 were ever said to have been affected with eczema. Gouty, strumous, and nervous states which are transmitted, predispose to eczema; eczema has also frequently been associated with asthma, affections of the liver, &c.

In Chapter IV the different forms of eczema are described, and we are told that eczema may be papular or squamous from beginning to end, the typical vesicular form being comparatively rare. Cases of papular eczema are often called lichen, strophulus, &c.

In Chapter VI the nature of eczema (whether constitutional or local) is discussed at length. Although educated at the Vienna School under the great Hebra, Dr. Bulkley has completely discarded his teacher's ideas as to the local pathology and treatment, and is convinced that eczema and many other diseases of the skin are constitutional diseases, and success depends in a great measure on careful constitutional treatment, aided, however, by local applications. Dr. Bulkley states that he has frequently seen cases of eczema disappear under constitutional treatment. Hebra and his school believe, on the other hand, that constitutional treatment alone never cured;

that constitutional and local treatment together cure, and also that local treatment alone cures. They inferred, therefore, that in the cases treated constitutionally and locally, it is the local treatment only which is curative. The author does not adopt the old humoral pathology to such an extent as to assert that the disease is due to a *materies morbi*, but gives some credit to the importance of local cell action. He, however, holds that there is such a condition as an eczematous diathesis and what is commonly called eczema produced by purely local causes, as irritation of insects, occupation, &c., is not eczema but dermatitis, that there is no more connection between the two conditions than there is between rheumatism and a sprained ankle; and that the success of the *local* school has been due to the fact of their not recognizing the difference between dermatitis and eczema. He admits that clinically these diseases cannot be distinguished, except by their different causes, and that their local pathology is identical. This, certainly, we think, is a distinction without a difference. Dr. Bulkley concludes that eczema cannot be both constitutional and local. His arguments in favour of the constituted character of the disease are very forcible, but still not completely convincing, especially that part where the chance of eczema being local is excluded by calling it dermatitis. Probably a view taking the happy mean between the local and constitutional schools would be nearer the truth, viz., that eczema is a disease which may be either constitutional or local in its origin and course.

Eczematous patients may be divided, says Dr. Bulkley, with tolerable accuracy into three classes: the gouty, the strumous and the neurotic. This corresponds to the three states of constitutional debility described by Mr. (now Sir) Erasmus Wilson, viz., assimilative debility, nutritive debility and nervous debility. Dr. Bulkley observes that he cannot understand how the influence of the gouty diathesis has been overlooked in connection with eczema by the local pathologists. The clinical signs by which the gouty state is manifested in eczematous patients are said to be: imperfect digestion, constipation, diarrhœa, imperfect urinary secretion and faulty cutaneous action; these states depend the one very much on the other. The most important of these symptoms are imperfect digestion and constipation. The second-class strumous is generally easily recognized. In Vienna, one-third of the children suffering from eczema, Neumann states, were found to be rachitic or strumous. The author draws attention to the fact that this condition exists in the aged as well as in children. The third, or neurotic class, includes all those who suffer from "nervous debility, neurasthenia, or lowered vitality of nerve action," and this condition is often induced by the gouty state. Besides the cases under these classes, others are seen where the eczema is connected with dentition, varicose veins, pregnancy, &c.

Among the local causes mentioned as causing eczema in persons predisposed to it, are atmospheric conditions, catching cold, bad air, burns, action of soap, water, scratching the skin, chemical irritants, as mercurial and sulphur ointments, &c.

Now, many of these causes produce an eruption which, according to the author, would be a dermatitis, and should, therefore, be ignored as causes of eczema. Still they are given, which shows how difficult it is to draw the line and keep to the purely constitutional theory. Of course it is said that these causes produce eczema only in those persons having the eczematous diathesis; but what is this diathesis which is only recognized by the appearance of an eruption, and how are we to say that it is not a dermatitis?

Dr. Bulkley believes that tobacco has some influence in producing or prolonging this disease, that is, if used at all in excess. The ill-effects are produced in three ways: 1st. By disturbance of digestion. 2nd. Depressing effects on the nervous system. 3rd. The irritating effects of the fumes, especially in eczema of the hands and face.

The author is evidently never at a loss to account for the causation of every case of eczema, and has no large class of cases, as Hebra had, whose causes are unknown. Dividing patients into the three divisions given above, there are few, even of ordinary people, who would not be included in one or other, especially when each division has such a wide range. Dr.

Bulkley is quite Abernethian in giving such prominence to disorders of the digestion.

Chapter VII is devoted to treatment, constitutional and local. Enemata and mineral waters to relieve constipation are disapproved of, pills of blue mass, colocynth and ipecac. being preferred. To relieve itching, chloral and bromide of potassium, alone or combined, are of the greatest service. Gelseminum is highly spoken of, in this connection, given in ten minim doses of the tincture, and increased and repeated every half hour till relieved. When speaking of local treatment it is very truly remarked that the greatest number of errors made are in the direction of over stimulating and over irritating applications.

Chapter IX., on the management of infantile eczema, is, perhaps, the best in the book, great stress being laid on proper constitutional treatment: Tonics and cod-liver oil for the strumous, with an occasional alkaline purge. For the apparently healthy child suffering from eczema, depurative remedies with alkalies have proved very valuable. The author remarks that children suffering from eczema are often apparently in the most rugged health, but he is confident that a careful medical investigation will always discover *something* to be corrected besides the disorder of the skin. With regard to local applications it is very truly remarked, that he is poorly able to treat infantile eczema, who knows only zinc ointment, which bears the palm for universality of use. Lard ointments are objected to in the treatment of infantile eczema, cold cream made from almond oil, spermaceti and bees-wax being much preferred. The products of petroleum have not sufficient consistency. Great stress is properly laid on the importance of keeping the applications continuously in contact with the eruption, day and night. Ointments should be applied on lint and not rubbed in. In nursing children the health of the mother should be attended to.

Chapter X and the three following chapters are devoted to regional eczema, as face and scalp, hands and arms, feet and legs, anus and genital regións. Chapter XV being taken up with eczema of the trunk and general eczema. Attention is drawn to the fact that eczema of the face and hands is constantly found to be associated with dyspeptic and nervous conditions. In eczema of the palms of the hands, soles of the feet and tips of the fingers, Dr. Bulkley has found the use of hot water a most important addition to the treatment. The water should be very hot, so hot that the part can be put in only for a few seconds; the affected part should be immersed thus several times, then dried carefully, and some ointment applied. In old, inveterate circumscribed eczema, Hebra's treatment by caustic potash, 5 to 20 grs. to the ounce of water, is advised. This, though painful, is often effectual. In the management of eczema and eczematous and varicose ulcers of the lower extremities, the use of the solid rubber bandages is unexcelled. The bandage may cause a little pain and heat, but the discomfort soon passes off. The most common and almost invariable symptom accompanying eczema of the arms and genital region Dr. Bulkley has found to be constipation, and this must be overcome if successful treatment is desired. Locally, very hot water is advised. When eczema occurs on the trunk, it often indicates "profound disturbance of the functions of nutrition," and, as might be imagined, local remedies have not much curative effect, and more attention should be paid to internal treatment. Arsenic, combined with other tonics, has been found useful, but should not be given alone. Cod liver oil is often beneficial. Beer and spirits in general eczema should be strenuously avoided.

Chapter XV is devoted to a consideration of diet and hygiene in connection with eczema. The author thinks, in common with many others, that articles of diet have a direct effect on the skin, for good or evil; he thinks no small share of the cases of eczema in private life are prolonged and perhaps caused by over-eating. This is especially the case in infants who are too frequently fed or whose mothers' milk is at fault owing to her partaking daily of beer, ale, porter and wine, or else large amounts of tea. Dr. Bulkley has noticed that eczema patients of all ages dislike fats as an article of diet, and from the favorable results he has obtained by the use of cod liver oil, he has long been convinced that the absence of fat is an important factor in causing eczema.

Tea, coffee, and fermented liquors should be avoided by the eczematous, also greasy soups. Sweet potatoes, cabbage, bananas and apples have a harmful effect on eczema, also salt food. Regular exercise in the open air is strongly advocated, especially long walks.

The last chapter (XVI) contains the formulæ for the various preparations used by the author, such as mixtures, lotions, ointments, &c. The book is well printed on thick paper, and is free from typographical errors. From its practical nature, easy style and original character, this work is sure to become popular, and take the first place among works on eczema.

The Physician's Clinical Record for Hospital or Private Practice, with memoranda for examining patients, temperature, charts, &c. Philadelphia: D. G. Brinton.

This is a handy little volume of the size of a small octavo volume, just fitted for the pocket. Almost its entire bulk is taken up with forms for clinical record. These are so ruled as to give space for pulse, temperature, respirations and other things generally required in such a record ; and in addition, a number of very good temperature charts, and (a new feature) a small pasteboard figure of the shape of the chest—a stencil, as it is called. From this an outline can at once be made on one of the blank pages, and special points concerning situation of tumors, areas of dullness, &c., can be noted thereon. For those who do not keep more extended notes of cases, one of these pocket records will be found exceedingly useful.

The Diagnosis and Treatment of the Diseases of the Eye.—By HENRY W. WILLIAMS, A. M., M. D., Professor of Ophthalmology in Harvard University, Ophthalmic Surgeon to the City Hospital, Boston, &c. Boston: Houghton, Mifflin & Co. Montreal: Dawson Bros.

This is an excellent and highly practical treatise by an author already well known from smaller works already published. All purely scientific and theoretical discussions have been purposely excluded, and the bulk having been thus materially diminished, it is made to contain, within very reasonable limits, all that is essential to the diagnosis, causation and treatment of eye diseases. All portions of the book seem to have been compiled with equal care, and the style is clear and logical. Special attention is given to those important affections of the deep structures of the eye, which are of such great diagnostic value to the physician in cases of suspected cerebral disorder. Color-blindness, and the method of testing for this defect are fully explained—a matter on which much observation has recently been bestowed. In conclusion, Prof. Williams' hand-book can be highly recommended as an admirable practical treatise on ophthalmic practice, and one extremely well suited to meet the wants of the general practitioner.

Books and Pamphlets Received.

ILLUSTRATIONS OF DISSECTIONS, IN A SERIES OF ORIGINAL COLORED PLATES. By George Viner Ellis and G. H. Ford. Vol. I. Second edition. New York: Wm. Wood & Co.

MARRIAGE AND PARENTAGE AND THE SANITARY AND PHYSIOLOGICAL LAWS FOR THE PRODUCTION OF FINER HEALTH AND GREATER ABILITY. By a Physician and Sanitarian. New York: M. L. Holbrook & Co.

A MANUAL OF ORGANIC MATERIA MEDICA. By John M. Maisch, Phar. D. Philadelphia: Henry C. Lea's Son & Co.

TRANSACTIONS OF THE MEDICAL ASSOCIATION OF GEORGIA—32nd Annual Session, 1881. Augusta, Georgia.

AN INDEX OF SURGERY. Being a concise classification of the main facts and theories of Surgery for the use of senior students and others. By C. B. Keetley, F.R.C.S. New York: Bermingham & Co.

PERCUSSION OUTLINES. By E. G. Cutter, M.D., and G. M. Garland, M.D. Boston: Houghton, Mifflin & Co.

A TREATISE ON HUMAN PHYSIOLOGY. Designed for the use of Students and Practitioners of Medicine. By John C. Dalton, M.D. Seventh edition, with two hundred and fifty-two Illustrations. Philadelphia: Henry C Lea's Son & Co.

A MANUAL OF DENTAL ANATOMY—HUMAN AND COMPARATIVE. By Charles S. Tomes, M.A., F.R.S. Second edition. Philadelphia: Presley Blakiston.

Society Proceedings.

MEDICO-CHIRURGICAL SOCIETY OF MONTREAL.

Stated Meeting, February 17, 1882.

GEORGE ROSS, M.D., PRESIDENT, IN THE CHAIR.

Dr. Osler exhibited a series of specimens illustrating certain points in the pathology of atheroma of vessels.

I.—*Atheromatous Plate and Ulcers on Arch of Aorta.*—The specimen was taken from a man aged 65, who died in the General Hospital after fracture of the left femur. Death was somewhat sudden and unlooked-for; the friends objected to the head being opened. Nothing of special note was found in the viscera; fat emboli were suspected, but none found on careful examination of the lungs. The heart was normal; valves a little stiff. The anterior wall of the arch of the aorta presented a flat plate about 10 × 6 cm., and from 3 to 6 times the thickness of the rest of the tube. The intima over this area was opaque, and presented irregular prominences. At one point, 2 cm. in front of the innominate, there was an oval-shaped loss of substance 8 × 4 mm., which opened into a small atheromatous abscess, the contents of which had in great part escaped. The increased thickness of the wall was due to a layer of brownish-yellow, firm, caseous matter, between the intima and the media; in places, this was 5 to 6 mm. in diameter, it was nowhere calcified. There was a second spot of softening in it which had not burst into the tube, but was separated by a thin brownish membrane. On squeezing from the outer side, a puriform fluid escaped. There were a few small spots of atheroma in the descending aorta. No satisfactory cause of death was found, and it seemed scarcely likely that the bursting of such a small abscess would produce immediate death. Unfortunately, the mode of death was not known, the patient being found dead by the night nurse. Such a spot might form the starting-point of an aneurism, as in the first specimen. Whether any symptoms follow this condition is not positively known; we certainly meet these ulcers in many cases, which, during life, have not afforded any evidence of their presence.

Dr. Girdwood thought it not improbable that the bursting of the abscess and discharge of its contents caused death, though, of course, it was impossible to say in the absence of an examination of the brain. He asked whether there was a murmur? Dr. Osler could not say.

II.—*Atheromatous Abscess and Aneurism of the Right Iliac Artery; general atheroma.*—This specimen was taken from an aged woman who had died from cancer of the cardiac end of the stomach. She had also dry gangrene of the toes of the right foot. Heart was in a state of brown atrophy, and valves were stiff. The aorta presented numerous calcareous plates, and towards its bifurcation was firm and rigid. The intima had many smooth, brownish-yellow calcified patches, and there were also several small atheromatous abscesses. The right iliac artery, at its origin, presented a firm, elastic tumour the size of a walnut, which almost obliterated its lumen. On opening the vessel, this tumour was found to be an aneurismal sac, communicating by a small orifice which was blocked with adherent clots. On section, the sac was found filled with a reddish thrombi in the lower, and pulpy atheromatous matter at the upper part. It was evidently a small atheromatous abscess converted into an aneurismal sac. The external iliac and femoral, with its branches, on being removed, were found to have thickened walls and in places calcified. Near the popliteal the lumen was greatly reduced, and an adherent thrombus almost obliterated the vessel. In several spots the calcified intima was elevated by a quantity of pulpy atheroma beneath it.

III.—*Bizzozero's New (?) Blood Element and its relation to Thrombus formation.*—The aorta in this specimen, which was obtained from a patient who died of extensive cancer of the stomach, presented an extraordinary condition. Just above its bifurcation there was tolerably advanced atheroma of the entire intima, patchy, and in places calcified; there was also a greyish-white irregular mass, 5 × 3 cm., somewhat flattened, but projecting from the intima about 1 cm., to which it was closely united. In the abdominal aorta there were six or eight smaller spots of a similar character attached to localized areas of atheroma, the appearance, when fresh, being very suggestive of a neoplasm, and these were thought at first to be secondary cancerous masses. On examination, the large spot was found to be composed of closely set small colourless bodies, about one-third or one-fourth the size of red blood corpuscles, discoid, and with a uniform greyish stroma. They appeared to be identical with the individual elements of Schultze's *granule masses*, which are so common in the blood of certain persons. In Dr. Wood's case of aneurism, the grey filaments on the walls were made up of precisely the same elements. A few colourless corpuscles and some fibrin fibrils also existed, but they were in trifling amount compared with the small elements. Dr. Osler remarked that these were the little bodies recently described by Prof. Bizzozero of Turin as a new blood element, but they had, in reality, long been known, having been described by Schultze in 1861. They occur in the drawn blood in the form of granular clumps, but he (Dr. O.) had shown, in a communication to the Royal Society in 1874, that in the circulatory blood the individual elements of the masses were isolated, and in the form of small discoids. An engraving was passed round illustrating them, as seen in a subcutaneous vessel of the young rat, which was the most favourable animal for the study of these bodies. In the case under consideration, these elements had apparently collected on an extensive area of atheroma, and had either multiplied there or the mass had been formed by their gradual accretion.

In comparative pathology, Dr. Osler presented the following specimens :—

Glanders.—1. The split head of a horse showing the nasal fossæ and sinuses. Horse had been ill for several months, but still in pretty good condition, but suffering from a chronic muco-purulent discharge from the nostrils. The specimen showed numerous ulcers, many of which could be seen from the external orifices ; glanders tubercles in the form of isolated neoplasms on the Schneiderian membrane. They were thickly set in the upper part of the septum, and some were as large as beans. 2. Diffuse infiltration of the mucosa, with a greyish material most evident in frontal sinuses and antra, but existed over the turbinated bones. 3. Stellate cicatrices of healed ulcers: there were numerous nodules in the trachea and a few ulcers; there were also some of the specific nodules of the disease in the lungs. Liver, spleen and kidneys healthy. The cervical lymph glands were much swollen and contained a few nodules, no cutaneous glanders. (farcy.)

Dr. Gurd asked with reference to its degree of communicability, and whether many cases in man had been met with here. The President believed that the liability to contagion in man was over-rated; at least there were many cases of glanders in horses and yet instances of infection of grooms and others were very rare. He had seen only one case; that of a groom who had taken charge of several glandered animals on board a river steamer. The stench from them was very great and he took the affection by inhalation of the poison.

Verminous Aneurism.—Portion of arteria colica artery from a horse showing a small aneurismal dilatation, the size of an almond, the walls thickened and covered with adherent thrombi among which were several specimens of the *strongylus armatus* or palisade worm. This parasite bores its way from the intestine, penetrates the artery and excites arteritis, with weakness of the walls, dilatation and thrombosis in the lining menbrane. It is a common affection among horses and according to Bollinger is the most frequent cause of colic in these animals. He states that of horses which are afflicted with internal disease, 40 per cent. suffer from colic; of any 100 diseased horses, 40 have perished from colic; and among 100 colic patients, 87 recover and 13 die. No epizootic or sporadic affection in horses is so common and so fatal.

Aneurism of Aorta. Perforation of Œsophagus.—Dr. Wood narrated the case—a female, aged 55 years, ailing for some days with dyspeptic symptoms. One evening, on going to stool, she complained of feeling sick, did not vomit, but fell over suddenly and died in a few minutes. There had been no apprehension of serious trouble, and nothing special could be elicited on careful examination of chest and abdomen. The autopsy by Dr. Osler revealed a large coagulum in the stomach, forming a mould of that organ. The source of the blood was not detected till the œsophagus was dissected, when a small aneurismal tumour, the size of a billiard ball, was found between it and the aorta, about two inches above the cardia. The aorta presented, in the lower thoracic portion, a small punched-out orifice, size of a five-cent piece, with a narrow zone of thickened translucent intima about it. This led directly into a small sacculated dilatation of the intima, not larger than a marble, which had ruptured and formed the main sac, spheroidal in shape, with walls composed of thickened media and adventitia. It contained fresh clots and thin mural thrombi. The perforation into the œsophagus was by a small orifice which was plugged with a clot. On the thrombi lining the sac there were curious-branched thread-like filaments well marked against the dark-red back-ground. These were composed of minute spherical bodies, identical with those found in the thrombus of the aorta in the case just described. No heart disease or atheroma of the aorta, except in the zone just about the orifice. The trouble had likely originated in a localized atheromatous process, with softening, rupture, and subsequent dilatation. The case was also interesting, as the patient had been treated four years before for pneumonic phthisis, but had unexpectedly made a complete recovery. The upper half of the right lung was firm, and contained much fibroid tissue, with several bronchiectatic cavities.

Dr. Girdwood remarked on the latency of many cases of aneurism and the varied symptoms produced by irritation or pressure. He narrated a case in point, in which digestive troubles were for a long time the most prominent feature in a case of abdominal aneurism. Dr. Mills asked if there had been any difficulty in swallowing, and suggested that auscultation of the œsophagns might have given some information in such a case. Dr. Wood had never been able to detect any abnormal physical signs in either chest or abdomen. He had not auscultated gullet.

Ammonia Poisoning.—Dr. A. A. Browne related the case, and presented the stomach and œsophagus. (*See page* 449.) The patient, aged 55, had been in the habit of taking bromide of potassium after drinking bouts. His bottle was accidentally filled with strong liquor ammonia, and he gulped down a mouthful directly from it. Great pain was at once experienced and profuse bleeding came on from the stomach, lasting twelve hours. The vomiting was frequent, but after the bleeding stopped only recurred on taking food. The patient lived four days and was sensible to the last. There was very slight affection of the mouth and fauces ; not much tenderness over stomach, chief pain being referred to chest. The amount swallowed could not be definitely determined. Autopsy revealed great engorgement of the tissues in the course of the œsophagus and about the fundus of stomach. The mucosa of fauces and gullet was of a deep yellow brown color looking dry and burnt. The cardiac end of the stomach and a patch at the fundus were chiefly affected ; mucous membrane much swollen, dark yellow, and in places looked sloughy ; deep congestion of the sub-mucous and muscular layers in this region ; rest of surface was unaffected ; mucous membrane of epiglottis and larynx were injected but not burnt.

The President said he had been called to see this case shortly after the accident, and had seen the patient on several occasions with Dr. Browne, and the points which struck him as most peculiar were the absence of laryngeal symptoms and the persistent pain in the chest.

Medico-Legal Case.—Dr. Girdwood then read a paper on "The Plantagenet Murder Case," which will appear next month.

Extracts from British and Foreign Journals.

Unless otherwise stated the translations are made specially for this Journal.

The Treatment of Consumption.—Dr. Robert Saundby contributes to the *Practitioner* (Vol. XXVII, No. 4) a very instructive article on the Treatment of Consumption, when chronic. Some very useful hints for the practitioner are to be found in this paper. He finds that the treatment of phthisis, based on the Listerian system, is of no great utility. Then taking up the symptoms separately he deprecates the use of the opirate linctus. "Cough mixtures and cough lozenges containing opium or morphia are poisons to consumptive patients."

This sounds very well, but as a matter of practice what is one to do with a case of phthisis where cough is the prominent symptom, where it occurs almost incessantly day and night. Every man has met with cases where morphia and morphia alone allays the distress and where all substitutes fail. However, it is well to begin with a very simple remedy. We are recommended to try barley water acidulated with lemon juice or citric acid, raspberry vinegar and water, and when the cough is troublesome and especially at night to advise the patient to hold camphor to his nose and mouth with his handkerchief, covering his head with the bedclothes. This simple expedient has proved very useful in many cases. Camphor may also be usefully employed in combination with steam by putting a lump of camphor into a jug or inhaler with half a point of boiling water. The use of this for a few minutes at bed time allays the irritability of the fauces and permits sleep. He finds that cödeia possesses the anodyne properties of morphia without its deranging effect upon the digestive organs. The formula employed is—℞ Codeiæ, gr i; Tr. Card. Co., ♏ x; Syrupi Tolutani ♏ xx; Aqua ad ʒi. M. Fiat linctus. Sig: To be taken when the cough is troublesome. Or, the lozenges of Cödeia may be used containing cödeia gr. ¼ each, made up with extract of licorice and compound tragacanth powder.

The dryness of the Mouth so frequently complained of by the phthisical is to be treated by the placing in the mouth of one of Wyeth's compressed tablets of chlorate of potash and borax. These are found to stimulate the salivary secretion and provide a medication suitable to the catarrhal condition of the mucous surface.

The Bronchitis of phthisis.—In mild cases inhalation of ten minims of turpentine in a jug with boiling water or when this proves too irritating a lump of camphor may be substituted. Externally the chest must be rubbed with liniment of camphor, or acetic liniment of turpentine, or in more severe cases a waistcoat should be made of spongeo-piline, fastening by means of tape shoulder straps and tapes to tie in front, and this should be worn constantly and kept wrung out of hot water and sprinkled with a few drops of turpentine. This waistcoat has the advantage, in addition to its counter irritant effect upon the chest, of keeping the patient in an atmosphere of steam and turpentine most likely to soothe the irritable condition of his bronchial tubes. I am glad to see repeated the opinion of Graves as to the efficacy of sulphur in bronchitis. Dr. Saundby thinks it next in importance to turpentine. On referring to Graves (Clinical Medicine, p. 231) I find that five to ten grains of sulphur taken three or four times a day is one of the best remedies that can be prescribed in cases of chronic cough, accompanied by constitutional debility and copious secretion into the bronchial tubes. * * * * As it has a tendency to produce elevation of the pulse, increased heat of skin and sweating, it will be necessary to temper its stimulant properties by combining it with cream of tartar, which is a cooling aperient, and has the additional advantages of determining gently to the kidneys. (Graves here quotes Baglivi: "In morbis pectoris ad vias urinæ ducendum est.")

Profuse Purulent Expectoration.—This is said to be best treated by large doses of sulphate of iron of which fifteen or twenty grains should be given daily, either in mixture or pill. Again to quote Graves, "the action of a chalybeate is not merely limited to strengthen the tone of the stomach and general system; it is also well calculated to arrest the superabundant secretion from mucous surfaces in many chronic fluxes, and hence its utility in gleet, diarrhoea, and chronic bronchitis." Dr. Saunby recommends, too, the use of an inhaler of his own design. It resembles the metallic chloroform inhaler, and enclosed in it is tow on which is sprinkled the particular substance to be inhaled. His favorite, is a one to twenty solution of carbolic acid.

Diarrhœa—In the treatment of diarrhœa he has abandoned all other means for the use of a lemonade made with sulphuric acid which the patient is to drink *ad libitum*. The formula is—℞ Acidi sulph, dil. ʒ ij; Tinct. Aurantii ʒ ij; Sacch. albi. q. s.; Aq. Fontanæ oj. M. Sig. To be drunk *ad libitum* every half hour till the diarrhœa has stopped.

CANADA

Medical and Surgical Journal.

MONTREAL, MARCH, 1882.

THE MEDICAL TARIFF.

It is but a few months since our Province was endowed with a tariff of fees for the medical profession. It emanated, as by law provided, from the Provincial Medical Board, and, after due delay, was sanctioned by the Lieutenant-Governor. One would have supposed that the rates thus fixed by a body of representative men from all the various districts of the Province would have been such as to commend themselves to the community at large. Instead of this having been the case, however, as soon as ever it was published in the daily papers, a perfect panic ensued. Condemnatory editorials were hurled at it in all directions, numerous letters appeared, all complaining of the high rates which had been fixed, and for a few days medical men, even in their daily rounds, heard little else but uncomplimentary remarks on the grasping greed of the grinding doctors. It required, however, only the assurance that we were *not* going to take our patients by the throat and demand instantaneous payment of treble our usual fees, for the matter to quiet down and be almost forgotten, like many another nine days' wonder. But it so happened that this explosion occurred shortly before the coming on of our Provincial elections. The opportunity was altogether too good a one to be lost by the politicians, and the consequence was that a warm feeling was easily fanned into a flame in the constituency represented by the Hon. Mr. Lynch, Solicitor-General, who was made responsible for the passage of the Bill. This gentleman was thus obliged by his wily opponents either to defend a measure which had been rendered highly unpopular or else promise that a relief bill should be brought in. He chose the latter course, and upon the hustings undertook to say that a measure for the partial or entire repeal of the obnoxious Tariff would be brought in at the earliest possible moment. To redeem this pledge, Mr. Lynch has now given notice of his intention to introduce a Bill concerning the Medical Tariff during the present session of our Provincial Legislature. We are given to understand that it is contemplated either to repeal the Tariff *in toto*, or else to do this for the whole of the country districts and allow it to remain in force in the cities. We are rather inclined to believe that, if the matter comes up for discussion, the opposition to the rates being so great, a demand will be made for complete repeal, *i.e.*, that the cities shall also be included. It may be looked upon, therefore, as pretty certain that after a remarkably brief existence, our tariff is doomed to a violent and ignominious death. It is to be regretted that sufficient time had not been allowed to have enabled us to see how this Tariff would have worked, for as it is, its premature strangulation has been decided upon purely through stress of a political emergency, induced by cleverly working upon a popular excitement. If it had been permitted to go on for a few years, and had been found to work badly, then its removal would have been founded upon justice and right, and would not have seemed so harsh a proceeding as the hurried immolation of the Board's first bantling.

The framing of a tariff of fees for the entire Province will necessarily always be a matter of difficulty, for what suits the cities will never suit the country districts, and what suits one city will not suit another; and even the rural districts themselves will be found to differ very materially in this respect. When, therefore, the general tariff is done away with, are there any other means which can be taken for the guidance and protection of the medical men? It has been suggested that we might follow the course taken in Ontario. There, each territorial division is represented by a Medical Association, which has the power of framing a tariff for that district, and which then becomes legal and binding. We have no such organization in existence in this Province, and we fear it is a plan which is not likely to come into effective operation in Quebec. The Medico-Chirurgical Society of this city long since framed a tariff for the guidance of its members. and it has no doubt been of much service, but it is not legal. We should be glad to give space to any of our readers who may desire to lay their views on this subject before the profession.

TORONTO UNIVERSITY.—The following are the Examiners in Medicine for the University of Toronto for the year 1882 :—

Medicine—Physiology and Pathology, Geo. Wilkins, M.D., University of Toronto, Montreal; Surgery and Anatomy, Irving H. Cameron, M.B., University of Toronto, Toronto; Medicine and Therapeutics, F. R. Eccles, University of Toronto, London; Midwifery and Medical Jurisprudence, D. B. Fraser, M.B., University of Toronto, Stratford; Clinical Surgery and Medicine, Chas. O'Reilly, M.D., C.M., McGill College, Superintendent General Hospital, Toronto.

This is the first time that a special clinical or practical bedside examination has been required at this University, and we are pleased to see that the choice of the governing body has fallen upon Dr. Chas. O'Reilly, an old student of McGill College, and one whose long service in direct connection with Hospital work renders him specially fitted for undertaking the duties of this important office.

Medical Items.

MEDICAL VACANCIES.—We have been informed that there is a good opening for a medical man at Gaspé Village, where an unopposed practice worth over eight hundred dollars a year is vacant. There is also a good opening at Bolton, E.T.

—Sir James Paget, in an article in the *Nineteenth Century*, thus illustrates the condition of English anti-vivisection law :—"I may pay a rat-catcher to destroy all the rats in my house with any poison he pleases, but I may not myself, unless with a license from the Home Secretary, poison them with snake-poison."

MEDICAL ÆSTHETICS.—The following from the *Medical Record* is being much passed from hand to hand in New York. It purports to be from the opera of "Patience":—

A New York medical man,
A very much advertised man,
A pills-in-variety, talk in society,
Each for himself young man.

A Philadelphia man,
An Index Medicus man,
A think-it-all-gammon, this talk of Buchanan,
Great-medical-centre young man.

A Boston medical man,
A hyper-historical man,
An ultra-persimmon toward medical women,
A Harvard-or-nothing young man.

A Chicago medical man,
A wide-awake, ethical man,
A good-as-the-rest-of-you, more-than-abreast-of-you,
Down-on-the-East young man.

A Toronto medical man,
A money grub, get all you can,
A societies shirker, night and day worker,
Stick-in-the-mud young man.

A Montreal medical man,
In-a-very-great-hurry young man,
A rhubarb-and-jalap, cab-at-a-gallop,
Case-in-the-straw young man.

—A man out West feared he was going to have the small-pox, and believing whiskey to be a preventive, he drank about three quarts of it. A coroner's jury, the next day, rendered a verdict "that he died from excessive prophylaxis."

RESECTION OF THE STOMACH.—After eating some fish, a young man in Geneva, Switzerland, was attacked with acute pains in the stomach. As they did not yield to the usual remedies, the attending physician, Dr. Wagner, inspired by the example of Billroth, promptly opened the abdominal walls, slit up the stomach, and removed some fish bones which were attached to its side! At last accounts the young man was progressing favourably. This incident, gravely given in the *Allgemeine Med. Central Zeitung*, June 4th, if true, is an astounding example of reckless surgery. But perhaps it is intended for what Artemus Ward called " a goak."—*Gaillard's Journal.*

—Dr. T. F. Houston writes:—For fresh cold in the head, accompanied with obstruction in the nasal passages:—

℞	Carbolic acid, - - - - - -	ʒ j
	Absolute alcohol, - - - - -	ʒ ij
	Caustic solution of ammonia, -	ʒ j
	Distilled water, - - - - -	ʒ iij

M. Make a cone of writing paper; put a small piece of cotton in it; drop on the cotton ten drops of the mixture, and inhale until all is evaporated. Repeat this every two hours until relieved.—*So. Med. Record.*

PODOPHYLLOTOXIN—the name given to the chloroform extract of the mandrake root—is claimed to be more reliable in its action than Podophyllin. As a cathartic, it is given to children under 1 year in doses of $\frac{1}{60}$ to $\frac{1}{30}$ gr.; up to 4 years, $\frac{1}{30}$ to $\frac{1}{15}$ gr., and above that age, $\frac{1}{15}$ to $\frac{1}{8}$ gr. It is readily soluble in rectified spirit.

JOHANN HOFF'S MALT EXTRACT—a liquid resembling in appearance British porter—has been sent to us from Germany pretty freely during the last few years. Our esteemed President (Dr. Andrew Fergus) brought it under my notice about twelve months ago, and acquainted me with the fact of its having—in many cases coming under his own observation—proved of service in restoring the energies of individuals suffering from faulty nutrition. Suffering at that time from an attack of illness which had not only reduced my strength, but brought on extreme exhaustion from inability to appropriate food, I tried the effect of Hoff's Malt Extract, in the usual dose of a wineglassful twice or three times a day. Its use was followed by marked effects:—(1) Food which had hitherto been found to pass the alimentary canal unchanged, digested properly. (2) There appeared an increased power of evolving animal heat and storing up fat.—*Dr. J. J. Coleman before the Philosophical Society of Glasgow.*

CANADA

MEDICAL & SURGICAL JOURNAL

APRIL, 1882.

Original Communications.

LEPROSY AND THE LEPER SETTLEMENT, MOLOKAI, SANDWICH ISLANDS.

By H. N. VINEBERG, M.D. (McGill), Portage La Prairie, Man.

On a sea-level plain, comprising about 20,000 acres, on the windward side of Molokai Island, hemmed in on one side by the waters of the Pacific, which, washing over the coral reef, form a foamy white line, and closed in on the other side by a perpendicular precipice 2,500 feet high, is what is known as the "Leper Settlement" of the Hawaiian or Sandwich Islands. Before taking my departure from these tropical isles, I paid a visit to this colony of misery. I left Honolulu on Monday evening in company with Dr. Neilson, the medical superintendent of the settlement, and Mr. Freeth, the superintendent of the Honolulu Water-Works, who was sent by the Board of Health to report upon the expediency of increasing the water supply of the settlement. The small coaster, the "Lebua," on which we took our passage, only touched on the leeward side of the island. This we reached about daybreak, after a night's not very gentle rocking in the cradle of the briny deep, during which we were frequently refreshed by the spray from the waves washing over the bow of the craft. There were a few natives living on the beach where we landed, with whom we breakfasted on "poi and fish," and from whom we hired saddle-horses to take us to the "pali" (precipice) overlooking the settlement, a distance of some ten miles. After riding about six miles, we came to the residence of Mr. R. W. Myers, the general superintendent of the settlement, an intellectual and highly-respected Hollander, but who had resided on the island for upwards of thirty years, and was the father of a large half-white family. We met with kind hospitality at his hands, and were made to partake of a more substantial breakfast than that we had already feasted on. Mr. Myers kindly accompanied us to the "poli," where we had to discard our horses, and make the descent of the perpendicular precipice as best we could, having at times to hang on literally with our "hands and teeth."

The view from the poli was one not easily to be forgotten, and which fully inculcated the meaning of a "living grave!" At our feet lay what appeared from that height (the grass being withered and dry) a sandy, arid plain, without a patch of green or a tree to relieve its barrenness. At either end of the plain were a number of small huts, most of which were white, some of a dark brown; beyond was the creamy surf line and the wild waste of waters of the Pacific, blending in the distant horizon with a wavy bank of fleecy white clouds. Just then not a living object could be seen moving about below, and the feeling of gloominess and depression with which the landscape and its associations impressed one is not to be expressed in words.

After several narrow escapes of going down faster than might be compatible with the process of respiration, we succeeded in reaching the plain beneath. There we were met by three of the colonists on horseback, with the disease in an advanced state, who had come to greet us—having previously heard of our intended visit—and exhibit themselves as objects of curiosity. They seemed well pleased with my close observation of them, but did not conceal their disgust at my friend Mr. Freeth, who lost no time in putting himself at a safe distance on their windward side. One of these had the "leonine expression" well marked. The skin of the face was extremely hypertrophied; the eyebrows were devoid of hair, and every feature of the countenance was uniformly enlarged. Though only about 15 years of age, he had the appearance of an octogenarian, whose irregular and dissipated life had left its marks on the face by knobby and tubercular projections, and deep furrows. He seemed quite happy, and took no small degree of pride in the fact of my taking more interest in him than in his companions. The colony is divided into two settlements, "Kalawao" and "Kalapapa," about two miles apart. At Kalawao are situated the hospital buildings, the doctor's house, the dispensary, a Catholic church, and the residence of the Catholic priest, Father Damiens. The hospitals comprised a dozen or so small wooden buildings, situated on an eminence, quite close to the beach, and were closed in by a fence. When the disease has made such sad havoc that the lepers are unable to attend to their own wants, they are transferred to these, and are there waited upon by their fellow lepers. The sight here was truly pitiful and revolting. Squatted or lying prone on their respective mats were the yet breathing masses of the loathsome disease, whose glistening and vacant stare, where the eye was not an ulcerous mass, had a ghastly and horrifying look. Father Damiens, who accompanied me through the hospital buildings, every now and then would say, "Doctor, you have not yet seen the *worst*. I will keep that for the last." We finally did come to the *worst*, in the form of what was once a Chinaman, but whom the disease had so transformed that all one could recognize was the form of a human being. It is impossible to give a true picture of the spectacle that was squatted before us. Take a human skeleton, with its fingers and toes amputated, put it on the floor in a sitting posture, with the knees well drawn up and the thighs flexed, envelop it loosely with a dark skin, completely covered with sores or scabs, place in each orbit a round, ulcerous body, in the mouth the stump of a tongue, and give to this a weak respiratory act, and you will have some idea of tho "leprous Chinaman." Father Damiens said to me, "John is much better than he was a fortnight ago! We thought then we would lose him by an exhausting diarrhœa, but by allowing him daily a little opium, to which he was accustomed, he has rallied, and is doing very well." The breathing skeleton moved its short stump of tongue, probably to express its gratitude to the father for his kind attention. There were over 40 patients in the hospitals. The total number of lepers in the settlement at the time of my visit was 723, of whom 440 were males and 283 females. Besides these, there were 60 "kokuas," the wives or husbands of lepers in the settlement, but who showed no signs of the disease themselves. Among the former were seven white people, who, different from the natives, fully realized their position, and looked upon death as a blessing and the only relief to their sufferings and misery. The natives appeared quite contented and happy, and as many of them had horses, they amused themselves by racing up and down from one settlement to the other. On our first night, while sitting on Dr. Neilson's verandah, we were serenaded by the band of the colony. The band consisted of a large and small drum, and three "penny whistles," the music of which one could scarcely distinguish from that supplied by so many fifes. They played very well, having belonged to the "Royal band" previous to their banishment. The two drum boys were each minus their four left fingers, and two of the "whistle boys" were wanting two and three fingers respectively of the right hand. On the second night we were serenaded by a band of choristers, but the cracked and husky voices of its diseased members were neither gratifying nor harmonious to the ear. The carpenter of the colony had his left hand entirely fingerless, but the heads of the metacarpal bones were enlarged, so that on bringing together that of the thumb and index finger a small opening was left, into which he would introduce, and so keep in position, the nail he wished to drive. It was highly interesting to note some of the ingenious expedients many of the fingerless unfortunates were driven to, but space will not permit me to give any more instances. The rations of food were ample and of good quality, being supplied by the Board of Health, and served out by Mr. Clayton Straune, the deputy superintendent, himself a leper. Each leper received weekly 21 lbs. *paioi*, the native food (the *arum esculentum* baked and slightly pounded), and from 4 to 6 lbs. of fresh beef. Other necessaries of life the lepers or their friends had to pay for, and could be obtained at cost price at a store in the settlement, kept by the Board of Health. When a fresh batch of exiles come to the settlement, they are cast upon the hospitality of those who have preceded them, until such time as their friends erect a hut for them, the result of which is that all the huts are filled to overcrowding. But this the natives rather like. Their chief complaint had been the want of water, and with a view to remedy that want the Board of Health had sent Mr. Freeth, who, after a thorough examination of the surrounding parts, came to the conclusion that an "artesian well" would be required. What action has been taken upon his report I am unable to say. The lepers from the various islands, after being certified as such by the Government physician of the district, are sent first to Honolulu, and when the number reaches 15 or 20, they are shipped in a schooner, kept for the purpose, to the settlement, Molokai. It occurred to me once to be present at the departure from the Honolulu wharf of the schooner with its living cargo. The lepers were sitting and lying about on the deck, and the wharf was thronged with the friends and relatives of the exiles. When the schooner weighed anchor, and was setting out into the stream, the loud and unearthly wailings of those on shore, and the husky cries and moans of those on board, were heartrending in the extreme. The schooner occasionally meets with adverse winds, and the lepers are exposed to a wet deck for two and sometimes three days before reaching their destination. Such was the experience of the immigrants who landed a day before my visit, one of whom died from the exposure an hour after landing, and another jumped overboard when a day out, and so ended his misery. The embryo Hawaiian Government is severely burdened by the expense of maintaining "the leper settlement," and though the state of affairs is not all one would wish, the government is doing all it reasonably can for the poor unfortunates. If a portion of the immense sums that have been collected from all parts of the civilized world to Christianize the Hawaiian race were devoted to ameliorating the condition of the lepers, more practical good, at least, would be obtained. The natives, as I have already said, appear tolerably contented, but the condition of the white lepers is very sad indeed. One poor fellow in particular was an object of pity and commiseration. He was of American extraction, and had resided in the settlement for six years. The disease had rendered him helpless, but he had no other attendance than that which a neighbor leper favored him with at times, and the frequent kind services of Father Damiens. His abode consisted of a small, low, dingy room, the only furniture of which was a roughly-constructed bed, on which the dirt-blackened clothes lay all in a heap, a rough deal table, a box, and a wooden chair. The sun's rays were pouring unmercifully through the uncurtained and dirt-begrimed window, and the heat of the room could only be compared to that of a heated furnace. A week or two before he had an attack of dysentery, and he told me he surely would have died from want of proper nourishment were it not for the Catholic priest, who used to bring him every day delicacies prepared by his own hand. He wanted to know if I was an American, and he thought, if I would only state his case to the United States authorities, they would see to his comfort for the short period he was destined to exist in this world. I informed him of my nationality and inability to move the U.S. Government on his behalf, but promised to make his case public at the first opportunity that presented itself.

Here let me say a few words about Father Damiens, the Catholic priest, whose name so frequently figures in this paper. When one sees a missionary at the head of a wealthy sugar plantation, and surrounded by all the luxuries of civilization, he may be pardoned if he has some suspicion as to the sacrifice and martyrdom of missionaries in general. But here was a case where the most worldly and cynical could cast no slurs. With youth, health, culture, refinement, and every prospect of advancement in the church, this man voluntarily exiled himself to this abode of misery eight years ago. During my stay of two days in the settlement I had good opportunities of making ob servations, and I noted that for every one, indiscriminately, he had a kind smile and a word of sympathy, and all—Catholics, Protestants and heathens—looked upon him as upon a common father. Miss Bird, herself a Protestant, in her book entitled "Seven Months among the Sandwich Islands," writes thus of him: "It was singular to hear the burst of spontaneous admiration which his act elicited. No unworthy motives were suggested, all envious speech was hushed; it was almost forgotten by the most rigid Protestants that Father Damiens, who has literally followed the example of Christ by 'laying down his life for the brethren,' is a Romish priest, and an intuition higher than all reasoning hastened to number him with 'the noble army of martyrs.'" When one takes into consideration that at the time of going to the settlement he had strong opinions upon the contagiousness of leprosy—which he still held,—one can readily conceive with what feelings he entered upon his duties.

The question of leprosy is growing to be a very serious one in the Sandwich Islands, and considering their proximity to the States and the inter-travel between the two places, it is one also which should engage the attention of this continent. The disease is spreading rapidly on the Islands, and the number in the settlement does not represent one-third of the lepers that are free and mixing with their fellow-beings, both colored and white. His Excellency, H. A. P. Carter, the Minister of the Interior, made praiseworthy efforts during last summer to weed out all the lepers that were free, and have them sent to the settlement for isolation, but in this he was thwarted by the natives themselves, and in a less degree by the head of the Government. For some inexplicable reason, a native would sooner undergo any other form of banishment than that to the island of Molekai. Instances are known where they have lain crowded in caves for years rather than allow themselves to be taken by the authorities and forwarded to the settlement. Some have become so desperate as to shoot at the official who tried to effect a capture. During my term of a year as government physician in the large district of Kuco, on the Island of Hawaii, only two lepers were brought to me by the deputy sheriff for examination and certificate. We knew of many more in the district, but they were never to be seen when the sheriff or his police were in the neighborhood.

It was in 1865 that the Hawaiian Legislature first passed an Act to prevent the spread of leprosy, and in the year following the "leper settlement" was established. I found it impossible to obtain from the authorities any figures on the subject, and those following were obtained from outside sources. Between 1866 and 1874, 1,145 were sent to the settlement, of which number 442 died during that period. At one time in 1875 there were 703. Through the kindness of Dr. Emerson, the former resident physician, I am enabled to give full figures for the year 1879:—

Number of adult males in the settlement January 1st, 1879..........	469
" " females " " " "	302
" children under 10 years—Males	14
Females	15
" births during the year	6
" lepers arriving during the year—Males...............	66
Females	31
" kokuas proclaimed lepers during the year—Males	8
Females	8
" deaths during the year—Males.......................	124
Females	79

The origin of the disease on the Islands is enveloped in considerable obscurity, but from all available accounts, traditional and written, it appears that the first case or cases were observed somewhere about 1840 and 1842. It is known by the natives as "mai alii" or "mai paki." "Mai alii" signifies *chief's disease*, and it received this cognomen from the tradition that the first case was recognized (1842) in a chief named "Maca," the uncle of the present Queen Dowager Emma. "Mai paki" means *Chinese disease*, and this epithet receives two explanations. One is (the most likely one) that the disease was first recognized by a Chinaman, who had seen similar cases in his own country; the other, that the Chinese imported the disease. I may say that the former explanation is that given by foreigners and intelligent natives and half-castes, while the latter is held only by the ordinary natives. An odd case, after the above, was observed here and there until 1857, when an epidemic of small-pox instituted throughout the Islands indiscriminate vaccination. The act was performed by any and everyone, and lymph was taken from arm to arm. Within a few years after this it was discovered that cases of leprosy were cropping up pretty thickly all over the Islands, and the disease has been gradually and steadily adding to the number of its victims ever since. There can be no doubt, I think, as to its propagation by vaccination. Most authorities on the subject admit that as one of the modes, and several cases on the Islands have been directly traced to that source. The older medical men on the Islands, who have had considerable experience with the disease, are very decided and unanimous upon this point. Cohabitation with a leper is also known to be a fruitful source of infection, and it would appear that when the disease is contracted in this way, syphilis forms an inexplicable factor, being, in the majority of cases, a precursor of the genuine malady. So much is this the case, that some of the older physicians of Honolulu regard leprosy as simply an advanced state of syphilis. Dr. McKibbin, surgeon to the Honolulu Hospital, and an active practitioner for over 20 years on the Islands, told me that he had seen, time and again, pure, unmistakable cases of syphilis followed by leprosy. Under an anti-syphilitic course the symptoms of the former would disappear, while those of leprcsy would only be confirmed. In the majority of his cases the symptoms of leprosy would only show themselves after the disappearance of the syphilitic symptoms, but in some they would go hand in hand, and modify one another to a more or less extent. The native custom of herding together, and eating with their fingers out of a common calabash, and smoking the same pipes, are other modes of spreading the disease. But, admitting this, it is difficult to explain the immunity from the disease many of the "kokuas" experience. I have already said that the term "kokuas" applies to the non-lepers in the settlement, who have followed to the place of banishment their wives or husbands, as the case may be, rather than break the conjugal tie. But it would be wrong to infer from this that the tie is very strong among the natives. At the time of my visit there were sixty kokuas, some of whom had resided in the settlement since it was instituted, but who showed no signs, subjective or objective, of the disease. I will give notes of a few of these cases.

No. 1.—Kuloa, aged 55, female; in 1854, married a leper, with whom she lived five years, and had four children. Has lived in settlement since 1866 with her present husband, and with whom she bas had also four children. All her children died before attaining the age of 12 months. Had syphilis two years after first marriage. Shows no signs whatever of leprosy, and is apparently in perfect health.

No. 2.—Kulchua, aged about 40, laundress for the hospitals for the past seven years. Lived as wife to a leper for 13 years. Has had four children, two of whom died at the respective ages of 2 months and 3 years. The second child is a leper, and is 15 years of age; the fourth is 12 years, and is quite healthy. Shows no traces of leprosy, and is robust and hearty.

No. 3.—Pukoku, aged 45, male; lived with a leprous woman for 12 years, and has resided in settlement 8 years. Has no suspicious symptoms of leprosy, and apparently is in the best of health.

But, on the other hand, it must be borne in mind that they do not all enjoy this immunity. A glance at the above figures for 1879 will show that in that year 16 were pronounced lepers by the resident physician. Several cases of cure of the disease are reported on the Islands, but as at that period the symptoms are very obscure, and often are not to be distinguished from those of syphilis and other skin diseases, much room is left for doubt. I saw several cases in the Honolulu Hospital of a doubtful nature, but who were undergoing the treatment of leprosy. Many of these, I thought, might safely have been put into the category of tubercular lupus of the face. I saw a couple of cases in whom the ulnar nerve had been stretched by Dr. McKibbin for contraction of the little finger and the adjacent one (an early symptom of leprosy), with marked benefit for the time at least. That was as much as the doctor expected. The treatment of the cases in the hospital was of an alterative nature, combined with local applications, chiefly caustics, to the patches of eruption, and the use of electricity in cases of defective enervation.

I am keenly alive to the deficiencies of this paper, but if it move a few charitably-inclined people to take an interest in the poor unfortunate victims on the Sandwich Islands, and awaken the profession to the danger of the disease invading this continent, it will have served its purpose.

VALEDICTORY ADDRESS

Delivered to the Graduating Class, 31st March, 1882,

By D. C. MacCALLUM, M.D., M.R.C.S., Eng.
Professor of Midwifery and Diseases of Women and Children, McGill University.

Gentlemen, Graduates in Medicine,—There occur periods in the lives of most men, when, having reached a certain point in their career, having accomplished a definite purpose, it is wise and salutary to take a retrospective glance over the work done and the causes which have led to ultimate success; and, further, to consider seriously the impending future with all its urgent demands, its grave responsibilities, and its varied possibilities. To each one of you this day is such a period. When you look back to the commencement of the four years or more which you have devoted to the study of medicine, you will readily recall the feeling almost of dismay with which you regarded the extensive curriculum of study presented to you. For medicine, in common with other sciences, has made wonderful progress in late years, and the difficulties of acquiring a thorough knowledge of it are rapidly increasing, Indeed it has become a serious question with thoughtful and observant members of the profession, more particularly with those engaged in teaching, whether the demands made on the student are not too onerous for the limited time allotted to him to fulfil them. It would really appear either that there should be a more restricted curriculum than the present one, or a longer time insisted on to master the subjects included in it. That you should, in the short space of four years, have fulfilled the demands made on you, and have acquired such an amount of professional knowledge as to have enabled you to pass successfully the rigid examinations to which you have been subjected, is in the highest degree creditable to you, and is an earnest that you are not wanting in those qualities which go far to ensure success in life. Your experience during these years will have impressed upon you the important truth that success is not due to a happy combination of fortuitous circumstances, but that it is the result of determined, persevering effort. Genius not infrequently attains its ends with apparently slight effort, but, as a general rule, that inborn aptitude to master certain departments of knowledge which is called *genius*, if not associated with a willingness to work, rarely accomplishes much. A man of average brain power, who pursues his object with singleness of purpose and with unflagging industry, will do more in the way of acquiring knowledge, and of adding to the sum of that already existing, than one more highly gifted by nature, but who is lacking in energy and perseverance. It is not the mere possession of talent that enables a man to secure a prominent position amongst his fellows. If he attain a front rank, it will be due mainly to his capacity for work. And the work, too, must be regulated, continuous, and directed towards a definite end. For labor is too often wasted when it is expended on a diversity of objects having no relation to each other, and not one of which is made the great aim of the worker's life. Another truth which you will have learned is, that mental labor is not altogether a task, but that in the pursuit of knowledge there is a pleasure which amply repays all the labor bestowed upon it. Although at times irksome, and attended by frequent discouragements, it affords the highest gratification to the noblest part of man's nature. In the cultivation of his intellect, in the storing of his mind with important truths, and in the effort to perfect himself in some honorable calling in life, man finds some of his highest and purest enjoyments. Apart from any consideration of the material advantages which may attach to a thorough professional education, or the fame and honor which may be the outcome of successful scientific investigation, there is in the acquirement of the one or the prosecution of the other that which eminently satisfies the thirst for knowledge, which is a leading characteristic of the mind of man. But with the satisfaction derived from present success, there is always associated a feeling that comparatively little has been accomplished, and this becomes a powerful incentive to further effort. And yet, as the eve approaches of a life honestly and devotedly spent in the cultivation of science, the most enthusiastic votary feels like Sir Isaac Newton, as if he had gathered a few of the pebbles only from the shores of the knowable, while the vast ocean itself stretches out before him unexplored. "I live joyless in my eighty-ninth year," writes the great Humboldt to his friend Varnhagen, "because of the much for which I have striven from my youth so little has been accomplished." So it is, and so it always will be. Despite his loftiest attainments, man always feels an intellectual want that must be satisfied, an intellectual void that must be filled. And, what is most singular, the more varied and profound his knowledge—the deeper he may have penetrated the arcana of Nature—the richer and more glorious the truths he may have brought thence, the more weak and ignorant does he appear to his own scrutinizing introspection. The general public, conscious of the vast distance that intervenes between their own acquirements and his, speak wonderingly of his great intellect and accumulated stores of learning. Whilst he, the scholar and wise man, according to the testimony of all, in view of the higher and still higher heights of truth remaining to be scaled, and whose outlines are appreciable to his exalted sense alone,—in view of the ever-widening and ever-lengthening vista that opens up before him as he pursues his travels into regions of thought and territories of investigation never before penetrated,—bewails his own littleness, his want of energy and mental vigor: for knowledge, as a rule, certainly has the effect of making its most favored votaries the humblest and least self-conceited of men. He regards the three-score years and ten allotted to man in this state of existence a mere fleeting point of time—all too short a period in which to grasp even a tithe of what presents itself for investigation,—and he therefore looks hopefully forward to an infinite future, where his soul may bathe without check or limit in the pure untroubled waters of truth.

That knowledge sometimes "puffeth up" its possessor is as true now as in the days of Saul of Tarsus, and probably more generally true now than at that time. If the *dictum* of that great and gifted mind were more generally known and received at the present day, and the conduct of men influenced by it, there would be fewer exhibitions of those pretentious and obtrusive claims of individuals to be regarded as burning and shining lights of science,—the ranks of scientists, as they call themselves, would be greatly thinned, and, I fear, that a goodly sized volume containing sketches more or less brief of the learned and distinguished men of this Dominion would shrink to one of very modest proportions. The *dictum* of St. Paul is: "If any man think that he knoweth anything, he knoweth nothing yet as he ought to know." Lay this, then, to heart; and whilst it need not prevent you from indulging a feeling of proper pride in accomplished work and its favorable reception by your fellows, it will save you from overweening vanity and a constant and restless craving for notoriety.

Your success in obtaining the degree of Doctor in Medicine and Master of Surgery of this University we may consider then as being due mainly to three causes,—*Capacity for work*, *Love of work*, *and Will to work;* the last being by far the most important. The professors in this Faculty, while rejoicing sincerely in your well-merited success, take no other credit in the result than simply that of having endeavored, as far as in them lay, to give proper direction to your studies and to strengthen and develop in you these all potent powers. And you have, therefore, the proud satisfaction of knowing that the honorable position in which you stand before your friends to-day is one which, in an important sense, you may be said to have attained *for* yourselves—*by* yourselves. Provided with the diploma which has just been placed in your hands, and with the power to claim all the privileges which it confers, you have now, especially, to enter into the struggles and contentions of life, and prove what there is of mettle in you. We would not that any one of you should prove a failure, and were it in our power to make you able and respected practitioners of medicine, good and upright men, loyal and patriotic citizens, willingly would we exert that power in your favor. But in this, also, we can only advise: we can only erect for your guidance a few finger-posts pointing the way of duty and responsibility. The power of making or of marring your own fortunes lies entirely with yourselves.

The great object of your life henceforth must be the prevention, alleviation, and cure of disease. And when you reflect that this involves the comfort and happiness of your fellowmen and the saving of human life,—preserving the bread-winner to those dependent upon him, the mother to the love and devotion of husband and children, the children to the yearning affection of parents,—you cannot but be strongly, even painfully, impressed with the magnitude of the responsibilities which will devolve upon you. Seek not in any way to weaken this impression, but let it have its full influence as an incentive to unremitting attention to duty. The way of duty in the profession of medicine is not always smooth and pleasant, but frequently rugged and wearisome. It can only be successfully followed by the exercise of patience, self-denial, energy and perseverance—qualities which you should carefully cultivate, for he only who possesses them is fitted to surmount difficulties or to shape events so as to favor the end he may have in view. At one time, cheered by success and the heartfelt gratitude of those whom you may have been the means of raising from a bed of suffering and disease, you will experience that sense of satisfaction, often amounting to exultation, which is felt by those who have accomplished a great and beneficent work, and you will rightly conclude that the ways of medicine are *sometimes* the ways of pleasantness. At another time, depressed and dispirited by failure in your efforts to save life, or by unmerited slight and the withdrawal of confidence by those who ought to consider themselves under obligations to you, you will again rightly conclude that the ways of medicine are *not always* the ways of pleasantness. But whatever your triumphs or your reverses, you must be equal to the former and rise superior to the latter. Undue elation and undue depression are equally proofs of weakness. The strong, self-reliant man, conscious of the integrity of his motives and his actions, courageously accepts whatever verdict may be passed upon them, and finds in the approval of his own conscience that which will sustain him under the most trying circumstances. So long as he feels confident that the end he has in view is laudable and good, he steadily pursues his course, feeling certain that the right thought and the right deed must ultimately prevail. The weak, shrinking man, on the other hand, has too often scant faith in his own judgment and convictions. Haunted by a constant dread of the adverse opinions of his fellows, he pursues a vacillating, hesitating course, and as the world smiles or frowns, so is he supremely happy or miserably wretched. But while *self-reliance* is always to be commended, as much cannot be said of *self-confidence*. The most disastrous events occurring in daily life are commonly the result of some serious blunder committed by a capable but too confident man. A serious blunder in the practice of medicine would be something akin to a crime. No matter then how thorough you may consider your knowledge, always act with an ever present conviction that it is quite possible to make a mistake. A certain amount of skepticism as to your own infallibility will prove one of the best safeguards against careless or precipitate action.

Although you are fully fitted by the course of studies which you have just completed to enter upon your life-work and assume its responsibilities, if you desire to excel you must exhibit the same capacity for, the same love of, and the same will to work that have so far crowned your efforts with success. The marked impetus which has of late years been given to experimental inquiry in all departments of medicine still continues. The restless, questioning spirit of the age has seized the master minds of the profession, and, as a consequence, great and important additions are constantly being made to our knowledge of the pathology, symptoms and treatment of disease. So numerous and active are the workers and so wide-spread their investigations, that you will find it no easy matter, even while using due diligence, to keep yourselves abreast with the results of their labors. This will be especially the case when your practice has become so extensive as to demand most of your time and attention. It is, therefore, of the highest importance, while you have the leisure, that you should lay broader and deeper the foundations of your knowledge by a careful study of the works of the classical authors in medicine, and build up and complete the superstructure as much as possible by additions from the works of the men of to-day. It is not to be expected, however, that professional studies should occupy your time to the exclusion of all efforts to increase and advance your culture in other ways. Medicine must certainly have the first place, and dominate over all other aims or objects, but at least a certain portion of your time must be employed in improving your mind in other directions. What you have to guard against is, that no other pursuit shall engage your attention to the neglect of professional studies. For, as Milton has well expressed it:—

> "Not to know at large of things remote
> From use, obscure and subtle, but to know
> That which before us lies in daily life,
> Is the prime wisdom! what is more, is fume
> Or emptiness, or fond impertinence,
> And renders us in things that most concern
> Unpractised, unprepared, and still to learn."

In all the relations of life be upright, honest and true. Never deviate from the line of rectitude and honor. To your patients be ever the earnest, attentive physician, willing to submit to any inconvenience, and to sacrifice time and leisure if the necessities of their case demand it. Act singly for their good and without the least consideration for self. Patients will not be slow in recognizing this, and they will give you credit for earnestness of purpose and feel grateful to you for your attentions. Their confidence in you will be strengthened, and when death invades and snatches away some loved member from their family circle, they will feel satisfied that all that devotion and skill could possibly do has been done to save the precious life.

To fellow-members of the profession be always considerate and generous—prompt to defend their professional reputation when thoughtlessly or maliciously assailed. Any attempt to improve your own position by detraction of a *confrère* would not only be unmanly and unprofessional, but would probably and justly fail. Always take a deep interest in the welfare of your country. Cultivate in yourselves and take every favorable opportunity to kindle in others a spirit of patriotism. Canada is a country of which her sons may well be proud. A not unimportant part of the greatest and most liberal empire the world has ever seen, with self-government secured to her, and with no old world class distinctions among her people, she is at present the freest, the happiest and the most secure place on the surface of the globe in which to dwell. Grateful, indeed, ought every Canadian to be for all that Britain, the grand old mother country, has done for this Dominion, and steadfastly should they resist any attempt to weaken the bonds which now unite the two. In no part of the empire does there exist a deeper feeling of loyalty and devotion to our Empress Queen than in this Dominion of Canada. When the tidings reached us of the late attempt upon her life, we, her loyal subjects in Canada, could scarcely realize its possibility. That there could exist a brain to conceive and a hand to carry out a murderous design against one whom the civilized world acknowledges to be peerless as a sovereign, peerless as a mother, and peerless as a woman, was beyond our comprehension, and it was with a feeling of relief that we learned that the brain and hand were those of one who cannot be held accountable for his actions. Thankful, fervently and profoundly thankful, are we for Her Majesty's providential escape, and that a national calamity has been thus averted. We hold her in reverence as the supreme head of the state, we honor her as the wise and constitutional ruler, but we love her for those qualities of heart which have made her, in good old expressive Saxon, the *sweet-heart* of her people. God save the Queen.

In conclusion, gentlemen, with a full and abiding sense of the responsibilities which now devolve upou you—with a firm determination to do your duty faithfully and honorably and to merit the affection and esteem of your fellow-men—with a high resolve to conquer a prominent position, or at least not to prove laggards in your profession—with feelings of charity and kind commisseration for the lowly and distressed, and with hearts overflowing with tender sympathy for all who suffer sorrow, pain or disease—go forth from this hall, and enter hopefully and cheerfully upon the work of your life, and may the blessing of Heaven rest upon your labors. Fare-ye-well.

THE INDUCED CURRENT FOR THERAPEUTIC PURPOSES.

BY L. E. FELTON, M.D., POTSDAM, N.Y.

(Read before the Medico-Chirurgical Society of Montreal.)

MR. PRESIDENT AND GENTLEMEN,—It is not my purpose this evening to discuss the merits of electricity as a therapeutic agent, but to give you the results of some of my experiments and investigations as to the best methods of inducing a current for therapeutic purposes. In the published works on Medical Electricity, the physics of the induced current is almost required, much of the little that is published being unscientific and inapplicable to medical induction apparatus. The reason of this is, because the writers began their investigations with electro-therapeutics instead of electro-physics. It is only by a thorough knowledge of the laws of electricity that one can hope to be successful in electro-therapeutics, and the time is fast approaching when only investigations based upon laws will be considered reliable.

Electricity is a force correlative with heat, light and motion, and its laws are as firmly established and as well understood as those of light, heat and motion. When in dynamic form or current, a complete conducting circuit must be formed. In the galvanic cell the force is generated at the surface of the zinc plate. The direction in which this force is exerted is from zinc to carbon within the cell, and from carbon to zinc outside the cell. At the zinc plate it is called E. M. F., throughout the circuit tension, sometimes called intensity or potential. Tension overcomes the R. of the circuit; it is the direct result of E.M.F., and with a large R. is directly proportional to it.

The form of machine best suited for generating the induced current for medicine is an induction coil, which consists of a coil, a current regulator, a current interrupter, and a galvanic cell. A coil should be made up of a bundle of soft iron wires, surrounded by one or more coils of insulated copper wire. If one end of this wire be connected with the positive and the other with the negative pole of a cell, a part of the electricity which flows through the coil will be stored up in the core as magnetism;

if either end of the wire be disconnected from the cell, the magnetism will be instantly transformed again into a current of electricity in the surrounding coil, if it form a circuit. This current is of but momentary duration, but has the power of overcoming many hundred times the R. that the cell which generates it has, depending upon the E. M. F. The laws which I have already given with regard to cells are equally applicable to coils. Electro-motive force is located at the point or points where energy takes the form of electricity. In the induction coil, in the convolutions forming the coil, each convolution having its own E. M. F., so that the E. M. F. of a coil is in direct ratio with the number of turns of wire without regard to its size. The E. M. F. of the coil varies as the number of turns of wire, the E. M. F. of each turn varies as the amount of energy from which it is derived, and that is the energy stored up in the core as magnetism. The amount of magnetism induced in the core depends upon the quantity of current flowing through the primary or battery wire, and upon the number of turns of this wire. The battery current depends upon the E. M. F. of the cell, its internal resistance, and the resistance of the primary wire. Thus we are enabled, by combining a coil with a single cell, to develop a tension that would otherwise require a large number of cells. It is held by many electrologists of authority that a different quality of current and different therapeutic results are produced by different sized wires. Based upon this theory, coils are sometimes made up of half a dozen different sizes, each size supposed to produce its special therapeutic effect and applicable to special cases. A coil that has an E. M. F. sufficient to produce a tension that will overcome the resistance of the body and furnish a sufficient quantity of current for therapeutic purposes will do all that a dozen wires can do. With the galvanic current, the same quantity passing through a circuit in a given time will produce the same effects without regard to the kind of battery used. So with the electro-magnetic battery, the same quantity of current at each interruption and the same number of interruptions per second will produce the same effect without regard to size of wire or kind of machine. Now a coil can readily be made of two wires, or even one, that will furnish a sufficient electro-motive force to give the desired quantity for therapeutic purposes, and with a proper regulator any desired quantity can be obtained. Where several sizes of wire are used, it makes a complicated affair for the physician, requires a larger number of connections to get out of order, and makes it more mysterious for the inexperienced.

The foregoing view is based upon an incorrect application of theory, and is opposed to Ohm's law. The only difference being a difference in the R. of the wire. With an external resistance *nil*, 100 turns of coarse wire would give a quantity only as much greater than 100 turns of fine wire, as the difference in the R. of the two wires; but with a great R. like the body, this difference cannot be considered. Writers tell you that coarse wire like large cells, gives a greater quantity of E., and that fine wire, like small cells, gives a greater intensity; that the one is applicable to one class of affections, and the other to another class. The mistake is due to a consideration of cells and coils with a small R. and applying the results to a large R. Intensity, as I have already told you, with a large R. is directly as the E. M. F. Q. is directly as the E. M. F., hence it must be directly as the intensity or tension, so that when we increase tension we necessarily increase quantity. The reason why coarse wire produces a milder effect is not because it has greater quantity and less tension, but because there being a less number of turns, the E. M. F. is less, the tension less, and the quantity less; the same number of turns of fine wire would produce precisely the same result.

In constructing a battery for any special purpose, it is necessary to know the resistance of the circuit and quantity required. The R. of the body varies so greatly that a battery for general therapeutic purposes must be made to furnish an E. M. F. that will overcome the greatest possible R., and then be supplied with suitable appliance to vary the E. M. F. and the R., and for the Q.

It is of the utmost importance that the strength of the current can be accurately regulated by the operator. Nearly all of the current regulators are based upon the following law: Where there are two or more circuits surrounding a magnetized core, a current will be induced in each inversely as the resistance. If a copper tube surrounds the core, and a great resistance (like a part of the body) be included in the circuit of one of these coils, the current would nearly all be induced in the copper tube. If this tube be arranged so that it will side on the core and a portion of the core be uncovered, a current will be induced in the coil surrounding that part of the core that has been uncovered by the tube. The tubes are generally placed between the core and the primary or battery coil, or between the primary and secondary coils. The last is objectionable, because the primary wire should be wound as close to the core as possible so as to magnetize the core as highly as possible. A compact coil cannot be made with a tube sliding within it. I overcome these objections by sliding a copper tube over the whole coil. The current is regulated to a nicety. The tube should not be made of brass, as the resistance is too great. The method of sliding the secondary coil over the primary is objectionable on account of the connections becoming broken while the coil is being moved, the result being to give the full force of the current induced in the primary wire, which, when applied to nervous patients, particularly if upon the head, is very pernicious. I would call your attention to batteries that have ornamental ferrules of brass or copper on each end of the coil; in some instances half of the coil being covered. The current is induced in these ornaments instead of in the wire, and the strength very much lessened.

To what are the therapeutic effects of electricity due? To polarization and molecular change, or to simple shock? That they are due to the former: that the current produces molecular change in the tissues that stimulates action there can be hardly a doubt. An evidence of this is that the constant current, from which there are no shocks, produces the same effects in even a more marked degree than the induced current. From the experiments of Prof. Blaserna, he has determined that the duration of the induced current at each interruption is about 1-1000 of a second. The chemical effects of a current of this duration must be very minute, but would be in a given length of time just in proportion to the number of interruptions in that time; that is, 1000 interruptions per second would produce 1000 times the chemical results that one would. Now if the therapeutie effects are due rather to the chemical effects of the current than to the simple shock, as I am led to believe by the results of the galvanic current as compared with the induced and the induced current with rapid vibrations compared with slow, we have reason to believe that the more rapid the interruptions the better the therapeutic results. The interrupters on nearly all of the induction coils are too clumsy to be called vibrators, but should rather be called oscillators. The springs are large and long, supporting on the free end a heavy iron armature and a large metal disk for the platinum. Such an interruptor can neither make rapid nor regular interruptions. A vibrator to make rapid interruptions must be constructed in accordance with the laws of vibration. These laws will be found fully discussed in works on acoustics. The vibrator must be made upon precisely the same plan as the organ reed which gives the highest pitch, as pitch depends entirely upon the number of vibrations in a given time. Temper, length and thickness, as well as uniformity, are important factors. It is highly important that no extra weight be put upon the free end, such as a heavy armature; the armature should be no thicker than the vibrator itself. The size of the vibrator depends upon the motive power that produces the vibrations, viz., the magnetism. From a long series of experiments I find that copper, zinc and silver, or copper and zinc, melted together, gives the best temper for rapid vibration. The tempering must be done by means of rolls, and it requires considerable skill to get the proper temper. I make the vibrator 1 inch long and about $\frac{1}{8}$ inch wide. On the free end I solder a piece of what is known as artists' tin-type, about 1-1000 inch thick, in such a manner that it makes an extension of the vibrator instead of thickening it; this is only about $\frac{1}{8}$ in. square, and forms the soft armature. A piece of platinum foil, about same size, is soldered on surface of vibrator, near middle, for contact with adjusting screw. The vibrations from this interruptor are very rapid, as shown by the pitch and quality of current. I am conducting a series of experiments to determine the number of vibrations that can be produced per second, the result of which will be given at some future time.

The idea advanced by many writers that slow interruptions of the induced current give better therapeutic results than rapid is wholly without foundation, and is not applicable to any case, except it be one in which you wish to produce as much pain as possible. It is, however, an acknowledged fact that slow interruptions of the galvanic current produce constrictions of paralyzed muscles when the induced fails. The reason for this seems to me very clear. Supposing the interruptions to be 1 a second with the induced current, we would have at each interruption a current lasting about 1-1000 of a second, and in another second another current of like duration. But with the galvanic battery, when the circuit is closed, the current passes until it is open again, and if of the same E. M. F. and R., we have several hundred times the quantity passing at each interruption as with the induced, and so long as electricity is just the same as long as it flows in the one case as in the other, it is safe to assume that the difference in therapeutic results is due to the difference in the quantity that flows at each interruption. Then it is reasonable to suppose that with a vibrator that will produce a large number of interruptions per second we should obtain results nearer like those of the galvanic current; this I have found to be the case, as I have repeatedly demonstrated in my experiments. In doing this, I make my slow interruptions in the induced circuit by removing the electrode, or using an interrupting handle.

The object of slow interruptions is to give the muscles time to contract and relax. With rapid interruptions there would be tonic contraction of the muscle. A shock sufficiently strong to produce a contraction is very painful, while a rapid succession of shocks will contract a muscle with little or no pain. The intervals of contraction and relaxation are far better made by the operator removing and applying the electrode, than by any automatic arrangement.

The plan of a vibrator is shown in Fig. 1; *e* is vibrator, having a soft iron armature *h* and platinum connection *f*; soldered to it *a* is adjusting screw having platinum point *g* for contact with *f*. When contact is made between adjusting screw and vibrator a current of electricity will "flow" from carbon through adjusting screw, which is connected with it and vibrator, to inner end of coil which is soldered to *d*, and through coil *k* to zinc. This current magnetizes the bundle of wires *l* and soft iron bar *i*; *i* attracts armature *h*, drawing vibrator away from adjusting screw, thus breaking the circuit and demagnetizing the wires and rod, which releases the vibrator, the elasticity of which causes it to fly back in contact with adjusting screw, thus breaking the circuit and demagnetizing the wires and rod, which releases the vibrator, the elasticity of which causes it to fly back in contact with adjusting screw, completing the circuit again. At each interruption we have a current induced, lasting according to the researches of Prof. Blaserna, about 1-1000 sec.

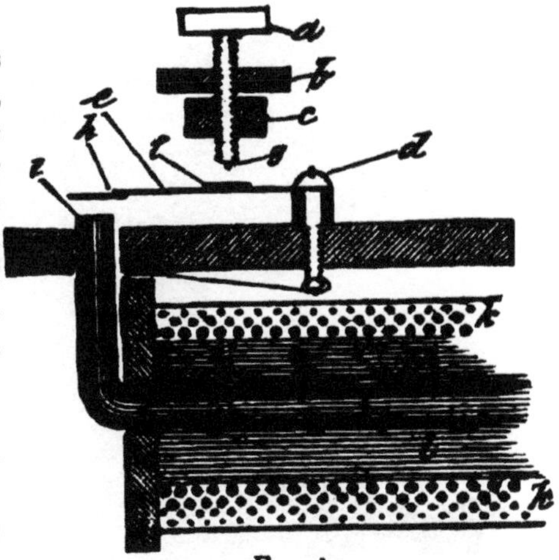

FIG. 1.

The next important part for consideration is the battery cell. The cell which gives the greatest E. M. F. is the Bichromate; the elements are Zinc and Carbon, and the Battery Fluid is a solution of Bichromate Potash and Sulpuric Acid.

The E. M. F. of this cell is a trifle over two Volts., and the internal resistance very much less than any other cell, being less than half an OHM. Hence it is best fitted for a Portable Battery, as a small cell may be used without materially increasing the resistance. There are, however, some decided disadvantages in the form usually employed—the Grenet. The Carbon plates are attached to a brass connection within the cell; the fluid very soon finds its way between them and oxydizes the brass, and breaks the circuit, and the current ceases. The same trouble occurs where the rod is screwed into the Zinc Plate, and also at the joint in the rod. Another disadvantage, the Zinc Plate is carried in the cell and is subject to the action of the fluid when carried. The plate being seldom cleaned and amalgamated, becomes coated with chrome alum, and produces an unsteady current.

I have devised a cell which overcomes all of these objections. The cell or jar *a* [*Fig.* 2] is hard rubber, all sides permanently closed when vulcanized. The negative element is a rod of carbon ⅜ in. in diameter, into one end of which is soldered a short piece of metal *e* for better con-

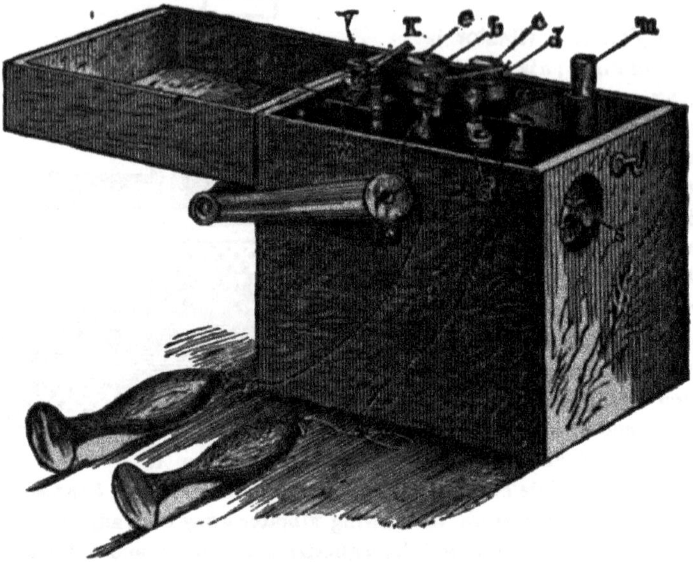

FIG. 2.

tact. Upon this end is fitted a hard rubber ferrule *b* secured by rubber cement so perfectly that no fluid can find its way through. The end of the ferrule is closed by a hard rubber disk, having a hole for *e*, secured in same manner. Upon lower end of ferrule is a screw fitted to a hole in one end of cell *a* and screwed in with cement. The carbon reaches nearly to bottom of cell, while end with ferrule projects outside, as shown in [*Fig.* 2.] A hard rubber neck is screwed into another hole in top and closed with stopper *c*. The connections are thus made outside of cell, so that there is no possibility of connection corroding or cell leaking whether upright or not. The cell is carried full of fluid; when used the stopper is removed, the zinc introduced and connections made with it. The zinc can be kept clean and amalgamated without trouble, and is not wearing except when in use.

I have adapted this cell to the galvanic battery. (*Fig.* 3.)

The cells B are of hard rubber, closed on all sides by vulcanising. The negative element is a rod of carbon ¾ inch in diameter, having a piece of metal *b* soldered into one end for connection. This end is filled with paraffine and fitted to a hard rubber ferule *c*, which is secured by cement and screwed into top of cell. By this means connection with carbon is made outside the cell and is protected from corrosion by fluid. A tube of hard rubber *e* is screwed into top of cell, into which the zinc elements are drawn when the battery is not in use, and through which the cells are filled and emptied. The ends of the tubes pass into holes in a platform of hard rubber *C*, shown in section 3 of engraving. These holes are covered by strips of rubber *h*.

The positive elements are rods of rolled zinc *f* supported by metal rods *g*,

(CASE REMOVED IN ENGRAVING.)

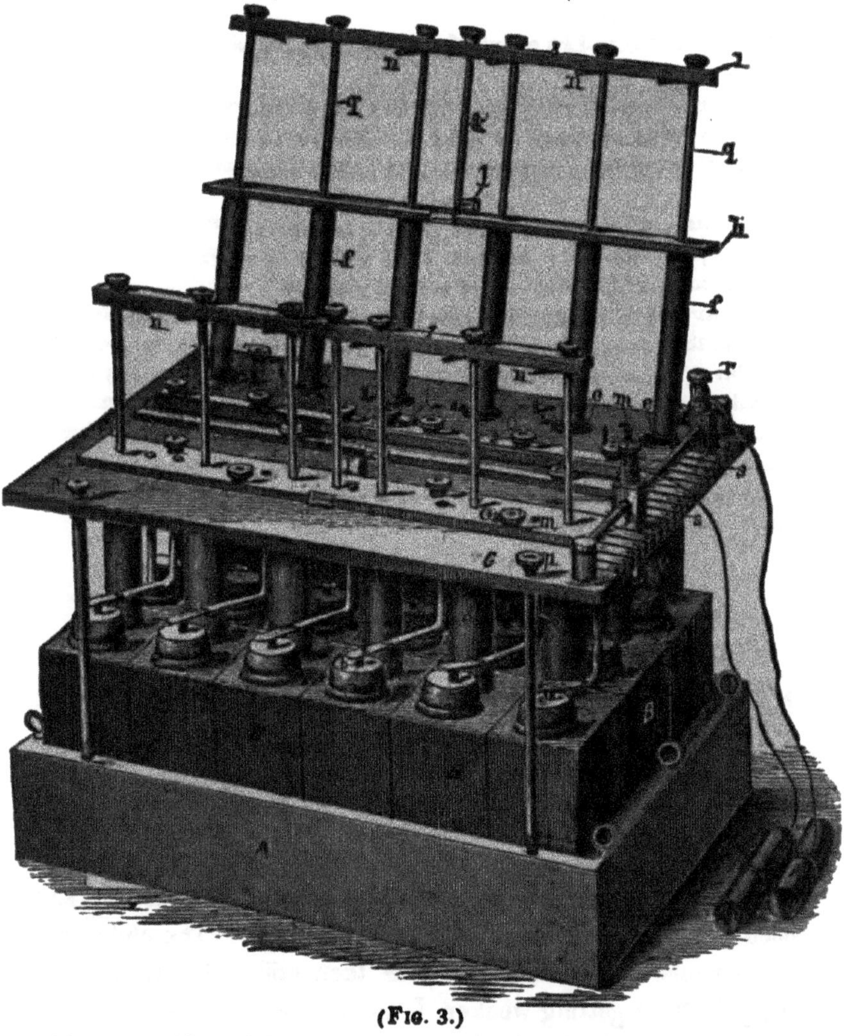

(FIG. 3.)

which are fixed in a bar of hard rubber *i* and slide through holes in *h*. They are arranged in sections of six each, and are supported out of fluid by rod *k*, which is notched for spring *l*. Connection with carbons and zincs is made by means of the angular rods *m*, which are each provided with a spring *o* firmly pressing upon metal *b*. The rod is firmly secured in the platform, projecting through it for contact with springs *n*. Each rod is connected by a wire to a corresponding metal clip *s*, which is numbered.

The binding posts for the cords, *r r*, which are in contact with the clips, slide upon a rod, so that any desired cell can be used first and the number increased from either way, one at a time, without breaking the circuit, until the desired number is obtained.

TO FILL THE BATTERY—Remove sections of zincs, as shown in engraving, and fill with funnel.

TO EMPTY CELLS—Lift off platform *C*, when the cells can be removed from tray *A*.

TO START BATTERY—Press upon spring *l*, when the section of zincs will slide into fluid; slide posts *r r* upon the clips *s s*, corresponding with the cell that you desire to commence with; then increase the number at pleasure.

TO CLEAN AND AMALGAMATE THE ZINCS it is simply necessary to remove a section, as shown in engraving. First section is supported in tubes; second section is immersed; third section removed.

THE ADVANTAGES presented in this battery are: The cells are absolutely tight, so that the fluid can neither leak nor spill, making it perfectly portable. The connections are made outside the cell, so that they do not corrode from contact with fluid. The carbons can not be broken. The zincs can be cleaned and amalgamated in a few minutes. Any section of zincs can be used at a time. Any particular cell can be brought into the circuit at a time. It is but a moment's work to start it. It is perfectly clean. It is particularly adapted for electrolysis.

SOME CASES IN PRACTICE.

BY JAMES DORLAND, M.D., MILWAUKEE, WIS.

No. 1.—*Suspended Animation in a Newly-born Child.*

Feb. 22nd, 1882, was called to attend Mrs. C. in confinement with her first child. Everything progressed favorably, and at 6.55 A.M. the head passed the perineum. Upon passing my finger in, found the cord once around its neck and pulsating vigorously. Attempted to put it over the head, but did not succeed, so left it alone, watching the pulsations. The child gave one convulsive movement and was then still. A minute after, the pulsations getting weaker, I again tried and succeeded in getting it over the head; it was still pulsating, and a pain coming on, the shoulders were born. A second or two later, found the pulsations in the cord had ceased; cut it at once and delivered the child. No hemorrhage from the cord, and no effort whatever at inspiration; there was a feeble fluttering at the heart. Sprinkled it with cold water, then hot, slapped it, and used every method known to me, including mouth to mouth inflation and taking the child and carrying it rapidly back and forward through the air, and allowing the head to hang down for a few seconds at a time. I also applied hot water cloths constantly, with alcohol, but for one hour could not get even a gasp, although the heart still beat feebly. Knowing that the air I forced into the lungs was devoid of oxygen, I bethought me it would be a good idea to use pure air, and thus give the lungs their proper stimuli. Getting the nurse to hold its nose, I put the nozzle of an ordinary syringe in its mouth, and, compressing the lips around it, forced in air. After repeating this three or four times at intervals of from four or five seconds, I had the satisfaction of seeing the child gasp, and by using it judiciously, at the same time keeping up heat artificially, at the end of two hours and five minutes we had the pleasure of observing regular respirations in the child. It had talipes calcaneus, but otherwise was perfectly healthy. It did well until on the morning of the 24th I was called hurriedly, and found its heart had ceased to beat, but that it was still breathing. Tried every method in my power, but could not revive it. This case proves what we can sometimes accomplish by perseverance, and that inflation by the mouth to mouth method cannot compare with the introduction of pure air. I have never seen that plan spoken of before, and from this time shall use it as a first and not a last resort. The family, as well as myself, feel perfectly satisfied that without the syringe the child would not have been restored.

No 2.—*Nerve-stretching for Sciatica.*

John S., aged 60, in November, 1879, contracted a cold, and the following day complained of intense pain along the course of the sciatic nerve, from its point of exit down almost to the knee. By chance I saw him that day, and ordered an opiate, with warm fomentations. He did not again consult me at that time, but I learned that he first consulted one, then another, but did not improve. He also patronized most of the travelling quacks that came to the city.

Jan. 1st, 1881.—I was asked to see him again, and upon examination, found him in the following condition : Able to walk, but only a short distance at a time ; then complained of pains all down the course of the nerve, severe at the knee, but worst at the dorsum of the foot, and of a peculiar stinging character. The muscles were very much atrophied, and the skin dry and harsh; his general health poor. Pressure at the exit of the nerve, and at several points in its course, produced severe pain. He had been treated in all manner of ways—the actual cautery, electricity, baths, tonics, &c.—but without the least apparent benefit. I told him there was a chance to cure him by stretching the nerve. He consented to a trial, but the day selected his sister carried him off and put him under the charge of a quack, who guaranteed a cure for $2.

On the 12th he sent for me to come and operate, which I did, Drs. Copeland and Robbins assisting. An Esmarch's bandage was put on, and the constriction applied as high up as possible. The operation was performed at the upper third of the thigh, using the biceps for my guide, and commencing my incision at the lower border of the glutens maximus muscle, making it six inches long. Dissecting carefully down, I had no difficulty in finding the nerve, which was divided high up. The nerve sheath was very thin, and at that point no apparent evidence of inflammation. I took up one branch with my finger and pulled on it until I felt something give way, which I supposed to be adhesions. Then I stretched the other, but did not feel any such sensation. I forgot to mention that before stretching I removed the constriction. The sheath was carefully replaced, a rubber drainage-tube put in, and the wound closed with four silver sutures and the interspaces supported with adhesive plaster. Not a drop of blood was lost until the sutures were put in, when about a teaspoonful came away. I finished the dressing with a thick roll of cotton, and held it in place by a few turns of a roller. Gave ¼ gr. morphia sulp. hypodermically.

Jan. 13th.—Pulse 108; temperature 100°; tongue coated, but moist. Wound closed externally by first intention. Slight discharge of bloody serum from the drainage-tube; by gentle compression, a little more came away. Had three small chills about four hours apart. Urine high-colored, but no albumen. Ordered quinine sulph. gr. iii every four hours. Syringed it out with a 3 per cent. solution of carbolic acid, and applied cotton dressing again, with a little more compression. *14th.*—Pulse and temperature about the same, but had no chills during the past 24 hours. Had felt no pain since the operation. I stretched the leg and flexed it on the thigh, and that on the abdomen. It produced very little pain. Ordered cinch. sulph., with mineral acids and bark, and to have electricity applied daily, together with friction of the limb.

From this time forward he progressed rapidly, with occasional twitches of pain, which, as the muscles regained their tone, grew less frequent, until, at the end of three months, he felt perfectly well, the leg being at that time the same size as its fellow. He has passed through the winter so far without any trouble whatever, and can be regarded as perfectly cured. He attends to his duties as road commissioner, which post he has now filled nine months, and it keeps him on his feet the most of the day. We did not get the specific effect from the stretching, for he had some twinges after; but I think it so changed the nutrition of the part, and broke up the adhesions, that electricity, with tonics, which had been tried persistently before without the least benefit, completed the cure.

No. 3.—*Foreign substance producing symptoms of Gall Stone.*

Dec. 11th, 1881, was called to see Mrs. N., aged 55, who had been suffering intense paroxysms of pain for the past six hours. A homœopath had been called in, but could afford no relief or give any satisfactory idea what was the trouble. The pain began at the epigastrium, and gradually grew worse. Upon examination, I found the pulse slightly accelerated, temperature normal, eyes becoming jaundiced, and an anxious expression of the face. Had vomited a great deal. Over the duodenum, and about the course of the common duct, was a place about 2½ inches long by 1 inch wide that was exceedingly sensitive to the touch, and from which all the pain seemed to emanate. No peritonitis, but slight tenderness, due to the pains and sympathy. Diagnosed it as gall-stone colic. Gave a hypodermic injection of morphia and antispasmodics, and ordered large linseed poultices over the spot.

Dec. 12th.—Patient had been easier since my visit; the paroxysms not so frequent; still great tenderness on pressure; the eyes deeper jaundiced, and the urine loaded with biliary acids. In addition, ordered saline cathartics, and left positive orders to keep everything that passed for inspection. She gradually improved until, on the 15th, she was feeling quite well; eyes clearing up, and urine a better color. Pain all gone, only the tender spot remaining on pressure. Felt sure the stone had passed, but failed to find it.

Jan. 19th.—Was called again, and found her in much the same condition as before. Ordered the same treatment. The eyes did not get quite so yellow, nor was the urine so heavily loaded. The pain began in the same spot. After her stomach had settled, gave a large dose of oil, as I felt sure the stone had lodged in the duodenum, part of which she retained. The following day she felt quite well, and upon examining the fæces I found a piece of walnut about $\frac{3}{4}$ of an inch long, nearly $\frac{1}{2}$ wide, and $\frac{1}{4}$ thick at the largest end, tapering to a thin point at the other. It gave evidence of having been in the alimentary canal for some time. Upon being questioned, she stated that she had not been feeling well for over a month before her first attack, and laid it to eating head-cheese, a food of doubtful composition. There is very little doubt but at that time the foreign substance was introduced, and that the sharp point of it caught at the orifice of the common duct. Since that time she has been in perfect health.

No. 4.—*Ununited Fracture of the Humerus.*

Chris. B., aged 20, in the spring of 1879, while riding on a car used in drawing stone out of a quarry, the cable broke and allowed it to descend with frightful velocity; he was thrown off, and suffered a fracture of the humerus at the juncture of the lower with the middle third. I did not see him until Jan. 3rd, 1880, about nine months after the accident, when I obtained the following history: The homœopathic doctors that were called in said it was a simple fracture, and treated it accordingly for nineteen weeks; from that time until he came under my care he had been to various surgeons, one of whom drove two ivory pegs in to create inflammation, which they did, but did not produce union, and were still in when I saw the arm.

He informed me that shortly after his fall he discovered that the radial artery did not pulsate, and when I examined him, no beating could be felt; but no doubt a small amount of blood still passed through. The forearm was at right angles to the arm, and firm fibrous union had taken place at the joint. The thumb was flexed on the hand, and the fingers flexed over the thumb, and held very firmly in that position. The hand was also flexed to its fullest extent towards the forearm. There was slight shortening of the arm. All the muscles from the shoulder down were very much atrophied, especially the interossei. The fingers could only be slightly straightened, the thumb still less, while it was very painful at the wrist to attempt to extend the hand. At the seat of fracture very little provisional callus was thrown out, and although the fracture was very plain, no crepitus could be made out, even with considerable pressure, when rubbing the ends together. I decided that union did not take place owing to some substance being between the ends of the bone, and thought most likely it was a piece of muscle. I told him it would have to be cut into and the ends wired together, which was done Jan. 9th, 1880, Drs. Senn and Bading assisting. The operation was performed bloodlessly, and an incision about four inches long made, commencing just below the insertion of the Deltoid, taking care to avoid the musculo-spiral nerve and superior profunda artery. No difficulty was experienced in reaching the anterior and lower fragment of bone, ripping up the periosteum, and sawing off the end, which was found rounded off to a sharp point, and quite smooth. A hole was then drilled through, and some silver wire inserted and held out of the way. The posterior fragment was much more troublesome to get at, but when raised, we found that it was a portion of the Brachialis Anticus muscle that prevented union. Upon loosening it from the bone, pulsation immediately returned in the radial artery, showing that the flow of blood had been stopped by the contraction of the muscles. The point of the fragment was in much the same conditions as the other. The periosteum was opened, and as small a piece as possible sawn off, a hole drilled through, and the two ends wired as firmly as possible together. The arm was then put up in a posterior splint, coming well around, and the patient kept in bed as quiet as possible. Two days afterwards he had a chill, followed by the symptoms of diphtheria, which soon developed into a case of medium severity. He had not been exposed, and the only way to account for it was that early in the morning I had performed tracheotomy on a child suffering from diphtheria, and had not time to change my clothes before operating on him. I put him on appropriate treatment, and in about a week he was fully recovered. Then I put him on bitter tonics and cod liver oil for some time, until his general health was fully up to a normal standard.

At the end of seven weeks he was able to come to the office, when electricity was applied daily to the muscles, and kept up until the end of the treatment. Union took place slowly, and was stimulated by driving in two nickel-plated nails, one in each end. They did excellent service. At the end of six months union had taken place, but it was not firm, and easily bent. It was now removed from the sling, and the motion produced irritation enough, so that at the end of another month firm union had taken place. Passive motion was used upon all the joints, and as the arm grew firmer, more force was applied. The elbow yielded considerably, as did the wrist, but the latter could not retain its extended position, and neither it nor the forefinger could ever be brought to a normal condition. He said his hand was so flexed shortly after the accident, but whether it was due to injury to the musculo-spiral at the time of accident, or gradual atrophy, I am unwilling to say, but I believe the latter. Sensation was not impaired, but owing to the feeble circulation the temperature was much lower than its fellow. He can cut his food and carry it to his mouth, chop wood, and has a very useful arm, with the muscles fairly developed.

This case is interesting from a medico-legal point. No doubt the muscle was between the ends of the bones immediately after the fracture, and I do not believe there could have been true bony crepitus at that time, and the absence of pulsation at the wrist should have made them search for the cause, and, if possible, remove it, thereby saving the boy a great amount of trouble and deformity. The case is now before the courts, but it is the company that is sued, not the surgeons.

QUARTERLY RETROSPECT OF SURGERY.

PREPARED BY FRANCIS J. SHEPHERD, M.D., C.M., M.R.C.S., ENG.

Demonstrator of Anatomy and Lecturer on Operative and Minor Surgery McGill University; Surgeon to the Out-Door Department of the Montreal General Hospital.

(*Continued from March Number, page* 479.)

Gastrostomy aud Œsophagostomy.—The operation of gastrostomy was first performed by Sédillot in 1849. Since then this operation has been practised a large number of times in England, America, and Germany. The first successful case occurred in the practice of M. Verneuil at the Hôpital de la Pitié, Paris, in 1876. The operation was performed for stricture of the œsophagus, in a boy 17 years of age, caused by swallowing a solution of potash. The previous operations had all been undertaken for malignant disease.

At a meeting of the Clinical Society of London in October last, Mr. Reeves read a paper on "Two cases of Malignant Stricture of the Œsophagus, in which Gastrostomy was performed, with a special reference to Œsophagostomy in narrowing of this tube." He said, in these two cases, he had performed gastrostomy in deference to the wishes of his colleagues, and went on to describe how he should act in suitable cases of stricture of the œsophagus. He said that malignant obstruction was most common in the upper part of the tube, and in such cases he considered œsophagostomy the preferable operation. Even when the stricture was low down, œsophagostomy is indicated as a preliminary and exploratory operation ; and, if a tube cannot be passed through the stricture, gastrostomy should be performed. Œsophagostomy is a much safer operation than gastrostomy ; never, in fact, having been fatal. Mr. Reeves said it should be performed on the left side of the neck by making an incision from half an inch above the episternal notch to the level of the upper border of the thyroid cartilage. The Surgeon should stand on the left side of the patient. If possible, a sound should be passed previous to the operation; and after the œsophagus is opened, a tube with a funnel-shaped end should be passed and tied in place, and nourishment administerod through it as soon as the effects of the anæsthetic have passed off. The operation should be undertaken early, before the obstruction is complete, and before the patient's strength is exhausted.—(*Lancet Report.*)

At the adjourned discussion on November 11th, Mr. Golding Bird presented brief abstracts of five cases of cancer of the œsophagus, in four of which gastrostomy was performed. In the fifth, the operation had to be abandoned owing to the occurence of œsophageal hemorrhage. He pointed out that gastrostomy was only a palliative operation and could not be judged of by bare statistics. One of his cases, a man aged 66, had lived five months, but symptoms had only existed two months before operation. In the others the histories were much longer. He said gastrostomy of itself was not a fatal operation, but that it was resorted to too late, and that the earlier operation was resorted to, the better the result. He believed in those cases which presented themselves for operation late in the disease, the stomach should be opened at the time of operation and nourishment given at once. He was distinctly opposed to œsophagostomy as a substitute. In four out of his five cases œsophagostomy would have been useless. Dilatation of a cancerous stricture high up might be fairly tried, but when in the chest it was his opinion that dilatation was more dangerous than gastrostomy itself. Mr. Durham advocated, where possible, feeding the patient through an elastic catheter, passed into the stomach through the mouth. The catheter should only be left in three or four days, and another then introduced. He did not think that Dr. Krishaber's method of passing the catheter through the nose so good, because more disagreeable. Dr. Krishaber, at the International Congress, stated that in œsophageal stricture the catheter could remain in for an indefinite period. Dr. Douglass Powell warned the users of catheters against the dangers of the passage of instruments from ulceration. Dr. Andrew Clarke, and the surgeons who subsequently spoke, almost all advocated the use of the catheter as long as possible.—(*Abstract of Report in British Medical Journal.*)

The prevailing opinion seemed to be that catheters should be used where possible, in stricture, to dilate it, and to feed the patient; also, the passage of a catheter in a cancerous stricture prevented the constant irritation of the stricture by food, and so temporarily arrested the growth. In cases where the stricture was low down it is probable catheterism would not be successful. Where the cancerous stricture was high up and a catheter could not be passed, it is probable œsophagostomy might prove a valuable operation; but where the cancer was low down and a catheter failed to pass, gastrostomy is indicated. It was the general opinion that the operation should be performed early, but that as a rule the patient would not consent till too late. Dr. Andrew Clarke brought out the fact that the passage of a catheter required a great deal of patience, and that if the operator persevered in his efforts to pass it, he was often in the end successful.

With regard to the operation of gastrostomy, several of the speakers advised, first, stitching of the stomach to the abdominal wall, around the opening, by two circles of sutures an inch apart, and leaving it thus for four or five days before the stomach was opened.

Dr. Carl Langenbuch (*Berlin Klin. Woch.*) regards the immediate opening of the stomach as unsafe. If there be urgency he would suggest the use of an aspirator syringe and injection of liquid food in this manner. Langenbuch thinks that as soon as the difficulties of swallowing are at all pronounced the first part of the operation should be undertaken, and that the surgeon should not wait till the stricture is impermeable. With regard to the second part, he recommends a very small opening into the stomach, so small indeed that a certain amount of force is required to get in the tube. The tube should be provided with a stop-cock, and so all escape is prevented. Before opening the stomach it should be fixed with a sharp hook to prevent puncturing the posterior wall.—(*Med. Times and Gazette.*)

Dr. P. Kraske, in the *Centralblatt für Chirurgie*, warns the profession against the danger of stitching the stomach to the wall of the abdomen some days before opening it, as the stomach contents are very liable to escape through the stitch punctures in the gastric walls. This occurs especially if there is any degree of tension. He reports a case where the escaped matter through the stitch punctures caused a fatal peritonitis. He therefore advocates immediate opening. Dr. Kraske thinks that this danger will have to be taken into account in considering the advisability of the first part of the operation being performed early in the case, as suggested by Langenbuch.

Dr. T. F. Prewitt, in a paper on gastrostomy, published in the *St. Louis Courier of Medicine*, gives a table of fifty-nine cases: forty were malignant, twelve cicatricial, three syphilitic, and in four nature of stricture not given. In the cases operated on for malignant stricture the patients lived fourteen days to six months, and one patient is still living. In the cicatricial variety six recovered, as also one where the stricture was of syphilitic origin. Peritonitis existed in only seven of the cases. Exhaustion alone is assigned as the cause of death in the large proportion of cases.

Mr. A. F. McGill, of the Leeds School of Medicine, reports in the *Lancet* for Dec. 3rd, 1881, two cases of gastrostomy. In both cases the operation was performed for malignant stricture of the œsophagus, about the level of the cricoid cartilage. In the first case the wall of the abdomen was incised and the stomach sewn to the edge of the wound by thirteen silver wire sutures; then the opening was made into the stomach four days after, the patient in the meantime having been fed with Slinger's nutrient suppositories. Four months after the operation the patient was still alive. In the second case the patient died on the seventh day from exhaustion.

Dupuytren's Contraction of the Fingers.—Dr. Myrtle, in the *British Medical Journal* of Dec. 3rd, 1881, contributes an article on the above affection, in which he denies its connection with gout for the following reasons :—1. It is never met with in women, and they are quite as much afflicted with gout as men. 2. Many of the worst cases he has seen (his own among them) have not been gouty themselves, nor have they ever had a gouty progenitor. 3. Gouty remedies have no influence over this affection. 4. That the very mode of dealing successfully with contracted finger, by division, with subsequent mechanical extension, is a plan which surgeons would not readily adopt in cases of enlargement, stiffening and contraction from gouty deposit. The general ignorance of the profession with regard to the pathological changes which cause this contraction appears to Dr. Myrtle incomprehensible, especially since the various writers on this disease have so clearly demonstrated that the contraction is due entirely to changes which have taken place in the bands of fascia of the fingers and palm; that the tendons with their sheaths, the joints with their covering and ligaments, are not implicated. He describes two forms of contracted fingers:—The one, traumatic, traceable to some local injury. The other, idiopathic, generally met with after middle life; one or more fingers may be affected, the third most commonly, and the forefinger and thumb being rarely implicated. Dr. Myrtle says there is only one method of treatment, viz., subcutaneous division of constricted bands with subsequent mechanical extension, as recommended by Mr. Wm. Adams. Every fibre of the tightened band must be divided separately.

Mr. H. A. Reeves (*Brit. Med. Jour.*, Dec. 31, 1881), cannot agree with Dr. Myrtle that gout and rheumatism are not frequent causes, and he differs altogether from the statement of Dr. Myrtle that it is never met with in women. He can clearly recall five cases, and is sure he has seen at least seven or eight in women. Mr. Reeves gives the causes as follows: 1, rheumatic and gouty diathesis; 2, injury; 3, occupation; 4, heredity; 5, neurosis. Occupation may claim a large percentage of cases, as it is not uncommon in boatmen, coachmen, sailors, bootmakers, writers, and even those who have for years carried a walking stick and borne their weight on it. Dr. Myrtle believes the contraction due to a hyperplasia of the fascia, while Mr. Reeves considers it to be inflammatory.

Mr. Southam, of Manchester, has also observed it frequently in women, and considers it commonly connected with a gouty diathesis.

Mr. Wm. Adams states (*Brit. Med. Jour.*, Jan. 21, 1882), that when he published his work on "Dupuytren's Contraction of the Fingers" in 1879, he had never seen a case in women, and since that time only one case has come under his observation, that of a lady aged 66, in whom both hands were affected. He says that the affection may be of more freqnent occurrence in females than has been supposed. Many cases have been sent to him as cases of Dupuytren's contraction which he excluded from that class, there being no puckering of the skin of palm or prominent fascial bands, but as a rule the fingers were contracted, because they were bent at the phalangeal articulations and could not be straightened. I have seen one case of genuine Dupuytren's contraction of the fingers in a woman aged 52, who had a decidedly gouty diathesis. The little finger and ring finger of the left hand were affected, and there was considerable puckering of the skin. I have seen but few cases at the Montreal General Hospital Out-patient department, and these all in gouty patients. I am inclined to believe that it is not a common affection in this country.

Treatment of Fissure of the Anus.—Dr. Mascarel proposes the following treatment, which he has used with much success in the case of those patients who fear the radical cure of fissure by forcible dilatation ;—1. An enema of warm water, to which a large spoonful of glycerine has been added, is ordered to be given daily. 2. After each motion, a small pledget of lint, saturated with the following ointment, is to be introduced into the anus: ℞ Glycerine, 30 grains; oil of sweet almonds, 30 grains; brown ointment (onguent de la mère), 60 grms. 3. After introducing the lint, care must be taken to smear the ointment well around the outside of the anus. 4. If there is great constipation, five centigrammes of powdered belladonna root should be given every night. In eight cases out of ten, fissure of the anus will be cured after three weeks or a month of this treatment. (*Le Progrès Médical*, July, 1881, quoted in *Practitioner*, Dec., 1881.)

I have found, where the patient will not consent to operative measures, or the pain of touching the fissure with a point of nitrate of silver, the application of an ointment of calomel gr. iv, opium and ext. of belladonna each two grains, to a drachm of simple ointment, as recommended by Mr. Allingham, prove often curative. The bowels, of course, should be kept open.

Treatment of Prolapsus Ani by Hypodermic Injections of Ergotine.—Dr. Vidal has treated successfully three long-standing cases of prolapsus ani in adults by means of injection of ergotine, a cure being effected in a few weeks. The author therefore recommends that this method should be adopted in similar cases. The method employed is to inject, by means of a Pravaz syringe, 15 to 20 drops of a solution consisting of one part of Bonjean's ergotine in five parts of cherry laurel water, every two or three days, through the anus, either into the sphincter or into the prolapsed portion of intestine. Severe burning pain follows the injection, tenesmus, lasting several hours, in many cases cramp in the neck of the bladder, and retention of urine for eight to ten hours. The author has not met with inflammation, abscess, or toxic symptoms in any of his cases. (*Der Praktische Artz*, in Nov. *Practitioner*.) Judging from the immediate effects of the operation, I think it would be hard, in this country at least, to prevail on the patient's submitting to a second injection; besides, it offers no advantages over Dr. Van Buren's method of treatment by actual cautery.

Hospital Reports.

Medical and Surgical Cases Occurring in the Practice of the Montreal General Hospital.

SURGICAL CASES UNDER DR. RODDICK.

I.—*Gunshot Wound of Foot.* (Reported by Dr. Henderson.)

On Dec. 3rd, 1881, Willie C., a well-nourished lad aged 15 years, while walking along with a man carrying a shot-gun with the muzzle directed towards the ground, it was discharged accidentally, the lad receiving the whole of the charge in his right foot, entering on its outer side about one inch in front of the malleolus, leaving a large circular, gaping wound one inch and a half in diameter; the charge then followed a straight course across the foot to its inner side, passing out just in front of the tubercle of the scaphoid bone. The wound of exit was much smaller than that of entrance, allowing only the introduction of the little finger, while three fingers could be passed into the other with ease. By means of the fingers it was found that a portion of the cuboid and all three cuneiform bones were very much shattered. The ankle joint and the bones of the metatarsus appeared to be uninjured, except the bases of the 4th and 5th metatarsal bones, which are both exposed. The flexor and extensor tendons of the foot were also uninjured. Bleeding was very free at time of accident, but very slight after removal to hospital. From the interior of the wound a quantity of *débris*, consisting of fragments of bone, blood-clots, shot, paper, shreds of wool and dirt, were removed with the finger; the wound was then thoroughly washed out with a one-to-forty solution of carbolie acid, and after passing strips of lint soaked in the same solution through the wound to serve for drainage, Lister's antiseptic dressings were applied. There was no swelling or deformity of the foot, and the motion of the ankle joint was free and painless.

Dec. 12th.—Wound was dressed daily up to the 9th instant, and then undisturbed for three days. To-day the condition is very satisfactory. There is no swelling or redness, and little or no pain complained of; the articular surfaces of the 4th and 5th metatarsal bones have come away, and a considerable quantity of shot, wool and fragments of bone again removed. The discharge is free, and quite devoid of offensive odor. Temperature, with the exception of the first two nights, has not been above 99°. An ordinary drainage-tube has been passed through the wound lately, instead of the strips of lint at first used.

Jan. 2nd, '82.—Since last note the condition of the wound has improved daily, healthy granulations forming in the interior, so that the drainage-tube can no longer be passed through; the exterior of the wound also presents a very healthy appearance. The discharge is still very free and perfectly sweet, and from time to time fragments of bone and bits of shot continue to come away. On one or two occasions the urine presented the dark, smoky appearance suggestive of carbolic acid absorption, but on omitting to inject the wound with the usual 1 to 40 solution this discoloration gradually disappeared.

Jan. 26th.—Antiseptic dressings discontinued to-day; wounds to be dressed with simple carbolic lotion dressings, and patient allowed up; discharge from wound almost entirely ceased.

Feb. 16th.—A small abscess formed in neighborhood of wound on inner side of foot; opened to-day and about an ounce of pus escaped, a small spiculum of bone also coming away with the discharge.

March 15th.—Patient discharged from hospital; interior of wound almost completely filled; no deformity, and motion of ankle joint is perfect. The general condition of the patient was excellent throughout, the temperature never going above 99°, except on the 18th January, when for three days it was somewhat febrile, owing to a rather severe attack of follicular tonsillitis, and on the occasion of the formation of the abscess on February 17th, when it once registered 103°.

II.—*Case of Abscess of Kidney—Nephrotomy—Improvement.*
(Reported by Dr. HENDERSON.)

Hattie S., aged 20; good family history and previous good health up to the age of twelve, when she had a severe attack of what was called spinal meningitis, since which she has never been strong. Six years ago she began to suffer from pain low down in the back, and extending down the thighs, neuralgic in character, and considered to be sciatica by the doctor in attendance at the time. Shortly after this she began to suffer from frequent and painful micturition, and the urine was found to contain at times small quantities of matter and sometimes appeared quite bloody. She was then examined for stone, but none was found. In the following year (now four years ago), these symptoms continuing unabated, rapid dilatation of the urethra was effected, and a number of small villosities were removed from the mucous surface of the bladder; weak injections of nitric acid were made use of for some time, but without marked benefit to the patient, the pain and frequency of micturition continuing off and on, sometimes better and sometimes worse, and the appearance of the urine very much the same. During the last fifteen months she has failed very much, losing flesh considerably. In July last she began to suffer from pain in right loin, and tenderness was marked in that region, but no swelling or fullness noticeable; she then also began to have repeated chills, with fever and frequent attacks of gastric and intestinal disorder. Last October Dr. Blackader, by whom she was being treated, found a well-defined tumour in right hypochondriac region, painful and tender on pressure. A hypodermic needle was used to explore, but no pus was reached. Since then she has been growing very much worse, and her symptoms greatly aggravated. Menses have been scanty aud irregular during the last 3 years, and since September last have ceased altogether.

On admission, March 6th, she was much emaciated, and in a weak condition. A distinct and well-defined fluctuating tumor, painful on pressure, was found occupying the right hypochondriac and lumbar regions, and extending to within two inches of the umbilicus; a fine aspirating needle was introduced by way of exploring, and pus was reached. There is great frequency of micturition, the patient requiring to perform the act almost every half hour; but total amount of urine is somewhat diminished (about 32 ounces daily). On standing, it deposits pus very heavily; no blood. Lungs and heart normal. Liver dullness not well defined.

On the day following admission, a transverse incision was made in the loin, midway between crest of ilium and the border of the ribs, and the abscess cavity punctured with a trocar and then freely opened. After securing the sac to the outer wound by means of silk sutures, about 20 ounces of putrid pus escaped; the finger was then introduced into the cavity and the substance of the kidney was found to have been greatly involved in the morbid process. There was no evidence of a calculus being present. The cavity was well washed out with 1 to 40 solution of carbolic acid and a large-sized drainage-tube applied, with Lister's antiseptic dressings.

March 17*th*.—Since the operation the wound has been dressed daily; the discharge has been quite free and devoid of odor. On the third day after operation the urine showed signs of carbolic acid absorption, having a decided smoky appearance; accordingly, instead of injecting the wound with carbolic acid, a solution of boracic acid was used, of the strength of 20 per cent, after which the smokiness rapidly disappeared and the urine appeared quite natural. On the first day after the operation the amount was very much diminished, the patient only passing ten ounces in the 24 hours, but the amount increased gradually from day to day up to yesterday, when 40 ounces were passed; the frequency of micturition has very much diminished, as has also the pain before the act. Her general condition has improved very much; she feels much stronger, and takes her nourishment well. There is complete absence of all chilly sensations, and the temperature has been below 100° ever since the operation.

March 24*th*.—Patient removed to her home to be treated privately; previous to doing so, the antiseptic dressings were removed and instructions given to have the wound dressed daily simply by washing it out with the 20 per cent solution of boracic acid, retaining the drainage-tube in position, and placing a large pad of oakum as an outer dressing. The wound at time of exit had contracted to very small dimensions, just allowing the free passage of the drainage-tube. The condition of the patient had very much improved, so that for the last five or six days she had been let up about the wards in an easy chair.

Reviews and Notices of Books.

A Practical Treatise on Hernia.—By JOSEPH H. WARREN. Second and revised edition. Boston: James R. Osgood & Co., 1882.

From the fact that this work is so soon in its second edition we should judge that it has been appreciated. It has been written chiefly to make known the author's favorite method of treatment of hernia by injection of oak bark extract. In this undertaking he has been more fortunate than Prof. G. Dorvell, of Texas, who wrote a book on hernia with the same object a few years ago, which has now passed into oblivion, though the peculiar method of treatment advised therein was worthy of a better fate. The method of curing hernia that the author advocates is that of the late Dr. Heaton, of Boston, who practised it with the greatest success for years, though as a secret operation. The method was not made public till 1877, when his book on hernia, edited by the late Dr. Davenport, was published. Dr. Warren, it appears, attended Dr. Heaton in his last illness. Dr. Heaton personally instructed him in the operation. Since Dr. Heaton's death Dr. Warren has endeavored to introduce Heaton's method of cure of hernia into the various centres of surgery both of America and Europe, and has communicated articles on the subject to numbers of medical journals.

The method consists in injecting the canal and tissues through which a hernia has passed with some astringent fluid. Dr. Heaton found that extract of white oak bark was the best fluid, and caused just sufficient irritation to produce closure of the canal by the production of inflammatory tissue. The fluid is injected by means of a syringe with a needle made out of a solid piece of metal bored and with the holes at the sides instead of, as in the ordinary hypodermic needle, at the end. This method is best suited to cases of reducible inguinal hernia. Dr. Heaton, in his book, affirms that it is perfectly harmless, and no serious results follow even if the peritoneum is injected. He, in many hundred operations, never had any fatal cases. After the patient has been operated on he should remain in bed for a week or ten days, with a bandage applied firmly to the part, and if there is any severe inflammation evaporating lotions of spirit and water should be used. Dr. Heaton was a most successful operator and his percentage of failures almost *nil*. Dr. Warren has improved on this method by, first, using a spiral or twisted needle with a somewhat blunt end, and secondly, employing a more concentrated fluid, that is, he evaporates the extract of white oak bark to the consistency of glycerine. Dr. Warren's book tells us very little more about hernia than can be found in any good text-book of surgery, and tells it to us in a manner which is very much more spun out. With regard to Heaton's operation, we much prefer the description as given in Heaton's work. It is more concise and much better arranged. Dr. Warren adds a number of cases, very few of which are given in detail. Cures are reported too soon; we should like to have the condition of more patients noted a year or so subsequent to the operation.

Other methods for the radical cure of hernia are fully described, more especially those of somewhat recent date. This part will prove useful to those interested in the subject. Why is it that writers on any part of the male form between the navel and the knees always feel obliged to write a chapter on varicocele? Dr. Warren is no exception to the rule. A dozen pages are added to the end of the work on private and press opinions. Some of the extracts from private letters are merely acknowledgments of the receipt of the book. The press opinions are of course eulogistic. There are some beautiful anatomical plates reproduced from Bourgery and Blandin which add much to the usefulness of the book. On the whole, Dr. Warren has written a very interesting book, and one which has involved a great deal of labor. We hold, however, that it would have been much more satisfactory if he had given an account of the special operation he advocates with a detailed account of cases operated on and the results after some length of time had elapsed. We see that in the quotation heading the introduction Dr. Warren has conferred the long delayed and much merited honor of knighthood on T. Spencer Wells; a baronetcy would have been a more suitable reward.

The Prevention of Stricture and of Prostatic Obstruction.—By Reginald Harrison, F.R.C.S., Surgeon to the Royal Infirmary, Member of Council, Liverpool University College, and one of the Professors of Clinical Surgery in its Medical Faculty. London: J. & A. Churchill.

Mr. Harrison takes exception to the teaching of Dr. Otis that the continuance of gleet is indicative of the existence of a stricture and that the cure of the former depends upon the removal of the latter. On the contrary, he maintains the pathology which we have been accustomed to believe in, viz., that a gonorrhœa leaves behind a chronic inflammation in a portion of the urethra, which is indicated by the presence of a gleety discharge, and which causes a granular condition of the mucous membrane. More solid infiltration of the neighboring strictures takes place, the secreting power of the membrane is lost, and with the disappearance of the gleet a stricture is found to have been formed. To prevent stricture, therefore, it is said we must cure the diseased state of the urethral lining, not simply dilate the canal by mechanical means. Injections by the ordinary syringe and internal medication are alike condemned as inefficient, and the means recommended consist in the thorough douching of the urethra with astringent solutions by means of a soft catheter and a Higginson's rubber syringe.

The equally important subject of prevention of the evils arising from prostatic enlargement is also treated of very suggestively. The first practical point made is that continued pressure upon the gland can hinder its enlarging in that direction. Thus, persistent catheterism is recommended from the very commencement of signs of tendency in the prostate to increase in size. This, though it cannot arrest the enlargement of the organ, will often prevent it from unduly encroaching upon the urethral canal. For this purpose olivary bougies, with a spreading bulb, have been found to answer best. A number of general rules are also laid down for the guidance of patients beginning to be affected in this way; and the employment of ergot of rye is said to have proved of assistance in maintaining the tonicity of the musculature of the bladder. This little *brochure* will be read with interest by all practitioners, and will be found to contain much useful and highly practical instruction.

A System of Surgery, Theoretical aud Practical, in Treatises by various Authors.—Edited by T. HOLMES, M.A., Cantab, Surgeon to and Lecturer on Surgery at St. George's Hostal. First American from second English edition, thoroughly revised and much enlarged. By JOHN H. PACKARD, A.M., M.D., Surgeon to the Episcopal and St. Joseph's Hospitals,

Philadelphia; assisted by a large corps of the most eminent American surgeons. In three volumes, with many illustrations. Vol. II. Philadelphia: Henry C. Lea's Son & Co. Montreal: Dawson Brothers.

The second volume of this great standard work contains the following sections: viz., Diseases of the organs of special sense; Diseases of Circulatory System; Diseases of Digestive Tract; Diseases of Genito-Urinary Organs. The revision seems to have been very efficiently carried out, and the illustrations are quite numerous. Two colored lithographic plates representing typical changes in the retina are also added. Amongst the names of the well-known American surgeons who have acted as revisors in the various departments are the following: Drs. Harlan, J. Solis Cohen, Lewis A. Stimson, J. H. Packard, Edwd. L. Keyes, J. William White, and Alex. J. C. Skene. Too much praise cannot be given to the publishers for the admirable appearance of the volume as regards binding and typography.

A Study of the Tumors of the Bladder.—With original contributions and drawings. By ALEX. W. STEIN, M.D., Surgeon to Charity Hospital, Genito-Urinary and Venereal Division, Professor of Visceral Anatomy and Physiology at the N. Y. College of Dentistry, &c., &c. New York: Wm. Wood & Co. Montreal: J. M. O'Loughlin.

This is a monograph of considerable value upon some rare forms of disease. The author has met with four cases of tumor of the bladder, in two of which he secured *post-mortem* examinations. These have been the foundation of his study of the subject. He has collected together the literature of these growths, and furnishes a complete bibliography of the published cases. They are classified and discussed *seriatim*, all important details concerning their nature, symptomatology, diagnosis and treatment receiving careful attention. The work contains several drawings of the original cases, as well as many others taken from the published observations of other writers. The volume forms a valuable contribution to the surgery of the bladder.

Favorite Prescriptions of Distinguished Practitioners, with Notes on Treatmeut.—By B. W. PALMER, A.M., M.D. New York: Bermingham & Co.

This is a handy little book, small enough for the pocket, in which are to be found three or four hundred prescriptions of various classes of diseases. They have been compiled from the published writings and private memoranda of the best known English and American authorities. From an examination of a number of them, we can say that the selections appear to have been very judiciously made. This little collection will, we are sure, be very welcome to all, especially junior practitioners, because, though perhaps knowing the best remedies to use in a given case, it is not always easy for one, without much experience, to compile at a moment's notice an entirely suitable formula for its administration. Failing this, he can, by the assistance of the "favorite prescriptions," fall back upon the formula which has been recommended by Barker, Bartholow, Gross, Loomis, Fothergill, Sims, or some of the equally eminent writers and teachers.

Books and Pamphlets Received.

A SYSTEM OF SURGERY, THEORETICAL AND PRACTICAL, IN TREATISES BY VARIOUS AUTHORS. Edited by T. Holmes, M.A. First American from second English edition, thoroughly revised and much enlarged by John H. Packard, A.M., M.D., assisted by a large corps of the most eminent American surgeons. In three volumes. Vol. III. Philadelphia: Henry C. Lea's Son & Co.

NERVOUS DISEASES: THEIR DESCRIPTION AND TREATMENT. By Allan McLane Hamilton, M.D. Second edition. Philadelphia: Henry C. Lea's Son & Co.

DISEASES OF WOMEN: A MANUAL FOR STUDENTS AND PRACTITIONERS. By Arthur W. Edis, M.D. With one hundred and forty-eight illustrations. Philadelphia: Henry C. Lea's Son & Co.

Extracts from British and Foreign Journals.

Unless otherwise stated the translations are made specially for this Journal.

Extract from a Lecture on Tubercle.—By Sidney Coupland, M.D., F.R.C.P., Physician to and Lecturer on Pathological Anatomy at the Middlesex Hospital.—*Gentlemen:* Having, in my last lecture, given you as explicit an account of the general pathology of tubercle as far as I understand it, I propose to-day, before leaving this subject, to recapitulate to you these facts in the form of a concise summary. In doing so, you must allow me to adopt a somewhat aphoristic and dogmatic method; for I feel that upon this subject, of all in pathology, it is necessary for us to have clear and definite ideas. There is hardly any pathological question that has been so swayed by every wind of doctrine as this of tubercle; not even the subject of inflammation has been viewed from so many standpoints and received so many and varied explanations. The conclusions I am about to give you do not claim to be anything else than the formulated expression of ideas gathered from time to time from various sources. They embody simply the essential points I have learned from others, confirmed, so far as opportunities have been given me, by my own *post-mortem* experience. Therefore, they are in no way original or novel. I hope they may be nearer the truth in consequence; as near, that is, as our present knowledge allows us to go. My sole aim is to teach you the facts which are established, and the inferences that appear to flow from them, in the simplest and plainest manner.

1. Tuberculosis is an infective disease to which man and the higher animals are liable.

2. It is characterized anatomically by the formation of minute nodules or "granulations," composed of elements like those met with in granulation tissue, the result of simple reparative inflammation.

3. These nodules, or elementary or primary "tubercles," may occur in an isolated manner, or, by their confluence, may form larger or smaller conglomerate masses.

4. The typical structure of each fully formed primary nodule consists (*a*) in a collection of lymphoid round cells, enclosed in a delicate fibrillar meshwork or stroma: (*b*) in an internal zone, more or less evident, of larger nucleated epithelioid cells; and (*c*) a central multi-nucleated or giant cell.

5. These "tubercles" arise apparently in connection with the lymphatic tissue that pervades the body. No region is exempt from them. They may occur in the substance of organs, in the bones and muscles, in serous membranes, as the pia-arachnoid, pleura, pericardium, and peritoneum; in synovial membranes; in mucous membranes (arising in the submucous stratum), as in

the mouth, pharynx, larynx, trachea, bronchi, intestines, and genito-urinary tract.

6. Being ill supplied with blood-vessels, they can only attain a certain size, and then perish. The central cells degenerate first, because they are the farthest removed from the nutrient blood stream, and mutual pressure due to their increasing growth hampers their vital activity. They become fattily degenerated, soft, opaque, caseous, forming "yellow" tubercles, which, when isolated, are larger and manifestly of older formation than the miliary translucent grey granules. Where such tubercles are confluent, larger and more irregular caseous masses are formed. Caseation may pass into cretification. On the other hand, there is no doubt that occasionally the tubercular nodules take on a fibroid change, passing from the stage of "granulation-tissue" to one resembling "cicatricial tissue."

7. Almost invariably there occurs, in the vicinity of the tubercular formation, some reactive inflammation. This may be protective by ultimately leading to encapsulation by fibrous tissue of the caseated tubercular focus; or, as more frequently happens, it aids in the disintegration of the surrounding tissues, and leads, with the necrosis of the tubercles themselves, to destructive ulceration.

8. Individuals who are prone to the development of tubercle are called "tubercular." The disposition may be inherited. Probably what we recognize as "struma" or "scrofula" is only one form of this: a tendency to tuberculosis of lymphatic glands especially; just as in phthisical subjects we have a tendency to pulmonary tuberculosis.

9. The tubercular manifestation is, in the majority of cases, at first local, *i.e.*, limited to one organ or tissue. It may remain so limited throughout life—may not even endanger life—or may lead to death by the local destruction to which it gives rise. On the other hand, it may be more or less widely diffused throughout the body of the same individual. This diffusion may be due sometimes to the simultaneous development of tuberculosis in many parts. More frequently it is due to secondary dissemination by a process of infection.

10. This dissemination takes place, as in cancer, in two ways,

viz., by direct extension, or infection of neighboring tissues by contiguity; and by general distribution of the tubercular virus through the medium of the blood-system (including lymphatics).

11. The tubercular virus seems to be most potent, or, at any rate, to retain its potency, *i.e.*, its infective property, in the caseous state.

12. Examples of the local extension of tubercle, or of propagation by contiguous infection, are seen (1) in the development of peritoneal tubercle from intestinal; (2) in the spreading of tubercle from one part of an organ (*i.e.*, lung) to another part; (3) in extension from lung to pleura; (4) in bronchial, laryngeal and intestinal ulceration excited by the passage over their mucous membrane of material expectorated from a phthisical lung; (5) in tuberculosis of bladder and vesiculæ seminales following upon renal or testicular tubercle, etc. The mode of its local extension approximates tubercle to the neoplasmata, viz., by its elements exciting in the tissue they infect changes leading to the formation of cell-masses resembling the primary focus.

13. The generalisation of tubercle is shown in the disease known as acute miliary tuberculosis, which is characterized by an eruption of miliary granulations in diverse organs and tissues. Its mode of occurrence may be (as above) compared to the general dissemination of secondary cancer, or, perhaps with equal truth, to the metastatic suppuration of pyæmia. With few exceptions, it appears to necessitate a primary tubercular focus to give rise to it. It is believed that the infective virus, whatever it be, enters the blood-stream at this local focus, and is thence widely disseminated, the resulting growths being for the most part miliary, grey, and translucent; life not, as a rule, being prolonged for a sufficient length of time after the occurrence of the generalisation to permit of the growths becoming confluent or caseous. As the membranes of the brain are generally involved in this widespread infection, death occurs early.

14. Lastly, tuberculosis is inoculable. In this respect it resembles pyæmia, and differs from the cancers; for there is reason to think that it may be and is communicated from one human being to another, *e.g.*, from husband to wife, and *vice versâ*;

and that it can be inoculated in animals from man (artificial tubercle). There is, further, a possibility, based on certain peculiar morphological resemblances of the formations, that bovine tuberculosis is communicable to man.

15. If the foregoing data be true, it follows that tuberculosis is an infective disease, probably due to the presence of a virus, which gives rise to the development of peculiar tissue-formations, capable of localized or general propagation in the body, and characterized mainly by their tendency to early disintegration.

16. Until the nature of the virus is known, it is impossible to formulate data concerning the conditions under which the disease arises in subjects free from inherited taint.

Cascara Sagrada for Constipation.—For the past two years I have been making constant use in my practice of the fluid extract of Cascara Sagrada (*Rhamnus Purshiana*) for chronic constipation. It always affords relief in even the most obstinate and inveterate cases, and often seems to effect a permanent cure. My methods of using it are as follows: For persons who do not object to the intense bitter taste of the medicine in plain water, I order a two-ounce bottle of the fluid extract, with directions to begin by taking ten drops in a wineglass of water before each meal. If within two or three days this does not produce a regular natural evacuation every morning, the patient is told to increase the dose by two or three drops every day until the required effect is produced; then to continue with that amount regularly three times a day for a week or ten days. At the expiration of this time, I advise that the dose be decreased again by taking one drop less every day, until it is reduced to nothing. Then, if the habit of soliciting a movement punctually at a regular time every morning is kept up, there is usually no more difficulty. In many cases the initial dose of ten drops three times a day is quite sufficient. Occasionally it is found too much, and five or six drops answers every purpose. In the more obstinate cases, however,—cases of patients who have accustomed themselves to take three or four compound cathartic pills, or some harsher quack concoction, every few weeks or days, "to keep their liver acting,"—the bowels sometimes require half a teaspoonful, and in rare instances even teaspoonful doses, three times a day to bring about regular alvine evacuaticns. Taken in this way before meals this medicine acts as a tonic to the stomach, increasing the appetite and improving the digestion, at the same time that it strengthens the peristaltic movements of the intestines and apparently stimulates the normal functions of the liver. But the cascara is one of the bitterest of medicines, and many persons, especially ladies and children, cannot take it unless it is first well disguised by elixirs, etc. For the benefit of these I have been accustomed to compound it as follows :—

℞	Ext. Cascara Sagrada, - - - -	f℥vj.	
	Glycerinæ, - - - - - - - -	f℥j.	
	Curacoa, - - - - - - - - -	f℥ij.	
	Syr. Glycyrrhiz. ad - - - - -	f℥vi.	M.

A teaspoonful of this mixture, which is comparatively palatable, will represent about ten drops of the cascara ; and a tablespoonful will represent half a teaspoonful of the same, which is usually all that the worst cases require, taking it three times a day. A solid extract of the same drug is now prepared, so that it can be ordered in proportionate doses in pill form for those who prefer pills to potions. These cascara preparations seem to me to act even better than the famous dinner pill, and other aloetic pills which have been so much in vogue for two generations at least. One thing is certain, they accomplish the purpose of a laxative most admirably, and usually—though not in every case—the dose can be diminished or even omitted altogether after a time, while other laxatives nearly always lose their effect, larger and larger doses becoming necessary.—*Dr. Boardman Reed in Medical Bulletin.*

Acute Follicular Tonsillitis.—Dr. M. Prince (*Boston Med. & Surg. Journal*, Feb. 2, 1882) discusses in an extended paper the question whether acute follicular tonsillitis is not at times a constitutional disease, and comes to the following conclusions : 1st, There is no constant relation between the local inflammation and the constitutional symptoms. 2nd, There is no constant relation between the local inflammation and the height of the fever. 3rd, There is no constant relation between the height of the fever and the remaining constitutional symptoms. 4th, The fever is often so high as to be far out of proportion to the local symptoms, which may be slight. 5th, With slight fever and slight local inflammation may co-exist severe constitutional disturbances. 6th, The disease occurs in an epidemic form when it is undoubtedly constitutional. 7th, There are strong, though not conclusive, reasons for believing it to be more or less infectious. 8th, The frequency with which it occurs in hospitals is such as to be best explained on the theory of a septic action on the system. 9th, It is probably often mistaken for diphtheria, from which it differs greatly in its course and symptoms. While Dr. Prince does not claim that every case of catarrhal sore throat is a constitutional affection, he claims that there is good reason to believe that there is a very frequent form of sore throat in which the follicles and mucous membrane of the tonsils are chiefly involved, which is the localized expression of an essential fever which has not been generally recognized.—*Chicago Med. Review.*

Mackenzie on the use of the Œsophagoscope.—The author's œsophagoscope (*Med. Times and Gazette*, July 16, 1881) is a skeleton speculum, which only assumes a tubular shape after introduction, by flexion of the instrument on the handle. To the upper end of the speculum is attached a laryngeal mirror. In fifty cases in which it was tried, the author succeeded in using it thirty-seven times. He relates three cases in which the instrument was of service in treatment. In the first, the author saw a ragged projecting growth in the gullet, about three inches below the cricoid cartilage, and removed a piece about the size of a cherry, which, on examination, was found to be of epitheliomatous character. The patient lived six months after the operation, which the author considers to have prolonged life for four or five months. Case two presented an oval semi-transparent polypus, about the size of a white currant, on the right side of the gullet, one inch below the cricoid cartilage. Complete recovery from the dysphagia ensued on removal of the growth. In case three, a flat lamella of bone, about four millimetres square, was seen about two inches below the cricoid cartilage, on the anterior wall of the œsophagus. It was removed with forceps, and complete recovery resulted.—*Lond. Med. Record.*

Nocturnal Incontinence of Urine in Children.—Few practitioners escape the care of frequent cases of children's nocturnal incontinence. It is one of the least dangerous, but at the same time one of the most annoying and persistent disorders of childhood, and any help we may get of a practical sort, especially in the way of prevention, will be welcome to our readers. A recent paper read before the Harveian Society by Dr. Tom Robinson has two homely hints that are of value, and to which we desire to call attention. "There is no doubt," he says, "that nurses and mothers are frequently to blame for this troublesome vice. Young children ought to be taken out of bed during the night and placed on a chamber, so as to excite their bladders to act." And again, "Fear will frequently prevent young people from rising in the dark to relieve themselves." If we instruct our patients to take up their children when they go to bed themselves, we shall do much, even in quite young children, to arrest the natural incontinence of infancy. And no parent should allow children to sleep without a dim but sufficient light, not only that they may readily find the chamber, or the water-closet, but that in case of fire or sudden illness darkness may not add its unknown terrors as a hindrance to their seeking aid, or the means of escape. If they sleep at a distance, or in different stories, the halls also should be lighted. —*Medical News.*

Do Pet Animals Communicate Contagious Diseases.—Dr. Wm. Bunce, of Oberlin, O., sends us a report of the following cases in support of the theory that pet animals may be the means of spreading fatal diseases. On May 1, 1881, he was called to see a boy 4 years old, of German

Nelson, W. M., Montreal, Q.
Phippen, S. S. C., Parkhill, Ont.
Porteous, Wm., Pembroke, Ont.
Renner, W. Scott, Jordan Station, O.
Ross, W. K., Goderich, Ont.
Rowell, Geo. B., Abbotsford. Q.
Smith, E. H., Prescott, Ont.
Smyth, Herbert E., Worcester, Mass.
Walker, Felix D., Launching, P.E.I.
Wilson, S. F., M.A., Springfield, N.B.
Wood, E. S., Faribault, Minn.

The following gentlemen, 27 in number, have fulfilled all the requirements to entitle them to the degree of M.D., C.M., from the University. These exercises consist in examinations, both written and oral, on the following subjects: Principles and Practice of Surgery, Theory and Practice of Medicine, Obstetrics and Diseases of Women and Children, Medical Jurisprudence and Hygiene; and also Clinical Examinations in Medicine and Surgery conducted at the bedside in the Hospital:—

Brown, Chas. O., Lawrenceville, Q.
Burland, Benj. W., Port Kent, N.Y.
Campbell, Lorne, Montreal, Q.
Cattanach, A. M., Dalhousie Mills, O.
Christie, Edmund, Lachute, Q.
Cousins, W. C., Ottawa, Ont.
Derby, W. J., North Plantagenet, O.
Duncan, W. T., Granby, Q.
Dunlop, H. A., Pembroke, O.
Dawson, R., B.A. (McGill), Montreal.
Gale, Hugh, Elora, Ont.
Grant, J. A., B.A. (Queen's), Ottawa.
Howard, Robt. J. B., B.A. (McGill), Montreal, Q.
Hurdman, B. F. W., Aylmer, Q.
Klock, R. F., Aylmer, Q.
McCorkill, R. K. C., Montreal, Q.
McDonald, A. R, Trinity, Texas.
McLean, T. N., Perth, Ont.
Musgrove, W. J., West Winchester, O.
Ogden, H. V., B. A. (Trinity), St. Catharines, O.
O'Brien, T. J. P., Worcester, Mass.
O'Keefe, Henry, Lindsay, Ont.
Rutherford, Clarendon, M.A. (Union), Waddington, N.Y.
Shaw, Alex., Seaforth, Ont.
Smith, E. W., A.B. (Yale), West Meriden, Conn.
Thompson, W. E., Harbor Grace, Nfld.
Thornton, H. W., B. A. (McGill), Montreal, Q.

Messrs. Howard and Campbell, natives of the Province of Quebec, have fulfilled all the requirements for graduation, but await the completion of four years from the date of passing the matriculation of the Provincial Board before receiving the degree. Mr. A. D. Struthers, who passed his examination last session, received his degree on this occasion.

The following have passed in Chemistry:—

Allan, J. H. B., Montreal, Q.
Barrett, Joseph, Prescott, Ont.
Cameron, D. A., Strathroy, Ont.
Doherty, W. W., Kingston, N.B.
Ferguson, W. A., B.A. (McGill), Richibucto, N.B.
Hallett, E. O., Truro, N.S.
Hutchison, J. A., Goderich, Ont.

Johnson, Charles H., Almonte, Ont.
Jolliffe, J. H., B.A., Cincinnati, Ohio.
Klock, W. H., Aylmer, Q.
Landor, T. J., London, Ont.
McClure, J., B.A. (McGill), ——
McKenzie, J. T., Plainfield, O.
O'Brien, T., Brudenell, O.
Ruttan, R. F., B.A. (Tor.), Napanee, O.
Sharp, J. C., Sussex, N.B.
Shibley, J. L., B.A. (Victoria), Yarker, O.
Shirriff, G. R., Huntingdon, Q.

The following have passed in Anatomy:—

Fairbanks, Chas. S., Oshawa, O.
Hutchison, J. A., Goderich, O.
Johnson, Chas. H., Almonte, O.
Jolliffe, J. H., B.A., Cincinnati, Ohio.
Landor, T. J., London, O.
McKenzie, J. T., Plainfield, O.
Park, James. Newcastle, N.B.
Sharp, J. C., Sussex, N.B.
Shirriff, G. R., Huntingdon, Q.
Smith, W. A., Montreal, Q.

The following have passed in Practical Anatomy:—

McKenzie, J. T., Plainfield, O.
O'Brien, T., Brudenell, O.

The following in Institutes of Medicine:—

Doherty, W. W., Kingston, N.B.
Fairbanks, Charles S., Oshawa, O.
Hutchison, J. A., Goderich, O.
Landor, T. J., London, O.
McKenzie, J. T., Plainfield, O.
O'Brien, T., Brudenell, O.
Sharp, J. C., Sussex, N.B.

The following have passed in Materia Medica:—

Landor, T. H., London, O.
Park, James, Newcastle, N.B.
Ross, L. D., Montreal, Q.
Sharp, J. C., Sussex, N.B.
Shirriff, G. R., Huntingdon, Q.
Smith, W. A., Montreal, Q.
Cameron, D. A., Strathroy, O.
Doherty, W. W., Kingston, N.B.
Fairbanks, Chas. S., Oshawa, O.
Ferguson, W. A., B.A., Richibucto, N.B.
Haldimand, A. W., Montreal, Q.
Johnson, C. H., Almonte, O.

The following have passed in Botany:—

CLASS I.—Wood (Prize), Harkin, Armitage, McMeekin, McGannon, Trapnell, and Irvine.

CLASS II.—Browning, Osborne, Robertson, McMillan (D. L.), Eberts, Hallett; Wilson, Hardman and Palmer (equal); Daly, Gustin, Baird; Carruthers and McLennan (equal); Johnson.

CLASS III.—Groves, Arthur, Hanna, Cattanach, McDonald (A. L.), McMillan (S. A.), Shaw, Brown, McDonald (H. J.), Corsan, Platt, Craig, Aylen, Erskine, Lynskey, McConnel, Cassidy, Dasé, Powell.

MEDALS, PRIZES AND HONORS.

The Holmes Gold Medal for the best examination in the Primary and Final Branches was awarded to R. J. B. Howard, B.A., Montreal.

The prize for the best final examination was awarded to H. V. Ogden, B.A., of St. Catharines, Ont.

The prize for the best primary examination was awarded to George A. Graham, of Hamilton, Ont.

The Sutherland Gold Medal was awarded to W. G. Johnston, of Sherbrooke, Q.

The Morrice Scholarship in Physiology was awarded to Wyatt G. Johnston, of Sherbrooke, Q.

The following gentlemen, arranged in the order of merit, deserve honorable mention:—

In the Final Examination—H. V. Ogden, B.A.; H. W. Thornton, B.A.; Rankin Dawson, B.A.; E. Christie, Alex. Shaw, and W. T. Duncan.

In the Primary Examination—G. Carruthers, G. B. Rowell, C. E. Gooding, W. G. Johnston, F. D. Walker, E. J. Elderkin, Alex. McNeill, W. G. Henry, and Arch. McLeod, B.A.

PROFESSOR'S PRIZES.

Botany—First prize, Edwin G. Wood, of Londesboro, O.

For the best collection of Plants—W. W. Doherty, of Kingston, N.B.

Practical Anatomy—Demonstrator's Prize, awarded to Geo. Carruthers, of Charlottetown, P.E.I., who was closely pressed by Charles E. Gooding, of Barbadoes.

MEDICAL FACULTY OF BISHOP'S COLLEGE.

The examinations in Medicine took place towards the end of last month.

The following gentlemen have passed the Primary Examination in Anatomy, Materia Medica, Physiology, Chemistry, Practical Chemistry and Practical Anatomy:—J. B. Saunders, Montreal, Q., first-class honors and Dr. David Scholarship (for highest number of marks in the primary branches); J. A. Caswell, Digby, N.S., first class honors; G. A. Balcom, Campbelltown, N.B.; E. Sirois, Montreal, Q., second class honors; W. D. M. Bell, New Edinburgh, O.; W. Pendergast, Montreal, Q.

The following gentlemen have passed the Final Examination

for degrees of C.M., M.D., in Practice of Medicine, Surgery and Obstetrics, Pathology, Medical Jurisprudence, Clinical Medicine and Clinical Surgery:—Heber Bishop, B.A., Marbleton, Q., first class honors and Wood Gold Medallist, (this medal is awarded to the graduate who has attended at least two six months' sessions at Bishop's College, and at the final examination has obtained the highest number of marks on all the subjects of professional examination); Ninian C. Smilie, Montreal, Q., first class honors and Chancellor's Prize; J. W. Cameron, Montreal, first class honors; Wm. D. M. Bell, New Edinburgh, Ont., and George A. Balcom, Campbelltown, N.B., second class honors; Walter Prendergast, Montreal.

At the special examination in Surgery, held subsequently, the Robert Nelson Gold Medal was awarded to H. Bishop, B.A. This medal (value $60) is presented annually for the best special examination in surgery, written, oral and practical, open to all candidates who have taken first class honors in all the subjects of the final examination, and who have attended at least two six months' sessions at Bishop's College.

In Practical Anatomy, the senior prize was awarded to E. Sirois, and the junior prize to R. C. Blackmer.

The prize in Botany was awarded F. R. England.

The following gentlemen receive honorable mention in the undermentioned subjects:—

Geo. W. Cameron, final examination; J. A. Caswell, primary examination; W. D. M. Bell, Medical Jurisprudence, Materia Medica; G. A. Balcom, Hygiene, Medical Jurisprudence; C. Lafontaine and Ernest Bronsdorph, Botany.

Medical Items.

THE USES OF MALTINE. BY J. K. BAUDUY, M.D.—"In all diseases of general debility, wasting or atrophic affections, and in nearly all varieties of indigestion, maltine is a therapeutic auxiliary, the most valuable I have as yet encountered, and I am daily more and more convinced of its advantages. With the long and very extensive practical experience I have had of its value, I would be at an infinite loss to replace it in my daily practice, now that my confidence in its real merits has been so fully established. As a nutritive tonic I use it exclusively in the place of cod liver oil, and alone or in emulsion with the latter I deem it a most important and therapeutic agent in pulmonary affections, and, as I have said before, in neuralgia, epileptiform complications, many varieties of paralysis, chronic and numerous other neurotic affections, I have found it a most important adjunct when combined with the standard remedies usually administered in such cases. In many perversions of nutrition, such as the atonic and nervous varieties of dyspepsia, maltine has a most happy effect, correcting functional gastric disturbance, improving digestion, promoting assimilation and *rapidly increasing bodily weight."—St. Louis Medical & Surgical Journal.*

A URETHRAL SYRINGE.—We would call the attention of physicians to the "Royal" Excelsior "P" Syringe, advertised in this Journal, which has been received with much favor by the medical profession, and the use of which is now directed in preference to any other Syringe by many eminent specialists. It has four advantages, viz., its greater capacity, its conical point, its ring handle, and the low price at which it is sold. Dr. E. Wigglesworth, of Harvard University, says: "I strongly urge it upon the profession as the best syringe in existence for the treatment of urethritis."

MILK FOOD.—We draw attention to the advertisement of the Anglo-Swiss Milk Food. It is claimed to be superior to any other farinaceous food for infants. As the highest authorities agree in condemning starchy food for young children, the Anglo-Swiss Condensed Milk Co. have overcome this objectionable feature of milk food by meeting an essential requirement in the method of preparing it. The Anglo-Swiss Milk Food is so prepared that when gradually heated with water, according to the directions for use, the starch contained in the materials used is converted, in a satisfactory degree, into soluble and easily digestible dextrine and sugar.

CANADA

MEDICAL & SURGICAL JOURNAL

MAY, 1882.

Original Communications.

THE VOICE IN DIAGNOSIS AND PROGNOSIS.

By T. WESLEY MILLS, M.D., L.R.C.P., Eng.

Assistant to the Professor of Physiology, McGill College; late Clinical Assistant at the Throat and Chest Hospital, London, Eng.

[Read before the Medico-Chirurgical Society of Montreal.]

MR. PRESIDENT AND GENTLEMEN,—While in more recent times the ear of the practitioner of medicine has been called into exercise for the diagnosis of disease in auscultation and percussion in a way and to a degree wholly unknown to a former epoch, it is very much to be doubted whether any very great advances have been made by the use of the sense of hearing outside of the region indicated; as a matter of fact, are we not in considerable danger of overlooking many helps to diagnosis that our ancestors were obliged to rely upon on account of their very imperfections in physical examination? Perhaps every experienced practitioner is guided in forming his opinions unconsciously by the voice of the patient, just as every one cannot but form some conclusions, it may be very vaguely, regarding the moral and intellectual character of those he meets by the qualities of that which we commonly summarize by the term "voice." But there has been, even by writers, very little clear analytical study of this subject as it applies to disease in general. Such study is valuable, inasmuch as it serves to direct the attention of the student, the beginner in medicine, to another field of exploration in our very imperfectly developed science, for, unfortunately for ourselves and our patients, a good deal of our procedure rests as yet on no strictly scientific basis. But in one part of the domain of medicine, during the laryngoscopic period, a good deal has been done in the direction indicated, and to the throat specialist almost entirely the credit of this advance in our knowledge is due. I regret that I have little knowledge of what the voice may teach in disease in general out of the region now referred to—so little, indeed, that I shall make no attempt to speak of it, but hope that the above suggestions may not be fruitless with those whose opportunities for observation in this direction are larger than mine ; I shall therefore call attention in this paper only to the voice as it relates to diseases of the air passages.

The ear, like its neighbour the eye, has a great capacity for discrimination when trained and urged to observation, but it has also an equally marked faculty for neglect, inadvertance. It often acts when roused by the eye to observe, and a physician's diagnosis frequently depends on this latter fact. When the eye has observed an actual lesion, the ear seems to perceive with double distinctness the alteration of voice dependent on the condition present. Sometimes, for example, a pair of enlarged tonsils alters the voice in a moderate degree ; upon opening the patient's mouth, and seeing them, the change seems then of a most decided character. This may be owing in part to psychological laws, but it is largely due to failure to cultivate the ear systematically in observing medical cases. Any one can observe, if he be not deaf, that marked muffling of the voice approaching extinction which is often present in acute tonsillitis, but it requires much more acuteness and discrimination to lead the observer to suspect the existence of a couple of slightly enlarged tonsils, nasopharyngeal growths, or moderate thickening of the nasal mucous membrane ; but such cases frequently occur. The patient may not have noticed it, the friends, even the mother, that acute observer of defects as well as perfections in the offspring, may have failed to observe the difference, so gradual may have been the change ; but none the less surely may that youth, destined for the pulpit, the bar, or the legislative hall, and the daughter with natural beauty, have their prospects diminished and usefulness impaired by what may now be a trifling, but curable, defect in some part of the upper respiratory passages, which also constitute the sounding-board in speech. When such a state of things is established, and permanent organic thickening exists, neither the popular trip to Florida, the south of France, &c., nor a consultation with a distinguished foreign specialist, will either cure the patient or remove from the family physician the blame that attaches to his neglect either to diagnose or have diagnosed for him the affection.

There is a lamentable and pernicious belief widely spread among the laity that nasal catarrh is a trifling affection, a sort of mild nuisance that it would be just as well to have abated, but which is not likely to lead to any serious consequences. Perhaps after it has existed for 5, 10 or 15 years the patient applies for relief, and expects to have it cured with all that readiness the quacks so glibly promise. But no! Nature is too just to herself, and will not be flattered into obliging either the patient or the quack. Parents often fail to seek relief for their children with nasal catarrh, enlarged tonsils, &c., from the belief that they will outgrow them. They may outgrow them, but generally they do not wholly, and more frequently, when they do outgrow the actual catarrh, it is to find that it has left a permanent and undesirable legacy of thickening of parts behind, upon the evils of which the limits of this paper will not allow me to enlarge. Would it not be well for family physicians to examine the nose, mouth and pharynx of the children of a family once or twice a year, even if no special complaint be made? It must be borne in mind, too, that these weaknesses are transmissable to offspring.

Occasionally the physician who sees much of throat and kindred affections is consulted by public speakers with complaint of a certain impairment of the voice. However they may individually express themselves as to the degeneration referred to, it is perceived, on listening to such cases, that the defect is due to obstruction of some kind *above the vocal cords.* Upon examination, the latter may be found nearly or quite healthy, but there is thickening or enlargement in some part of the path the sound takes on its way outward. This may be due to somewhat enlarged tonsils, thickened palatine folds, relaxed velum, or nasal thickening. Or the case may be different: the speaker may have chronic throat affection, severe enough at times to render his duties harassing, if not positively painful; he consults for the case, and the examining physician may be the first to have clearly detected that there is an imperfection of voice which, indeed, others may have felt after a fashion, but could not analytically account for. I have such a case now under treatment. The patient had no distinct notion of having had nasal catarrh; he did not recognize that slight but characteristic lack of resonance which is wholly different from any of the peculiarities of voice produced by affections of the vocal cords; in fact, in this case, the vocal cords were not seriously at fault. The prognosis as to complete recovery of good voice when due to a considerable degree of paresis of the velum, or to much thickening of the nasal mucous membrane, is bad; but by persistent treatment, much improvement may be effected; and what is of great importance in all such cases, the individual may be taught, by a little training, how to use the portion of the sounding-board that remains intact to the greatest advantage. Of course to impart this knowledge successfully implies an accurate and practical knowledge of voice production both in speaking and singing, and some acquaintance with the science and art of music; in fact, without a quick ear and some skill in elocution, possibly also a little ability to sing, it is difficult to understand how a physician can effectually deal with the troubles experienced by public speakers and singers, for very often the cause of the whole matter lies in some faulty use of the voice, and the diagnostician must be enough of a musician and elocutionist to be able to detect the error. If this cannot be made out in the office at the time of consultation, it may be necessary to actually hear the patient during the performance of his functions in public.

Very frequently in diagnosing affections of the vocal cords that are concerned in faulty voice production, it may be necessary to put the patient through a series of vocal gymnastics with the mirror *in situ*, as only then, it may be, will the special weakness be discovered. Fortunately public speakers and singers are generally anxious to co-operate with the practitioner, and have considerable control over the vocal organs. In the case of singers, extreme relaxation of the velum and uvula, or, as perhaps describes it better, paresis of the velum, together with a relaxed, pallid, almost œdematous look of the part, is a more serious matter as regards the voice than has been generally recognized even by specialists. Allow me to illustrate that by a case I have at present under treatment. Mr. ——, a young man following a confining occupation during the day, used the vocal organs excessively during the evening; for many months he sang almost every night, kept very late hours, and indulged beside in various kinds of dissipation. At length he almost lost his voice, and was obliged to desist from singing. For months after his vocal break-down, he felt a distressing aching in the throat after using the voice, even in conversation for a few minutes; and all attempts at singing produced an aggravation of this feeling amounting to actual pain. He has had severe naso-pharyngeal catarrh, and this, I have no doubt, hastened the failure in the larynx; the nasal thickening is considerable. His ordinary conversational tones betray weakness, and close attention discovers the nasal muffling. Upon placing the mirror *in situ*, and asking the patient to phonate, no special failure in the indaptation of the cords is visible, but as he ascends the scale in a singing voice, a certain degree of general weakness of the muscles controlling the cords is apparent; but this is not all, nor in his case the chief cause of his difficulty in voice production, for as he reaches the upper register it becomes apparent that the lagging velum is the chief factor in the difficulty, it failing to rise sufficiently, and, in addition, is too bulky on account of the paresis, and thus spoils the shape of the sounding chamber. What is the prognosis? With reformed habits and appropriate continued treatment, the larynx will regain in all probability most of its lost power, though the muscles are possibly somewhat atrophied. There will be likelihood of relapses, especially as the case is complicated with naso-pharyngeal catarrh. With regard to purity of tone and perfection of resonance in certain notes, less may be expected, as he is not likely to recover wholly from the effects of the nasal thickening. However, youth favours him. In this case the history and the voice suggested in a striking manner what the laryngoscope and rhinoscope revealed.

A reference to two other cases will illustrate another phase of the subject. I am indebted to Dr. Roddick for seeing them in the first instance.

Miss ——, æt 16, came under my observation a few months ago. Her voice attracted my attention at once. To say that it was hoarse very imperfectly described it. In the course of a short conversation it would be now gruffly harsh, then sliding into a high pitch, then again almost merging into a whisper, while occasionally a word was lost altogether; presently a sentence was spoken as well as could be desired; but there was an uncertainty about the action of the larynx that had anything but a soothing effect on the listener. Upon inquiry I found that this condition had existed, with improvements and exacerbations, even total aphonia at times, for two years; the only actual history of injury to the larynx was exposure, during a ride of seven miles on a wintry day while the patient had Measles. Cases of laryngeal weakness after severe attacks of the Exanthems, especially if convalescence has been interfered with by cold, &c., seem frequent, and may be a factor in favouring onsets of hysterical aphonia or weakened utterance. The aphonia in this case occurred when the patient caught a cold. There was a fairly marked hysterical temperament, but this was evidently not quite the usual form of laryngeal hysteria. She had been treated by several physicians, but her throat had never been examined laryngoscopically. The case interested me a good deal. From her peculiarities of voice, I did not expect to find the usual laryngoscopic appearances of hysterical aphonia. There was uncertainty enough in the voice to admit of the existence of a foreign growth in the larynx, though this was rather inconsistent with the fact that she could sing songs of certain range fairly well—in fact, that she could sing better than she could converse. The case proved to be one of a class occurring in hysterical people, viz., *paralysis of the internal tensors*, and the mirror discovered the characteristic *elliptical opening between the vocal cords* when the patient was asked to phonate. Under treatment, especially if naso-pharyngeal catarrh be absent, the prognosis is hopeful, but with this complication there will probably be frequent relapses. Much might be done in these cases, I think, by carefully prescribed vocal exercises. But that imp, *Hysteria*, is very slow to take advice, and seems to find considerable delight in upsetting our best concerted plans. In the present case the said imp nipped everything in the bud, for the patient would undergo no treatment whatever. While conversing with this girl her sister was present, and from her constantly half opened mouth, her obstructed speech, and the weakening of her voice, I was led to make some inquiries. She was of a similar temperament, but to a comparatively slight degree. She had had acute tonsillitis several times, and diphtheria three or four years previously ; she was aware that she had nasal catarrh, and wished treatment. An examination revealed the existence of such nasal obstruction as had caused her to sleep with the mouth open, in consequence of which she was then suffering from *Pharyngitis Sicca.* There was rather imperfect approximation of the vocal cords on phonation, and evident weakness of the muscles governing them. There was a pallor of the pharynx, velum and larynx that pointed to weakness of the parts, and which, in a tubercular subject, would have been very suggestive of approaching *Phthisis Laryngea.* It was extremely interesting to notice the resemblance between this girl's throat and that of her sister. There was the same pallor, the same weakness of muscles, &c. A favourable prognosis was given ; she came under treatment, and the result seemed satisfactory to her, though she lacked that perseverance which is essential to cure in all chronic affections, to which rule those of the throat form no exception. But the so-called Hysterical Aphonia is not to be treated with levity, inasmuch as competent observers have noticed that many such cases have afterwards been attacked with phthisis, and it seems fair to conclude that the throat trouble is only one form of that weakness which leads to such disastrous degeneration afterwards. Here, again, the laryngoscope may paint its warning picture and lead to frequent and careful inquiries, and still more careful examinations of the chest.

Speaking of phthisis, I would beg leave to express a conviction I have in regard to this matter, viz., *that the laryngoscope is not generally used early enough in this disease.* If it be true that a stage of catarrh or a stage of extreme anæmia precedes the formation of tubercles in the larynx, then to discover this is to avert perhaps those ulcerations which lead to such a distressing existence and painful end. It is at the early period, before ulceration is established, that astringent applications may be of service; but to use them, as is often done, when the case is far advanced, has seemed to me to hasten the very condition they are intended to avert.

But there is another interesting class of cases in which the diagnosis is suggested by the voice, and which lie quite out of the domain of hysteria. They are marked by general weakness of voice, failure on prolonged exercise of the function, inability for successful use in the higher register, &c. An examination reveals the fact that while the vocal cords approach each other fairly in one part, they do not do so equally throughout. A case may make the matter plainer. Mr. ——, æt. 59, many years ago—more than twenty—after a day's shouting as an officer at a grand review, lost his voice, and seems to have suffered also from either paralysis or spasm of the pharynx. His voice has remained as I have described above. Upon examination, it is found the cords do not approximate anteriorly. The prognosis in such a case is, at his age, unfavourable, but not hopeless, and in younger persons must, of course, be much better—indeed, may be said to be good.

The connection between disease of the pharynx and that of the larynx, as suggested by the last-mentioned case, but especially so in the case of Granular Pharyngitis in public speakers, as clergymen, is of special interest. It has been noticed that a clergyman, without any actual laryngitis, but with Chronic Pharyngitis, may find himself, after a third service on Sunday, hoarse and even almost aphonic; and it has been suggested that this condition of things is owing to nervous influence leading to incoordination in the action of the laryngeal muscles, causing, in fact, spasm not only of the pharynx, but of the larynx. This explanation is, I believe, correct, and two cases I have under treatment seem to furnish demonstration of it. Both are clergymen in active duty. One has Follicular Pharyngitis well marked; the other relaxed pharynx and bronchial irritation. The first case reports that sometimes when preaching there is a sort of spasm in the throat, as he himself expresses it, by which a single word only, it may be, is lost, strangled as it were. The other expresses it somewhat differently. "I sometimes feel as if I could not get the words out." In both cases there is *spasm of the tensors*. Now, neither of these men suffer from chronic congestion of the cords—in fact, in the first instance, the cords are in good condition. The practical part of the matter is that it must be evident that a granular pharyngitis may be responsible for an amount of irritation that one who had not experienced it himself or given special study to the matter would scarcely credit; it is, in fact, a potent explanation of those break-downs to which clergymen with disordered throats are subject.

A word in regard to the *voice* in that rare affection—rare, at least, in a high degree of development—due to *spasm of the tensors*. The utterance is unlike anything else known. It is, in fact, a sort of stuttering, so that Dr. Prosser James seems to have meant this affection when he described "Stammering of the vocal cords"; but there is this difference: while the stammerer does get out all the words in some fashion, the subject of this spasm loses a great many of them altogether. When in London I heard unexpectedly a preacher with this affection to such a degree that I wondered his auditors could put up with his efforts, for truly the words seemed to play a regular game of "hide-and-seek" with his vocal cords; at first, at least a quarter of them were lost; but during the delivery of the sermon, not so many. This affection is easily recognized by the utterance; but the treatment of bad cases seems to be very unsatisfactory. Except in mild forms of it I have no experience whatever.

Another source of voice impairment, as well as sore throat, arises from adhesions of the pillars, or extensive thickening of them, due either to ulcerative inflammation or the incautious use of caustics; and here permit me to refer to the extensive use of strong caustics, in former years at least, and, it would seem, during the acute stage of tonsillitis and pharyngitis. Such treatment, even with nitrate of silver in strong solution or the solid form, is very apt to entail permanent weakness of the throat, which may even extend in its effects to the larynx. I have seen a subacute laryngitis caused by the application of the nitrate of silver to the pharynx when none of it dropped into the larynx, and in all cases the use of this remedy should be preceded by testing its toleration by touching only a small portion of the diseased part. Dr. Solis Cohen of Philadelphia has made a similar observation.

Another lesson is strongly impressed by a case which forms but one of many. A public speaker lost his voice, or nearly so, and regained it under rest and treatment, the laryngoscope never having been used; he again lost it, and completely, being quite unable to speak except in a whisper. He was treated by several physicians, none of them having seen the vocal cords, till he fell into the hands of the President of this Society, who used the laryngoscope, and having discovered the condition of his larynx, very kindly passed the patient on to me for treatment. This man has a large growth on one of his cords, and may never recover useful voice, but if his condition had been discovered early, a small growth might have proved but a minor matter. Should we not lay down the rule that in all cases of aphonia and all cases of hoarseness or other impairment of voice lasting longer than ten days, the diagnosis should be made by the laryngoscope? And if an ordinary examination does not suffice, let all the skill and care that we can command be brought to bear on the case.

It will be concluded, from the tenor of my paper, that I call attention to alterations of voice chiefly as *suggestive* in the diagnosis. There are cases, however, occurring every now and then in which the diagnosis is difficult, and every help is needful. Let me conclude this paper by illustrating this by a case for which I am indebted to the kindness of Dr. Gurd.

Mr. ——, æt. 39, has had lung affection for some years. Now there is evidence of extensive degeneration in both lungs, high temperature, extreme wasting, &c. The patient has throat affection, with the following characteristics: Ulceration of the velum and between the palatine folds, the patches large, irregular, with no special tendency to bleed; on one side deep sloughs, on the other a dirty grey colour, without such marked excavation. The epiglottis is thickened to two or three times its natural size, and bent over, so that it it is impossible to see the vocal cords well. There is ulceration of the same dirty hue on the pharyngo-laryngeal folds. No history of syphilis can be gained. Is it syphilitic ulceration, is it tuberculous, or is it the one modified by the other? The ulcers are not the lenticular ones occurring on the back of the pharynx, described by Dr. Morell Mackenzie as characteristic of phthisis. If it be tubercular, with such extensive disease of the larynx, why is the voice not more affected? The voice is not absent, nor is there that sense of escape of air so often present in advanced ulceration in phthisis. The voice does not suggest extensive loss of tissue; it is hoarse, very hoarse at times—indeed it suggests the voice of syphilis, which is rancous and obtrusively harsh to a degree unequalled in any other affection. Yet it is difficult to conclude that it is a case of syphilitic ulceration with such extensive lung disease and with no specific history. But the onset of the throat affection was sudden and its progress rapid (5 to 7 weeks), and this is in favour of syphilis rather than phthisis. It is erroneous to draw conclusions from the action of iodide of potassium, for other forms of ulceration are benefited sometimes by it, while occasionally syphilis seems to be made worse. I have not made a positive diagnosis, but state the case to show how voice may assist in the diagnosis, or, at least, make one cautious.

It is scarcely necessary to add that to conclude, because a man has disease of the lungs, that his throat affection is tuberculous; while it may be considered a fair *inference*, cannot be called *diagnosis*.

CLINICAL REMARKS ON CASES OF INHERITED SYPHILIS.*

Delivered in the Summer Session Course, at the General Hospital, April 21st, 1882.

By WILLIAM OSLER, M.D., M.R.C.P., Lond.
Professor of the Institutes of Medicine in McGill University, and Physician to the Montreal General Hospital.

Gentlemen,—In the out-door department and on the surgical side you will have many opportunities of seeing acquired syphilis in its recent forms. The inherited disease presents many manifestations which come under the physician's care, and at the present time I have three examples in my wards which we may study to-day with advantage. And first a word of caution. Do not use the term syphilis before your patients, particularly as in the case just to be brought in of a mother and her child. Many a poor woman has lived in blissful ignorance of the precise nature of her child's affection until an incautious word has suggested to her the cause, and then, for her, "farewell the tranquil mind." We shall use the old term *lues*.

Case I.—M. O., æt. 6 weeks. Admitted on 12th inst., with snuffles and skin eruption. Mother has been married two years; family history good; has no signs of disease; nipples were sore, but not specific; had one miscarriage at 7 months; the father of the child, she says, is healthy (?).

The *child was born healthy*, had no snuffles and no skin trouble; in two weeks began to snuffle; at four weeks spots appeared on the body and about the buttocks; on admission had an eruption on the buttocks, groins, genitals, face and nose. The eruption consisted of irregular blotches, and about the anus some soft mucous patches, and here and there a pustule. The patches were erythematous, and the scrotum also was swollen and sore. About the mouth the skin was rough, raw and red, but no pustules nor papules could be seen; on the arms and hands papules now exist. On the 14th inst. was given gr. ½ Hydrarg. cum Creta, t.i.d., and a piece of mercury ointment about the

* Reported by Mr. C. E. Cameron.

size of a pea was rubbed into the skin at night. Since that time the child has improved; the eruption about the face has faded, leaving a reddish coppery stain; the buttocks have also improved in condition; the nostrils are still stuffed, but not so much as when first seen; no distinct mucous patches are to be seen inside the mouth.

Now, gentlemen, I would ask you to make a careful study of the child. Do not suppose that it is only in hospital practice that you will find these cases; lues is no respecter of persons, and there is no station in life in which you may not expect to meet it.

Within the womb the fœtus may be blighted and abortion occur at the fifth, sixth or seventh month. If it affects the child in utero, as a rule it kills there, and the child is born dead; if not affected in utero, the child is born healthy, and in about two weeks it begins to snuffle, and a rash appears upon the buttocks: there may be also a rash about the mouth, and this may become general. About the buttocks there may be soft, raised, injected spots—mucous patches. The above appearances are characteristic.

To *treat* this condition give mercury, the mercury and chalk powder in gr. ½ doses three times a day, and rub in a little of the mercury ointment every night, or the latter may be spread on the child's flannel roller; or you may give corrosive sublimate, gr. ½ in ℥vi. of water, and of this give ʒi every three or four hours. These cases, as a rule, do well.

Infantile lues may lead to characteristic appearances in the child; the eruption causing fissures about the mouth, which, when healed, leave scars which radiate from the angle of the mouth to the cheek. In the infant before you the present rash is healing, but during the first year there may be occasional skin eruptions, or mucous patches in the mouth. If the child survives the first year the disease usually remains latent, but as puberty is approached again declares itself, as you will see in the next cases to be brought in. Now that the patient has left the room, we may ask the question, Who is responsible for this—the father or the mother? The latter, so far as we can gather, seems healthy; has had no skin eruptions, or throat trouble. The husband is away, and though she says he is healthy, and never had any particular disease which she knows of, I am inclined to think that he is at fault. What about the woman herself? Is she syphilized? Most writers think that a woman who has borne a syphilized child is contaminated in some degree, though showing no positive signs. A strong proof is the fact, that you cannot innoculate her with syphilis. If the child you have just seen were given to a healthy nurse, with its condition of lips, it would give the woman a chancre of the nipple. This is sometimes known as Colles's law.

The next cases illustrate some interesting later manifestations.

CASE II.—Girl, æt. 13, showing severe ulceration of throat.

History.—Mother healthy; no symptoms of lues; father has no evident disease, (?) but is dissipated. This child is the last of seven; several of the others died early, one with blisters; all had stuffed noses; four out of the seven died within the year; one lived to five years and the other to six years. This girl was born healthy, and remained so till two years ago, and then became blind; cured by Dr. Buller; last year got deaf; this also cured; has had sore throat for six months, not much pain, but some difficulty in swallowing.

Present Condition.—Small; well nourished; has not the syphilitic countenance. *Teeth*—Upper central incisors are eroded at the neck, not dwarfed, a little honey-combed, but are not Hutchinson's specific teeth. In the *mouth* nothing is seen on the tongue or cheeks, but in the throat there is extensive disease; the uvula and velum are gone; there is a cicatrix on the posterior wall of the pharynx, linear in direction; the mucous membrane of the right side is much thickened, especially below the orifice of the Eustachian tube; as low as can be seen in the pharynx on the posterior walls are cicatrices with reddish fleshy outgrowths; nothing else noticeable. *Eyes* are apparently clear, but on careful inspection both corneæ are seen to be slightly turbid and hazy. She has had interstitial keratitis, a common affection in secondary syphilis, which comes on usually between the twelfth and sixteenth year, is specific, and if properly treated, generally curable. Secondary acquired lues in man rarely destroys the structures of the throat. In the inherited form the throat affection is apt to be more intense and phagadænic, as in this child. *Ear* trouble is not uncommon in inherited lues. In this instance it may have extended from the pharynx; but middle ear disease may occur with throat complications. In this case the disease in the pharynx is not progressing. She is on potas. iodid., grs. x, t.i.d. To do any good, these cases require early and energetic treatment, as the ulceration is rapid and destructive.

CASE III.—Girl, æt. 23, admitted Feb. 10th with Bright's disease, dropsy of the legs and face. Family history uncertain. This girl presents, as evidences of inherited disease, large tibial nodes, onychia, and a suspicious-looking spot of ulceration on her forehead *Nodes* are, in acquired pox, common on the forehead, clavicle, tibiæ, &c., and are the result of specific periostitis, caused by virus in the blood. They may be absorbed, or go on to the formation of bone. They are also important features in inherited syphilis. Nodes produced in the congenital form differ from those produced in the acquired, inasmuch as they affect more often the bones of the upper and lower extremities, are generally symmetrical, are much larger, and may occur over the whole extent of the bone; they are rarely painful, and often disappear under treatment.

The tibiæ of this girl are enlarged, thickened, and misshapen: almost a uniform node from ankle to knee. The fibula on the left side is thickened, especially about the lower part. I remember, on several occasions, hearing Mr. Hutchinson call attention to the fact that these large nodes were often mistaken for Rickets. I pass around one of his plates illustrating this form of node. *Teeth*—Lower incisors eroded at the root; upper ones well formed, nothing suggestive about them. *Nails* of the thumb, ring and little fingers of right hand are mal-formed, rough, dry, discoloured, scaly, and are typical instances of *Onychia sicca*, or psoriasis of the nails.

You noticed that I examined the teeth of these two cases with special care. I did so because these organs sometimes give valuable or even positive evidence of inherited syphilis. Mr. Jonathan Hutchinson first called attention to this fact, and I have here for your inspection his Plates illustrating the subject. The teeth in case II. would be called by some "specific," but they are not so, and I gladly take this opportunity to impress upon you the characters of the teeth which this profound observer has been led to regard as distinctive. At the Congress last year he complained very justly that men had not sufficiently studied his writings on the subject, and were too apt to regard any malformed teeth as syphilitic. The facts are briefly these: 1, Teeth giving information are the permanent ones. 2, The specific ones are the upper central incisors. 3, Characters are: dwarfed, stunted in length and breadth, and narrower at the cutting edge than at the root. Anterior surface has usually the enamel well-formed and not eroded or honeycombed; the cutting edge presents a single notch, usually shallow, sometimes deep, and in that notch the dentine is exposed.

Other irregular teeth, eroded at the surface, are indications of an early *stomatitis*, an inflammation of the mouth, perhaps from mercury, or associated with convulsions.

Children who have been the subject of syphilis frequently grow with a very characteristic physiognomy, recognizable at a glance. The following are chief points in a *Syphilitic countenance:* 1, forehead prominent, especially the frontal eminences; 2, saddle-nose, bridge being defective, owing to early coryza and inflammation; 3, often striated lines from corners of mouth, and the skin is colourless and muddy.

CASE OF CEREBRO-SPINAL MENINGITIS.

BY G. W. MAJOR, B.A., M.D.

May H., aged 13 years, born prematurely, of a delicate and highly nervous nature, lived five years in India, where she contracted malarial fever of a severe type, and was, in consequence, sent to this country. On the 17th ult., showed symptoms of slight coryza, and was kept in the house. On the 18th and 19th she seemed in her usual health, appetite unimpaired, and spirits remarkably good. On the 19th, retired at 9 p.m. On the following morning (20th), I saw her for the first time, and found her condition as follows: Complained of severe pain in the head, of a neuralgic character; pulse 120; temperature 102°F.; skin very dry. Child lying quietly; pupils dilated, but contracting to light; and in rather a stupid sleep, but easily roused. Intense intolerance of light. Temper very irritable and rebellious, constantly refusing to take her medicine, which was a mixture of Pot. Chor., Tr. Aconit. and Ammon. Acet. Condition remained much the same during the day and early evening. Later the pain in the head became greatly aggravated, and vomiting occurred at intervals of an hour or two.

21st—Vomiting still continues; temperature 103°F.; pulse 120. Headache still more severe in type. Skin now moist. Creeping pain in spine, and slight tendency to contraction of muscles. Child declared to be in a dangerous condition. Bromide ordered. Rebelled against all medicine, but would take nourishment in small quantities.

22nd—Made an early visit; found child lying on her side, her body curled up. On attempting to turn her on her back, complete opisthotonos ensued, giving rise to great agony; temperature 103°F.; pulse 140, but varying from 120 to 170 at very short intervals. Dr. Fenwick saw her with me at noon, and ordered ergot in addition to the bromides. Child was now constantly drawn up in opisthotonos. A hypodermic of ⅓ gr. morphia at 7 p.m. gave relief and sleep for seven hours; it was again repeated at 2 a.m., with but partial success; at 6 a.m., another, but with no result. At noon Dr. F. ordered chloral hydrat. by the bowel; the first dose was successful, and gave relief for four hours, when a second was administered.

23rd, 5 a.m.—Child suffering great agony; ordered chloroform to be administered, which was kept up until 3 a.m. on the 24th, when death ensued.

Nutritive enemata were in use from the 21st, and were well retained. Vomiting was only a symptom for 24 hours. Constipation was marked. On the 21st, an enema of turpentine and castor oil produced a large evacuation. The urine was voided constantly and involuntarily from the afternoon of the 21st.

During the illness the child was obstinate and rebellious, contrary to her usual custom. Three weeks before she would suddenly jerk the hand across from her mouth on taking food, and would raise the elbows to a level with the chin.

The autopsy, by Dr. Osler, revealed the following conditions: The *brain* contained an excessive amount of blood; the dural sinuses and all the veins and arteries were engorged. Some of the veins of the pia were as large as quills; the blood in them was clotted. At the base, there was exudation about the chiasma and inner parts of Sylvian fissures; none on pons or medulla. No lymph in the course of the middle cerebral arteries, which, with the strio-lenticular vessels, were removed and carefully searched for small tubercles, but without positive result. On the surface, much lymph beneath the arachnoid on either side of the longitudinal fissure, more on the right hemisphere, where it covered the hinder end of 1st frontal, the upper parts of asc. parietal, asc. frontal, and the superior parietal lobules. On the left side it was less extensive. Moderate serous exudation in the ventricles; walls not softened; fornix and septum firm; velum and choroid plexuses intensely congested. *Spinal cord*—Vertebral veins engorged. Vessels of the pia deeply congested, the entire membrane reddish in colour in anterior aspect. On posterior surface, from the cervical enlargement to the cauda equina, a thick layer of fibrino-purulent exudation extended beneath the arachnoid, producing, at spots, irregular bulgings. It was creamy, greyish-yellow in colour, and in places ensheathed the posterior roots. There were no tubercles. *Lungs* healthy, no caseous masses; no miliary tubercles. *Heart* contained clotted blood; abdominal viscera normal.

SKIN DISEASES AT THE MONTREAL DISPENSARY.

UNDER THE CARE OF R. L. MACDONNELL, B.A., M.D., M.R.C.S., ENG.

During the last few months the cases of skin disease treated at this institution have been numerous, and many of them being of interest, I venture to place upon record a selection of them in the pages of the CANADA MEDICAL AND SURGICAL JOURNAL.

Syphilitic Skin Diseases.—Should we treat primary syphilis by mercury, or should we wait for secondary symptoms? Of the benefit of the former plan I have not a doubt, and have always given the antidote as soon as there was the least uncertainty in my mind as to the purely local character of the sore. Here, then, are the notes of two cases—the husband treated with mercurials, the wife let alone until the secondary stage.

L. L., an ice-cutter, æt. 30, presented himself on the 27th January, 1881, with a remarkably well defined hard chancre on the glans penis. Protiodide of mercury was given at once, and has been taken faithfully until a few weeks ago. About four weeks after the appearance of the chancre there was a papular rash upon the trunk. This disappeared in less than a week. It was noted on the 12th Feb., 1881, that, with the exception of slight induration at the seat of chancre, and some few brown stains upon his skin, there was no trace of the disease. He had been warned to avoid giving the disease to his wife, but in spite of this, when he returned on the 26th March the thin cicatricial covering of the chancre was found abraded. On the 27th July, his wife, a healthy young woman, came to the Dispensary and told me that in the beginning of April—*i.e.*, four weeks after the abrasion above mentioned—she had a chancre about the vulva, and for the last two months had an eruption, with sore throat. The skin of the trunk, arms and legs was covered with an cothymatous eruption. In this case the poison had a three months start of its antidote, consequently it was a much more difficult one to manage than that of the man. Until August 24th the eruption did not improve. At date (Feb. 24th, 1882,) the body is covered with the brown stains of the disease. Mrs. L. also suffered from sore throat and from falling out of the hair.

In the next two cases no history could be obtained.

A girl æt. 16, who was anæmic, and whose menses had not yet appeared, showed me a periosteal node upon the left tibia which had come on a few weeks ago, and which was very painful. On the inner side of the left knee there was a round ulcer, the size of a sixpenny piece There was another upon the abdomen, and two or three symmetrical scars upon the legs. These ulcers, she told me, had been coming and going for years. The presumptive proofs of syphilis were: 1st, the presence of brownish scars, produced by sores which occurred without any such cause as burns, injuries or bed-sores; 2nd, the number of the ulcers; 3rd, their site; 4th, the colour of the scars. After a short course of iodide of potash and iron, the ulcers healed rapidly and the nodes disappeared.

An unmarried woman, who gave her age as 40, but whose appearance implied greater antiquity, came to the Dispensary on the 12th Oct., 1881. Twelve years ago there was a sudden suppression of the menses, followed by neuralgia and headache. About the same time an eruption appeared upon the side of the nose and upon the right cheek, which went on to ulceration. Denies syphilis. All these years she had been under treatment more or less, but the disease steadily advanced. She was in two hospitals, and in one she had been put under ether and burnt with the actual cautery four times. On the 12th October she presented the following appearance: On the left cheek there were three large ulcers, covered with greenish-black crusts, while the rest of that side of the face, the forehead, the top and right side of the scalp was one large unsightly cicatrix. Above and behind the left ear there was a large ulcer, discharging most fetid pus. The hair was almost all gone. Complained of pains in the head, worse at night. She told me that she had never had any internal treatment. Prescribed 15 grains of iodide of potash, to be taken three times a day. No local treatment beyond the use of soap and a weak carbolic lotion. She began to improve immediately, and in six weeks all ulcers had healed. At present there remains but a slight ectropion of left lower lid, the result of the contraction of a cicatrix upon the cheek.

A case came under Dr. Shepherd's care, showing how easily syphilis may be simulated. A hysterical girl, about 16 years old, who had been taking iodide of potassium for a year, came to the Dispensary to get more of this costly medicine. She had an ulcer on the leg, and had enlarged post-cervical glands. After the application of a parasiticide ointment the glands resumed their normal size. The ulcer proved hard to heal, and it was thought it was irritated by the girl herself. She went to the Montreal General Hospital, where it healed eventually.

Psoriasis.—Several cases of psoriasis have been under treatment at the Dispensary lately. Under all circumstances a difficult disease to manage, it is especially so in out-door practice, owing to the lack of perseverence on the part of the patients and the irregularity of their attendance. For cases of this kind, an ointment of 20 grains of chrysophanic acid to an ounce of lard has been found useful; but the frequent recurrence of the disease convinces me that we have not yet found a remedy to thoroughly control it. Here is a case in point.

Mrs. B., æt. 38, came to the Dispensary on the 21st Sept., 1878. Psoriasis in patches about both elbows, both knees, chest, back, and at the root of the hair. No history of syphilis. No syphilitic scars. General health excellent. Began using a 20-grain ointment on the 27th September, taking care to apply it to but one or two patches at a time. The improvement was rapid. In January, 1879, she told me that she had gone on using the ointment for two months, until all the skin was clear. In July, 1879, she reappeared at the Dispensary, with the psoriasis as bad as ever. Towards the end of the month she was again better, and I lost sight of her until October, 1881. The disease extended over more than one-half the scalp and forehead. The 20-grain ointment was again applied, and in a month she was well again.

This case illustrates the fact that the ointment is certainly effective, but that it has no power in preventing a recurrence. The disease in this case might probably have been eradicated had she been treated during the intervals with arsenic and other tonics, and had she been able to keep her hands and arms, where the eruption began, out of soap-suds and water. In the other cases of psoriasis met with at the Dispensary, the 20 or 30-grain ointment has been successful in restoring the healthy action of the skin. I have found it always a trouble to get the patients to report themselves. As soon as slight relief is afforded they never come near the place again.

An obstinate case of psoriasis is at present under treatment. Chrysophanic ointment (30 grains to the ounce of lard) having caused much irritation and done little good, I applied a 20-grain to the ounce ointment of pyrogallic acid with very good effect.

It caused less redness, and the skin is clearing up, patch after patch.

Herpes Zoster affecting the Superficial Cervical Plexus.—(In private practice.)—A young lady, aged 20, of very nervous temperament, complained, on the 16th April, of pain in the right side of the neck, under the occipital bone, and thought that she had an ordinary stiff neck. On the following day the pain was much more severe, and a crop of vesicles appeared, dotted along the course of the nerves forming ascending division of the superficial cervical plexus. Several vesicles extended along the course of the occipitalis minor, and behind the ear the skin was red and hot, and exquisitely tender on pressure. Around the neck there was a half collar, formed by three or four large blisters. The pain preceding the eruption of herpes was very great, and to procure sleep a quarter of a grain of morphia had to be given for three nights in succession.

BI-MONTHLY RETROSPECT OF OBSTETRICS AND GYNÆCOLOGY.

PREPARED BY WM. GARDNER, M.D.,

Prof. Medical Jurisprudence and Hygiene, McGill University; Attending Physician to the University Dispensary for Diseases of Women; Physician to the Out-Patient Department, Montreal General Hospital.

Nitro-Glycerine in Puerperal Convulsions.—W. E. Green, M.R.C.S. of the Isle of Wight, reports a case of puerperal convulsions in which this remedy was administered with apparently most satisfactory results. The uterus was empty, the convulsions had ceased, but unconsciousness remained, the pulse was quick and of high tension, the face and eyelids puffy, the legs œdematous, the feet cold, and the urine highly albuminous. There was a history of scanty urine and anasarca for months previous. A mixture containing eight minims of a solution of nitro-glycerine (1 per cent.) in an ounce of water was precribed, with instructions to give a teaspoonful every hour. The first dose was given to the patient two hours and a half after the commencement of the attack, the coma at that time being as profound as at any time. Within ten minutes of taking it, she regained perfect consciousness, and asked questions about her confinement and child, of which till then, she had been oblivious. Four or five doses were given; the pulse was then soft and quiet. Recovery was tedious; it was necessary to wean the child, and it was six weeks before albumen completely disappeared from the urine. Mr. Green was induced to use nitro-glycerine in this case from the marked evidences of arterial tension, as indicated in the pulse and by the cold extremities. These and other symptoms pointed to the case as identical with uræmic convulsions, in which nitrite of amyl and bleeding are both beneficial, the effects of the amyl being, however, apt to be transitory. The value of nitro-glycerine in angina pectoris has been pointed out by Dr. Brunton and Mr. Wm. Murrell. Experience of the value of the remedy in reducing arterial tension and of its power of keeping up the effect determined Mr. Green to use it when he met with a case of uræmic convulsions, and by it to bleed the patient as it were into his own blood vessels by dilating them. The rapid recovery of consciousness in the case related appeared to verify the theory and justify the practice.—(*Brit. Med. Jour.*, April 22, 1882.)

Treatment of Cancer of the Uterus, by W. H. Baker, M.D., Instructor in Gynæcology, Harvard University, Boston.—The author of this paper is much in favor of the early, complete, and repeated (if necessary) removal of malignant disease of the uterus. In this he is only in accord with nearly all the leading gynæcologists of the present day. The method of operation which he follows and which he believes to be superior to any which he has seen described, does not differ very much from parts of other operations, but he believes unites the advantages of several, and discards objectionable or unimportant features. He divides operative cases into two classes:—1st. Those where the disease is limited to parts which can be entirely removed; these are cases in which cure or long respite may be reasonably hoped for. 2nd. Where the disease has so infiltrated the parts about the uterus that it is impossible to remove more than its superficial and most vascular portions, as a relief from hemorrhages or sloughing tissue, with its offensiveness and deleterious septic influence. In a suitable case of the first class, when the disease is limited to the cervix, the patient being in the Sims' position, the cervix is seized with the vulsellum forceps and dragged as nearly to the outlet as possible. The portio vaginatis is then cut into anteriorly with the scissors, and the supra-vaginal cervix anteriorly is separated from the bladder with the scissors and tearing with the forefingers. This part is similar to Schrœder's method for the removal of the uterus by the vagina. The same incision is then made into the vagina posteriorly, and the supra-vaginal cervix separated from the peritoneum up to the level of the internal os uteri. The peritoneum is not purposely opened as in Schrœder's method, but it is accidentally cut into at times during the operation. The anterior and posterior incisions are now connected with lateral ones, and the supra-vaginal cervix separated on the sides in the same manner as was done in front and behind. The uterotome is now substituted for the scissors and a funnel-shaped portion of the body of the uterus cut out. In this procedure there is a resemblance to Sims', but it differs in that the base of the cone-shaped portion to be removed is situated at the level of the internal os uteri at the junction of the peritoneum to the body of the uterus, both before and behind, and the apex of the cone extends nearly or quite to the fundus of the uterus. It is thus possible to remove more of the uterus than by Sims' method. The entire cervix, both infra and supra-vaginal, and the same time nearly or quite one-half—the most important half of the body of the uterus is removed. This method secures removal of the glandular structure, which is first affected in cancer of the body of the uterus, whether of primary origin or the result of extension from the cervix. If the vaginal tissues either anteriorly or posteriorly be involved they are to be cut through into the peritoneum or bladder, as the case may be, if necessary, and removed, the edges being brought together by sutures of silver wire, thus closing the opening into the peritoneum or vesical fistula thus created. The patient is to be kept in bed for two weeks, kept on a nourishing liquid diet, and protected from distension of rectum or bladder, and guarded from any efforts at straining. After convalescence monthly examination of the parts for several years should be practised. If any outgrowths appear, they are to be removed with the cutting curette, and the base seared with the thermo-cautery. Dr. Baker has seen no advantage from the administration of arsenic as recommended by Sims, Goodell and others. Chian turpentine did no good.

In the second class of cases the curette, followed by the thermo-cautery, is recommended and used by Dr. Baker. During four years he has treated 47 cases of uterine cancer. Of these 12 were operated on with the hope of entire removal; of these 9 are living, 7 are well at periods of 29, 27, 22, 21, 18 and 11 months respectively after the operation. Of the three who died, one was unwilling to follow up the treatment, which promised as much for her as for the others who survive. Of the thirty-five remaining cases, ten were operated on to ameliorate the symptoms. In one of the cases, by repetition of the operation three times at intervals of some months, the patient lived three years and five months, and was kept free from many of the sufferings which make life with this disease so intolerable. Of the remaining 9, 6 lived 18, 10, 9, 8, 7 and 6 months respectively; 2 are still living after 12 and 8 months; the remaining one was discharged from hospital four months after the operation, and has not been heard of since.—(*American Journal of Obstetrics*, April, 1882.)

Hospital Reports.

Medical and Surgical Cases Occurring in the Practice of the Montreal General Hospital.

MEDICAL CASE UNDER CARE OF DR. MOLSON.

Case of Sarcoma of the Jejunum—(Reported by Dr. J. A. MacDonald, House Physician.)

J. B. B., French-Canadian, aged 41, plasterer, admitted into Hospital March 4th, 1882, to be treated for general dropsy; says he was a healthy man till present trouble began. Six months ago, after exposure to cold, had general pains in body and an attack of vomiting, with constipated bowels; was better in three or four days, and attended to his work as usual. No headache, and noticed nothing peculiar about his urine. From this time till eight weeks ago went about his work, but every two or three weeks would have an attack of vomiting, lasting three or four days. Bowels were very constipated. Appetite poor, and patient lost flesh slowly. All this time he did not suffer from headaches, and noticed nothing wrong with urine. No disturbance of vision. Eight weeks ago abdomen began to swell rapidly, followed in a few days by great swelling of feet, legs, arms and face, and says that at this time urine was scanty and high-coloured, but without blood. He now suffered constantly from headaches. Constipation continued, but bowels would act with a purgative ; vomiting frequent, but not constant, and without reference to food. For the last two weeks has suffered greatly from shortness of breath. Since his trouble began, six months ago, would have occasional attacks of chilly feeling, followed by feeling of heat ; this always occurred toward night.

On admission, patient so weak that he cannot sit up in bed, and is evidently dying. Temperature 101°F. ; pulse very weak, 120 ; respirations 40. Is a large, pale, cachectic-looking man. Arms, face, trunk and legs very œdematous. Abdomen full, dullness in both flanks ; cannot palpate on account of the thickness of the walls with the anasarca. Large bubbling râles over front of both lungs ; cannot examine back. Heart sounds scarcely audible. In 24 hours, passed 75 ozs. urine, which contains a very small trace of albumen, very little deposit, and no casts. Skin acting freely. To have Infus. Digitalis, Liq. Am. Acet. āā ℥ss, 4 q.h. From the time of his admission till his death, March 8, nothing special to note. Temperature from 99°F. in the morning to 101°F. in the evening.

Autopsy by Dr. Osler.—General anasarca ; left arm more swollen than the right. Abdomen protruberant ; when opened coils of intestines matted together by tolerably firm, but separable adhesions ; a large mass filled the left half of the cavity, from the ribs to the crest of the ilium. The omentum was closely adherent to it, as were also several coils of the small bowel and the descending colon. It was readily peeled out of its bed ; the left kidney was firmly attached to it behind, and the colon and sigmoid flexure to the left border. On dissection, the tumour proved to be an enormous growth, involving about 18 inches of the jejunum, which tunnelled the mass in a curved direction. The walls of the gut were infiltrated with the neoplasm, being in places 6 to 8 inches in thickness, of a greyish-white colour, and firm. The lumen was expanded and the mucosa represented by blunt valvulæ conniventes; about the centre of the canal there was a transverse depressed ulcer almost encircling the tube. There was a large ischio-rectal abscess, communicating by a round orifice with the upper part of the rectum. The walls of this were much thickened and infiltrated with the new growth. It had no direct contact with the jejunal mass. The *kidneys* were enlarged, and presented innumerable secondary masses. So far as Dr. Osler's examination has gone, he believes it to be a primary large round-celled sarcoma of the jejunum with metastases in kidneys.

MEDICAL CASES UNDER CARE OF DR. OSLER.

Cases of Tubercular Meningitis.—(Reported by Dr. J. A. MacDonald.)

Cases I and II illustrate well the common forms of this affection. Cases III and IV are of interest, from the existence of tubercles—extensive in IV—without special head symptoms.

Case I.—*Chronic Phthisis—Tubercular Meningitis—Cheyne-Stokes Breathing.*—E. S., aged 31, admitted Feb. 3rd, 1882. On admission, complained of cough, shortness of breath, night sweats, and loss of flesh. Gives a well marked history of slowly advancing phthisis. Slight consolidation in left apex; a little more advanced in right. Had an ischio-rectal abscess six months ago; fistula still discharging.

April 1st—Nothing special to note up to this time. For a few days patient has been complaining of headache and lassitude, and now lies in bed all day. Temperature 101°F. Disease in lungs progressing slowly. *13th*—Still complains of headache. *15th*—Patient passed stools and urine in bed last night. To-day the patient is delirious, not noisy or talkative, but as he lies in bed answers questions in a fairly rational manner. He is sullen and contrary; refuses to take his medicine. Abdomen markedly retracted. Temperature 101°F.; pulse 95. *16th*—Drooping of right upper lid to-day. Lies in same condition as yesterday. Passes stools and urine in bed. Occasional long, sighing respirations. *17th*—Patient quite heavy and stupid to-day. Cannot be roused. Eyes examined last night; no neuritis. Marked Cheyne-Stokes respiration. Next day, same condition. Death on the 19th. No autopsy, as body went to the college.

CASE II.—*Basilar Meningitis.*—S. M. F., aged 4½ years, admitted to Hospital April 24th, 1882, in a perfectly unconscious condition. Lies with eyes wide open, face turned towards left. Breathing quietly and regularly, 25 to the minute. Temperature 99°F.; pulse 120. Child is a thin, spare lad, face pale. No evidence of paralysis. Eyes open equally; pupils dilated and equal. Conjunctiva slightly injected. No plantar reflex. On tickling soles of feet, the legs are drawn up very slowly. Hands appear to have much less sensation than legs. Abdomen not retracted. *Tache cerebrale* well marked. Nothing abnormal found in lungs. The following is the only history that can be obtained: Has been ill two weeks; friends could not say what the trouble was. Six days ago, noticed continual tossing of left arm and leg; this lasted three days. Three days ago had a fit, and that morning became unconscious, and has remained so ever since.

April 25th.—Child is much brighter to-day; spoke to the nurse several times. Ptosis of left upper lid. Sighing, irregular respirations. Pulse 130. *26th*—Child became comatose during the night, and died this morning.

Autopsy showed matting and opacity of membranes at the base; not much exudation. Numerous tubercles on arteries of perforated spaces and branches of the middle meningeal. Fluid in ventricles, central softening. Two caseous masses in lungs. No general eruption of miliary tubercles.

CASE III.—*Chronic Phthisis—Tubercles in Occipital Meninges—No head symptoms.*—C. L., æt. 36, admitted into Hospital with well-marked phthisis for the first time, Jan. 16th, 1882, and was discharged unimproved, March 3rd, 1882.

April 23rd.—Patient readmitted into Hospital in a very weak state; had been in fairly good condition for a week after his discharge, when he began to loose flesh rapidly; cough very bad, and expectoration abundant. At present patient is emaciated to an extreme degree; speaks in a low, hoarse whisper, and is unable to swallow on account of the soreness of throat, which has come on in the last two weeks; extensive disease in front of both lungs; large cavity in right mammary region; marked retraction of abdomen, with some tenderness in umbilical region. Mind quite clear; no symptoms of meningeal or brain trouble. Died April 26th, the third day after his admission. Mind remained clear till death. Refused all nourishment on account of the difficulty in swallowing.

At the autopsy an extensive cavity was found in right side, occupying nearly the whole of the upper lobe; smaller one in left apex. No peritoneal tubercles. Mesenteric glands much enlarged. Extensive ulcerations in ileum and cœcum. One ulcer had perforated, and the contents of the gut had passed into the pelvis. In the brain no basilar meningitis; no effusion into the ventricles. The meninges of both occipital lobes on the upper surface a little thickened, and on removing the pia mater from these regions many tubercles were found on the vessels, particularly those in the calcarine fissures; some were as large as peas, and were imbedded in the brain substance.

CASE IV.—*Diarrhœa—Diphtheria—Chronic Tubercle of Brain and Meninges—No head symptoms.*—J. E., æt. 2½, a feeble and emaciated child, admitted with diarrhoea, which had existed for several days, and which improved with treatment. No chest symptoms. On April 8th took diphtheria of severe type. Throat symptoms improved by the 12th, but the child did not rally, and died on the 16th. There had never been any head symptoms further than heaviness and stupidity during the attack of diphtheria.

At the autopsy, brain only examined. No basilar meningitis. On the cortex, vessels full; no lymph, no ventricular effusion or softening. On both hemispheres, in parietal lobes close to the longitudinal fissure, small tubercles adherent to the membranes and imbedded in the substance; none of these were larger than peas. On the inner faces of the hemispheres, occupying the *precuneus* and convolutions of *cuneus*, were numerous coarse tubercles, isolated and in groups. These were most abundant on the right hemisphere, and in the *precuneus* of this side there was a mass the size of a quarter dollar, the membrane adherent to it and thickened.

Reviews and Notices of Books.

The Illustrated Quarterly of Medicine and Surgery.—Edited by GEORGE HENRY FOX, Clinical Professor of Diseases of the Skin, College of Physicians and Surgeons, New York, and FREDERICK R. STURGIS, Professor of Venereal Diseases, Medical Department, University of the City of New York. Vol. I. Nos. I and II. New York: E. B. Treat & Co.

This *American Quarterly* marks quite a new departure in the Medical journalism of the United States; indeed, as far as we know, there is nothing similar to it in any country. The intention is to give illustrations of large size and artistically executed of a great number of important and unique medical and surgical cases, such as are continually presenting themselves to the eminent practitioners of a great city like New York. The idea of the publication has no doubt originated from the great success which was achieved by the two illustrated serials already produced by Dr. Geo. H. Fox, viz., those on Skin Diseases and on Venereal Skin Affections. The size, get-up and general appearance of the *Illustrated Quarterly* is very similar to those just mentioned. Each number of the journal is to contain four quarto plates, on cardboard, 10 x 12 inches, with twenty-four or more quarto pages of accompanying text. Woodcuts are also interspersed where found necessary. It consists thus entirely of original matter.

The first two numbers, January and April, have now appeared, and enable us to judge of the merits of the work. The large illustrations in No. I are devoted to the following cases:—Dr. Post, Restoration of the upper lip; Dr. Parker, Fibrous tumour of the face; Dr. Little, Separation of the lower epiphysis of the femur; Dr. Sexton, Facial paralysis in connection with aural disease. Besides which, other cases are illustrated by excellent woodcuts. In No. II, the following cases have artotypes attached: —Dr. Isaac E. Taylor, Ovarian pregnancy; Dr. Sabine, Plastic operations for loss of nose, lower eyelids, &c.; Dr. Gibney, The pathological anatomy of a case of spinal caries with paraplegia; Dr. VanWagenen, A case of skin-grafting for a burn.

These artotype illustrations are most excellent pieces of work —perfectly accurate, of course, as they are photographs, and very well coloured by hand. The letter-press, paper, and other typographical work also leave nothing to be desired. We are satisfied that there will be a large demand for this really valuable periodical, because in a few years each subscriber will find himself in possession of a complete picture-gallery of an immense number of the rarest and most unique cases in all branches of medicine and surgery. The long list of eminent names given as collaborators ensures a never-ending supply of such material. We wish the *Illustrated Quarterly* much success, and shall always look with interest for its arrival.

The subscription price is $8.00, which may be paid quarterly. Considering the great amount of skilled labour needful for producing such artistic plates, this must be considered very reasonable.

Illustrations of Dissections in a series of Original Colored Plates, the size of life, representing the Dissection of the Human Body.—By George Viner Ellis, Professor of Anatomy in University College, London, and G. H. Ford, Esq. (Reduced on a uniform scale, and reproduced in *fac-simile* expressly for Wood's Library of Standard Medical Authors.) Vol. I. Second edition. New York: Wm. Wood & Co. Montreal: J. M. O'Loughlin.

This is the first volume of the new series of Wood's Library for the present year. There are twenty-eight colored lithographic plates of dissections of various important regions of the body, including the head, neck and upper extremity. The reduction from life-size has been well executed, so that the outlines are very distinct, and all the parts can be seen quite clearly. If exception should be taken to them on any point, it would probably be that in some of the examples so many structures are brought into view that upon the small scale it cannot avoid making it look somewhat confused. It will no doubt prove a very welcome addition for all students of anatomy and of surgery.

A Manual of Organic Materia Medica, being a guide to Materia Medica for the vegetable and animal kingdoms. For the use of students, druggists, pharmacists and physicans.—By JOHN M. MAISCH, Phar. D., Professor of Materia Medica and Botany in the Philadelphia College of Pharmacy. With many illustrations on wood. Philadelphia: Henry C. Lea's Son & Co. Montreal: Dawson Bros.

An excellent concise description of all the organic drugs of the United States and British Pharmacopœias. It is claimed to contain in concentrated form "what may be considered the *essential* physical, histological, and chemical characteristics of the organic drugs, so as to render the work a useful and reliable guide in business transactions." The name of the author and his previous association with the large National Dispensatory are, of course, ample guarantee for the accuracy of the descriptions and the care with which they have been compiled. A few useful drugs which are not found in the pharmacopœias but which are employed in certain localities with success, are also very properly introduced. Upwards of two hundred wood cuts are used for illustration. It is a very handy volume, and will no doubt be widely availed of by those for whom it has been more especially intended.

Marriage and Parentage, and the Sanitary and Physiological Laws for the production of children of finer health and greater ability.—By a Physician and Sanitarian. New York: M. L. Holbrook & Co.

The first thing that strikes one on looking at the title page of this book is the absence of the author's name. It is probably not a wise father who is ashamed to own his offspring, and it would *primâ facie* appear as though in this case hiding under an *incog* betrayed a consciousness of the defects which might be found to exist in the production. The subject treated of is necessarily one of importance to every nation, but at the same time it is beset with difficulties, and it would require a very clear mind to grapple with these and be able to suggest practical means for their removal. We find nothing of that kind here. The principal point dwelt upon is that science, having done so much for the improvement of the domestic animals by careful selection of sires and dams in the hands of judicious breeders, should also be allowed to arrange the pairing of the human family in some way so that the results should be the improvement of the race. That like produces like, and that the direst results are brought about by hereditary taints, every one admits; but we look in vain for the real remedy for this state of things. A number of chapters are given relating to marriage and constitutional diseases, &c., with reference to their transmissibility. They contain numerous quotations and illustrations from Darwin, Hæckel and other scientists, but very little that is either new or original.

An Index of Surgery, being a concise classification of the main facts and Theories of Surgery. For the use of senior students and others.—By C. B. KEETLEY, F.R.C.S., Senior Assistant Surgeon to the West London Hospital, Surgeon to the Surgical Aid Society. New York: Bermingham & Co.

This compendium or compact note-book of surgery will probably find a good many admirers amongst students going up for their final examination. If it is made simply to supplement the reading from text-books and other treatises, its employment can only be productive of good. It has evidently been carefully prepared, and by one who fully appreciates the proper method for a book of this kind. It is arranged in alphabetical order the names of important diseases and important parts of the body, and under each heading is given in as few words as possible all that it is essential that a well-informed student should know about the affection in question. Every attempt to assist a student in the arduous work of preparing himself thoroughly for his searching examinations is a good work done, and the *Index* certainly belongs in that category.

Books and Pamphlets Received.

ON THE MORBID CONDITIONS OF THE URINE DEPENDENT UPON DERANGEMENTS OF DIGESTION.—By Charles Henry Ralfe, M.A., M.D London: J. & A. Churchill.

DE LA LITHOTRITIE RAPIDE.—Par le Dr. Peliquet. Paris: Adrien Delabage et Emil Lecrosnier.

ELEMENTS OF PHARMACY, MATERIA MEDICA AND THERAPEUTICS.—By Wm. Whitton, M.D. London: Henry Renshaw.

TRANSACTIONS OF THE MEDICAL SOCIETY OF THE STATE OF PENNSYLVANIA at its 32nd annual session, held at Lancaster, May, 1881.

THE TRANSACTIONS OF THE AMERICAN MEDICAL ASSOCIATION. Instituted 1847. Vol. XXXII.

Extracts from British and Foreign Journals.

Unless otherwise stated the translations are made specially for this Journal.

Criminal Abortion.—Dr. Thomas reported a case as follows: While visiting a patient in the upper part of the city, Dr. Nicoll, his assistant surgeon at the Woman's Hospital, came for him in great haste, saying that he had had an unfortunate occurrence in the hospital. Dr. Thomas went with him immediately, and found that the alarm was concerning a patient who was admitted with the following history: A German woman, the mother of three or four children, was admitted, so exceedingly blanched from prolonged hemorrhage that she could scarcely move about the ward. She said that she had had a miscarriage six or seven weeks previously, and that the after-birth could not be got away. The physicians who attended her for the retained placenta had passed instruments, but had failed to remove it, and she had nearly bled to death, and came into the hospital for the purpose of having the after-birth, or what remained of it, removed. Dr. Thomas saw the patient at the time of her admission, and recommended to Dr. Nicoll that he dilate the os and empty the uterus. Accordingly, Dr. N. introduced one or two sea-tangle tents on the next day; but before passing the tents, he introduced Sims' flexible probe, and found that it passed in *four* inches. After the dilatation, Dr. N. introduced Dr. Thomas' small wire curette, and removed quite a large piece of placenta. With the finger he touched more, and then introduced a pair of curved forceps, seized it and withdrew it. The portion came into the vagina readily, and he then discovered that he was still drawing something out, and to his great surprise he found that he had a foot or more of intestine between the woman's thighs. Dr. Thomas found a tampon in the vagina, and when it was removed, a piece of the omentum and a coil of intestine came out. He found it impossible to return the gut and the omentum to the abdominal cavity. The patient was in collapse. He at once began laparotomy, and as soon as the abdominal cavity was opened, it was seen where the hernia had occurred. Taking hold of the intestine, he readily drew it back into the uterus, and thence into the abdomen, and then found the explanation of the case which, up to that time, had been mysterious. In the anterior wall of the uterus was an opening sufficiently large to admit his thumb. It was evidently an old wound. The portion of the intestine that had escaped into the uterus was very dark, but it was decided that the chances were in favour of its being restored. The opening in the uterus was closed with three or four silver sutures, the abdominal wound was closed, and the patient put to bed. Within 24 hours peritonitis developed, and the woman died. The case was remarkable in several respects. In the first place, it was very evident that nothing which Dr. Nicoll had done had made the opening in the uterus. The opening was not a recent one, and the probe which he introduced probably passed through it into the abdominal cavity. Besides, the probe used was not able to produce such an opening. The tents used were the ordinary sea-tangle tents made by the instrument makers, and could not have passed so as to disappear through the external os. Again he saw the intestine within fifteen minutes after it came down, and certainly within that time it could not have got the blackened colour it presented. The curette could not have made the opening, because it is not able to inflict such a wound. Besides, there was exudation of lymph upon the edges of the wound in the wall of the uterus; all of which proved that the uterus had been full of intestine ever since the miscarriage.

Dr. Mundé referred to a case somewhat similar to the one last reported by Dr. Thomas, and communicated to him by Dr. Baldwin of Columbus, Ohio. A multiparous woman became pregnant, and had an abortion produced at about the third month of utero-gestation. Within a week after, she was suddenly seized with abdominal pain, fell into collapse, and died within 24 hours. At autopsy, the uterus was found enlarged, it contained a few fetal bones, and there was a hole in the side of the organ large enough to admit the index finger, and under the layers of the broad ligament was a mass of fetal bones. The report gave no history of placenta. The questions were, whether this opening in the uterus was made by the abortionist, whether the fetus could have passed between the layers of the broad ligament and become macerated within a week, or whether there was extra-uterine pregnancy, and the opening in the wall of the uterus was of gradual formation.

Dr. Thomas referred to a remarkable case reported by Douglas of Dublin, in which the uterus ruptured during labour at full term, and the child was delivered through the vagina. The woman began to improve, and continued to do so steadily; and there was only one peculiarity in her case after recovery, and that was that she passed all her fœces through the uterus. It was recognized that a portion of the intestine had been dragged into the uterus and permanently opened into the uterine cavity. The more curious part of the case was, that after a time fœcal matter ceased to pass through the uterus, and the patient ultimately got perfectly well.—*American Journal of Obstetrics.*

Percussion as a Therapeutic Agent in Nervous Diseases.—By Dr. J. Mortimer Granville. With the cognisance of the leading physiologists and neurologists in England and on the continent, I have for some years past been employing carefully graduated and precisely applied percussion as a therapeutic agent in the treatment of nervous diseases and disturbances, on a principle of which the following statement, published by me in February, 1881, may be taken as a brief exposition :—

" As far back as 1862-3, I was, in the course of certain clinical studies of mental and sensory phenomena, induced to believe that many forms of the sensation we call 'pain' were, in fact, unnoccessary, and might be interrupted by appropriate mental and physical methods and appliances. My first observations were made in connection with the paroxysmal or recurrent pains accompanying the uterine contractions in the natural process of parturition. On May 4th, 1864, Dr. Graily Hewitt was good enough to communicate the results of my experiments and to show certain apparatus to the Obstetrical Society of London. In a paper 'On the application of extreme cold as an anodyne in the pain attendant on parturition,' a short abstract of which will be found in the *Lancet* of July 9th, 1864, I contended that the sensations of pain experienced by the parturient woman were not invariably synchronous with what, for want of a better name, we term the 'pains' of her labour; and from this and other premises—for example, the circumstance that the sensation is commonly 'referred' to some region more or less remote from the contracting uterus, or the dilating external passages, in which the real seat of the pain might have been supposed to be located—I deduced that the pain attendant on labour is neuralgic in its character. I had constructed small boxes or chambers of such sizes and shapes as to admit of their being conveniently applied to the supposed seats of the pain. These were filled with freezing mixture, and the effect of sudden contact in some thirty cases was to arrest the sensation of pain without in the least degree lessening the force of the uterine contractions. The experiment was, of course, simply interesting as bearing on the nature of the pain, as this process was too troublesome to admit of its adoption in practice; albeit some of the persons on whom I had the opportunity of trying my method experienced such striking relief that, on subsequent occasions, I believe they asked that the measure might be repeated. Having thus far persuaded myself that this form of pain was neuralgic, and that if the nerve affected could be strongly impressed, so as to change its *state of irritation*, the pain would cease, I proceeded to try the effect of rapidly tapping the skin over the fifth nerve in ordinary facial neuralgia with a Bennett's percussion hammer, using the ivory pleximeter as a shield. The results obtained by this method were very remarkable. Still, I simply thought of arresting the morbid action by shock. Later on—it is only possible to sketch the outline of the inquiry—I was led, by the light thrown on Newton's doctrine of concords and discords by Grove's generalisation as to the correlation of forces, and, more recently, by Professor Tyndall's beautiful series of experiments with sensitive flames and musical burners, to believe that the results of the tapping were not, like the interruption with shock produced by the sudden application of cold, due to a mere arrest of the painful state of irritation into which the nerve had been thrown, but were, in fact, brought about by the extinguishment of some morbid—that is, either inordinate or disorderly—set of vibrations by the superimposition of another, incompatible or discordant, set of vibrations mechanically produced. With this notion I set to work to devise an instrument which should give a known number of blows per second, and thus admit of this new phase of the inquiry being pushed further. . . . .

" The sensation produced by the application of the instrument over a healthy nerve, so situated as to be readily thrown into mechanical vibration, closely resembles the effect of a weak dose of the interrupted current of electricity, and if it be prolonged the vibration will extend its area, exciting first formication or tingling, then a sensation of numbness, and finally some twitching of the superficial muscles. A nervous headache, and even migraine, may be induced by the application of the percuteur to the frontal ridges or the margins of the orbit. By the interposition of a thin plate of metal, or even stiff paper, the vibration may be readily propagated through a considerable region of the surface of the body, and in time the deeper muscles will frequently begin to act. I have even produced an involuntary movement, not unlike tendon-reflex, by applying the percuteur for some time over the ligamentum patellæ or the margin of the patella. Still more notable has been the fact that, by laying a sheet of paper over the abdomen, and moving the percuteur slowly in large circles round the umbilicus, the intestines have seemed to be excited to vermicular movement, and the bowels commenced to act. These results have not been constant, but have occurred with sufficient frequency to indicate that the experiments already made are worthy to be repeated. . . . .

"I will take leave to say that I think these results go to support my theory that it is by the introduction of discord into the rhythm of the morbid vibrations of the painful 'state' the change which brings relief in neuralgia is effected. To apply the percenteur with a high rate of blows per second will aggravate the morbid state when that is itself a series of rapid vibrations; and in the same way a low speed of percussion increases, instead of relieving, the pains of a low-pitched and slow 'boring' or 'grinding' sensation. Acute or sharp pain is, I believe, like a high note in music, produced by rapid vibrations, while a dull, heavy, or aching pain resembles a low note or tone, and is caused by comparatively slow vibrations. A slow rate of mechanical vibration will therefore interrupt the rapid nerve-vibration of acute pain, while quick mechanical vibration more readily arrests the slower. The aim—if I am right in my conjecture—should be *to set up a new set of vibrations which shall interrupt or change the morbid set by introducing discord.* This is the principle. Failure in the application of this principle will, I believe, be found to explain the failure to put an end to the pain; and I have, accordingly, set as much scientific value on my failures as on my successes."

My method is, it will be seen from these extracts, based upon the hypotheses (1) that all nerve action, whether normal or morbid, is vibratile; and (2) that it is possible to influence and control abnormal vibrations—in the manner above described—by mechanical vibrations propagated to the nervous structures, in *particular* directions and at *known* rates of speed. It is not my present purpose to discuss these hypotheses, or the method in detail; but I am anxious to re-state, and now affirm, certain propositions, founded on experience, which, in previous intimations of the progress and success of my experiments, I submitted tentatively. They are these.

1. I have rarely failed, in a fairly large number of cases—many of them of several years' standing—to bring the cerebro-spinal and, sometimes directly at others in secondary circuits, the sympathetic, ganglia under control, by the application of my percuteur over, or in mechanical relation through the adjacent tissues with, those ganglia.

2. I have in no instance failed to produce activity of the bowels, even in cases of previously obstinate constipation; and in many instances I have succeeded, within a short period, in restoring the periodic evacuation of their contents without recourse to drugs. This success alone places the method on a footing of value in daily practice.

3. I can now, in result of my more recent experiments, propagate the vibrations I produce along the trunks and into the branches of most of the principal nerves, from their centres of origin, or call them into action, reflexly, through the afferent nerves connected with those centres. In limited paralyses, and even in circumscribed scleroses, this power is of the highest therapeutic importance.

4. I can nearly always arouse torpid centres to action, and thus pave the way for their restoration to states of normal activity. Since it is physiologically certain that nutrition depends on exercise, and every part of the organism feeds in proportion as it works *healthily*, it is a great thing to be able to act thus directly on the nerve-centres which are the seats of energy.

5. I can subdue the exaggerated reflex irritability of revolting subordinate centres, and replace them under the control of the higher centres, even in cases of lateral sclerosis.

Applying these facts—for such they undoubtedly are—to the needs of special nervous states, the practitioner will have no difficulty in perceiving that my method has great and obvious uses. I am anxious not to overstate the results I am obtaining, but they are such as to show that the physiological process of mechanical vibration is likely to prove a potent agent in the treatment of a wide range of maladies now the most intractable. It will afford me much pleasure to show the process to any medical man who will call on me. It is impossible at present to describe its details in writing; but I will gladly aid anyone in its application. My method has nothing in common with the "muscle-beating" and shaking to which you directed attention in your last issue. It is a system which must be approved and practised by the profession exclusively. Nothing do I so much dread as its falling into unprofessional hands. I have been engaged upon it since 1862, shortly after which date some of the results were communicated to the Obstetrical Society.—*Brit. Med. Journal*, March 11, 1882.

Self-Mutilation in China.—Dr. R. J. Jamieson, of Shanghai, has recently presented to the Museum of the Royal College of Surgeons a pair of feet, to which the following remarkable history is attached. Some months ago, a Chinese beggar excited much pity, and made a very profitable business in the streets of the foreign settlement, Shanghai, by showing the mutilated stumps of his legs, the feet belonging to them being tied together and slung around his neck. Warned frequently by the police, he was knocked down one day by a carriage when scrambling out of the way of a constable. He was brought into the hospital, under Dr. Jamieson's care, being slightly injured; and on recovery from his bruises, he sold his feet to his medical attendant, which otherwise would have been confiscated by the police. He admitted that, for the purpose of making himself as attractive as possible to the charitably disposed, he had, about a year previously, fastened cords around his ankles, drawing them as tight as he could bear them, and increasing the pressure every two or three days. In about a fortnight the bones were bare, and he had no more pain. At the end of a month and a half the bones were quite dry; and by this time, according to his account, he was able to remove the feet by partly cutting and partly snapping the bones. The feet were quite black and mummified; on the wounded surface of the right foot the upper aspect of the astragalus was seen, no trace of the malleoli remaining; but the external malleolus lay in its normal position in the left foot, and it had evidently been removed by cutting and snapping, as the patient affirmed. The stumps were perfectly healed, and conical;

the ends of the tibiæ and fibulæ were apparently fused, and both stumps were covered in with a good cicatrix, puckered at the centre, and admitting of a very considerable amount of pressure before pain was produced. Such instances of self-mutilation appear to be frequent in China; and, when performed for such a motive as in Dr. Jamieson's case, they throw a light on that singular mixture of courage, deceit and sacrifice of almost anything to advance low enterprise, which characterize the lower orders of that country.—*Brit. Med. Journal.*

On Abuses of the Jacket-Treatment of Spinal Disease.—The writer, while acknowledging fully the debt European surgery owes to Dr. Sayre for the able advocacy of his treatment, and granting that it is due to his exertions that in England it has come into such general use, considers that in many cases the jacket is hastily and needlessly applied, and that its employment is often actively harmful. He divides the cases in which the jacket-treatment is abused into two classes—*A*, Those due to a wrong selection of cases; *B*, Those due to wrong methods of application of the jacket. In class *A* the following are given as improper instances:

1. *Simple rickety spines*, often mistaken for cases of commencing caries.

2. *Cases of simple lateral curvature*, in which the disease is perpetuated by the use of rigid support.

3. *Certain cases of true spinal caries.*—In infants, during the early progress of the disease, the older plan of rest and horizontal position succeeds better than does any attempt to immobilize the spinal column; it is free from the risk of preventing due development of the trunk. But the jacket may be used from the first in older children with or without confinement to bed.

4. Cases in which the lungs or heart are affected, in addition to the affection of the spine.

5. Cases in which the carious spine is associated with any high degree of paralysis, incontinence of urine, etc.

In class *B*, the following are the chief instances of misapplication of jackets:

1. *Undue heaviness*, many jackets being far too thick and strong.

2. *Use of the swing.*—This apparatus is considered to be, for children, useless, if not harmful, the object of extension being to allow the body to hang as straight as it may while avoiding all risks of disturbing any adhesions between consolidating vertebræ, and to bring the chest-walls into a condition of extreme inspiration. It is held that these objects are best attained by holding the child by the arms, with the feet on the floor, or by the use of an inclined plane.

3. *Bad fitting and bad shaping of the jacket.* More especially neglect of the inspiratory position of chest-walls, insufficient hold of the jacket on the pelvis, and inaccurate fitting to the spinal curve or angle.—*Walter Pye in Amer. Jour. of Obstetrics.*

Partial Resection of the Lungs.—Abdominal surgery is every day achieving fresh successes, and while ovariotomy remains, and probably will remain, its greatest triumph, the later successes have been neither few nor small. So recently as the close of 1879, Professor Nussbaum, of Munich, said in a public lecture, "So soon as the physician diagnoses with certainty a cancer of the pylorus, the surgeon will allow but little time to pass before he excises the cancerous growth." The words seem almost prophetic, for within a year and a half we have from Dr. Wolfler an account of several such operations, some of them successful, performed in the clinic of Professor Billroth. The operation is now recognized, the cases suitable for it described, and the method of performance fully detailed. With regard to abdominal surgery generally, we may say that operations which a very few years since would have been scouted as utterly beyond the pale of rational and justifiable surgery, have been performed with a success which more than justifies the boldness of the operators. The question very naturally suggests itself, how far the thoracic organs lie outside the domain of surgery. The successful treatment by free incision and drainage of pleuritic and pericarditic effusions, whether serous or purulent, is the last advance in this direction; but in the localized catarrhal pneumonia, the phthisical cavity, and the limited pulmonary tumor, there seems to be a field for further advance, although it is admittedly beset with difficulties of diagnosis for the physician, of technique for the surgeon. As a contribution to the subject, Dr. Schmid, of Berlin, details (*Berliner Klin. Wochenschrift*, No. 51, 1881) the result of certain experiments he has performed on the dog. These results are put forward in the most modest possible manner, with full knowledge of what they do and what they do not prove. The operation performed by Dr. Schmid consisted in the resection of apex of the lung on one side. On the day before tne operation one side of the dog's chest was shaved and thoroughly cleaned, and the animal was operated upon while under the influence of morphia and ether. A portion of the fourth or fifth rib was excised subperiosteally, the portion being made as large and as far from the sternum as possible. A lobe of the lung was now drawn through the opening, or as much of it as possible. This was transfixed with a double catgut thread below the part to be excised, and a part of the lung, including the wedge to be excised, was then ligatured. The wedge was excised with scissors, all the larger bloodvessels and bronchi ligatured, and the edges of the lung brought together with catgut sutures. The double catgut ligature round the base of the lobe was now removed, and after seeing that no hemorrhage occurred, the part was returned into the thorax and the external wound closed. Almost no antiseptic precautions were adopted throughout, with the exception of disinfection of instruments, sponges, etc., with salicylic acid. The operation was performed eight times in all, and succeeded in three cases, while in five death occurred. The first dog operated on died within half an hour from carbolic poisoning, the spray having been used; while the other four died within two to five days from purulent pleurisy, evidently the result of septic infection. There was no hemorrhage or gangrene in these cases, and in only two was there a slight local pneumonia. Several of the animals had subcutaneous emphysema. In no case was there loss of blood from the lungs. Two of the successful operations were on the same animal. Dr. Schmid has performed the same operation, *post-mortem*, on the healthy and the phthisical human lung. He finds the great difficulty lies in getting the lung drawn through the opening, more especially when there are extensive adhesions. The operation, he believes, however, is perfectly practicable, and with the choice of suitable cases, and the use of all antiseptic precautions, he considers that the operation is one that can justifiably be attempted on the human body. The results of incision and drainage of phthisical cavities have not as yet proved very encouraging, but it must be admitted that the procedure has not yet had a fair trial. Any advance in the treatment of this terrible malady, before which, in the great majority of cases we stand so hopeless and helpless, will be welcomed by us all. Whether such an advance is possible, can be determined only by the skilful diagnosis of the physician, the bold and careful operating of the surgeon.—*Med. Times and Gazette.*

How the Fibrinous Clot of an Aneurism is Formed.—The old and long-accepted view that laminated aneurismal clots are formed by a retarded blood-current depositing its fibrin in successive layers, and the late theory of Broca, by which clots were classified as vital, active, or fibrinous, in contradistinction from those that were passive or mechanical, have been re-examined by Dr. H. D. Smith of New Orleans, with special reference to a case of fusiform aneurism of the femoral. He had been much struck on previous occasions with the irregularity in the disposition of the fibrinous layers, differing as they did much from types that have been described. In this present instance he found abundant evidence to prove that the original fibrinous deposit, which measured only 2¼ inches in diameter, had been separated from the wall of the vessel, allowing the blood to pass behind it. The laminæ also were not concentric, but imbricated, as a rule, and it was plain that the blood-current wave had swept in different directions, at different times. The appearances called to mind the arrangement in the corollary petals of a flower like the rose, rather than the coatings of an onion, which has been the object so often selected for comparison.

The cause of these peculiar deposits he traces to various conditions, and even to the position of the patient. When the fibrin is deposited between the clot and the sac, ridges and columns are formed, which at first are rectangular to the sac, but subsequently are pressed down by the onward current of the blood, which, in passing, deposits another series. The blood-corpuscles are thought to be active agents in the organization of the thrombus. Each change in the form of the tumour necessitates a change in the manner in which the fibrin is deposited.—*Annals of Anatomy and Surgery.*

Puerperal Infection in the Male.—During (*Centralblatt fur Gynækologie*, August 6th, 1881,) a severe epidemic of puerperal fever in Pollenza, a woman in childbed was attacked by a fever. A few days after the last paroxysm, when the patient left perfectly well, her husband attempted to have sexual intercourse with her, but intense pain in the frenum compelled him to desist. He stated that he was sure something must have been torn at the time, but had not noticed any bleeding. In a short time the pain subsided. Twenty-four hours later, however, a chill occurred, followed by fever, with remission of of all the symptoms on the following morning. In the evening the chill and fever recurred. On the third day, the right inguinal glands became swollen. The fourth day Lapponi diagnosed erysipelas of the skin of the penis, lymphangitis and lymphadenitis. The erysipelatous inflammation continued to spread and the skin became gangrenous at several points. On the sixth day the patient died with septicæmia. Although not able to discover any laceration, Lapponi still assumes that the point of infection was a slight tear of the frenum, which the patient suffered during the unsuccessful attempt at sexual intercourse.—*New Eng. Med. Mo.*

Genital Irritation.—At a recent meeting of the New York Neurological Society (*American Journal Neurology and Psychology*), a paper entitled "The Effect of Genital Irritation in the Production of Reflex Nervous Symptoms" was read by Dr. L. C. Gray, of Brooklyn. His conclusions were as follows:—1, That there is no proof that genital irritation can produce a reflex paralysis. 2, That while it is probable that the slight nervous disorders, as incontinence, retention, difficult micturition, erratic movements, and slight nervous disturbances, can be produced by genital irritation, the proof is not yet complete. 3, That operations for the removal of genital irritation may be beneficial even in organic nervous disease. 4, That we should, therefore, remove such genital irritation, if it exists, in any case whatsoever, and thus give our patients the benefit of the doubt. 5, That in all cases of nervous disorders, with accompanying genital irritation, we should not regard the latter as the cause of the former until all other probable or even possible causes have been rigidly excluded. 6, That operations upon the genitals, even when there is no genital irritation present, may prove to be a useful therapeutic measure in certain cases.

Salicylate of Soda in Acute Tonsillitis.—From the close connection which has long been recognized between rheumatism and certain forms of tonsillitis, Dr. Jos. W. Hunt has been induced to try this remedy, and the results have been most favorable. In his hands it has acted almost as a specific in acute tonsillitis. Provided that there is no actual formation of pus, most decided relief is afforded in about twenty-four hours—*i.e.*, the swelling and angry-looking condition of the tonsils are reduced, pain diminished, and the patient can swallow with comfort, while the temperature becomes normal, and the pulse is reduced in frequency and improved in quality. Since he has used this drug he has had no single case go on to suppuration; nay, more, where it has appeared, from the state of the tonsils and the brawny and infiltrated condition of neighboring parts, that suppuration must ensue, it has been arrested by this treatment. The doses used have been fifteen grains every four hours for an adult, and about ten grains every four hours for a child. He has met with no unpleasant symptoms from its use, beyond a little tinnitus and occasional vertigo. When the brunt of the attack has fallen upon one tonsil, a relapse in the other, when the salicylate has been discontinued, is not uncommon, but this speedily yields to the same treatment. One or two medical friends, who have used the salicylate at his suggestion, have expressed themselves in equally favorable terms.—*Lancet*, March 11, 1882.—*Medical News*.

How to apply the Soda Remedy in Burns and Scalds.—It is now many years ago (see the *London Medical Gazette* of March, 1844) that the author of this paper, while engaged in some investigations as to the qualities and effects of the alkalies in inflammations of the skin, etc., was fortunate enough to discover that a saline lotion, or *saturated* solution of the bicarbonated soda in either plain water or camphorated water, if applied speedily, or as soon as possible, to a burned or scalded part, was most effectual in immediately relieving the acute burning pain; and when the burn was only superficial, or not severe, removing all pain in the course of a very short time; having also the very great advantage of cleanliness, and, if applied at once, of preventing the usual consequences—a painful blistering of the skin, separation of the epidermis, and perhaps more or less of suppuration. For this purpose, all that is necessary is to cut a piece of lint, or old soft rag, or even thick blotting paper, of a size sufficient to cover the burned or scalded parts, and to keep it constantly well wetted with the sodaic lotion so as to prevent its drying. By this means, it usually happens that all pain ceases in from a quarter to half an hour, or even in much less time. When the main part of a limb, such as the hand and fore-arm or the foot and leg, has been burned, it is best, when practicable, to plunge the part at once into a jug or pail, or other convenient vessel filled with the soda lotion, and keep it there until the pain subsides; or the limb may be swathed or encircled with a surgeon's cotton bandage previously soaked in the *saturated* solution, and kept constantly wetted with it, the relief being usually immediate, provided the solution be saturated and cold. What is now usually sold as bicarbonate of soda is what I have commonly used and recommended; although this is well known to vary much in quality according to where it is manufactured—but it will be found to answer the purpose, although, probably, Howard's is most to be depended on, the common carbonate being too caustic. It is believed that a large proportion of medical practitioners are still unaware of the remarkable qualities of this easily applied remedy, which recommends itself for obvious reasons.—*F. Peppercorne in Popular Science Monthly for March.*

The Treatment of Syphilis without Mercury.—A NEW ABORTIVE REMEDY.—Dr. J. Edmund Guntz of Dresden, in a work just published by him, makes some novel announcements regarding the treatment of syphilis. If true, they are of the highest importance, for he claims to be able "not only to do away with mercury in syphilis, but, in a large proportion of cases, to abort the disease." It is now over twelve years since Dr. Guntz wrote on this subject. He is therefore not a novice in the matter. In 1869 he advocated the use of bichromate of potassium as being a useful drug in treating syphilis. He could not prove any very great advantages for it, however, at the time. It acted slowly, and was apt to disturb the stomach, but being convinced that there was something in the drug, he set to work to find some way of getting more into the system without producing functional disturbance. For a time he combined the bichromate with the nitrate of potassium, and gave pills containing 1-16 gr. of each three times a day. With these pills he produced "remarkably favourable results." Yet the action was slow, and when a prompt amelioration of symptoms was needed, as in malignant cases, the remedy would hardly meet the expectations. From the favourable results obtained by giving the various minerals in solutions with carbonic acid water, our author was led to attempt administering chromium in the same way, and with, as he now claims, very great success. He found that much larger doses could be taken in this form, and that a profounder impression on the system could thus be made. As a maximum dose he was able to give 3½ grains (.3 grammes) daily of bichromate of potassium in about 600 grammes of carbonic acid water, this being divided into five doses. Larger amounts provoked vomiting. This "chromwater," as he calls it, could also be given daily for weeks and months in all forms of syphilis without detriment to to the health.

Having described his method of giving the drug, Dr. Guntz discusses its action upon the initial stage of syphilis and upon the disease itself after its full development in the system. In estimating the possible value of any drug as an abortive of syphilis, the numerous sources of error are referred to. The existence of and difference between true chancre and chancroid are admitted. The following are his statistics: Within one and a quarter years the author treated 194 cases of chancre. For comparative study he selects only 85 of these, since in the others there were sources of error. In 14 of these 85 cases the sores were cauterized. The remainder were treated with nothing but the chromwater; and in 47 of them constitutional syphilis failed to appear. In order to avoid every possible chance of mistake the author excludes 10 of this 47. Even then there were left 37 patients, or over one-half, who, when given chromwater alone, developed no after-symptoms. It is not stated, however, how long they were watched, except that 18 were under observation for 159 days. Still more favourable results took place with the 14 cases in which the initial lesion was cauterized. Of these only two developed symptoms of constitutional syphilis. Of the 85 patients therefore presenting, as Dr. Guntz asserts, initial lesions of syphilis, 49, under the "chromwater" treatment, remained entirely free from the disease. This is certainly a very extraordinary showing, and will be received with a great deal of incredulity. If this new agent is given after constitutional symptoms make their appearance, its action is to ameliorate the disease and hasten its course. It is efficient even in cases where mercury fails, and it acts more pleasantly and promptly. In fact, the disease is "in the shortest time definitely cured." The author has, for several years, used the chrome salt exclusively in the treatment of syphilis, and has given it in more than a thousand cases. He thinks that the day of mercury is over. He has recorded the histories of a large number of his cases.

Dr. Guntz has also used his chromwater with the best results in diphtheria. He suggests that the drug acts by reason of its powerful oxidizing properties. Without committing himself to any germ theory, it is thought that there is certainly a specific poison which develops in the various contagious diseases. And in chromium we have an agent that is inimical to the syphilitic poison, while it does not harm the system itself, but rather benefits it. The importance of Dr. Guntz's claims, and the caution with which they should be received, are alike apparent and need no comment.—*N. Y. Medical Record.*

The Tomato as a Dietary.—The profession and the public are by no means agreed as to the dietetic value of the tomato. The classical authorities on food, such as Pavy and Chambers, dismiss the claims of this vegetable very curtly, simply placing it among the auti-scorbutics, and allowing it little, if any, nutritive power. The public, on the other hand, believe this ally of the potato to be not only a highly nutrient vegetable, but a stomachic, a cathartic, and generally a potent blood-purifier. That the tomato is thought too little of by the profession generally is true, but it may be doubted whether it possesses those wonderful alterative powers ascribed to it by the Americans, many of whom persuade themselves that they are never in health except in the tomato season. This fruit (as it may also be called), however, exhibits one remarkable property in connection with plant diseases, which suggests its use as a germicide and a protector against those disorders, so many of which we now know derive their origin from bacteria and allied germs. If a tomato shrub be uprooted at the end of the season, and allowed to wither on the bough of a fruit tree, or if it be burnt beneath, it will act not only as a curative, but protective, against blight and similar attacks. This hostility to low organisms is due to the presence of sulphur, which is rendered up in an active condition in the decay or burning. Remembering that digestion also splits up the tomato into its chemical constituents and releases sulphur, probably in a nascent condition and probably in the intestinal canal, it may have as great potency there as experiments prove it to have outside the body. Summer diarrhœa, English cholera and typhoid fever are all due to low organisms. As the diarrhœal and typhoid seasons are luckily contemporaneous with the fruiting of the tomato, it is not unreasonable to assume that tomato-eaters would be more than ordinarily likely to escape such diseases. It is worth noting that typhoid fever is most prevalent among the poor, to whom this expensive vegetable is almost unknown. Sailors, too, just after landing, are particularly liable to typhoid, and in them we may always assume a more or less scorbutic condition. But the question of the protection against disease by certain diets, and by such habits as the use of alcohol, tobacco and opium, has as yet been hardly inquired into.

Experiments are now being made on the tincture of the tomato which will help in determining its therapeutic value. Meanwhile, eaten cooked with hot meats, and in the form of salad *after* a cold lunch, it is a pleasant and useful addition to our ordinary regimen. The fruit-acids it contains, combined with the mechanical effect of the seeds and skins, render it to some extent an enemy to scurvy as well as a laxative, and the sulphur, with its known power over septic conditions, would probably contribute to make its use a protection against the poison germs of those diseases, like typhoid, that find their way into the system primarily by the alimentary canal. One caution is needed to the lovers of this esculent. The taste for it being an acquired one, it is the more likely to be indulged in to excess, and we have known almost as many *tomato-maniacs* as *ostro-maniacs*. All kinds of raw fruit, it should be remembered, except used with care, are liable to irritate, and we have known an instance where a person, working hard all day on raw tomatoes only, was seized with inflammation of the bowels, which proved fatal in a few hours. As an article of diet, then, two or three tomatoes will be found as effective as, and certainly safer, than a dozen.—*Australian Medical Journal.*

Mitral Presystolic Cardiac Murmurs.— From a careful clinical study of the varieties, mechanism, and clinical significance of mitral presystolic murmurs, in the *American Journal of Medical Sciences* for April, 1882, Prof. Austin Flint draws the following conclusions :—

1. There are two varieties of this murmur, which are dis-

tinguished by differences in quality and in mechanism. One variety is a rough, and the other is a soft, murmur.

2. The roughness in the first of these varieties is characteristic, and may be distinguished as vibratory or blubbering. The softness of the second variety is bellows-like, like other soft cardiac murmurs. It may vary in pitch and intensity, but as a rule, it is low and weak.

3. The rough murmur is due to vibrations of the curtains of the mitral valve, caused by the passage of blood from the auricle to the ventricle. The soft murmur, like other bellows murmurs, may be due either to contraction of the orifice through which the blood passes, or to roughness of the surface over which it flows.

Hysteria.—When called to treat a young girl with an hysterical attack, there are three things which you had better do: 1st, Institute at once firm pressure in the neighbourhood of both ovaries. This is very apt to quiet the patient at once. 2nd, Administer an emetic. I have found that a woman who is well under the action of an emetic has not the opportunity to do anything else than be thoroughly nauseated. Give a full dose of ipecac with one grain of tartar emetic. 3rd, And this method of controlling the spasm will often act charmingly: take a good-sized lump of ice and press it right down on the nape of the neck. This produces quiet by its powerful impression upon the whole nervous system.—*Dr. Goodell in Clinical News.*

Gezow's Corn Cure.—The following formula, which produces a clear, light, green solution, was recommended by Gezow, a Russian apothecary, in the *Zeitschrift für Russland:*

Extract of cannabis indica,	5	parts.
Salicylic acid,	30	"
Collodion	240	"

Mix and dissolve.

It is applied with a camel's-hair pencil, so as to form a thick coating, for four consecutive nights and mornings. The collodion at once covers and protects the corn from friction. The Indian hemp acts as an anodyne, and the acid disintegrates the corn, so that after a hot bath on the fifth day, it will come out, adhering to the artificial skin of collodion on the toe. This causes no pain, and is said to be very effective.—*New Remedies.*

CANADA

Medical and Surgical Journal.

MONTREAL, MAY, 1882.

CHARLES DARWIN.

On the 20th ult., the scientific world was bereft of its brightest ornament, its most distinguished member. For nearly half a century the name of Charles Darwin has been associated with a series of memoirs on natural history, subjects of extraordinary excellence. From the early papers on coral reefs and volcanic islands to the "Habits of Earth Worms," published a few months ago, the patient observer, the skilled experimenter, the philosophical thinker, has been apparent to all. But it is not so much as a naturalist that his name is famous in outside circles. The theory of natural selection, as elaborated in the "Origin of Species," published in 1850, while it shocked the sensibilities of the public, at once was accepted as a working theory by a considerable number of biologists, with whom it has steadily increased in favor. There are now very few distinguished men (of whom Principal Dawson is one), who do not acknowledge it in some form or other. Its influence has been enormous, and, chiefly through the writings of Herbert Spencer, the evolution philosophy has become the creed of modern science. The storm of opposition has now virtually spent itself, and even the "Queen of Sciences" has in many quarters adapted itself to the new conditions, and the very pulpits which were loudest in denunciation of the iniquity of the theory and its inconsistency with religion, have recently acknowledged the possibility of its truth. The attitude of Mr. Darwin during the controversy was characteristic of the man. Leaving the war of words to the rank and file, he quietly set to work to collect and arrange various facts bearing on the habits of animals and plants and the variability of species, and science has reaped a rich heritage in such volumes as the "Fertilization of Orchids," "Animals and Plants under Domestication," "The Descent of Man," "Expression of the Emotions in Man and Animals," "Climbing Plants," &c. With a comfortable fortune, he resided in his quiet British home, rarely visiting the haunts of men, but delighting all whom he happened to meet by the modesty and native integrity of his character. His family forms a striking illustration of the laws of heredity; the father of Dr. Robert Darwin, F.R.S., was the noted son of the still more noted Erasmus Darwin, author of "Zoönomia" and other well-known works Three sons survive him, all of them rapidly rising to eminence in their respective professions. Robert (M.B. of London), has been associated with his father in several of his recent works.

McGILL UNIVERSITY.

ANNUAL DINNER OF THE MEMBERS OF THE GRADUATES' SOCIETY.

The annual University dinner, under the auspices of the Graduates' Society, was held in the Windsor Hotel on the 2nd inst., and both from the number of those present and from the high order of the intellectual proceedings, the gathering was a most decided success. About eight o'clock the President (Dr. Osler), the invited guests, and the members of the Society, about 130 in number, entered the dining-room and took their seats. On the right of the President sat Principal Dawson, LL.D., F.R.S., C.M.G.; Mr. John H. R. Molson, Mr. G. W. Stephens, M.P.P.; Mr. S. Haight, and Rev. James Roy, and on his left Hon. P. J. O. Chauveau, Hon. Justice Mackay, Mr. R. A. Ramsay, Rev. W. H. Drewett (of Manchester, England), Rev. Dr. Stevenson, and Dr. J. Clarke Murray. The vice-chairs were occupied by J. Hall, Jun., Mr. C. H. McLeod (Vice-President), and Dr. F. W. Kelley.

In proposing "The University," the President said he felt highy honored to have the privilege of proposing this toast on such an occasion, and in doing so would give, in a few words, the history of this University, of its early trials, and of the men who so nobly encouraged its career, of its founder, and of those who in the past had borne the burden and the heat of the day, who had sown the seed from which they had reaped the harvest, and who had long entered into their rest. He felt honored, because he felt that this was a festive gathering to celebrate the coming of age of their University. McGill University was in the 50th year of its existence, or more correctly its 50th session. A University, like some other things, came to maturity slowly, and he thought they might safely say that their University was to-day coming of age. In this connection it might be interesting to ask the parentage of this Institution; who fathered her? Why, the merchants of Montreal; she was born, so to speak, in the Chamber of Commerce. She had been reared, wet and dry nursed, by merchants; all her little early difficulties and troubles had been treated by the Corn Exchange. To whom did she first lisp forth her early prayers? To the merchants of Montreal. They had seen her safely through the teething, the measles and the several other critical periods of her existence. Moreover, they saw her through the critical period of puberty, and he believed that period was the time at which they sought the aid of their noble Principal; he was the doctor called in, and he reared her through that critical period. In looking over the history of the institution briefly, he did it with a medical eye, and just at that time there were indications of commencing maturity, and it was very fortunate for this institution and this city that they called in so skillful a physician. He might say in this connection that this University was a child of trade; founded, as he said, by the merchants of Montreal, she owed her continued existence almost exclusively to these gentlemen. There was nothing in the whole history of Montreal to which the merchants of Montreal could look forward with so much pride as McGill University. The coming of age of this University brought with it additional responsibilities. In the first place, the University should be a teaching place where the youth could go and seek information in all departments of knowledge, where men could be educated to fill any calling in life. To do this they required a staff of the ablest men they could get—not only the ablest men that the country possessed, but the best that money could get, the best talent that they conld get irrespective of nationality. He hoped that by the time of the next jubilee—namely, the centennial dinner—their University would be known not only as a centre where men could come and get education, but a centre where men could find the means of extending the limits of knowledge. The graduates of McGill University should look forward to the time when she would have her laboratories and the necessaries to give to students opportunities of individual and private research. Referring to the large amount of work done by the professors, Dr. Osler said that the man who gave twelve or thirteen lectures a week could not be expected to devote much time to original work with any proper degree of enthusiasm. He would give them "The University."

The toast was received with the greatest enthusiasm.

Hon. Justice Mackay responded. He alluded especially to the financial difficulties which had lately beset the University, and to the exertions that are being made to prevent the usefulness of the Institution becoming crippled. He thought the appeal for help to the citizens a very wise step, and spoke hopefully of what had already been accomplished and would be likely still to result therefrom. Special mention was made of the recent very handsome donation of $30,000 from Mr. W. C. MacDonald, and of the approaching completion of the great Redpath Museum.

Rev. Prof. Clark Murray also responded for the University. He dwelt particularly upon the changes recently made in the curriculum, stating his firm belief that they were in the best interests of coming students and of the efficiency of the University teaching.

Rev. E. J. Rexford, as a Representative Fellow, addressed words expressive of the affection and gratitude entertained by graduates towards their University.

Prof. Moyse proposed "Our sister Universities," which was responded to in an eloquent speech by the Hon. P. J. O. Chauveau. The hon. gentleman, at the conclusion, took occasion to recommend very strongly the establishment of a *pensionnat* for students such as they have already at Laval.

Principal Dawson then proposed "The University and Montreal." He spoke of the founder, James McGill, as "a giant in his day," and alluded feelingly to many others upon the now long list of benefactors. He referred to the love of fame inherent in man, and contended that no more lasting monument could a man raise for himself than an endowment, a chair, or a scholarship, and finally compared the University to the peaceful St. Lawrence —always flowing onwards, and bestowing benefits throughout its course.

Mr. Geo. Hague responded for the citizens, and strongly urged the necessity of providing the $150,000 asked for, showing how easy it would be for such a wealthy city to find so small a sum for such a great purpose.

The Rev. Dr. Stevenson then proposed "Canada." In a most eloquent and stirring address he drew a picture of this great country as it is and is bound to become. Its climate, its scenery, its perfect freedom, its peaceful admixture of two great nationalities, its boundless capabilities,—all these were touched upon with a master hand.

This toast was most suitably responded to by Dr. Louis H. Frechette, the crowned poet of the French Academy, of whom this Canada is so justly proud. On resuming his seat Dr. Frechette was greeted with loud cries of *Soixante-dix*, in response to which he repeated the words of his poem "1870." This stirring recitation by the talented author was warmly applauded. Mr. Eugene Lafleur then sang "*Sol Canadien.*"

Prof. J. E. Robidoux then proposed "McGill in Parliament," which was responded to by Mr. G. W. Stephens, M.P.P.

The toast of "The Ladies," who have been largely benefactresses of McGill University, was duly honoured, and a very successful meeting came to a close.

COLLEGE OF PHYSICIANS AND SURGEONS, PROVINCE OF QUEBEC.

The semi-annual meeting of this College (the Provincial Medical Board), was held in the old Government House (Laval Medical School) Notre Dame street, Montreal, on the 10th May,

Dr. R. Palmer Howard, President, in the chair. The attendance of governors was good, only six being absent. After the opening of the meeting resolutions of condolence with the families of the late Drs. Munro and Bibaud, of Montreal, and Dr. Dubé, of Rivière-du-Loup, were passed, and copies ordered to be sent to the relations of deceased. The President announced that at the present session of the Legislature the College had obtained important amendments to its Act, having especial reference to the penal and prosecuting clauses of the Act. These amendments were drawn up by the Hon. Mr. Mercier, and before presentation to the Legislature were submitted to and approved by the Governors of the College representing Montreal and Quebec. The tariff which had become law only last year was abolished, but the right to make a tariff was still possessed by the College.

The Board of Preliminary Examiners reported that the following gentlemen had successfully passed the required examination, and been admitted to the study of medicine:—Alfred Letourneau, H. Ernest Choquette, Albert Rolland, Ovide Ostigny, Charles Collett, John L. Duffett, Touissant Charron, Charles Pilon, F. Marquis, Jules Laberge, L. J. Hercule Roy, Alfred Poole, Alex. Boucher, A. Faucher de St. Maurice, Aquilas Cheval, Auguste F. Schmidt, Wilbrod Henault, Henry Dauth, Anaclet Bernard, James B. Gibson, Hercule Roy, Eugene Mackay, Arthur Delisle, Joseph Rodier, A. N. Worthington, Charles Rochon and L. J. N. Delorme. Twenty-one candidates were rejected. The assessors of the various schools reported favorably on all the examinations. The question as to the right of Dr. Keyes, of Georgeville, P. Q., to register his Eclectic diploma, granted in 1868 by the Province of Ontario, came up for discussion. The Secretary read the opinion of the Hon. Dr. Church, Q.C., a member of the College, affirming Dr. Keyes' right to register; also an opinion obtained by the College from W. H. Kerr, Q.C., to the same effect. The subject was deferred to another meeting for discussion and action.

Mr. C. E. Lamirande, the detective officer of the College,

presented his report for the past six months, showing that during that time he had taken out twenty-two actions; of these, eleven had resulted favorably to the College, four had been dismissed, and seven were still pending in court. He reported having compelled two persons to properly qualify themselves by taking out the license, and to having collected a considerable amount of arrears of contribution. The collection of the contributions was placed in Mr. Lamirande's hands. The committee to whom had been referred the charges against Dr. A. M. Ross, and who reported at the last semi-annual meeting that the Act gave them no power to act, again reported that in accordance with the instructions given them they suggested that the following be inserted in the Medical Act, with a view of meeting such and similar cases:—"Any registered member of the medical profession who shall have been convicted of any felony in any court of law, or who shall have been guilty of infamous or disgraceful conduct in any professional respect, shall be liable to have his name erased from the register, and in case of a person known to have been convicted of felony or who has been guilty of infamous or disgraceful conduct in any professional respect shall present himself for registration, the Registrar shall have the power to refuse registration. The Provincial Medical Board may, and upon application in writing of any three registered members of the profession in this province, shall cause enquiry to be made in the case of any person alleged to be liable to have his name erased from the register under the provisions of this section, and on proof of such conviction or of such infamous or disgraceful conduct as aforesaid, shall cause the name of such person to be erased from the register."

The following gentlemen were appointed a committee to arrange a new tariff of fees, and to be ready to report at the September meeting of the College: Drs. Lemieux and Parke (Quebec), Drs. Lachapelle and F. W. Campbell (Montreal), Dr. Perreault (Longue Pointe), Dr. Prevost (St. Jerome), Dr. Ladouceur (Sorel), and Dr. Worthington (Sherbrooke).

The President suggested that it would be as well to confine

the new tariff to a few items, and to have the fees for operations, &c., a matter for arrangment.

The following women, after examination, were found qualified and received the Midwifery Diploma of the College : Mrs. Mary Davies, Mrs. Mary Böhme, Mrs. Jessie McNab, Mrs. Margaret Miller, Mrs. Elizabeth Sutherland, Mrs. Sophie Husson,, and Miss Emily Harris.

The following gentlemen presented diplomas from the Universities named, and, after being sworn, received the license as member of the College :

McGill University—A. A. Henderson, M.D., Ottawa ; Wm. Stephen, M.D., Montreal ; Alex. D. Struthers, M.D., Freligbsburg, Q. ; Hastwell W. Thornton, M.D. ; New Richmond, Q. ; Alex. H. Dunlop, M D., Pembroke, Ont. ; Robt. H. Klock, M.D., Aylmer, P.Q. ; Wm. G. Duncan, M.D., Granby ; Wm. B. Burland, M.D., Port Kent, N.Y., U.S. ; R. C. McCorkill, M.D., West Farnham.

University of Bishop's College—Walter J. Prendergast, M.D., Montreal ; Ninian C. Smillie, M.D., Montreal ; James L. Foley, M.D., L.R.C.P., Lond., Montreal ; William D. M. Bell, M.D., Ottawa.

Victoria College—Fred. St. Jacques, M.D., St. Anne des Plaines ; J. Bpte. LeRoy, M.D., Montreal ; Jos. H. Gauthier, M.D., St. Pie ; Felix P. Vanier, M.D., St. Martin ; Samuel K. Kelly, M.D., French Village, Kingsey ; J. Bpte. Maillot, M.D., Memramcook, N.B. ; Alex. Snyck, M.D., Wright ; Horace Manseau, M D., Montreal ; Napoleon Dubeau, M.D., St. Gabriel de Brandon.

Laval University (*Quebec*)—Albert Marois, M.D., Joseph A. Marcoux, M.D., Auguste C. Hamel, Laval University, Montreal ; Isaie Cormier, M.D., Montreal ; Joseph Cuerrier, M.D., Coteau Landing ; Ovila Maillet, M.D., Montreal.

Dr. Larocque, Health Officer of Montreal, appeared before the College and advocated the Public Health Bill now before Parliament. A resolution heartily endorsing it was unanimously passed, after which the College adjourned.

Obituary.

HORATIO YATES, M.D.

We regret to chronicle the death of this eminent physician of Kingston. Dr. Yates was one of the most prominent physicians of that city, and his name was known and respected throughout the profession. The following particulars are taken from the *Queen's College Journal* :—

" Dr. Horatio Yates, son of Dr. Wm. Yates, of Sapperton, Derbyshire, Eng., was born in 1821, in Otsego County, N.Y., and came to an uncle in Kingston at 12 years of age. Five years later he was articled to the late Dr. Sampson as a medical student, attended the courses at the University in Philadelphia, and took his degrees there in medicine in 1842. Thence he went to London and spent a year at St. George's Hospital. Since then he has been employed here in an active and successful practice of his profession to the present time. He was much devoted not only to science, but to works of charity, and the poor always received medical services and medicine at his hands without stint. In 1854 he undertook a reform of the Kingston Hospital, which had become completely demoralized. He found, on his return to Kingston after a long absence from sickness, the building in a state of complete dilapidation, the fences gone and the little remaining furniture utterly worthless. The wards contained less than a dozen patients, and the medical services performed by an inexperienced young man at a petty salary. The Hospital was being managed by a committee of the City Council, good men in their way, but who knew nothing and cared less for hospital work. In order to achieve his purpose, he became a city alderman, got placed on the Hospital Committee, and soon assumed full charge, medical and financial, assisted by Drs. Dickson and Strange, who cordially co-operated in the work. His first act was to advance from his own pocket many hundred dollars to pay off executions against the Hospital and to purchase necessary supplies ; next he sought and obtained a new charter, which he himself had drawn up, placing the charter in the hands of life governors and a few *ex-officio* governors. The new board relieved him of personal supervision, and has to this day managed the Hospital with great success. He was for many years chairman of the Board. In the establishment of the Medical Faculty of Queen's University in 1854 he took an active part, and chose for himself the chair of science and practice of medicine. Until the change to the Royal College he had for some time been Dean of the Faculty.

" In the fall of 1873 he was appointed Surgeon in A Battery, which position he occupied until recently, when he resigned and came to Kingston to resume the practice of his profession. The reason he accepted the position in the first place was with a view to recuperating in health and securing a cessation from his arduous duties. His last residence here has been very short."

Dr. Yates had as a young man been threatened with pulmonary disease ; but his final illness was very short, as he died a few days only after having been taken with pneumonia. His genial social qualities, combined with much ability, had made him very popular, and he will long be missed in his chosen city.

—We regret to hear of the death of Dr. Fred. Wright, of Toronto, son of Dr. H. H. Wright, Lecturer on Medicine at the Toronto School. Dr. Wright graduated in 1872 at the University, and after two years in the hospitals of Europe, returned to his native town, and was appointed joint Lecturer on Histology at the Toronto School.

Medical Items.

THE MEDICAL ASSOCIATION OF ONTARIO.—The second meeting of the Ontario Medical Association will be held in Toronto on June 6th.

—John Campbell, M.D., McGill, has been admitted L.R.C.P., Edinburgh, at the examinations held in April.

—Rankine Dawson, B.A., M.D. (McGill, 1882), has been appointed surgeon to a section of the Canadian Pacific Railway.

—J. Williams, M.D. (McGill, 1881), has been appointed City physician to Charlestown, Mass.

—The Canadian students attending at Edinburgh have formed themselves into a club, and have obtained rooms at the Literary Institute.

—We are pleased to notice that James Robertson, M.D. (McGill), of Montague, P.E.I.; P. McLaren, M.D. (McGill), of New Perth, P.E.I.; and J. Gillies, M.D. (McGill), of Summerside, P.E.I., have been elected to the Local Assembly of Prince Edward Island.

McGill Graduates Society.—The annual meeting of the McGill Graduates' Society was held on the 2nd inst., in the Natural History Society's Rooms, when the following officers were elected for 1882:—President, J. S. McLennan, B.A.; Vice-Presidents, J. Hall, B.A., B.C.L., W. A. Molson, M.D., J. McLeod, M.A.; Secretary, W. McLennan, B.C.L.; Treasurer, H. H. Lyman, M.A. Non-resident Councillors—Rev. J. Taylor, B.A., Quebec; Brown Chamberlain, D.C.L., Ottawa; J. A. Grant, M.D., Ottawa; Chas. Gibb, B.A., Abbotsford; J. Stewart, M.D., Brucefield, Ont. Resident Councillors—R. L. Macdonnell, M.D., A. McGowan, B.C.L., J. R. Dougall, M.A., F. Kelly, Ph.D., Rev. E. J. Rexford, B.A., C. H. Chandler, M.A.

—Among the widespread and steadily increasing race of bores, a high place must be claimed for those fussy and objectionable people who, under cover of social relations, persist in endeavoring to obtain a medical opinion without payment of a fee. An old lady the other day asked an eminent London surgeon, who was seated beside her at a dinner table, what was the best "cure for corns." To this the surgeon replied: "You can adopt no better plan, my dear madam, than to grease the corn over night with a tallow candle, when I venture to say you will find the corn kicking about the bottom of your bed next morning." The old lady was profuse in her thanks, but the surgeon cut them short by adding, "I should say, my dear madam, that it would still be on your foot."

CANADA

MEDICAL & SURGICAL JOURNAL

JUNE, 1882.

Original Communications.

REMARKS ON OPTIC NEURITIS.

By F. BULLER, M.D., M.R.C.S., Eng.,
Lecturer on Ophthalmology in McGill University; Attending Physician to the Ophthalmic and Aural Department, Montreal General Hospital.

(Read before the Medico-Chirurgical Society of Montreal.)

It is not my intention to go deeply into the subject of optic neuritis; in fact it would be trespassing too much on the patience and good nature of this Society were I to attempt any such exploit on the present occasion. Nevertheless, having seen in the past six years quite a considerable number of cases in which optic neuritis formed a prominent symptom of other morbid conditions, I will try and make use of them in such a way as to illustrate some of the points of interest in this complicated and difficult chapter in neural pathology. I have only to mention the theories that have been advanced in explanation of optic neuritis, to justify the expressions I have made use of in speaking of the subject as a difficult one, and to show furthermore that there is still much to be learned before we can say our knowledge of this affection is satisfactory and complete.

These theories are four in number. They all, however, start on the common basis, viz.: that the affection is caused in some way by, and is an expression of an abnormally increased intracranial pressure, leaving out of the question, of course, the comparatively rare instances in which the condition is due to disease situated on the side of the optic chiasm.

4 peripheral

The first was advanced by Von Grafe, who held that abnormal and excessive intra-cranial pressure so acted on the cavernous sinus as to cause a stasis in the ophthalmic vein, and hence the swelling and venous engorgement about the optic papilla. This theory is now generally admitted to be incorrect.

The second seems to offer a satisfactory explanation of a certain number of cases, and still finds some supporters. According to this theory, fluid from the arachnoid space finds its way into the nerve sheaths, and thus causes choking of the lymph vessels in the optic papilla. According to this theory, sheath dropsy is the cause of the papillitis.

The third, as I understand it, teaches that the irritation of the brain, induced by certain intra-cranial lesions, causes a disturbance in the vaso-motor nerves, which govern the blood vessels of the papillæ, and thus give rise to the effusion into these structures.

The fourth assumes that with every case of papillitis there is œdema of the brain substance, that is, interference with the lymph circulation. By direct continuity this obstruction or interference extends to the intra-ocular portion of the nerves, and occasions the swelling, etc., of these parts.

However plausible each of these theories may seem, facts have been observed in connection with different cases of optic neuritis which cannot be explained by any one of them. How, for instance, account for the occasional occurrence of monocular papillitis under apparently identical conditions with those that induce the ordinary symmetrical disease? Or, if œdema of the brain is essential to the production of papillitis, how explain a case described by Hughlings Jackson in which there was atrophy of the brain? Some of these mysteries we cannot yet solve; but I strongly suspect the difficulty will ultimately be found to lie in our defective knowledge of the process of nutrition as occurring in the brain and the structures so closely connected therewith as are the optic nerves.

If my memory serves, I once heard H. Jackson say he could quite believe the papilla forms a sort of indicator for the condition of the brain, even where no actual disease of the optic nerve can be said to exist, and I often think there is a good deal of truth in this remark when I see a dull, turbid-looking nerve in the eye of some unfortunate who has been burning the candle at both ends. The conditions giving rise to optic neuritis are so various in regard to the nature and extent of the primary lesions that we cannot look for any constant set of symptoms indicative of this change. Violent and persistent headache, giddiness, vomiting, and epileptiform attacks occur probably only when the intra-cranial disease has progressed so rapidly that the brain has not had time to become tolerant of the irritant. On the other hand, there are many cases in which a dull, heavy feeling in the head, slight headache, with some obtuseness of the intellectual faculties, and loss of memory, may be the only symptoms noticed. This is true of a case recently in the Hospital, who came to me on account of catarrhal deafness, and merely incidentally one day mentioned that he thought his sight was failing. This led me to make an examination of the eyes, and I discovered a well-pronounced double optic neuritis, with considerable diminution of acuity of vision in one eye, and to a less degree in the other—R. 20/50, L. 20/30. A chart of the visual fields made with Carmalt's Perimeter shows that both are contracted, the left moderately, with pretty good central vision, the right reduced to an exceedingly small area, and the sense of color obliterated. In the left eye the color sense, though impaired, is still fairly good. This man was some four weeks under treatment in Hospital, and during this time his vision did not undergo further deterioration. His history was not conclusive of syphilis, though there was pretty strong presumptive evidence that way. He had no symptoms of brain trouble beyond slight dullness, and some pretty constant headache, though never at all severe.

Another case still in Hospital came to me last November complaining of pain in the eyes, when used as they had been a good deal in reading and sewing late at night. Her story was just that of a person suffering from asthenopia after over-use of the eyes, except that she occasionally lost her sight altogether for a few moments or minutes. Vision, when first examined, was normal in both eyes. A few days later she came again, saying she could not see so well. I then found vision barely 20/20 with one eye, and only 20/30 with the other. This led me to make an opthalmoscopic examination, which resulted in the discovery of double optic neuritis. I then made further enquiries, and found that for several months she had suffered from intense headache, chiefly in the left temple, and thought to be ordinary neuralgia, but she had also had two or three fits, evidently epileptiform. She was sent to Hospital and placed under treatment, and although the head symptons are greatly mitigated, the nerve affections has gone on to atrophy, and terminated in total blindness.

The disease, as far as the eyes are concerned, has run a rapid course, more so I think than can be explained by a tumor of the brain, unless it presses on the optic tracts or chiasma. Optic neuritis from cerebral tumor is known to exist in some instances for a very long time before blindness ensues, and on the other hand there may be symptoms of cerebral tumor for many years before papillitis occurs. This woman may have had neuritis for a much longer time than we are aware, but still the fact of rapid failure of vision remains the same. The case is one in which there is strong reason to suspect constitutional syphilis, and with this in view mercury was used energetically from the commencement; indeed the drug was pushed farther than I intended, for the mouth became decidedly sore, probably from want of care and cleanliness on the part of the patient. I make it a rule always to stop short of this result in the treatment of these cases, for I am quite certain actual mercurialization cannot be desirable in any instance. Tumors of the cerebellum are well known to be a frequent cause of optic neuritis, but Hughlings Jackson says he has never seen it associated with cerebellar abscess. Now it so happens that I have only seen one case of cerebellar abscess since I have been in Montreal, and in that instance there developed a double optic neuritis some three weeks before death. I have already mentioned this case in a paper on mastoid disease in a brief note as follows:

Case XV.—J. L., æt. 23, French-Canadian; mill-hand; chronic purulent middle-ear disease since childhood. During the past ten years the discharge was only occasional and scanty. The hearing power was entirely destroyed. Came to Hospital in June, 1879, on account of intense pain in the back of the head, which had persisted ever since an attack of ear-ache the previous autumn, brought on by working in the cold and wet. There was also great tenderness over and behind mastoid, *but not a trace of swelling*; scanty purulent discharge from the ear and nearly complete loss of the drum-head. The patient walked like a drunken man, and suffered excruciating pain from slight movement, such as driving in a cab; vomited occasionally without any apparent cause. Examined when first seen there was no sign of optic neuritis. A few days after admission an ophthalmoscopic examination was made, and double optic neuritis discovered. Diagnosis—Abscess of cerebellum, secondary to chronic middle ear disease. Died July 13th, twenty-five days after admission. The *post-mortem* revealed an abscess half the size of a hen's egg, in left lateral lobe of cerebellum. Unfortunately, I was absent from Montreal when he died, and did not witness the *post-mortem*. No minute examination of the bone was made, and therefore the connection between the abscess and the disease of the ear was not discovered, though there can be no reasonable doubt that the two conditions stood in the relation of cause and effect.

This patient, when interrogated as to his vision, claimed to see quite well, but was too ill to undergo an accurate examination, or to give reliable answers. The pupils, however, were equal, active, and not at all dilated. There is no reason to doubt the abscess had existed for many months, and thus, perhaps, approximated in its local effects the action of a slowly-growing tumor. I am not sufficiently familiar with abscess of the cerebellum to say whether a delay in the fatal issue is usually of considerable duration.

I may here mention another case of mastoid disease of a subacute character, in which the patient had pretty severe brain symptoms. After these had lasted some weeks, I was asked to make an ophthalmoscopic examination, and found well-marked double optic neuritis, without discoverable impairment of vision. This case ultimately made, I believe, a complete recovery, and is probably unique of its kind.

Sometimes we meet with neuritis for which no cause can be assigned beyond the possible injurious influence of exposure to cold or wet. In 1878, I treated a youth, 19 years of age, at the General Hospital, who belonged in this category. There was no history of syphilis or injury, nor any symptoms indicating brain trouble. He attributed his eye trouble to working in a cold, draughty shop, and being often suddenly chilled after becoming heated at his work. The eye presented the ordinary characters of a moderately developed neuro-retinitis, with great impairment of vision. Under the use of mercury and iodide of potassium, in pretty full doses, the nerves cleared up, and vision was considerably improved when he left the Hospital. I have not seen the case since, though he promised to come as an out-patient if vision was not in a satisfactory condition. It has been said that very great swelling of the optic papilla, amounting to more than four dioptries, is diagnostic of brain tumor, and that white spots about the macula, having a stellate arrangement like the well-known picture of Bright's Retina, indicates a chronic meningitis.

Some time ago I treated a young gentleman for optic neuritis, with swelling amounting to five dioptries, and about the macula the exact picture of Bright's Retina, the entire disease disappearing under the use of mercury inunctions and iodide of potash, in very large doses, for a month or more; about 300 grains of potash were taken daily. Although the optic nerves are now decidedly atrophic in appearance, vision remains almost unimpaired. In this case the disease was undoubtedly some form of brain syphilis. The visual trouble had been preceded by several weeks of intense headache, which also speedily subsided under treatment.

The more I see of optic neuritis, the more I am convinced that Hughlings Jackson struck the key-note of its treatment when he said the only remedies we can rely upon are mercury and iodide of potash in full doses. Doubtless there are many cases which will terminate disastrously, no matter what plan of treatment is pursued; but, on the other hand, a fair proportion will yield to these drugs, and if taken in time an otherwise incurable blindness may be averted by inducing absorption of the products of inflammation before they have induced hopeless degeneration and disorganization of the nerves.

Many cases are no doubt of syphilitic origin, in which we can get no history sufficiently definite to warrant a positive diagnosis of syphilis, such, for instance, as the one from which the right optic nerve now in my possession was taken.

The patient, a robust young man, employed as a commercial traveller, was brought from a provincial town about 200 miles distant in a condition of unconsciousness, which had lasted for several days. No definite history of the case could be obtained, and there was much obscurity as to the real nature of the case. Three or four days after his arrival in Montreal, I was asked to make an ophthalmoscopic examination. I found the patient in a comatose state, but had no difficulty in making out a commencing doubleoptic neuritis. The patient died the same day, and the autopsy revealed several rather large syphilitic gummata in the brain and a greatly swollen condition of the optic nerves, with the characteristic ampulla-like enlargement close behind the eyeball. The chances are that an early diagnosis and energetic treatment would have saved this patient's life.

There is a peculiar group of cases in which neuro-retinitis seems to be induced by menstrual disorders. Of these, the few I have seen have occurred in connection with suppression of the menses. The last patient of this class under my observation was a young woman about 20 years of age, who had not menstruated for more than six months. During all this time she had suffered almost constantly from headache, often very severely. For three months she had noticed an increasing impairment of vision, and latterly was scarcely able to read ordinary print. I found double neuro-retinitis, without hemorrhages, or white exudations in the retina. There was neither anæmia nor debility. I commenced treatment by the local abstraction of blood by means of the artificial leech, then the rapid induction of slight mercurialization—this to be kept up for several weeks,—together with potassium iodide in moderate doses three times daily.

I have since been informed that under this treatment a complete recovery was made.

Two other cases in which atrophy of the nerves had made considerable progress before a similar treatment was adopted did not terminate so favourably. The atrophic process not being arrested, complete loss of vision ensued.

In view of the importance of optic neuritis, both as a symptom and as an affection which often requires to be treated *per se* with as little delay as possible after its existence has once been discovered, I cannot refrain from urging most strongly the propriety of making a careful ophthalmoscopic examination from time to time in all cases of obstinate or persistent headache, and especially if other features in the case render the occurrence of this serious and important lesion a matter of probability. Although, in treating optic neuritis, we must be guided to a great extent, in the choice of the various measures to be employed, by the particular circumstances connected with each case, we have in mercury and iodide of potash two remedies of immense value when properly used, in a large proportion of these cases. If mercury is to be of any service, it must be used with tolerable freedom, and the same holds good of iodide of potash, but admits of being emphasized still more strongly. Without intending to lay down any hard and fast rules, I may say the plan I generally adopt is as follows: Secure physical and mental rest as far as possible by making the patient stay in bed in a quiet, dimly-lighted apartment; carefully regulate the diet. Use mercury, in the form of inunction twice daily, about a drachm of the strong ointment each time. Keep the mouth scrupulously clean, and as soon as the gums show the action of the mercury is unmistakeable, diminish the quantity used just to the extent of keeping up this action and no more; this must be continued from four to six weeks. About the third day of the mercurial inunctions, commence with iodide of potash, say three or four grains for the first dose, and increase by one grain each dose, at the same time increasing the quantity of water in which it is dissolved. A drachm of the salt will require to be dissolved in about a tumblerful of water, otherwise gastric disturbance will be likely to occur. I never stop short of 30 grains three times daily, and have several times given more than two drachms thrice daily for a long time without causing inconvenience and with most satisfactory results. If symptoms of iodism present themselves, the quantity administered must be reduced to such an extent as may be necessary for their removal.

THE ÆTIOLOGY OF TUBERCULOSIS.

AN ADDRESS DELIVERED BY DR. ROBERT KOCH BEFORE THE PHYSIOLOGICAL SOCIETY OF BERLIN.

TRANSLATED BY W. D. OAKLEY, M.D, (McGILL).

The discovery made by Villemin that Tuberculosis can be conveyed to animals has, as is well known, received frequent confirmation, but apparently well founded contradictions have also been made to it, so that until a few years ago, it remained undecided whether Tuberculosis were an infectious disease or not. Since, however, the inoculation in the aqueous chamber of the eye, performed firstly by Cohnheim and Solomonson, and later by Baumgarten, and further the inhalation experiments of Tappen and others have confirmed without doubt the contagious nature of Tuberculosis, a place amongst infectious diseases must in future be assigned to it.

If the importance of a malady be measured by the number of victims who perish by it, then all diseases, including the most dreaded infectious diseases, such as Pestilence, Cholera, etc., must pass into the background when compared with Tuberculosis. From statistics we learn that 1-7 of mankind die from Tuberculosis, and when nearly the mid or reproductive ages are taken into consideration, a third, and often more than a third, of these are carried off by Tuberculosis. The public have therefore sufficient reason to devote their attention to so fatal a disease, wholly apart from the fact that other circumstances, (of which merely the relation of Tuberculosis to the Perlsucht of domestic animals will be mentioned,) claim the interest of the sanitary authorities.

In the study of infectious diseases one great object of investigation with reference to the public well-being, is the elucidation to their ætiology; therefore it is our urgent duty, making use-of the light shed by previous investigations, to seek out the cause of Tuberculosis. It has been repeatedly attempted to isolate the morbid agent or germ of Tuberculosis but hitherto without success. The various staining processes which, in so many cases, have led to the discovery of Pathological micro-organisms, have completely failed in this instance. Again, the experiment of isolating and cultivating the Tubercular virus, could not, up to the present moment, be regarded as successful, so that Cohnheim, in the latest edition of his lectures on General Pathology designates "The discovery of Tubercular virus as a problem which, "up to the present day remains unsolved."

In my researches into Tuberculosis I adhered at first only to the known methods without succeeding in attaining any enlightenment as to the cause of the disease, but I was led through some chance observations to forsake these methods and to adopt others, by the aid of which I was finally enabled to attain positive results. The object of the investigation was directed to proving the presence of foreign parasitic organisms which possibly could be regarded as the causes of the disease. This proof I was able to obtain through certain special methods of staining, with the help of which, Bacteria—heretofore unrecognized—were found in all Tubercular organs. It would take too long to describe the way by which I arrived at this new mode of procedure, and therefore I will pass on at once to the description of the results I obtained. The objects to be examined were prepared in the usual manner for examining Pathological Bacteria: namely, either spread out on the cover slip, dried and heated: or, after hardening in alcohol, cut into sections. The cover glasses, or sections were placed in the following staining fluid: 200 Ccm. of distilled water were mixed with 1 Ccm. of a concentrated alcoholic mythelene blue: this solution must be well shaken, and then must be added 0.2 Ccm. of a 10 p.c. solution of caustic potash. This mixture should give no precipitate after standing for days. The objects to be colored remain in the same

NOTE.—These two objects, cover-glasses and sections, refer to the material used.—That is a soft material such as pus, caseous matter, &c., is spread on a cover-glass while a tissue is made into sections, and then both heated alike.

from 20 to 24 hours, though by warming the staining fluid to 40° C. in a water bath, this time can be shortened from half an hour to one hour. After this a concentrated aqueous solution of Vesuvin (Bismark Brown)—which must be filtered each time before it is used—is then poured upon the coverslips, and washed off after one or two minutes. When the cover slips come out of the mythelene blue the stratum adhering to each appears of a dark blue colour, but through the treatment with Vesuvin, the dark blue color is lost, and each appears of a faint brown.

Under the microscope all the tissue elements, particularly the cell-nuclei, and their detritus appear of a brown colour, while the tubercular Bacteria, on the contrary, appear of a beautiful blue. All other Bacteria I have as yet examined,—with the exception of Lepra-bacteria,—take a brown colour by this staining process. The contrast in color between the brown-coloured tissues and the blue Tubercle Bacteria is so striking that in spite of the very small number in which the latter often exist, they can be detected with the greatest certainty, and as such be recognized. The sections are to be treated in a similar manner. They are taken from the mythelene-blue solution, are placed in the filtrated solution of Vesuvin, and remain in it from 15 to 20 minutes; they are then washed in distilled water until the blue color disappears and a brown color, more or less deep, takes its place. After that they are freed from water with alcohol cleared up in oil of clove, and can then at once be microscopically examined in this fluid, or else finally preserved in Canada Balsam. In these preparations also the tissue elements appear brown, and the bacteria in tubercles blue.

The Bacteria which are rendered visible by this method, present an appearance peculiar in many respects. They have a staff-like shape, and thus belong to the group of the Bacilli. They are very thin, and as long as a quarter, or one half of the diameter of a red blood corpuscle, though they can attain a greater length, even to the complete diameter of the blood corpuscle. As regards their shape and size, they possess a striking similarity to the Lepra-bacilli, but they can be distinguished from the latter by being a little thinner, and more pointed at the ends. The Lepra-bacilli also stain by Weigert's methods of staining, but the Tubercular-bacilli do not. On all points where the Tubercular process is of fresh origin and is advancing rapidly, the bacilli are present in great quantities; they then form ordinarily, small groups closely pressed together and often arranged in bundles, which frequently lie in the interior of cells, and in some places give exactly such pictures as the Lepra-bacilli. On the other hand there are abundant bacilli which lie free: especially at the edge of large caseous deposits there are almost exclusively groups of bacilli which are not enclosed in cells. As soon as the acme of the tubercular infection is past, the bacilli are not so numerous, and they are then found only in small groups, or even singly, at the edge of the tubercular deposit along with bacilli which are weakly stained and scarcely recognizable; apparently, these have either begun to die, or are already dead. At last, they may wholly disappear, though it is only very seldom that they are completely wanting, and then only in the places where the tubercular process has come to a stand still.

When giant cells appear in the tubercular tissues the bacilli generally lie in the interior of these structures. In tubercular processes which are slowly advancing, the interior of the giant cells is generally the only place where the bacilli can be found. In this case the majority of the giant cells enclose either one or a few bacilli, and it makes a striking impression to find over large areas of the section, ever-recurring new groups of giant-cells, almost every one of which contains in the wide interior space, surrounded by brown-stained nuclei, one or two exquisitely fine, blue-stained staves, seated almost in the centre of the giant-cell.

It is also possible to recognize the Bacilli unstained. For this purpose it is best to choose such places as contain the Bacilli in large numbers: we can take a little substance from a grey miliary nodule in the lung of a guinea-pig which has died of artificial tuberculosis, and examine it in distilled water or blood serum—to avoid the currents in the preparation it is better to use a hollowed slide, under these circumstances the bacilli appear as very fine rods with a molecular movement. Independent movement is entirely wanting in them.

Under certain circumstances, which we will mention later, the Bacilli form spores, even in the animal body; the simple rods then contain from two to four spores which are arranged longitudinally, at regular intervals.

With reference to the presence of the Bacilli in the different tubercular diseases of man and animals, I have investigated up to the present the following cases:—

I. From man: 11 cases of Miliary Tuberculosis. The Bacilli here were never absent in the miliary tubercles of the lungs, often indeed they could not be found in nodules of which the centres did not stain, but in such cases they were found in small groups at the edge of the tubercle. In young tubercles, whose centres were still non-caseous, they were found in great quantities. They were also found in the miliary tubercles of the spleen, the liver and kidneys, and especially abundant in the grey nodules of the Pia Mater in Basilar Meningitis. In caseous bronchial glands, also, which in several cases were investigated by me, dense groups of Bacilli were found, and among them, many containing spores; here they were generally found in the miliary tubercles, embedded in the gland tissue.

II.—*Twelve* cases of caseous Bronchitis and pneumonia, in which cavities were present. The presence of the Bacilli was here generally limited to the edge of the caseous infiltration, and they were often present in great numbers. Also in the interior of the infiltrated portion of lung nests of the Bacilli were sometimes to be seen. In the cavities they were especially abundant. The well-known small caseous masses consist almost entirely of masses of Bacilli. Among those Bacilli which were met with in the cavities and in the softened caseous deposits, sometimes many were found which contained spores. In the large cavities they were mixed with other Bacteria, though from the difference in staining they were easily to be distinguished from these; tubercle Bacteria staining blue, and the others, as already mentioned, brown.

III.—*One* case of solitary Tubercle of the brain, the nodules being larger than a hazel-nut. The caseous mass of the tubercle was enclosed by a tissue rich in cells, among which, many giant-cells were embedded. The greater number of giant-cells contained no parasites, but here and there groups of giant-cells were seen, each of which contained one or more Bacilli.

IV.—*Two* cases of Intestinal Tuberculosis. In the tubercular nodules which were grouped around the intestinal ulcer, the Bacilli could be very easily seen, and they were principally contained in the smallest and most recent nodules. In the mesenteric glands in these two cases, the Bacilli were present in great numbers.

V.—*Three* cases of freshly extirpated bronchial glands. Only in two of these could the Bacilli be seen, enclosed in giant-cells.

VI.—*Four* cases of fungous inflammation of joints. In two cases the Bacilli were found in giant-cells which were arranged in small groups.

Then follows a list of affected animals in which the bacilli were found.

By the regularity of the presence of the tubercular bacilli, it may appear strange that they have not been discovered ere this time, but this can be explained by the fact that the bacilli are extraordinarily small structures and very few in number, especially where their presence is limited to the interior of giant-cells, so that, in the absence of special staining re-action, they would not be seen by the most attentive observer. If they are present in greater quantities they are so mingled with and covered by a fine granular detritus than their detection is even rendered in the highest degree difficult. It is true there exists some assertions as to the presence of micro-organisms in tissues which have undergone tubercular changes. Schüller, in his paper upon Scrofulous and Tubercular Joint diseases, mentions that he has constantly found Micrococci. Doubtless in this case, as also with regard to the very small moveable granules found by Klebs in Tubercles, the appearance must have been produced by something else than the Tubercular Bacilli seen by me, which are immovable and rod-shaped. Further Aufrecht, as he says in the first volume of his Pathological Reports, has found in a number of rabbits which he had infected with Tubercular substances, three cases in which in the centre of the tubercular nodules—

along with two different varieties of micrococci—there were also short rod-shaped structures, whose long diameter only exceeded the short diameter by half. The tubercle bacilli, on the contrary, are at least five times as long as they are thick, or even still larger in proportion to their thickness; besides, in pure tuberculosis they are never mixed with micrococci or other Bacteria. It is therefore extremely improbable that Aufrecht has seen the real Tubercle Bacilli; were this the case, he would probably have found the bacilli in human tubercle, and in the lungs of the Perlsucht, and the striking relation between the Bacilli and the giant-cells could not have escaped him.

On the ground of my abundant observations, I regard it as proved that in all Tubercular affections of men and animals, the Bacteria, designated by me as Tubercle Bacilli, which through their characteristic properties are differentiated from all other micro-organisms, are constantly present.

(To be continued.)

AN ABNORMALITY.

By J. J. GUERIN, M.D., Montreal.

I was called last evening to attend a Mrs. R— in labour. On arriving, found the os dilated to the size of a silver dollar; the membranes had not yet been ruptured, but the head was pressing down forcibly. The pains were vigorous, and within three-quarters of an hour the membranes were torn and the head was on the perineum; after a few more pains, the child came into the world still-born. The first thing that struck me was the small size of the child, it having the appearance of a fœtus between the sixth and seventh months, notwithstanding the fact that the mother protests her belief that she has been in the *family way* during the last ten months.

The mother is a well-developed, powerfully-built woman, of English extraction. She menstruated normally about the 15th of last June, after which she says she felt that she was pregnant. Two months later, when her husband was coming home one evening, he was attacked and severely beaten at his own-door, before her eyes This naturally terrified her considerably, and the next day she says her menses returned, but only remained for twenty-four hours. Two months later one of her boarders, who worked in the St. Lawrence Sugar Refinery, was killed, having been suffocated while at work in one of the filters. When she saw him brought home she was greatly shocked, and for several months would not enter the room which the man had previously occupied. The woman seemed to have a presentiment that these frights were going to have an injurious effect on her child, for she drew my attention to the fact that she was not as large as she generally was when her children had come to full time, and as soon as the child was born she inquired if it was perfect. The father is a powerfully-built German, quite healthy. They have had two children, both of whom are healthy and strong. The infant which was just born presented the following peculiar abnormalities: Length, 15 inches; appears generally undeveloped, but more especially on the left side. The left side of the forehead was flattened, and the left side of face wore a blank expression, as though all the muscles were in a state of paralysis. There was inability to open the left eye, but the child was able to move both arms and legs. There is double hare-lip and cleft palate. The left forearm is of a most rudimentary character, thus bringing the hand very close to the humerus, and giving an appearance as though the wrist articulated with that bone; however, the elbow and a very small forearm can be felt. The hand articulates with the internal surface of this undeveloped forearm, and attached to the hand are four fingers, but no thumb. The right side of the head is fuller and rounder than the left; the right eye is more prominent than the opposite one, and was kept constantly open. There was a peculiar blueish appearance of the skin on the right side of the face and head, which was not perceptible on the left side. The thumb of the right hand is rather sessile, being attached to the hand merely by integument. The right testicle is present in the scrotum, but the left is conspicuous by its absence.

QUARTERLY REPORT ON PHARMACOLOGY AND THERAPEUTICS.

By J. STEWART, M.D., BRUCEFIELD, ONT.

THE TREATMENT OF DIABETES.

I.—*By Codeia.*

Dr. Shingleton Smith, at the last meeting of the British Medical Association, related the particulars of three cases of diabetes, which all exhibited marked improvement while taking Codeia, which improvement ceased when the Codeia was withheld, and was renewed on its repetition. Morphia had been given in two of the cases, but the result was not nearly so marked as when the Codeia was administered. Dr. Smith did not find any unpleasant effects following the use of Codeia. The skin continued moist and the bowels regular. Its use is not followed by headache. It can be given in very large doses without producing the physiological effects of opium. As much as 10 grains three times a day can be used by a diabetic without giving rise to any inconvenient symptoms.

Dr. Smith read a paper before the New York Academy of Medicine last February on the treatment of diabetes by means of Codeia. He gave the details of three well-marked cases of diabetes occurring in hard-worked men. The improvement followed quickly after the administration of the drug, and progressed steadily until all the symptoms, including the presence of sugar in the urine, had completely disappeared. More than a year has elapsed since the disappearance of the sugar from the urine. One point of interest was the fact that in these three cases the patients were hard-working men mentally, suffered from disturbances of digestion and mental depression, and led a sedentary life, with but little muscular exercise. Dr. Smith gave an account of a man, who, when he first came under his observation, in 1873, had lost 50 lbs. in weight. His urine had a sp. gr. of 1·044, and contained sugar in great abundance. He was placed upon Codeia, restricted diet, and the free use of claret with his meals, and in eighteen months he-gained in weight thirty-five pounds; the specific gravity and quantity of the urine had reached the normal; sugar had disappeared, and at the present time he was in excellent condition.

Dr. Wm. Squire says that he has seen a case of diabetes where three and a half ounces of sugar were excreted daily, completely recover where Codeia in full doses was one of the means employed.

II.—*By Bethesda Water.*

Dr. Murrell reports a case of *diabetes mellitus* treated by these waters, and although the patient died from acetonæmia, he considers that he was much benefited by their use, and urges a more extensive trial of them in *diabetes* and Bright's Disease. The spring is in Wisconsin. An analysis of the water shows that it contains seventeen grains of carbonate of lime and twelve of carbonate of magnesia to the gallon, besides chloride of sodium, sulphate of potash, alumina, silica, and some gaseous constituents. These waters have been recommended for several years by many American physicians. The patient is directed to take from eight to ten tumblerfuls daily for ten days, and then half the quantity for the next fifteen, thirty or sixty days.

III.—*By Chloride of Ammonium.*

Adamkievics, acting on the theory that protein, the fundamental sustenance of the organism, may be regarded as the resultant of sugar and ammonia, has made a series of experiments upon diabetics in the hope of reducing the morbid production of sugar by administering to them ammoniacal compounds. From his first series of experiments, made on healthy men he draws the following conclusions :—(1.) Ammonium chloride is decomposed in the intestine of the healthy man; the greater part of the resulting ammonia is absorbed and probably reappears in the urine in the form of albumen. (2). Ammonium chloride acts exactly like sodium chloride; it is dehydrated in the tissues, and favors the decomposition of albumen. (3). The decomposition of albumen and the excretion of ammonia do not proceed *pari passu.* In the second series of experiments made on diabetics, he remarks that (1) ammonia is quickly metabolized in them, and its assimilation coincides with the metabolism of the abnormal sugar, so that in slight cases the sugar may disappear from the urine. (2). So long as the sugar is not completely metabolized, the ammonia absorbed does not increase the quantity of water or urea excreted ; but so soon as the sugar disappears, both water and urea at once increase. This he takes to be a convincing proof that a part of the ammonia is converted into urea and is excreted as such.

Explanation of the Mode of Action of Bromide of Potassium, Atropin and Cinchonidin in the Cerebrum.

Dr. Albertoni, of Genoa, has arrived at the following conclusions as the result of an extended series of experimental investigations into the action of the above drugs on the cerebrum :

I.—The continuous use of bromide of potassium in dogs reduces the excitability of the brain in such a marked manner, that it no longer responds to electric irritation. One large dose is sufficient to deaden the activity of the cerebrum to electric irritation. After the continuous use of bromide in dogs, it is impossible to induce through electric irritation of the brain movements of the muscles of the face and extremities.

II.—Atropine increases the excitability of the cerebrum, and induces an increased susceptibility of it to electric irritation. The variations in the irritability and development of the cerebrum explains satisfactorily the following interesting facts :—(1) The slight action of atropine in childhood. (2) The cerebral symptoms induced by atropine in dogs are more severe than those in sheep. (3) The complete failure of atropine to have any influence over pigeons. The brains of pigeons are not irritable like those of sheep. Small doses of atropine induce an increased circulation through the brain by the action of the drug on the inhibitory influence of the vagus. Medium-sized doses bring about contraction of the vessels of the brain, and dilatation of the vessels of the rest of the body. The contraction of the cerebral vessels ceases when the cervical sympathetic is cut. This action of the atropine takes place through the vaso-motor centre.

III.—Cinchonidin increases the frequency of the fits in epi-

In typical hemicrania, he has had also great success with the nitro-glycerine. He is of the opinion that many cases can be permanently cured by means of it. It is only in the *anæmic* variety of headache that it is useful.

Korcynski reports five cases of angina pectoris where the use of nitro-glycerine was attended by the most gratifying results. In speaking of its use in this formidable malady, he says that it is immaterial what induces the angina ; its relief by nitro-glycerine is generally certain. Cases associated with or due to chronic valvular disease, atheromatous condition of the blood-vessels, degeneration of the muscular tissue of the heart, are all readily relieved by this drug. If the attacks are due to deficient or perverted cardiac innervation, they are not only relieved for the time, but can be permanently prevented by the continuous administration of the nitro-glycerine. Workmen employed in handling nitro-glycerine, even in the form of a weak solution or pill mass, are affected by it very unpleasantly. It causes headache, flushing of the face, nausea, sleeplessness, &c.

LITERATURE.

S. Smith—Codeia in Diabetes. (*Brit. Med. Journal*, Sept. 17, 1881.)

A. A. Smith—Clinical Observations on Diabetes Mellitus. (*New York Med. Record*, Feb. 25, 1882.)

Murrell—Bethesda Water in the Treatment of Diabetes Mellitus. (*Brit. Med. Jour.*, Nov. 26, 1881.)

Albertoni—Untersuchungen über die Wirkung einiger Arzneimittel auf die Erregbarkeit des Grosshirns nebst Beiträgen zur Therapie der Epilepsie. (*Archv. fur Exp., Path. und Pharma., Band* 15.)

Seeligmüller—Geistesstörung durch Iodoformintoxication. (*Ber. Klin. Wochensch*, No. 19, 1882.)

Schuster—Zur Frage von der Iodoformvergiftung. (*Ber. Klin. Wochensch.*, No. 20, 1882.)

Napier—On the use of Chrysophanic Acid internally in Psoriasis. (*Lancet*, May 20.)

Hammond—Some of the Therapeutical uses of Nitro-Glycerine. (*New York Med. Record*, Oct. 22, 1881.)

QUARTERLY RETROSPECT OF SURGERY.

PREPARED BY FRANCIS J. SHEPHERD, M.D., C.M., M.R.C.S., ENG.
Demonstrator of Anatomy and Lecturer on Operative and Minor Surgery
McGill University; Surgeon to the Out-Door Department
of the Montreal General Hospital.

Acute Traumatic Malignancy.—Mr. Richard Barwell, in the *British Medical Journal* of Feb. 11th, 1882, describes several cases of malignant disease rapidly following injury, to which he gives the name—Acute Traumatic Malignancy. He thinks that "under the stimulus of severe irritation, the tissue-elements which, under favourable circumstances, would assume only the additional activity necessary to repair, may take on a more prolific cell-germination, culminating in a rapid form of malignant disease in one of those forms, be it named myeloid or round-celled sarcoma, or encephaloid cancer, which consists of little else than heaped up cells and their progeny."

The first case is that of a boy aged 17, who, whilst playing football, fell on his shoulder and disabled it. This occurred on April 24th, 1875. A week after the shoulder began to swell rather rapidly, and on May 19th Mr. Barwell saw him, and then there was a swelling most marked in front, which was soft with some ovoid patches harder than the rest; the swelling did not rotate with the bone. On May 25th the shoulder was considerably increased in size, the skin a little tense, surface white and waxy, and large veins coursing over the growth. The texture was soft and doughy, with a sense of false fluctuation. An exploratory puncture was made and a shred of tissue removed, which, under the microscope, was seen to be made up of large cells with brilliant nuclei. Excision was advised, but was not consented to for a month. It was performed, and a round-celled sarcoma removed. The disease returned shortly after, and the boy died in about three months.

The second case was that of a stevedore aged 65, who came into Hospital for bruise of left side, due to injury from falling down the ship's hold 18 days previously. He died two weeks after admission, and the *post-mortem* disclosed malignant disease of the left pleura and lung. The new growth was an oval-celled sarcoma.

Mr. Barwell also mentions a case of malignant disease following fracture of the fibula, which many years ago was under the care of Mr. Lloyd, of St. Bartholomew's Hospital. Mr. Barwell thinks in these cases there must have been tumour diathesis, and that the local injury was provocative of a neoplasm.

Mr. H. B. Walker (*Brit. Med. Journal*, April 1, 1882), also cites several cases of acute traumatic malignancy which have come under his observation.

I remember last summer seeing an example of this affection in the Montreal General Hospital. A girl aged 18 was admitted for ununited Colles' fracture. It appears that some weeks before she had broken her right radius about an inch from the wrist, and it had been put up in the usual way, but soon after became painful, and on examination, the seat of fracture presented considerable swelling, rather soft in character, and fluctuating. The lower end of the upper fragment was expanded, and cracked when pressed. The swelling increasing, she was recommended for admission to hospital under Dr. Roddick. On admission, the tumour was incised and found to be myeloid in character, and the arm was amputated below the elbow. The case did well, the stump healing rapidly. This is the only case I can recollect having seen. The fact that malignant disease may follow injury or irritation has long been known, as, for example, epithelioma of the lip and tongue following the continued use of a short clay pipe (in those probably having the tumour diathesis), chimney-sweep's cancer following irritation from soot, blows on the breast, and probably repeated attacks of mastitis, causing malignant disease, &c. It is probable that an injury which in some would produce merely an ordinary inflammation, in others would, owing to certain misplaced germinal cells being stimulated by the increased nutrition into embryonal activity, cause a malignant growth. The additional point, however, which Mr. Barwell wishes to bring forward is that such growths occasionally assume an acute form.

Mr. Butlin, in a letter to the *British Medical Journal*, March 18th, 1882, directs attention to the fact that many cases of sarcoma of the bones, apparently directly due to injury, are already on record, and gives several references; and he himself has seen at least six cases which have pursued an acute course, and a still greater number a chronic course. He agrees with Mr. Barwell in believing that there is a distinct tumour diathesis, and says the evidence in favour of this theory is as strong as that which supports the belief in a strumous or rheumatic diathesis.

Mr. Harrison Cripps relates two cases of malignant disease following traumatism which came under his notice when registrar of St. Bartholomew's Hospital, and remarks, with reference to a traumatic causation, that thousands of blows may be struck on bones without causing acute pyæmic necrosis, just as we see that similar injuries are rarely followed by malignancy. He goes on to say that in cases of acute pyæmic necrosis, the primary subperiosteal abscess often teems with minute organisms, and yet there has been no lesion of the skin by which such bodies could have been admitted from the external air. Thus he is driven to the conclusion that the poisonous organism must have been circulating in the blood, in which it is innocuous; but when the extravasation caused by the blow allowed it to become stationary, it multiplied, producing all its poisonous effeots. He asks whether the explanation of traumatic malignancy might not lie in some organism accidentally circulating in the blood, becoming the cause of active disease by infecting the cells of a part, when left stationary, by effusion into the tissues.—(*Brit. Med. Journal*, May 6th, 1882.)

Abortive Treatment of Buboes.—Dr. Morse K. Taylor, assistant surgeon U.S. army, in a paper in the April number of the *American Journal of Medical Sciences*, says that for nearly seven years he has treated commencing buboes by simply injecting the glands with a solution of carbolic acid. He has treated nearly 150 cases of various forms of lymphadenitis arising from specific and non-specific causes; and where he has seen them before the formation of pus was well established, he has not failed to arrest the process immediately, and allay the pain in a few minutes. Ten to forty minims of a solution of 8 to 10 grains of acid carbolic to the ounce of water is injected. Some care is required to insure certainty in reaching the central portion of the gland, and Dr. Taylor has found it better to wait until the gland has attained some size, and its stroma has become sufficiently distended to admit of free permeation of the injection to all parts of its structure. He also advises numbing the skin of the gland with ether spray before injecting, so that the gland may be firmly held to determine its size and to ascertain the depth to which the needle must penetrate to reach its central parts. The average time patients treated by this method have had to forego their usual avocations has not exceeded three or four days. Some twenty cases (successful) are given in detail. When pus has already formed, Dr. Taylor aspirates and then injects carbolic acid solution, and applies compression by means of a bag filled with shot or sand, with an intervening layer of oakum or absorbent cotton. Under this treatment the bubo rapidly disappears, and there is no need of the knife or poultices. For the axillary and cervical regions, he finds that compression can be most easily kept up by means of a potato trimmed to fit the location and enveloped in a strip of thin muslin.

I have several times arrested suppuration in buboes by accurately applied strips of belladonna plaster. This relieves the pain, and often, by the pressure which is used, arrests suppuration. Dr. Taylor's plan, however, is so simple, that if others find it as successful as he, it bids fair to become a recognized and favourite form of treatment.

Treatment of Fractured Patella.—Mr. Jonathon Hutchinson holds that in fractured patella the separation of the fragments is not caused by the muscles: repeated observation has convinced him that it is always caused by, and in proportion with, the effusion into the joint. If there be no effusion there is no separation. Mr. Hutchinson says that when the muscle is at rest it is always relaxed, and when relaxed there is no reason why the upper fragment of the broken bone should not come easily down to the other, and, in fact, that it always does so when there is no effusion. Spasm of the muscle may of course cause separation at the moment of the accident, but as soon as the limb is in bed at rest its agency ends. If the effusion is the cause of the separation of the fragments, get rid of it as quickly as possible ;

the effusion may be blood or synovia or a mixture of the two. If it occur immediately after the injury it is probably blood, and these cases, Mr. Hutchinson says, are most difficult to treat, for blood is more slowly absorbed than synovia. The treatment of both kinds of effusion is the same, viz: a vigorous application of cold. The ice-bag and spirit lotion are the best measures according to Mr. Hutchinson, who says that if by these means you can get rid of the swelling in 8 to 10 days you will have a good chance of bony union. When the effusion has been subdued the bones should be brought together with oblique strips of plaster fixed in the notches of the splint. The limb should be extended from first to last on a well-padded back splint, and the leg kept elevated; after being bandaged the limb should not be touched for from six weeks to two months, when the patient should be allowed up, using a patellar apparatus, however.

Mr. Christopher Heath while agreeing with Mr. Hutchinson as to the cause of the separation of the fragments (*British Medical Journal*, March 25th, 1882,) carries the treatment further than Mr. H., and does not hesitate to aspirate the knee-joint, both in cases of fractured patella and injury of the joint without fracture. If the joint be aspirated a few hours after the accident, the blood being still fluid, can be readily withdrawn. Having emptied the joint Mr. Heath does not hesitate to apply at once a plaster of Paris bandage over an envelope of cotton-wadding, and he allows the patient to go about with crutches as soon as the plaster is dry. If he sees the case before there is effusion, he at once applies a plaster of Paris bandage, and allows the patient to move about.

This method of treatment which Mr. Heath adopts is certainly a great improvement on the old one of clumsy apparatus, and prolonged rest in bed, when atrophy of the quadriceps is certain to ensue, and it is some months before use of it is regained. The most successful result of fractured patella I have ever seen was in a case where before effusion took place the leg was put up in a plaster of Paris bandage, and after a couple of days the man allowed to go about with crutches. The bones were separated by a very short interval, and of course the union was fibrous, but the man had perfect use of his joint. Dr. Hamilton of New York uses a back-splint of leather or gutta-percha, or gum shellac cloth (the latter preferred). It should reach from the middle of the thigh to two or three inches above the heel; a roller of cotton is then turned round the leg and splint to within three inches of the knee, and another from the upper end of the splint to within three inches of the knee. While an assistant approximates the fragments, the surgeon should make two or three turns with a third roller around the limb and splint, close above the knee, after which the roller descends below the knee, and a number of circular turns are made close below the lower fragments, which turns should approach each other in front till the whole patella is covered. The heel is left elevated or suspended. Dr. Hamilton does not believe in evaporating lotions, but says the swelling usually goes down in a day or two, and then the patella bandages should be tightened daily as required by overstitching the oblique turns. At the end of four weeks the apparatus should be removed and the limb bent gently daily, after which the splint shonld be re-applied and the patient allowed to go about with crutches.

With regard to the union of the fragments, some surgeons deem it necessary to always get bony union, and Mr. Lister frequently wires the fragments together. Now the belief is getting abroad that bony union after all is not the most desirable, but that patients who have good fibrous union have better use of their limbs than those with bony union, and besides the tendency to refracture is less. Mr. Hutchinson says he is by no means an enthusiast as to bony union. Dr. Hamilton decidedly prefers ligamentous. Mr. Heath remarks that the reason bony union is less advantageous than ligamentous is that the patella contracts adhesions to the external condyle. No doubt we are more apt to have ankylosis with bony union than with ligamentous, and for this reason the great Pott abandoned apparatus; he considered that position alone approximated the fragments sufficiently.

Iodoform in Surgery.—Iodoform has now taken a recognized place as one of the most valuable antiseptics. It may be used in the form of powder or iodoform wool. As a powder it is most useful in the treatment of local sores, sinuses, &c. Its powers of lessening suppuration are remarkable, and under its influence an unhealthy sore soon takes on a healthy action. The iodoform wool is difficult of preparation. It is made by heating eight parts of iodoform with 88 of ether; in four pints of this mixture half a pound of absorbent cotton is soaked for a short time, and the wool is afterwards placed in a drug press; when dry the wool contains about 10 p.c. of iodoform, and is ready for use. The objection to the wool is that an irritating powder is spread over the room, and its odour is very disagreeable to many people. The former tendency is overcome by adding a little glycerine to the ether, and the latter is modified by the addition of eucalyptus oil. The wool should be stored in air-tight boxes. It is very useful as a dry antiseptic dressing and is much used at present in Germany. After an amputation the stump may be dressed, after sewing the wound with catgut or silver wire, and inserting a drainage tube, by properly applied pads of this wool kept in position by gauze bandages, the dressing may often be left on for ten days without change, and the drainage tube and stitches (if of silver wire) removed in the first dressing. The wound is, in a large percentage of cases, found to have united by first intention.

This mode of dressing gives us all the requisites for the rapid healing of wounds, viz., rest, elastic pressure, antisepticism, and drainage. Before applying the wool pads, iodoform may be dusted on the wound. In Germany, where it has been used most freely and in large quantities, some cases of poisoning have occurred, characterized by elevation of temperature and an erythematous eruption, and albumen in the urine. The Germans use it in wounds of the mouth, and pack it in cavities in the form of a paste made with resin. Some fatal cases have been described by H. Henry. According to Mikulicz of Vienna, the use of iodoform gives brilliant results in strumous diseases, and also in lupus after the epidermis has been removed with caustic potash. I have found it of the greatest benefit in gangrenous and sloughing wounds seen after crushing injuries; also in foul ulcers of the leg. The best way to treat foul ulcers is to dust on iodoform powder thickly, cover this over with oiled silk, over this place a pad of absorbent cotton, and bandage carefully and firmly. Here, again, we have the benefit of elastic pressure, with asepticity. In the treatment of soft chancres, its superiority to every other application is generally admitted, and its application is quite painless. Its odour is objected to by many, but it may be controlled by keeping a tonga bean in the box containing the powdered iodoform. Mr. W. Whitehead (*Brit. Med. Jour.*, March 11, '82,) first dries the sore and then applies with a camel's hair pencil a solution of iodoform in ether. The ether rapidly evaporates and leaves the iodoform uniformly spread over the surface of the sore. This process may be repeated several times, and when the application is dry, it may be painted over with collodion, and a pinch of absorbent cotton is applied over this. Mr. Whitehead has had great success by this method. The solution of iodoform he sometimes uses is one part to two of ether and collodion ten parts. The dressing is renewed in 24 hours.

Mr. Lennox Browne says a solution of iodoform in collodion may be made without the addition of ether, by shaking up one part of iodoform with ten of collodion. The iodoform should be added to the collodion, and not the collodion to the iodoform, to obtain a clear solution. He uses it in glandular enlargements of the neck.

Colectomy.—Mr. John Marshall, F.R.S., in a clinical lecture delivered at University College Hospital on April 27th, 1882, gives an interesting account of the above operation. It was performed in a case of "chronic intestinal obstruction, the seat and cause of which could not be ascertained, even under the influence of an anæsthetic, but which was discovered, on a median abdominal section, to be due to a circumscribed cylindrical growth, situated in the descending colon. Whereupon this growth was forthwith removed, through a left lateral abdominal incision, by resection or excision of the diseased part, together with small adjoining portions of the intestines. The two free ends of the bowel were then attached to the lateral wound in the abdominal walls, more or less after the manner adopted in colotomy, whilst the median abdominal section was closed by the usual deep sutures." The patient, unfortunately, only survived the operation three days, dying from a low form of peritonitis. Mr. Marshall remarks that he should approach another case of the same kind hopefully, and would make use of the left lumbar incision, as holding out greater chances of success.

Mr. Bryant, at a meeting of the Royal Medical and Chirurgical Society of London, on March 28, '82, reported "a case of excision of a Stricture of the Descending Colon through an incision made for a left Lumbar Colotomy." The operation was performed on a lady aged 50, who had suffered from complete obstruction for eight weeks. The stricture could not be felt from below. The bowel was removed by simply pulling the segment strictured through the wound and stitching each portion of the bowel, with its two orifices divided, to the lips of the wound. The stricture was of the annular kind, and involved about one inch of the bowel, and it was so narrow as only to admit the passage of a No. 8 catheter. A discussion ensued, in which it was stated that this was the first operation of the kind in British surgery. The majority of the speakers favoured abdominal incision to the left of the left rectus muscle, as being more likely to lead to a correct diagnosis in obscure cases.

Gastro-Enterostomy.—Dr. Anton Wölfler, in the *Centralblatt für Chirurgie*, describes an operation to which he gives the above name. A man, aged 38, had been the subject of gastric cancer for six months, and was admitted to Billroth's wards on the 27th of September last He was weak and much emaciated, and for three months had vomited the greater portion of his food. Under chloroform, a tumour the size of an orange was felt in the pyloric region, and from the circumstance that it was movable in all directions, Dr. Wölfler was induced to make an exploratory incision, when he found cancer of the pylorus (freely movable), but in addition, the hepatico-duodenal ligament and head of the pancreas were infiltrated with the new growth. As a resection of the pylorus seemed impracticable, and as he did not wish to close the abdomen without accomplishing anything, the establishment of a nutrient fistula in the small intestine was the only thing to be thought of. The objections were obvious enough, viz., the due admixture of bile and pancreatic juice is prevented when the fistula cannot be established at the upper accessible portion of the duodenum, and the condition of the patient with such a fistula is always more or less deplorable. Accordingly, Dr. Wölfler determined to set up a direct communication between stomach and small intestine. The stomach was opened by an incision two inches in length in its greater curvature, a finger's breadth above the insertion of the gastro-colic ligament. He then made an incision the same length in a coil of small intestine (opposite the attachment of the mesentery), and stitched the edges of the wound on the gut to those of the gastric aperture. Strict antiseptic precautions were used, but no spray. The progress of the case was in every way satisfactory; the vomiting ceased, and the patient was able to eat solid food at the end of eight days without discomfort. The external wound healed by first intention Four weeks after, the patient was well and was passing firm, brown-coloured stools. Prof. Billroth performed a similar operation a few days later for extensive pyloric carcinoma, but bilious vomiting setting in the day after the operation, the patient only lived ten days.—(*Edinburgh Med. Journal*, April, 1882.)

Early Treatment of Prostatic Obstruction.—Mr. Reginald Harrison, of Liverpool, advises the early use of instruments in prostatic disease (*British Medical Journal*, March 18). To dilate the passage, he uses specially adapted bougies. The instruments are gum-elastic, two to four inches longer in the stem than usual, with an expanded portion an inch from the tip, which is made to enter the bladder. In this way the prostate is subject to pressure on the insertion and withdrawal of the instrument. As a rule no irritation is aroused. By the use of these dilators Mr. Harrison asserts that the enlargement of the prostate is so moulded as to prevent obstruction. In a few persons it becomes necessary to establish a state of instrumental toleration. In some individuals the intolerance is entirely due to the presence of unnatural quantities of uric acid in the urine.

In case of difficulty in the passage of instruments where there is *Retention of Urine* Mr. Harrison advocates tapping of the bladder from the perniæum through the hypertrophied prostate. He has devised a special trocar and cannula. The trocar is hollow, and when the bladder is reached urine flows through it. The trocar is then withdrawn and the cannula tied in. The cannula is arranged with a stop-cock, so that the urine may be turned off or on at will. A case is related in which the urine was passed through this prostatic cannula for six weeks, with the greatest comfort, at the end of that time the urine began to pass through the natural passage. The cannula was then withdrawn and the puncture rapidly healed, and urine was passed as usual through the penis. In fact nearly all the functional symptoms of enlarged prostate ceased to exist, and on examination through the rectum the gland was found to be much smaller, having rapidly atrophied after having been punctured with the trocar.

On Digital Exploration of the Bladder through incision of the Urethra from the Perinæum.—At a meeting of the London Royal Medical and Chirurgical Society, held April 11th, 1882, Sir Henry Thompson reported a case in which he had successfully removed a tumour of the bladder (in a man) through a perinæal section of the urethra. The patient has been operated on some time previously for stone (by lithotrity) but without complete relief to his symptoms; subsequently some phosphatic deposit was removed by the lithotrite, at this time he seized what at first felt like a calculus, and practically crushed it under pressure, but it was evidently fixed, giving the impression of partially imparted stone. As little benefit followed this operation it was decided to open the bladder. This was done by perineal section, and on introducing his finger into the bladder and pressure being made from above the pubes Sir Henry recognized a tumour about the size of a chestnut growing from the opposite wall, coated with phosphatic matter. The mass was easily twisted off with a pair of forceps and very little bleeding followed. The patient speedily recovered and had no return of the bladder symptoms subsequent to the operation. Regarding this and other cases Sir Henry advised that in certain cases of hematuria which was clearly vesical and was not explicable except by the hypothesis of impacted calculus or vesical tumour, an incision of the membranous portion of the urethra from the perineum, for the purpose of exploring the bladder, should be made. In a paper in the *Lancet*, of 7th May, 1882, Sir Henry remarks that it is only during the last few years that he has gradually realized the fact, that it is possible, in not a few cases, to explore through a small perineal incision the whole or nearly the whole, of the internal surface of the bladder with the index finger—a necessary condition, of course, is that the bladder should be empty, and that firm pressure should be made with the right hand above the pubes. The method of operating the author describes as follows: The central incision should always be adopted, and a medium grooved staff, and a long, straight narrow-bladed knife, with the back blunt to the point, should be used. Having placed the left index finger in the rectum, the knife may be introduced edge upwards, about three quarters of an inch above the anus, with or without a small preliminary incision in the skin, until the point reaches the staff about the apex of the prostate gland, where it divides the urethra for half an inch or so and is then drawn out, cutting upwards a little in the act, but so as to avoid any material divison of the bulb. The left index finger is now removed from the rectum and following by the groove of the staff, slowly passes through the neck of the bladder as the staff is withdrawn, when exploration is made. This operation is often of benefit in old cases of cystitis, and, as well as satisfying the surgeon as to the exact condition of the bladder, often relieves symptoms where no lesion can be made out.

Splenectomy.—Mr. Warrrington Haward at a meeting of the London Clinical Society held on March 24th, 1882, read an interesting paper describing a case in which he had excised the spleen. The patient was a woman, aged 49, who for eighteen months had suffered pain in the left side of the abdomen, and for ten months had been conscious of an abdominal tumour, which had been steadily increasing in size, and which distressed her by its weight. When admitted into St. George's Hospital, she was rather a stout woman of good complexion, she did not look at all anæmic, and although the number of white blood corpuscles was increased she did not show any other signs of leucocythemia excepting a very enlarged spleen. The spleen occupied the greater part of the abdomen, and extended from the ribs to the groin, and from the loin to three inches beyond the middle line; no other glandular enlargements were present, nor was there ever any dyspnœa, palpitation, or hemorrhages. Pulse, temperature, and respirations were normal. It having been determined to remove the spleen, Mr. Haward performed abdominal section. An incision was made in the middle line from two inches below the ensiform cartilage to within two inches of the pubes. The enlarged spleen at once presented, and was found free from adhesion. The enlarged vessels at the hilus were clamped and ligatured in separate portions with carbolized silk, and the organ was removed without difficulty. While the wound was being closed the patient became collapsed suddenly, but was revived by artificial respiration and the injection of ether. Five hours after the operation vomiting came on, and persisting with great frefuency, rapidly exhausted the patient, who died the evening of the operation. The spleen presented to the naked eye the appearance of simple hypertrophy. The fatal result was not caused by hemorrhage, but seemed to be due to disturbance of the great sympathetic plexuses, and the consequent shock of vomiting.

In the discussion which followed, Dr. Stephen MacKenzie raised the question whether removal of the spleen in leucocythemia was justifiable, quoting Mr. Collier's tables, which show, that though the spleen has been excised successfully in several cases, in no case has the operation succeeded when performed for leucocythemia. Dr. MacKenzie thought possibly the operation was jutifiable when the blood disease was not advanced, and the subject was a young one, as there were grounds for believing that the spleen was primarily at fault. Mr. Lucas thought a less serious operation, as ligature of the splenic artery, might be adopted if the affection were a simple hypertrophy. It would seem that for the present surgical interference in leucocythemia is narrowed down to splenectomy in selected early cases in young subjects, or perhaps to the substitution of some less formidable operation as ligature of the splenic artery.—(Report in *British Medical Journal.*)

Surgery of the Kidney.—The operations of nephro-lithotomy, nephrotomy and nephrectomy are now considered by the surgical world to be justifiable operations. It has been established beyond doubt that *nephro-lithotomy* is a most successful operation in properly selected cases, viz., where the stone is of moderate size and single, and the kidney has not become disorganized. It is a most scientific procedure to perform this operation where stone has been certainly diagnosed by needle exploration, or where the pain and other symptoms lead one to believe there is a stone present. If left, the stone is certain to disorganize the kidney, cause much suffering, and probably death. The operation of incising the kidney (*nephrotomy*) has not proved a dangerous one, and it has been frequently demonstrated that the kidney can be easily explored through a lumbar incision, and even cut into with great safety. In cases of strumous or calculous pyelitis, the sacculated kidney can be drained through a wound in the loin and the patient freed from the danger and pain of retained matter. Nephrotomy, as an operation, is merely palliative, and, as Mr. Lister suggests, should only be performed where the patient is too weak for nephrectomy.

Dr. Roddick lately, at the Montreal General Hospital, performed nephrotomy in a girl suffering from scrofulous pyelitis of right kidney. The incision made was the transverse one, as in lumbar colotomy, the enormously distended kidney, which could be esily felt as a fluctuating tumour, was reached without difficulty, and about 20 ounces of foetid pus evacuated ; a drainage tube was introduced after washing out the sac with a 1 to 40 solution of carbolic acid. The operation was performed under the spray. The third day after the operation the girl had suppression of urine and symptoms of carbolic acid absorption, but after this had passed away (boracic acid being substituted for the carbolic acid) the girl improved rapidly, and was sent home some eighteen days after the operation, where I have heard she has since died, her improvement being only temporary. The relief afforded by the operation was decided, and I think this operation may be fairly considered to have been successful.

Nephrectomy, or removal of the kidney, is a much more formidable operation than the foregoing. The dangers are much greater, many cases having been followed by suppression of urine, which by some has been attributed to the use of carbolic acid, either as spray or injection. It has also proved fatal from hemorrhage and wounds of neighbouring organs, as lung and pleuræ. It has not yet been fully determined in what cases it should be performed, or at what period. Nephrectomy has been performed for tumour, cancerous disease, strumous and calculous pyelitis. Lately Dr. Barlow and Mr. Godlee read, at the London Clinical Society, notes of a case of nephrectomy performed for calculous pyelitis. The existence of the stone had been previously diagnosed by needle puncture. The kidney was removed by abdominal section, under antiseptic precautious. After the operation, a morphia suppository was administered and the patient passed off into a quiet sleep. Next morning the temperature was high, urine suppressed, and the patient was in a semi-comatose condition, from which she never recovered. Mr. Golding Bird and Dr. Goodhart, before the same Society, reported a case of nephrectomy for scrofulous pyelitis of the right side only. The incision was made in the right loin and the kidney removed. The patient died of collapse shortly after the operation. The operation was difficult, and part of the 12th rib had to be removed. Mr. Howard Marsh also reported a case of exploration of the kidney and partial excision, where the patient died in thirty hours of suppression of urine.

These cases are instructive ; in one apparently the morphia suppository had something to do with the fatal result. It also seems that partial excision of the kidney is quite as, if not more, dangerous than complete excision. Suppression of urine seems to be a very common complication. It is a question whether before nephrectomy is performed, a preliminary nephrotomy should not be tried. Now the loin is the most favourable position for nephrotomy and perhaps the most difficult incision for nephrectomy, so this would be an objection. Some hold that if a preliminary nephrotomy is performed, it much increases the difficulty of a subsequent nephrectomy. Again, it is important, in considering the advisability of performing nephrectomy, to find out whether the pyelitis is confined to one kidney, or, rather, whether the other kidney is healthy. Strumous pyelitis is rarely confined to one kidney, and therefore excision of the kidney must be a defective operation, as the pyelitis is only a small part of a general disease. These are some of the difficulties in the way which make one hesitate to perform nephrectomy. Having, however, decided on the operation, which is the best incision, through the loin or abdomen? Certainly the abdominal incision gives the operator more room, and the surgeon sees what he is doing. I have frequently excised the kidney on the dead subject, and have been often amazed to find how much more easy it was to remove a kidney through an abdominal incision than through the lumbar one. Removal through an incision in the loin is very difficult, especially the ligaturing of the vessels entering the pelvis of the kidney, besides, in some people, the distance between the last rib and crest of the ilium is very short; in these cases, of course, the 12th rib has to be excised, or a T incision made, both of which procedures increase the risk of the operation. The only objection to the abdominal incision is that two layers of peritoneum are wounded; but now-a-days we are not so fearful of wounding that structure as formerly. There is another danger to which I have previously called attention,* and which may be more easily avoided by the abdominal incision, and that is where the renal artery is multiple, and enters the kidney in all parts, and also where it is double, one entering the extreme upper end the other the extreme lower end of the kidney, no artery entering the pelvis at all. Many more operations are necessarp before we can decide when and how to perform nephrectomy.

* Brooklyn Annals of Anatomy and Surgery, Vol. III, 1881.

Reviews and Notices of Books.

A Treatise on Human Physiology, designed for the use of Students and Practitioners of Medicine.—By JOHN C. DALTON, M.D., Professor of Physiology and Hygiene in the College of Physicians and Surgeons, New York; Member of the New York Academy of Medicine, &c. Seventh edition. With 252 illustrations. Philadelphia: Henry C. Lea's Son & Co. Montreal: Dawson Brothers.

This text-book of Physiology has always been a great favorite. The clear descriptions, the easy mode of writing, the handsome black-ground woodcuts, have each had their share in winning this popularity. It having now reached its seventh edition is proof enough of the value placed upon it by the profession. Several important additions and alterations have been made in this latest edition. "In the section of Physiological Chemistry, the most important alterations relate to the classification of the albuminoid substances, and particularly to the prominence given to the Ferments as a special group. In the department of the Nervous System, more extended consideration has been given to the localization of function in special parts of the cerebro-spinal axis." "In the present work, as a general rule, topics which are uncertain or incomplete have been treated with comparative brevity, a greater space being devoted to those which are demonstrated by satisfactory evidence."

A System of Surgery, Theoretical and Practical, in Treatises by various Authors.—Edited by T. HOLMES, M.A., Cantab, Surgeon and Lecturer on Surgery at St. George's Hospital. First American from second English edition, thoroughly revised and much enlarged. By JOHN H. PACKARD, A.M., M.D., Surgeon to the Episcopal and St. Joseph's Hospitals, Philadelphia; assisted by a large corps of the most eminent American surgeons. In three volumes, with many illustrations. Vol. III. Philadelphia: Henry C. Lea's Son & Co. Montreal: Dawson Brothers.

The issue of the third volume of Holmes' Surgery completes

the work. It contains the articles upon the following subjects: viz., Diseases of the Respiratory Organs; Diseases of the Bones, Joints and Muscles; Diseases of the Nervous System; Gunshot Wounds; Operative and Minor Surgery, and miscellaneous subjects. As in the foregoing volumes, the names of the writers are those well known to the profession in their several departments. The revision by the American collaborators has been carefully performed, only such portions having been added as were called for by reason of more modern views thereon having been distinctly brought forward since the previous edition. The rapid completion of this elaborate and extensive work is highly creditable to the publishing firm, and they have spared no expense upon the typography and binding, both of which are of the highest quality.

A Manual of Dental Anatomy, Human and Comparative.—By CHARLES S. TOMES, M.A., F.R.S. With 191 illustrations. Philadelphia: Presley Blakiston. Montreal: Dawson Bros.

A most complete handbook, containing full descriptions of the natural formation and evolution of the teeth in the human being from the earliest period of fœtal life. The physiology and structure of all the various portions of which the dental apparatus is composed are fully discussed. A large portion is devoted to a description of the different kinds of teeth found in the different classes of animals, and to the important bearing that these have upon classification. It is complete and thorough in every part, and is fully illustrated with excellent woodcuts.

Percussion Outlines.—By E. G. CUTLER, M.D., Assistant in Pathological Anatomy, Harvard Medical School, Pathologist to the City Hospital, &c., and G. M. GARLAND, M.D., Assistant in Clinical Medicine, Harvard Medical School, Professor of Thoracic Diseases, University of Vermont. &c. Boston: Houghton, Mifflin & Co.

The object of this work, intended for the use of all practical students of medicine, is to give accurate information concerning the exact position of the various internal organs with reference to the surface of the body, and to show to what extent this can be determined by means of percussion. It is illustrated by means of a series of excellent lithographs, showing both the anatomical boundaries of these various parts and also the outlines of these as determined by actual percussion. Very great care seems to have been taken both in the completion of the letter-press and in the preparation of the plates. It will no doubt prove a very useful handbook to those engaged in studying this, one of the most useful arts which an accomplished physician can possess.

Books and Pamphlets Received.

HOMŒOPATHY. WHAT IS IT? A STATEMENT AND REVIEW OF ITS DOCTRINES AND PRACTICES. By A. B. Palmer, M.D., LL.D. Detroit: Geo. S. Davis.

ELECTRICITY IN SURGERY. By John Butler, M.D. Boericke & Tafel, New York and Philadelphia.

A MANUAL OF OBSTETRICS. By H. F. H. King, M.D. Philadelphia: H. C. Lea's Son & Co.

ON DIET AND REGIMEN IN SICKNESS AND HEALTH, AND ON THE INTERDEPENDENCE AND PREVENTION OF DISEASES AND THE DIMINUTION OF THEIR FATALITY By Horace Dobell, M.D. London: H. K. Lewis.

Society Proceedings.

MEDICO-CHIRURGICAL SOCIETY OF MONTREAL.

Stated Meeting, May 26th, 1882.

GEORGE ROSS, M.D., PRESIDENT, IN THE CHAIR.

A letter from Dr. O. C. Edwards, tendering his resignation as Secretary of the Society, was read.

Moved by Dr. F. W. Campbell, seconded by Dr. Roddick, and unanimously resolved—"That this Society accepts with regret the resignation of Dr. O. C. Edwards. In doing so, it desires to place on record its full appreciation of the valuable services he has performed during the four years he filled the position which he now resigns. In parting with him the members of the Society desire to express the hope that in his new home in the North-West he may meet with that success which his professional skill and kindness of disposition fully merit; and that a copy of this resolution be sent to Dr. Edwards, and published in the English daily papers."

It was then moved by Dr. Trenholme, and seconded by Dr. Buller, that Dr. Edwards be elected a corresponding member of the Society.—*Carried.*

Pathological Specimens.

Dr. Roddick exhibited a bladder in a state of acute inflammation, taken from a patient who had recently died in the hospital. The patient was admitted with complete paraplegia, the result of a fall into the hold of a ship. Death occurred on the sixth day from pneumonia. Dr. Roddick thought the condition of the bladder in this case pointed strongly to the necessity for frequent catheterization in all similar cases; he believed that the cystitis was due simply to over-distension, and in such cases where the use of the catheter was rendered difficult owing to priapism, tapping the bladder would be indicated.

Dr. Gardner exhibited a quantity of semi-solid, jam-like substance removed from the interior of the uterus of an unmarried woman 30 years of age; she had never menstruated, and had always enjoyed good health up to six months ago, when she began to fail, but had no definite uterine symptoms until two weeks ago, when there was pain and tenderness in the left iliac region. A tense pyriform mass was evident in abdomen, corresponding to a 5½ months pregnant uterus; the pubic hair was fairly developed, but the breasts were *nil;* per vaginam, the uterus was found large and the cervix presented a nipple-like prominence, with a depression in the centre. Ether was administered, and after incising the prominence, the os was dilated with the fingers. A quantity of dark, semi-fluid, bloody matter first escaped, and subsequently about 1½ pints of the substance exhibited came away. The cavity of the uterus was smooth; the attachment of the growth was from the fundus; to the finger, it felt very much like broken down placenta. A microscopic examination was not made, but Dr. Gardner believed the growth to be of a sarcomatous character.

Dr. Buller showed a microscopic specimen of a substance taken from the ear of a lad who came to him with his ear blocked up with what appeared to be cerumen and epithelium; on its removal, the membrana tympani and auditory canal were red and thickened. Insufflation of boracic acid and oxide of zinc was used, and the boy improved for a time, but soon returned in the same condition as before ; the ear was again cleaned out, and this time a strong solution of nitrate of silver was used. In two weeks the boy again returned, and was treated as on the first occasion. A week later, he came back again ; this time the ear was fuller than ever, and the substance more tough and firm. Dr. Buller, now believing that the growth was fungoid in character, after cleaning out the ear, injected a quantity of rectified spirits, which he allowed to remain for five minutes, and then introduced a plug of cotton wool, after which the boy recovered completely. The specimen presented a number of small, black globular bodies embedded in epithelium, and is known as *Aspergillus nigricans*. It is of rather uncommon occurrence. Rectified spirit, in the treatment of such cases, is very effectual, and gives rise to little or no inconvenience. Dr. Buller then read a paper on "Optic Neuritis." (*See page* 641.)

Dr. Proudfoot stated that he had a case of optic neuritis, associated with suppression of the menses, in a female 30 years of age, whom he was treating with bichloride of mercury, with evident benefit. He thought a good deal might be said *pro* and *con* in regard to the various theories given in explanation of optic neuritis. He was inclined to favor the theory of œdema of the brain, but thought it strange that in hydrocephalus, papilitis is rare, possibly from expansion of the bones.

In reply to Dr. Fenwiek, Dr. Buller said that mercury and iodide of potassium were not given because of supposed specific origin of the disease, but from their tendency to reduce inflammatory action.

Dr. Roddick asked if it was advisable to give mercury in later syphilitic conditions, and not rely more on iodide of potassium. In diseases of the rectum, much harm may be done by mercury, whereas the iodide is highly beneficial. Dr. Buller, in reply, said that mercury was bad in ulcerations, from its tendency to break down tissues, and that is just why oculists use it, to break down the new tissue and then promote its absorption by iodide of potassium.

Dr. Shepherd said that he had found mercury very useful in tertiary symptoms, in combination with iodide, after the latter had failed when given alone.

Cases in Practice.—Dr. Proudfoot mentioned having lately removed scales of molten lead from the cornea from the eyes of a young man; he recovered, with perfect vision in the one eye and only slight opacity in the other. Dr. Buller thought this might be explained by the extreme thinness of the scales; the heat was not sufficiently concentrated to cause deep injury. Dr. Shepherd mentioned a case of Phtheiriasis palpebrarum in a young man, in whom there were no traces of the parasite in other regions.

The meeting then adjourned.

Extracts from British and Foreign Journals.

Unless otherwise stated the translations are made specially for this Journal.

Treatment of Acute Rheumatism by the Salicylates.—The Medical Society of London has done good service to the cause of therapeutics by eliciting, through discussion, the opinions and conclusions of those who have had the largest experience of the salicylates in the treatment of acute rheumatism. All the speakers agree that the fever and the joint-affection are alleviated by the administration of the salicylates, and that so far this method is superior to other plans of treatment. On the question of relapses, of cardiac complications, of the dose of the drug which is most efficacious, the opinions are in striking contrast. Dr. Broadbent, with Dr. Coupland and others, believes that relapses, as shown either by a renewed rise in the temperature, or by an accession of joint-pain, are perhaps even more common under the new than under the old method of treatment. The explanation is, however, to be found in the rapidity with which all the acute symptoms subside under the salicylate: patients are thus not so careful of themselves as when they have gone through the sufferings of an unalleviated attack. Dr. Coupland, moreover, believes that the withholding of the drug renders the patient more liable to relapses than if its administration be continued, while he finds that the relapses may occur in spite of tolerably large doses having been given; as many occurring under doses of 60 grains in 24 hours as under smaller doses. Dr. Douglas Powell supposes that relapse will follow upon any exposure, exercise, or improved diet, so long as the tongue remains coated and the secretions disordered, whatever be the treatment adopted. The joint-inflammation and the pyrexia are not the essential features of acute rheumatism, any more than pyrexia and diarrhœa form the essential points in enteric fever. Dr. Broadbent and Dr. Fagge agree in anticipating that as the salicylates are brought to bear upon rheumatic fever in the first days of its existence, a notable diminution will occur in the proportion of cases in which cardiac lesions are manifested. At present Dr. Broadbent finds that his cases have presented about the usual proportion of cardiac complications; he also finds from experience that the salicylic compounds have no influence whatever upon pericarditis, and only a very slight effect upon endocarditis. For this reason he discontinues the administration of salicylic compounds the moment that he recognizes any cardiac inflammation. In no case has any permanent cardiac weakness been left behind, as a result of salicylate treatment. Dr. Gilbart Smith is of opinion that so far as hospital statistics are concerned, there is no evidence to show that the introduction of the salicylate treatment has led to any diminution in the amount of cardiac complication in acute rheumatism. Dr. Douglas Powell, on the other hand, thinks that the treatment tends to prevent and to alleviate when already present the heart-affection. Dr. Maclagan is similarly of opinion that this method of treatment diminishes to some extent both the frequency and the danger of heart complications; and the particular series of cases upon which Dr. Coupland based his observations showed in like manner that the percentage in which pericarditis appeared was below the average. The latter observer, however, states that no definite influence upon the cardiac or other complications can be observed, and that both pericarditis and endocarditis may be observed whilst the patient is under the influence of the remedy.

As regards the dose of the drug and the toxic symptoms which may arise during its administration, Dr. Isambard Owen shows that with different dosage there is practically no difference in the total duration of the illness. Dr. Broadbent gives 20 grains of salicylic acid in combination with soda every hour for six hours, repeating it on the second day. The further administration of the salicylic compounds has been in the same dose perhaps thrice a day, or, if the temperature has not absolutely gone down, four times a day for some days afterwards. In only very few cases did any unfavourable symptoms set in which could be attributed to the drug—delirium, sullenness, giddiness, deafness, etc.; in the majority of these cases he attributes the symptoms to impurities in the salicylate used. Dr. Coupland has throughout endeavoured to give as small an amount of salicylate of soda as was possible, the usual quantity being 15 grains every four or six hours; relapses are, as far as possible, guarded against by continuing the administration long after the subsidence of the primary fever. Dr. Coupland finds also that the toxic effects are serious in proportion to the largeness of the dose, and perhaps also to the state of impurity of the drug, and in this latter point he is confirmed by Dr. Fowler, who shows that no such toxic symptoms occur in the case of patients treated with the acid obtained from oil of wintergreen. Dr. Maclagan, regarding acute rheumatism as a malarial fever, maintains that the salicylic compounds must be given in full and frequently repeated doses; in fact, that the larger the quantity that can be thrown into the system in a given time, the more rapid will be the destruction of the poison. Salicin is looked upon by Dr. Maclagan as equally powerful with salicylate of soda, whilst its use is infinitely preferable, inasmuch as it produces none of the deleterious effects of the salicylates; so that in several cases full doses of salicin have been given with the best results to patients suffering from the depressing and disturbing action of salicylate of soda. Dr. Bedford Fenwick, after a free purge, gives 20 grains of salicylate of soda every hour for six hours, adding digitalis and brandy to each dose if the heart-sounds are feeble and dull, and suspending the treatment if faintness or vomiting occur. The after treatment consists in giving half-drachm doses of citrate of potash every six or eight hours, until saliva becomes alkaline to test-paper.

The *modus operandi* of the drug in cases of rheumatism is explained by Dr. Latham thus: Salicylic acid enters into chemical combination with the antecedents of lactic acid and glucose, to whose presence in the circulation the disease is due. The presence of the excess of lactic acid in the blood is due to the inaction of an "inhibitory chemical centre," whose function it is to control the nutrition of the muscular and other tissues. Relapses will occur if the administration of the remedy has been suspended after the symptoms are relieved, but before the "inhibitory chemical centre" has recovered its tone. Dr. Maclagan, as we have hinted, regards the rheumatic poison as malarial, *i.e.*, due to minute organisms. The local joint and heart affections are the result of the action of these organisms on the fibrous textures of the joints and heart. The salicylic compounds produce their anti-rheumatic effects solely in virtue of their destructive action on these organisms.—*The Practitioner.*

Torsion of Arteries.—At Guy's Hospital, the London correspondent of the *Boston Med. & Surg. Journal* says that all the surgeons use torsion to the exclusion of the ligature, except in very small vessels wherein it is difficult to isolate the vessel from muscular fibres. They give a very large statistical showing in its favor. He has seen every kind of amputation there except of the hip-joint. and never a ligature applied to a large vessel. They use no transverse forceps, but seizing the cut end of the vessel with strong forceps, twist it until it is felt to "give way," that is, the two inner coats break. He has often seen six and sometimes ten complete turns given to the femoral artery. Mr. Bryant said: "Doctor, theoretically the twisted end ought to slough off, but practically it never does. We have to talk to our students about secondary hemorrhage, but we do not show it to them." Mr. Lucas told him that for a long time they have ceased to dread or look for secondary hemorrhage.

CANADA

Medical and Surgical Journal.

MONTREAL, JUNE, 1882.

THE ONTARIO MEDICAL ASSOCIATION.

The second annual meeting of the above Association was held in Toronto on the 7th and 8th days of June. The attendance of members numbered over a hundred, and the greatest interest was manifested in the proceedings. About twenty papers and reports were read, most of them by country members. None were of special merit; in fact, as a rule, it may be said the papers were rather below than above the average. No papers but those on that one topic, which is so dear to the ordinary practitioner, and in which so many are or would like to be amateur specialists, elicited any discussion. Of course we refer to gynecology. Ontario seems at the present time to be suffering from a severe attack of laceration of the cervix, and her medical men are vigorously applying the now very fashionable remedy—Trachelorhaphy.

Discussion was rather discouraged than otherwise. Papers were rapidly read, one after the other, and no opportunity for discussing them offered. The acoustic properties of the hall were such, that unless the reader of the paper had a remarkably clear delivery, or the listener remarkably sharp ears, very little could be heard.

The proceedings were opened on the morning of the 7th with an address by the President, Dr. Covernton, on State Medicine and Hygiene, in which he strongly urged that it was quite as important that special hospitals should be established for the purpose of isolating cases of diphtheria, scarlet fever, and other contagious diseases, as it was to have them for small-pox. He also advised that the bodies of persons dying of infectious diseases should be burnt or otherwise destroyed. The President remarked that very little doubt now remained that earth worms conveyed infection to the surface of the ground. The importance of physicians reporting to the Central Board of Health all cases treated by them during the year was insisted on; also that the officers of the Local Boards of Health should be medical officers. After alluding to the discoveries of Pasteur in regard to chicken cholera, charbon, &c., he expressed a hope that soon all infectious diseases would be produced in a modified form, so that people might be protected from their ravages by inoculation of the poison in a diluted condition. Next the discoveries of Klebs in reference to the effect of water washing away ague germs were alluded to, and the importance of Koch's investigations concerning the existence of a tubercle bacillus was discussed. Finally, this most eloquent and instructive address concluded with a few well chosen remarks on the necessity of educating the public on health matters generally, and the hearty co-operation of the members of the Association in this great work was solicited.

It being now 12 o'clock an adjournment took place, and on reassembling at 2 p.m. a number of papers were read.

The first paper was read by Dr. Worthington, of Clinton, on *Diphtheria*. The principal treatment advised was the application of cold externally and internally, supporting the patient with free use of brandy, beef tea, milk, and quinine gr. ii every two to three hours. It was also advised that the throat should be brushed with acid carbol. 1-80, and sometimes a spray of nitric acid used. Dr. Worthington held that cold applied to the throat best controlled the inflammation in the larynx and lowered the temperature. A number of cases were detailed.

Dr. Philip, of Brantford, next read a paper on the *Antiseptic Method of Treating Phthisis*, in which paper he adopted the views of Dr. McKenzie, of Edinburgh, viz., the use of continuous inhalation of carbolic acid. Dr. Philip held that if the disease was of septic parasitic origin, then this method of treatment was the most rational one. The inhaler should be used 8 to 10 hours a day. Dr. Philip has drawn his deductions from too few a number of cases, and the improvement in those cases was not sufficiently detailed. The special inhaler was shown.

Dr. Stewart, of Brucefield, then exhibited a case of *Locomotor Ataxia*, in which the sciatic nerve had been stretched, with the usual result of relief of the pain, but not of the ataxic symptoms. Dr. Stewart read a most scientific and able report of the case. Before the nerve was stretched the patient had severe paroxysms of pain every twenty-four hours, generally confined to one limb, and often to one spot, the dorsum of the foot. The strange thing about the case was that after these attacks the limb atrophied within twenty-four hours, often measuring from 1½ to 2 inches less in circumference. This symptom Dr. Stewart has not seen noticed in works on the subject. There was also loss of sensation in the limbs, and no plantar reflex. If the limb was pricked with a needle it took five or six seconds to feel it. After the stretching, patient had no pain for three weeks, and now has pains only at long intervals of six weeks and more. Has some plantar reflex, and can feel the prick of a needle in two seconds. The ataxic symptoms are not affected. This is the fourth case in which Dr. Stewart has stretched the sciatic for locomotor ataxia. In three the pain was relieved, but not the ataxic symptoms; in the fourth, both pain and ataxic symptoms relieved, and patient now well.

After Dr. Stewart had exhibited his patient, Dr. Avery, of the Michigan State Board of Health, was introduced to the meeting, and made a short address; after which Dr. Fenwick, of Montreal, President of the Canada Medical Association, assured the members of the Ontario Medical Association that the Dominion Association did not look on them with any antagonistic feelings, but, on the contrary, wished them well in the good work they were doing, and hoped that the other Provinces would follow their example. Dr. Fenwick, after alluding to the good fortune of Ontario in having lately instituted a Board of Health, thanked the meeting for the kind way in which he had been received.

Dr. Curry, of Rockwood, then read a paper on the *Science of Medicine*, in which he dwelt on the great importance of reflex action, and the wonderful influence the sympathetic ganglia had on disease. After some allusion to the pineal gland and other structures, the reader concluded a novel and original paper, the pathology of which was, however, rather obscure.

Dr. Temple's paper on *Laceration of the Cervix Uteri* was the next one presented. He believed this operation had a brilliant future before it. The men who oppose the operation do so on *a priori* grounds, having had no experience in its performance. Dr. Temple does not believe that every case of laceration needs sewing up; most of the minor cases of laceration will get well of themselves. According to the greatest authorities (as Emmet, Thomas, &c.) 32–33 per cent. of women delivered suffer from laceration of the cervix. After detailing the symptoms and consequences of rupture of the cervix, mentioning, among others, pelvic cellulitis, prolapsus uteri, and last, but not least, cancer, the reports of a number of cases were read in which the reader of the paper had performed Emmet's operation with perfect relief. In one case the ruptured cervix had caused prolapse of the uterus, so that it protruded beyond the vulvæ several inches; after the operation had been performed all the symptoms were relieved, and of course the prolapse as well. Now the uterus was reduced to its normal size.

(The discussion on this paper was postponed till other papers on the same subject had been read, and will be given in the report of the second day's proceedings.)

A paper was read by Dr. Powell, of Edgar, on *Hemorrhage after Tonsillotomy*. He said few people understood how to quickly and surely stop the bleeding after this operation. He mentioned his personal experience as a patient, how he had been operated on, and the surgeon who operated on him (Dr. Lefferts, of New York), having left the dispensary, severe bleeding came on. No one seemed to know what to do. One advised iron, others astringent gargles, and one suggested tying the carotid artery, and it was only after loosing between five and six pints of blood than another surgeon arrived, who easily arrested the hemorrhage by pressure of a pad of cotton applied with a forceps. Dr. Powell advises the use of the tonsillotome in children and adults where the gland protrudes, the blunt-pointed bistoury where the gland is sessile.

Dr. Dupuis, of Kingston, related a case of dislocation of both bones of the forearm backwards successfully reduced after six weeks, and others after two and three weeks. Nothing new was advanced in regard to the treatment or pathology of this accident. As more mistakes occur in diagnosing this accident than any other, Dr. Dupuis advises that in all cases of difficulty the assistance of other surgeons should be sought to divide the responsibility.

At the evening session Dr. Daniel Clarke read a most interesting paper on the Therapeutics of Insanity, in which he recommended chloral, bromides and hyoscyamine, after which Dr. Oldright explained some fallacies regarding *Measurements in Surgical Practice*, showing how that when the lower limb was abducted and flexed it apparently was shorter by from half an inch to an inch than the other. That before measuring, both limbs should be in the same plane. He exhibited a simple instrument by which this could be made certain. This consisted of a thin stick of wood, with cross piece of cardboard on the top. The stick should be placed in centre of pubes, and the cardboard cross piece should reach from one anterior superior spine to the other. In this way any obliquity of the pelvis could be discovered, and any fallaceous measurements corrected.

Dr. R. W. B. Smith, of Sparta, read a paper on *Alcohol in Disease*, which was listened to with great interest, after which some valuable contributions on State Medicine were presented by Dr. Yeomans, of Mount Forest, on the *Relation of Local Boards to the Provincial Board of Health*, and Dr. Playter, Toronto, on *Some Points in Vital Statistics in Ontario*. That the recent establishment of a Board of Health has stimulated the profession of Ontario into taking a greater interest in health matters than heretofore, is evinced by the increasing numbers of papers read on State Medicine.

Dr. Ryerson, of Toronto, read a paper on *Adenoma of the Roof of the Pharynx*, and exhibited a patient suffering from this affection. He advised removing these growths from behind with a scoop, which he showed the members; also the galvanic cautery proved often useful. He drew attention to the fact that this affection was often mistaken for enlarged tonsils, and was principally confined to young people. This affection generally leads to deafness, and the children suffering from it have a peculiar stupid expression. Numbers of plates exhibiting the growths *in situ* were exhibited.

Dr. Osler remarked that Dr. Ryerson had neglected to mention the use of an instrument which every surgeon carried about with him, and which was most efficacious in removing these growths from behind. He referred to the finger, and mentioned several cases where it had been used with the greatest success.

It being now 10 P.M., the meeting adjourned till the next morning, when Dr. Palmer read a paper on *Hygiene in Schools*, which chiefly treated of myopia in children, produced by bad light, badly constructed desks, badly ventilated rooms, &c., and and over-study in those predisposed. He concluded by hoping the Provincial Board of Health would give attention to this matter, and bring about such changes as were necessary to protect the health of juvenile scholars.

Dr. Macdonnell, of Brechin, next read a paper on the use of Calcium Chloride in Phthisis. He instanced several cases in which the above remedy proved highly beneficial and probably curative; especially in cases of broncho-pneumonia, which do not yield readily to potassium iodide, is the effect of this remedy most useful. It is also useful in buboes and glandular enlargement. Dr. Macdonnell did not attempt an explanation of the *modus operandi* of this remedy, nor from his description was it perfectly clear in what special affections of the lungs was calcium chloride curative. Potass. iodide seems to have been a favorite remedy with Dr. Macdonnell and his brother practitioners before calcium chloride was introduced, and was given in heroic doses for lung affections.

Dr. Holmes, of Chatham, was now called upon to read his paper on Trachelorhaphy. Nine cases of successful operation were reported. To prevent this accident, Dr. Holmes advised that in cases of labor, where the cervix was thin, the patient should be cautioned against bearing down, and when the os was completely distended chloroform should be given. After the reading of the paper was concluded a lively discussion ensued.

In answer to Dr. Mullin, of Hamilton, Dr. Holmes said that laceration of the cervix occurred in 33 p. c. of deliveries.

Dr. Temple, of Toronto, in this operation said he prefers the scissors to the knife, as then there is less hemorrhage. He gives no anæstethics when operating. The cervix should be protected from injury during the first stage of labour, and gr. ¼ of morphia should be administered hypodermically to relax the os when rigid.

Dr. Zimmerman inquired in what number of forceps cases laceration occurred. Dr. Holmes replied that three out of the nine cases operated on by him were lacerated by the forceps.

Dr. Gardner of London wanted to know in what class of cases during labor laceration occurred. Dr. Holmes replied, where there was a rigid os and strong expulsive pains.

Dr. Macfarlane of Toronto held that in many cases the cervix and perineum will be ruptured in spite of all precautions, and that meddlesome midwifery is bad midwifery. Where rupture occurs, he does not operate, but trusts to nature and rest. Thirty-three per cent he thought a too great percentage of lacerated cases. Subinvolution is, in his opinion, more often caused by letting the patient up too soon than by laceration of the cervix.

After a few remarks from the President and Dr. Bray of Chatham, Dr. McFayden said the reason older men had not seen more laceration was because they did not examine patients properly. This should, first of all, be done with the finger, and afterwards the woman should be examined in the Simms' position, with a duck bill or Simms' speculum.

Dr. Albert McDonald of Toronto remarked that if the laceration was slight, operation might be avoided. He also advised sewing up the cervix and perineum at the same time, if necessary.

Dr. Mullin of Hamilton said he had attended all kinds of people with small and large heads, and he had not seen many cases of laceration. He remarked that the gentlemen who had read papers had not spoken of their own experience as to the frequency of laceration. Now some women he had attended in seven or eight labours, and according to the percentage given, each should have lacerated her cervix twice. Well, all he would say, that if his patients have had laceration, he has not found it out, and they have gone on bearing children as usual. He should like to see statistics giving the frequency of laceration, and how many cases get well without operation.

Dr. Canniff did not think that laceration of the cervix is a frequent accident, and he did not care, as long as his patients remain well, whether they have or have not rupture of the cervix.

After a few remarks from other members, the discussion was closed, and the meeting adjourned till the afternoon.

On reassembling, Dr. Ghent read a paper on *Diphtheria*. He always treated his cases by insufflations of equal parts of sulphur and powdered borax. This powder was blown into the throat every 1 to 4 hours, according to the severity of the case. The treatment was commenced by a dose of calomel and Dover's powder, followed by castor oil. The room should be fumigated with sulphurous acid, by heating sulphur on coals. By this method of treatment, Dr. Ghent says the patch disappears in 24 hours, and the glands give no trouble, nor are the cases followed by paralysis. Dr. Ghent has treated one hundred cases in this way and has not lost one.

After a short discussion, in which Drs. White, Osler and the President took part, Dr. McKelkan of Hamilton read a paper on the *Treatment of Diphtheria*. He said that by experiment he found that the membrane was dissolved by Liquor Calcis in 25 seconds; he therefore used it in cases of diphtheria in spray of Liq. Calcis, to which is added Permanganate of Potash gr. ii to 1 oz. of Liq. Calcis. He also gives this internally in doses of half a drachm every half hour. By this treatment he found many severe cases recovered, though some died.

After a few remarks by Dr. MacDonald of Hamilton, Dr. Osler said that diphtheria was a self-limited disease. Many cases get well without treatment; others, again, have no hope of recovery from the first.

Dr. Holmes divided cases into laryngeal and non-laryngeal. The first class were generally fatal, and the latter, as a rule, terminated favorably. His treatment was pure air, nourishment, with tinct. of iron, chlorate of potash and quinine internally.

Dr. Riddell of Toronto was now called upon to read his paper on *Coroners and their Duties*. He said that as his paper was a long one, and the hour was late, he would not read it; but on the President putting it to the meeting, it was decided that Dr. Riddell should proceed, which he did.

The various reports were then presented: Dr. Geikie, on the International Congress in London; Dr. Fulton, on Medicine, Pathology and New Remedies; Dr. Roseburgh, on Ophthalmology. The report of the Elective Committee was then read and adopted unanimously:

President—Dr. Macdonald, Hamilton.

1st Vice-President—Dr. Stewart, Brucefield.

2nd Vice-President—Dr. Dan. Clarke, Toronto.

3rd Vice-President—Dr. Dupuis, Kingston.

4th Vice-President—Dr. Harrison, Selkirk.

General Secretary—Dr. White, Toronto.

Treasurer—Dr. J. E. Graham, Toronto.

Corresponding Secretaries—Dr. Wm. Graham, Brussels; Dr. Burt, Paris; Dr. Coburn, Oshawa; Dr. McIntosh, Vankleek Hill.

Committee on Credentials—Dr. Beeman, Centreville: Drs. Burns and Payne, Toronto.

Committee on Public Health—Drs. Playter, Allison, Oldright, and Yeomans.

Committee on Legislation—Drs. Spohn, Sloan, G. Wright, Covernton, Mallow and Macfarlane.

Committee on Publication—Drs. Cameron, Burns and Fulton, with the Secretary and Treasurer.

Committee on By-Laws—Drs. A. H. Wright, Moore, Tanner, Cotton and Bowlby.

Committee on Medical Ethics—Drs. O'Reilly, McKelcan, Carney, C. K. Clarke, and Sinclair.

Dr. Riddell then presented the report on Necrology. He had only one death to report, viz., that of Dr. F. H. Wright, son of Dr. H. H. Wright of Toronto.

Dr. Avery of Michigan then offered the following resolutions, which were passed:

"This Association approves of the action of the Provincial Board of Health of Ontario to co-operate to the full extent of its powers with the National State and Local Boards of Health in the United States and in the Dominion of Canada in the attempt to prevent the introduction and spread of smallpox by the inspection and vaccination of immigrants, and the disinfection of their baggage and clothing, and by notification to all Boards of Health interested of the entry or proposed entry within their jurisdiction of immigrants suspected of carrying within them the germs of any disease dangerous to the public health. That in this attempt to lessen the spread of smallpox and other communicable diseases on this continent, it is desirable that all Health Officers and Boards of Health under whatever governmental control shall earnestly and faithfully co-operate, and to secure this co-operation at the earliest possible date we bespeak and invite the individual efforts of every member of this Association."

A discussion now ensued as to whether it was advisable that the Association should move round from place to place annually or remain in Toronto permanently. Finally the members decided to hold the next meeting in Toronto.

At the evening session, Dr. Canniff moved—"That in the opinion of this Association the formation of a Medical Library and Museum would prove beneficial to the profession of this Province, and that the following committee be appointed to consider the feasibility of such a scheme, to report to the next meeting: Drs. Cameron, Holmes, Fulton, Reed, Davison, Powell, and the mover." *Carried.*

Dr. D. Clarke moved that the secretary, Dr. White, receive a gratuity of $100 for his valuable services during the past year. *Carried.*

The President elect, Dr. Macdonald, was then installed, and made an appropriate speech, thanking the Association for the honor conferred upon him, and prophesying a brilliant future for the organization.

After passing some formal resolutions the meeting adjourned.

F. J. S.

THE ROYAL SOCIETY OF CANADA.—His Excellency the Governor-General has been pleased to establish a National Literary and Scientific Society, the first meeting of which was held in Ottawa on the 25th ult. Four sections have been formed, two of Literature, French and English, one of Chemistry and Mathematics, and another of Geology and Biology, the number in each being limited to twenty members. A large number of valuable papers were presented, and the gathering may be considered a great success. An Association of this kind will do much to stimulate research and bring men into contact with each other. Strong hopes are entertained that the Government will give a grant sufficient to cover the publication of a quarto volume of Transactions. The medical members are: Dr. Bucke (English Literature), Professor Girdwood (Chemistry), Dr. Grant (Geology), Professor Osler (Biology), and Professor Robert Bell (Geology).

NOTICE TO GRADUATES OF BELLEVUE HOSPITAL MEDICAL COLLEGE.—A second decennial revision of the catalogue of Alumni of this College is being prepared for publication, and we are requested to ask that all graduates send their present address at once, on a postal card, to the Historian of the Alumni Association, Bellevue Medical College, New York.

—We regret to see announced the death of Surgeon-Major Hughes, Professor of Midwifery in Grant Medical College, Bombay. Dr. Hughes was a native of Toronto, and graduated at the University in 1868. He went to India in 1870, and since 1874 had been in Bombay, where he enjoyed a large practice, and occupied the Chair of Midwifery in the College. His death was from blood poisoning, caused by a small puncture received while performing a trifling operation.

Obituary.

GEO. W. CAMPBELL, A.M., M.D., LL.D.

It is with no ordinary feelings of sorrow and deep regret that we find ourselves called upon to record the death of our oldest surgeon, Prof. Geo. W. Campbell. On the 30th March last Dr. Campbell attended the annual convocation of McGill University, and took leave of his friends and colleagues, as he was leaving for England the following day. No one who saw him that day, no whit less cheerful and active than usual, for one moment dreamt that this city would so soon be shocked by the telegraphic news of his death in a far-off country. But so it was. For some years past Dr. Campbell suffered from bronchitis, and was obliged to retire from active practice and give himself more rest. He had also suffered from slight attacks of pneumonia. When in London, pneumonia again set in, but being somewhat better, he went to Edinburgh, where, however, more serious symptoms showed themselves, and he expired on the 30th May.

In losing Dr. Campbell, an immense loss has been sustained by the whole of this community. The Faculty of Medicine loses its Dean—its tried and trusty general, who has directed its operations with a master hand for many years. The Hospital loses its senior consulting surgeon—him whose opinion always carried the weight of experience and mature judgment. Our greatest financial institutions lose one who has been found worthy to fill posts of the highest trust and confidence. The general public lose one to whom they could always go for sympathy in distress and relief in extremity. His friends—and their name, indeed, is legion—lose a warm-hearted, true and generous friend. His professional brethren in this district lose their chief—that chief who, from his personal and professional worth, retained for so many years the loyalty and devotion of all.

One, indeed, has gone from amongst us, of whom it has been a common remark that, "take him for all in all, we shall not look upon his like again." This feeling has been produced by the rare combination of good and attractive qualities which found themselves so happily associated together in our estimable Dean. As a professional man—and he was that before all things—in how many ways was he an example to us all,—able, skillful, devoted, untiring towards his patients—courteous, generous and invariably considerate towards his *confrères*—energetic, zealous and enthusiastic in all touching the progress of the medical art and science—always upholding, by word and deed, the dignity of that profession to which he was proud to belong—kind and encouraging to every brother honestly practising his profession in a straight path, but an uncompromising foe to every kind of professional dishonesty or hyprocrisy. No wonder that there gradually grew up for such a man a feeling of rare warmth and affection, a feeling which we know to be shared by all within our ranks. No matter how else divided, on this point there was unanimity, viz., that in Dr. Campbell we recognized a noble example, whom to imitate was to do right.

With Dr. Campbell has passed away one of those links, now so few, which joined the present generation of medical practitioners to a past one. Possessed of the best technical education which was afforded at that day, Dr. Campbell came to this new country to make his own way in the world. How well this was accomplished, and what well-merited success he met with, is known to all. Whilst thus pursuing his way to name and fame, no selfish aims were ever allowed to obstruct his exertions in the common cause. Endowed with great strength of character, combined with an excellent judgment in all the ordinary concerns of life, he always interested himself in every scheme tending to the promotion of the general good. Firm and fixed in his endeavors to attain an object once definitely settled upon as being desirable, his great influence was naturally always sought for and highly prized.

Not only was Dr. Campbell deservedly looked up to as the leading surgeon of the city, but he was held in the warmest estimation as a citizen. His voice and influence were always to be counted upon to assist in any good work, and many an undertaking to-day in flourishing condition, and on a firm basis, owes the success of its early efforts to the assistance then lent it by this public-spirited man. The greatest of our public charities, the Montreal General Hospital, always claimed and received a large share of his fostering care. In every matter connected with the medical management of this large Institution, the advice of Dr. Campbell was looked for, and time and attention to its interests were given ungrudgingly and without stint. It is not for us to speak of the many marks of the esteem in which he was held amongst our merchants and laymen—the many posts he has held, of themselves, speak for this. He was for many years Director, and lately Vice-President of the Bank of Montreal, and also Director in the City Gas Company, the Montreal Telegraph Company, and many others. He will long be remembered amongst his fellow-citizens as a clear-headed and judicious business-man, possessing qualities in this respect sufficiently uncommon amongst medical men.

For nearly half a century Dr. Campbell's name has been identified with the Medical Faculty of McGill University, and it is largely due to his ability as a teacher of surgery that that school attained the high degree of popularity which it has so long enjoyed. As its Dean, he always possessed the fullest confidence of his colleagues, and, under his able management, its policy was always dignified and liberal, whilst internal dissensions were entirely unknown.

Dr. Campbell did not write much for the medical journals. "Deeds, not words," was his motto. But his work as a successful teacher, and as a member of the Corporation of the University, led to the appropriate bestowal of the honorary degree of LL.D. His style of lecturing was free from all oratorial effort, but it was clear, forcible and impressive. Hundreds of practitioners throughout this continent and elsewhere owe the foundations of their surgical knowledge to Dr. Campbell's early teaching.

As the acknowledged head of the profession in Montreal, he was often called upon to entertain strangers and professional visitors, and most worthily did he perform this duty. His house always held for such, a warm welcome, and we know that the news of his death will bring sorrow to many who have there received a true warm-hearted Scotch reception. He was an excellent host; his pleasant, cheery manner, his sparkling reminiscences, his stores of learning always bright, his animated conversation, made an evening spent in his company always something to be remembered. He took great pleasure in seeing his friends around him, and all know well the kindly and generous hospitality which for years has been dispensed from his house by himself and his talented family.

Dr. G. W. Campbell was born in Roseneath, Dumbartonshire, Scotland, in the year 1810. He entered early upon his medical studies, which he pursued in the Universities of Glasgow and Dublin. After graduating with distinction, he came to Canada in May, 1833, and settled in Montreal. His marked ability soon placed him in the front rank amongst his compeers, and gave him a large share of city practice. The success following him naturally led to his being very frequently called in consultation by his *confrères;* and for a great many years before his death very few cases of any importance were treated in this city without the advice of Dr. Campbell having been obtained. His grand knowledge of pathology, naturally clear insight into the varying shades of distinction between clinical conditions apt to resemble each other, made him our expert in diagnosis. Surgery was always his *forte*, and his great reputation was chiefly made by many successful achievements in operative work. In 1835 Dr. Campbell was appointed to the Chair of Surgery in McGill University, which position he continued to hold with credit to himself and great advantage to the school until 1875—exactly 40 years—when, owing to failing health, he resigned. He was made Dean of the Faculty in 1860, taking then the place of the late Dr. Holmes. The duties of this office he fulfilled even after his resignation of the Chair of Surgery, and it was only in March last that Prof. Howard was appointed Acting Dean in order to relieve him of some necessary work and supply his place during temporary absences.

The example of such a man as Dr. Campbell cannot fail to be productive of great good. An accomplished physician and skillful surgeon, an upright, honorable citizen, a kind and considerate friend to the poor, a loved and honored counsellor of the rich, zealous in business but scrupulously honorable, a firm protector of the dignity of his profession, and, above all, a thoroughly consistent Christian gentleman.

Medical Items.

—Professor Hüter of Griefswald, the celebrated German surgeon, died last month, aged 44, of kidney disease.

—Mr. H. P. Gisborne has been appointed Canadian agent, with his head-quarters in Toronto, for Messrs. Reed & Carnrick, manufacturers of Maltine, and also for the New York Pharmacal Association, manufacturers of Lactopeptine.

MEDICAL CANDIDATES FOR PARLIAMENTARY HONORS.—There seems to be an unusual number of medical men brought out as candidates for Parliamentary honors in the approaching Dominion elections. The names of those already announced are as follows: Dr. Wilson, East Elgin; Dr. Landerkin, S. Grey; Dr. Sproule, E. Grey; Dr. Sullivan, Kingston; Dr. St. Jean, Ottawa; Dr. Platt, Prince Edward; Dr. Ferguson, Welland; Dr. Chamberlain, Dundas; Dr. Sloan, E. Huron; Dr. Springer, South Wentworth; Dr. Samson, Kent; Dr. Bergin, Stormont; Dr. Bowlby, N. Waterloo; Dr. Gravel, Beauce; Dr. Lesage, Dorchester; Dr. St. George, Portneuf, Que.; Dr. Borden, Kings, and Dr. Forbes, Queens, N.S.

OBSERVATIONS ON THE DIGESTIVE FERMENTS.—By WILLIAM ROBERTS, M.D., F.R.S.—" If properly prepared, malt extracts are rich in Diastase, and have a high power in digesting starchy matters. But you will be surprised to learn, as I was, that a large proportion of the malt extracts of commerce have no action on starch. This is owing to a high temperature having been used in their preparation. Any heat above above 150° Far. is destructive to Diastase in solution, so that if the extract be evaporated, as is directed by the German Pharmacopœia, at a temperature of 212° Far., it is necessarily inert on starch. Out of fourteen trade samples of malt extract examined by Messrs. Dunston and Dimmock, *only three* possessed the power of acting on starch. These brands were MALTINE, Corbyn, Stacey & Co.'s Extract, and Keppler's Malt Extract."—*Brit. Med. Journal.*

CANADA
MEDICAL & SURGICAL JOURNAL

JULY, 1882.

Original Communications.

THE ÆTIOLOGY OF TUBERCULOSIS.

AN ADDRESS DELIVERED BY DR. ROBERT KOCH BEFORE THE PHYSIOLOGICAL SOCIETY OF BERLIN.

TRANSLATED BY W. D. OAKLEY, M.D., (McGILL).

(*Continued from page* 655.)

To prove Tuberculosis to be a parasitic disease, caused by the growth and multiplication of the bacilli within the body, it is necessary, in the first place, to isolate the parasites and to propagate them for a long time in pure culture until they become free from every accidental disease product with which they might be associated; and, in the second place, to reproduce the entire phenomena of Tuberculosis—which we know can be accomplished through the inoculation of tubercular substances of a natural origin—by the inoculation of the isolated and artificially cultivated Tubercle Bacilli.

Passing over many initial experiments which led to the elucidation of the problem, only the completed methods will be here given. Their essential feature is the use of a stiff, transparent culture-material, which, even at the breeding temperatures, remains unaltered in consistence. In an earlier publication I have stated the advantages of this method in bacteria investigations. By its use the pure culture of the Tubercle Bacillus, not an easy matter, was accomplished.

Serum from beeves' or sheep's blood was obtained as pure as possible and placed in a flask, the mouth of which is closed with a wad of cotton, and then heated one hour daily to a temperature of 68°C. By this means it is possible—not always, it is true, but still in most cases—to completely sterilize the serum. It is hastily heated to 65°C. for several hours, until it becomes stiff and firm. After this treatment the serum is of a yellowish or amber colour, is completely transparent, or only slightly opalescent, of a jelly-like consistence, and shows, even when kept for days, not the slightest development of colonies of bacteria. However, should the temperature rise over 75°, or last too long, it becomes opaque. In order to obtain a large surface for cultivation purposes, the serum should be allowed to stiffen when the flask is held in an inclined position. For a culture which would be accessible to direct microscopical examination, a little serum may be allowed to stiffen in a watch-glass or concave slide. To this jelly-like substance the tubercular material is to be transferred in the following manner.

The simplest way, and the way which is successful, almost without exception, when the animal has just died of tuberculosis or has immediately previously been killed while suffering from that disease, will be first described. The skin over the breast and belly is cut with instruments which have shortly before been heated to redness. The ribs are then divided with scissors or forceps which have been similarly treated. The anterior wall of the thorax is then removed without opening the abdominal cavity, the lungs being thus to a great extent laid bare. These instruments are exchanged for others also previously heated, and single tubercular nodules are dissected out and tranferred to the jelly surfaces as quickly as possible by means of a platinum-wire fixed into a glass handle, and which has been quite recently heated to redness. Of course the stopper of cotton is to be raised only momentarily. In this manner a number of flasks, from 6 to 20, should be provided with tubercular material, because even with the greatest care not all the flasks will escape accidental contamination. Caseated lymph-glands are quite as suitable as lung tissue, but pus from broken down lymph glands is not so good, because it contains few or no bacilli.

The cultivation of the bacilli from material taken from human tuberculous lungs or the lungs in perlsucht is much more difficult. I repeatedly and carefully wash in such cases the portions of tissue with a solution of bichloride of mercury, after having used all the precautions above-mentioned on their removal from the body. Then I cut away, by means of properly heated instruments, the superficial layers until such a depth is reached as one would consider free from the presence of the bacteria of putrefaction. The flasks which have in such manner been provided with tubercular material are placed in the breeding apparatus and kept at a constant temperature of 37° or 38°C. In the first week there should be no appreciable change; but in case contamination of the culture has occurred, a change does take place. This can be recognized by the appearance of white, grey or yellowish spots, and the jelly also becomes liquified. This is due to a growth of bacteria, and proceeds from the tubercular substances introduced or arises remotely from them. The growth advances rapidly, and on account of impurity the experiment fails. The true products of the growth of the tubercle bacilli cannot be seen by the unaided eye until the second week after planting, usually on the tenth day. Then appear very small points like dry scales, which vary in number and extent according as the tubercle mass, when introduced, was broken, or, by rubbing, was brought into contact with a greater or less extent of the jelly surface. These points lie around the smaller fragments of tubercle in smaller or larger circles. If there were but few bacilli in the tissue introduced, it is almost impossible to have removed them from the tissue to the jelly, consequently when they multiply they can be seen within the tissue itself when sufficiently transparent—as in scrofulous gland tissue—appearing dark by transmitted and white by reflected light. By the aid of a lens of slight power—30 to 40 diam.—they can be seen at the end of the first week. The organisms appear as very fine structures, generally of a spindle or S shape, or other similarly curved figures. Spread upon a slide, stained, and examined with a high power, the characteristic extremely small bacilli are seen. The growth of these colonies advances gradually during three or four weeks. They grow larger, form smooth masses generally somewhat smaller than a millet seed, which lie loosely on the surface of the jelly, but never penetrate into it independently, or cause it to become fluid. These colonies form such compact masses that the separate scales can easily be lifted from the stiffened serum by means of the wire, and it is only possible to crush them by using a certain amount of pressure. This extremely slow growth—which cannot be obtained at all except at breeding temperatures—and their peculiar dry, hard, scaly quality are characters presented by no other known variety of bacteria, and renders the confusion of the culture products of this bacillus with that of other bacteria impossible, so that only a slight experience enables one to recognize any accidental impurities in the culture. The growth of the colonies, as mentioned above, ended after a few weeks, and further increase does not occur, apparently because the bacilli are deficient in all power of independent motion; they spread out on the jelly surface merely by the pressure of growth, and, consequently, these slow-growing cultures reach only slight dimensions. In order to keep such a culture progressing, some of the bacilli must, some time after planting—from 10 to 14 days—be conveyed to new jelly. This is done as follows: Some of the scales are removed by a platinum wire—which, of course, has been previously heated so as to thoroughly disinfect it—to a fresh flask containing sterilized, stiffened serum, and pressed into and spread about the surface as much as possible. Then, as before, fresh scaly masses make their appearance and spread more or less over the new surface. In this way are the cultures changed or repeated. Other substances having similar properties can be used as well as stiffened serum to nourish the tubercle bacilli. For example, a sort of jelly prepared with Agar-agar, which remains hard at breeding temperatures, and to which some meat infusion and peptone has been added. On this, however, they do not grow in such characteristic forms as on blood serum.

At first I had only cultivated the bacilli from the lung tubercles of guinea-pigs, which had been infected with tubercular material. The bacilli, coming from different sources, were thus compelled to undergo a sort of intermediate culture—that is, in the body of the guinea-pig. In this way, and also in the conveyance from flask to flask, errors could arise should, accidentally, other bacteria be introduced, or if the animals used for experiment should become affected with spontaneous tuberculosis. This latter not seldom occurred. To avoid these sources of error, especial precautions were necessary, suggested by the results of observations upon spontaneous tuberculosis (*spontantuberkel*)—which constituted the most important source of error. Among hundreds of guinea-pigs occasionally just purchased, which were killed in other investigations, not a single one have I found tuberculous. The spontaneous tuberculosis was manifested in single isolated cases, and never before three or four weeks after the animal began to live under the same conditions as those which had been inoculated with the disease. In the cases of spontaneous tuberculosis, the bronchial glands were found invariably very much swollen and broken down, and generally also large caseous deposits in the lungs broken down in the centre, so that, as in human lungs, cavities had been formed. The development of tubercles in the abdominal cavity was far less frequent than in the lungs. The enlargement of the bronchial glands, and the evident commencement of the process in the respiratory organs, leaves no room for doubt that spontaneous tuberculosis in these animals is caused by the inhalation of a few or possibly only one single infectious germ, and which, on that account, has taken a very slow course. The tuberculosis caused by inoculation progresses in an entirely different manner. The animals were inoculated on the belly, in the vicinity of the inguinal glands. These first begin to swell, and thus give an unfailing sign of the success of the infection. This tuberculosis runs a course incomparably more rapid than the spontaneous, because at the outset a large quantity of infectious material is introduced into the body, and, on *post-mortem* examination, the spleen and liver are more severely affected than the lungs. It is therefore not at all difficult to distinguish the spontaneous from the inoculation tuberculosis in animals used for experimental purposes. When therefore several from a number of guinea-pigs, bought at the same time, inoculated in the same manner and with the same substances, isolated in an especial cage, become, after a short interval, without exception, simultaneously diseased in the manner just described, which is characteristic of inoculated tuberculosis, we are entitled to assume that the production of the tuberculosis can only have been due to the action of the substance which has been inoculated.

In the manner just detailed, proceeding with all possible precautions—such as disinfection of the point of inoculation and the use of previously heated instruments—four to six guinea-pigs were always inoculated with the substance to be tested. The result was invariably the same. In all animals inoculated with fresh material containing the tubercle bacilli the small inoculation wound was almost always adherent on the following day. It then remained for about eight days unaltered. Then was formed a nodule, which either increased in size without breaking down or more frequently developed into a smooth, dry ulcer. Even in two weeks the inguinal, and sometimes also the axillary glands, were swollen to the size of a pea. From this time on the animal rapidly emaciates and dies in from four to six weeks, or is killed in order to avoid complications from the later-appearing spontaneous tuberculosis. In the organs of all these animals, especially in the spleen and liver, were the well-known characteristic tubercular lesions. That the infection of the guinea-pigs was caused by the inoculated substances only is shown by the facts, that not one single animal became sick after the inoculation—of 1st, material from scrofulous lymph glands; and 2nd, from fungous masses of diseased joint, in both of which substances no tubercle bacilli could be found; and 3rd, with tubercular material soaked in alcohol for two months. On the other hand, animals inoculated with material containing the bacilli, without exception, became in a high degree tuberculous four weeks after infection.

From guinea-pigs which had been inoculated with tubercular substances from the lungs of an ape, with miliary tubercles from human lungs and brain, with caseous material from human phthisical lungs and nodules from the lungs of perlsucht cattle, was the culture of the bacilli effected in the manner above described. From this culture was it demonstrated that not only were the disease-phenomena produced, precisely similar in the animals though infected with material from such various sources, but also were the culture products derived from the diverse sources just enumerated, identical even to the smallest detail. In all 15 pure cultures of tubercle bacilli were made, of which four were obtained from guinea-pigs which had been inoculated with substances from tuberculous apes; four in the same way from perlsucht, and seven from human tubercular products.

It may be objected that the bacilli might possibly undergo some change within the bodies of the guinea-pigs, this change being possibly a modification (gleichverden) of originally differing organisms towards uniformity, or a morphological assimilation of the bacilli contained in such diverse substances. But this objection was provided for by the cultivation of bacilli taken directly from the diseased organs of both man and animals suffering from ordinary or spontaneous tuberculosis.

Such experiments were frequently successful. Pure cultures were obtained from two cases of human miliary tuberculosis, and from one case of caseous pneumonia, also human; two also from the contents of small vomicæ in phthisical lungs, one from caseous mesenteric, and two from freshly extirpated scrofulous glands—all human; moreover, two from perlsucht lungs of cattle, and two from the lungs of guinea-pigs affected with spontaneous tuberculosis. The results of these direct cultures were identical with those derived from the organs of guinea-pigs which had been inoculated with tubercular material from these same sources, the bacilli being quite unaltered by their intermediate culture in the bodies of the guinea-pigs. With these facts before us, it can not be doubted that the bacilli of these different tubercular processes are the same.

With reference to this question of cultivation, it must be mentioned that Klebs, Schüller and Toussaint have also cultivated organisms obtained from tubercular masses. All these investigators found that the cultivation fluid, after being mixed with tubercular material, became cloudy in two or three days, and contained numerous bacteria. In Klebs' experiments small staff-like bodies, having the power of a rapid motion, were observed. Schüller and Toussaint obtained micrococci. I have repeatedly convinced myself of the fact that, being wholly without the power of movement, the tubercle bacilli grow in liquids with great difficulty, and also never make the same cloudy. Moreover, if a growth does not take place at all, it can be recognized only after three or four weeks. The above-mentioned investigators must therefore have observed other organisms than the tubercle bacilli.

So far it has been proven by my experiments that the presence of these characteristic bacilli is invariably connected with tuberculosis, and that these organisms can be obtained in tubercular organs and isolated in pure culture. An important question still remains to be answered: Whether the isolated bacilli, when introduced into the animal body, are capable of producing the entire pathological process—tuberculosis? To exclude every source of error on the experimental answering of this question is the point of difficulty in the elucidation of the nature of the tubercular virus. To that end a series of experiments, varied in every conceivable way, were undertaken, and which, on account of the importance of the subject, will be separately described. The first were experiments in the simple inoculation of the bacilli in the manner previously detailed.

First Experiment.—Of six guinea-pigs bought at the same time and kept in the same cage, four were inoculated on the belly with a bacillus cutting-product derived from human miliary tuberculosis, and cultivated 54 days, with five renewals or changes. The two remaining animals were not inoculated. In the inoculated animals the inguinal glands became swollen after 14 days. The place of inoculation became an ulcer and the animal emaciated. After 32 days one died, and after 35 the rest were killed. All—the one which died and those which were killed—showed a high degree of tuberculosis in spleen, liver and lungs, the inguinal much swollen and caseated, and the bronchial glands slightly enlarged. The uninoculated animals showed no trace of the disease in lungs, liver or spleen.

When one reviews these experiments, keeping in view the

very different methods of inoculation, namely, through simple inoculation into the subcutaneous cellular tissue, by injection into the abdominal cavity or anterior chamber of the eye, or directly into the blood stream, it is seen that of a large number of animals, all, without exception, became tuberculous, and, indeed, there were not merely a few single nodules formed, but the extraordinarily large number of tubercles resulting corresponded with the great number of infectious germs introduced. In other animals it was possible, by the injection of as small a number as possible of the bacilli into the anterior chamber, to produce exactly the same tubercular iritis as in the well-known experiments of Cohnheim, Solomonsen, and Baumgarten, which were so important in the solution of the question of the inoculability of tuberculosis.

Two sources of error in these experiments must be referred to, viz.: Firstly, the possible mistake of this artificial tuberculosis for the spontaneous disease; and secondly, the accidental and unlooked-for infection with tubercular virus of the animals used in experiment. But these possible errors must be excluded for the following reasons: 1st, Neither spontaneous tuberculosis or any accidental infection produce such enormous eruptions of tubercles in so short a time. 2ndly, The control-animals which were treated in exactly the same manner as the infected ones, except that they were not inoculated with bacillus cultures, remained sound. And 3rdly, In the many guinea-pigs which were in the same manner inoculated and infected with other substances in other experiments, this typical appearance of miliary tuberculosis never appeared. This appearance can then only be produced when the body is infected with a great number of infectious germs.

All these facts taken together justify us in saying that the bacilli appearing in the tubercular structures are not only an accompaniment of the tubercular process, but actually cause it, and that in the bacilli we have before us the essential tubercular virus. The possibility of assigning definite limits to the disease called tuberculosis is also apparent, but which up to the present time could not be strictly done. A sure criterion was wanting, and consequently many regarded miliary tuberculosis, phthisis, scrofula and perlsucht as essentially the same disease. Others, with apparently just as much right, held that these pathological processes were different.

In the future it will not be difficult to decide what is tubercular and what is not. It is not the peculiar structure of the tubercle, not its nonvascularity, nor the presence of giant-cells which will determine the tubercular nature of a growth, but proof of the presence of the tubercle bacilli: either by staining reactions or by cultivation in stiffened blood-serum. Accepting this criterion as the only positive and decisive one according to my investigations must miliary tuberculosis, caseous pneumonia, caseous bronchitis, intestinal and glandular tuberculosis, the perlsucht of cattle, and spontaneous and inoculation tuberculosis be regarded as identical: my investigations in scrofula and fungous joint-affections are not sufficiently numerous to be decisive. However, a large proportion of these are undoubtedly purely tubercular and perhaps all are to be looked upon as tuberculosis. The discovery of the bacilli in the caseated glands of a hog, and the tubercular nodules of a chicken leads us to believe that tuberculosis is much more wide-spread than is generally supposed, and it is very desirable to thoroughly explore the territory of this disease in connection with the domestic animals.

The parasitic nature of the tubercular virus having thus been rendered certain, in order to complete our knowledge of this disease, two questions must be answered—Where do the parasites originate, and how do they gain entrance into the body?

With reference to the first question, it is necessary to decide whether the infectious material develops only under such conditions as are provided by the animal body, or whether, as can the splenic fever bacillus, it can pass through its development-process in any place free in nature.

The results of several experiments showed that the tubercle bacillus can grow only at the temperature of 30° to 41° C. Under 30° and at 42°, not the slightest growth took place during three weeks time, while on the other hand the bacillus anthracis grows actively between 20° and 42° or 43° C. On the ground of this one fact, the first question can be answered. In temperate zones, at no time does there occur at least two weeks of a continuous temperature of over 30°. It follows therefore, that the tubercle bacillus in its process of development is limited to the animal body, and is, moreover, not an accidental but a pure parasite, and can only originate in an animal organism.

The second question—How do the parasites enter the body?—must now be considered. The great majority of all cases of tuberculosis begin in the respiratory tract, and the infectious material first becomes apparent in the lungs or bronchial gland. It is therefore very probable that the bacilli are inhaled clinging to particles ot dust. The way and manner in which they become mixed with the air is no longer mysterious, when we consider the quantity of bacilli in pulmonary cavities which, mixed with other contents, are expectorated and everywhere disseminated.

In order to obtain an idea of the number of bacilli in tubercular sputa, I examined the expectoration of a great number of phthisical patients, and found that though in many of them no bacilli were present, in about 50 per cent of such cases extraordinary numbers were discovered, some of them containing spores. I will merely remark that bacilli were never found on examining the sputa of nonphthisical patients. Animals were also inoculated with fresh bacilli-containing sputum, and became tuberculous with as much certainty as when inoculated with the substance of fresh miliary tubercle.

Moreover, such sputa after drying does not lose its virulence. For example, four guinea pigs after inoculation with sputum, two weeks old, four after inoculation with sputum, eight weeks old, became tuberculous in precisely the same manner as after inoculation with fresh tubercular material. It can therefore be inferred that sputum which has dried upon the ground on the clothes, &c., retains its virulence for a long time, and should it enter the lungs as dust is capable of causing tuberculosis. It is probable that the tenacity of this virulence depends upon the spores of the bacilli, and it may here be stated, that the spore development of this bacillus takes places within the animal body and not outside it, as in the case of the bacillus anthracis.

To enter upon a discussion of an acquired or inherited predisposition to tuberculosis—though a most important factor in the ætiology of this disease—would lead us too far into the realm of speculation. In this direction thorough investigation must be made before a judgment is pronounced. I will now call attention to only one fact which serves to explain many puzzling phenomena, and it is, the especially slow growth of the bacilli. For this reason, probably, they are not able—as is the quick-growing bacillus of splenic fever—through any slight injury to infect the body. If one wishes with certainty to render an animal tuberculous, he must bring the infectious material into contact with the subcutaneous cellular tissue, the peritoneal cavity, the anterior chamber, or, in short, into some protected position wherein it can grow and get firmly established. Infection though surface wounds of the skin, which do not penetrate into the subcutaneous tissue, is only exceptionally successful—the bacilli being cast off before they can obtain a firm footing in the tissue.

Thus is explained why, in dissection of tuberculous cadavers, infection does not occur even though slight wounds on the hands come into contact with tubercular substances—small, slight wounds not being suitable for the entrance of the bacilli. The same considerations serve to explain the adhesion of the bacilli when taken into the lungs. The retention of the organisms would be favoured by such conditions as stagnant secretion, laying bare of the membrane from loss of epithelium, &c. Otherwise it would be scarcely possible to understand why tuberculosis is not oftener acquired, though every man. especially in the more thickly populated districts, comes into contact more or less with the disease.

Let us now ask ourselves of what further importance are the results of these investigations? In the first place, it may be regarded as a triumph of science that it is now possible to produce complete proof of the parasitic nature of a human infectious disease, of the disease, indeed of all others, the most important. Up to the present, such complete evidence existed only in the case of Splenic Fever, though in a number of human infectious diseases—Relapsing Fever, Wound-infection diseases, Gonorrhœa and Leprosy—a parasite accompanied the manifestations of pathological progress, but causal relations between the parasite and the symptomatic phenomena have not been directly proven. It is a reasonable expectation that the elucidation of the ætiology of tuberculosis will furnish new points of view for the consideration of the remaining infectious diseases, and that the methods so useful in the investigations into tubercular ætiology may also be usefully applied to the elucidation of others, especially to those—as Syphilis and Farcy—which are more closely connected with tuberculosis, and constitute with it the infectious tumour diseases (Infections-Geschwultst Krankheiten) of Cohnheim.

To what extent pathology and surgery can utilize the knowledge of the parasitic nature of tuberculosis, it is not my task to inquire; whether, for example, the finding of tubercle bacilli will be of advantage in diagnosis; whether the sure recognition of many local tubercular diseases will affect the local treatment of the same, or whether therapeutics will be in any way improved by greater knowledge of the life-conditions of the bacillus. My investigations were undertaken in the interest of hygiene, which will, I hope, receive great benefit.

One has been accustomed until now to regard tuberculosis as the outcome of social misery, and to hope, by relief of distress, to diminish the disease. Clear rules for the warding off of tuberculosis have not been possible heretofore. But in the future struggle against the dreadful plague of the human race, one will have no longer to contend with an indefinite something, but with an actual parasite, whose life-conditions are for the most part known, or can easily be still further investigated. That this parasitic organism only finds conditions suitable for its existence in the animal body, but cannot, as the Bacillus Anthracis, outside of it, exist under ordinary natural conditions, bids us hope for results in battling against tuberculosis. Above all, so far as lies in man's power must be closed those sources whence come the materials of infection, and of these sources certainly the chief is the sputa of the already phthisical. Sufficient care has not heretofore been taken in the collection and removal in an uninjurious condition of such sputa, and there are no great difficulties to interfere with its proper disinfection, by which a great part of the infectious matter is rendered innocuous. Certainly care must be bestowed upon the clothes, beds, &c., which have been used by the tuberculous.

Another source of tubercular infection is undoubtedly furnished by the domestic animals. Especially does this hold good of perlsucht. With regard to the injuriousness of the flesh and milk of perlsucht animals, the position of the sanitary authorities must now clearly be indicated. Perlsucht is identical with the tuberculosis of man, and communicable to him. On this account it is to be treated as all other infectious diseases communicable from animals to man. Be the danger from the use of perlsucht milk or flesh great or small, it exists, and must be avoided. It is known that splenic fever flesh has been eaten by many persons and for a considerable time without any injury. But from this no one would draw the conclusion that trade in such flesh is to be permitted. With reference to the milk of perlsucht cattle, it is worthy of remark that the invasion of the milk-glands by the tubercular process has been observed by veterinary surgeons, and it is therefore very probable that the tubercular virus is directly mixed with the milk.

The consideration of this subject from other points of view may lead to the suggestion of other measures aiming at the limitation of the disease. When the conviction that tuberculosis is an exquisitely infectious disease has taken root among physicians, then will be fully elaborated, by means of discussion, the most efficient rules of warfare under which to contend with our common enemy.

CLINICAL REMARKS ON LEUCOCYTHEMIA.

Delivered in the Summer Session Course, at the General Hospital, May 17th, 1882.

By WILLIAM OSLER, M.D., M.R.C.P., Lond.

Professor of the Institutes of Medicine in McGill University, and Physician to the Montreal General Hospital.

Gentlemen,—There are certain diseases which affect principally the blood and the organs of the hæmato-poietic system. Of these the principal are:—

1. *Anæmia.*
2. *Chlorosis.*
3. *Leucocythemia;* and
4. *Lymphadenoma*, or *Hodgkins' Disease.*

These are characterized by profound alterations in the constitution of the blood, and certain of them are accompanied by definite changes in those organs of the body which we regard as the blood-making ones. The form of anæmia which particularly belongs to this class is that known as *pernicious* or *essential.*

Of the affections characterized by an alteration in the structure and appearance of certain of the blood-forming organs, the most important are *leucocythemia* and *Hodgkins' disease.* In these affections, either the spleen alone, the lymphatic glands alone, or the spleen with the lymphatic glands are affected. In the former we have, in addition to the changes in the spleen and lymphatic glands, a special alteration in the blood, characterized by a great increase in the colourless elements. Hence the term, Leucocythemia, or Leukæmia. In Hodgkins' disease there is no such increase in the number of colourless corpuscles, though the characters of the changes in the organs may be identical; hence the term Pseudo-Leukæmia is sometimes applied to it. I have here to-day, owing to the kindness of Dr. Lapthorn Smith and of the patient himself, an exceedingly interesting case illustrating a disease met with but rarely in this country,

* Stenographical report by James Crankshaw, Esq., B.C.L.

and yet one which it is very important for you to know accurately and well. The history of this case is as follows:

— Vervais, æt. 39, has been a healthy man. Has been a moulder, but for the past eight years kept an hotel. Always lived in Montreal. Never had ague. Mother died at age of 80; father dead of an accident. Got hurt 17 years ago in the left side; strained while lifting. Ill now for 13 months; began with swelling of hands and legs, which continued for five or six months; then the belly began to swell. Had pain in belly, and noticed a swelling in left side. Occasional vomiting in morning. Never passed blood in stools, or vomited it. No palpitation at heart. I saw him about New Year's in consultation with Drs. Hingston and Trenholme, and we found great œdema, with ascites and enlargement of the spleen. Since that time he has been under the care of several physicians. The chief symptoms have continued to be: dropsy, for which he has been tapped three times, weakness, and shortness of breath on exertion. Within the past month the patient has improved, and I see a great change for the better in him.

We will now examine the patient and ascertain the symptoms he presents. The first thing you notice is that he has an enlarged abdomen, with slight dropsy of the feet and legs; this is not nearly as much as it was when I saw him last. His face does not present a specially cachectic appearance. He is looking now much better than a month ago, but has not got quite so good or healthy a look as when I saw him first about the New Year. The breathing is, you notice, a little short. The pulse is about 108. On examination we find the following: The abdomen is uniformly distended, not more on one side than the other, and measures about 45 inches. A few large veins are seen, but they are by no means prominent. On palpation, the abdominal walls yield; they are not tense; there is no increased sense of resistance until the fingers reach the left side of the abdomen. You then feel a distinct solid mass. It is firm, hard, and reaches below the level of the crest of the ilium. There is a definite edge, and at about the level of the navel and at a distance of three inches to the left you feel a distinct notch at this edge.

This resistant mass can be felt well into the left hypochondriac region, and far back into the left lumbar region. On percussion there is a dull note, while over the greater portion of the abdomen, a flat, tympanitic note is obtained. In the umbilical and the hypogastric region there is a distinct wave which can be seen and felt on percussing one side of the abdomen. So that we find here a large collection of fluid in the abdomen, and evidences of a tumour in the left side. The liver cannot be felt below the ribs; its upper limit of dulness is half an inch below the nipple. The chest is well formed. The apex beat is in the fourth interspace, and just within the nipple line. On auscultation, a soft, systolic murmur is heard. The lungs appear normal. The lymph glands are not enlarged.

Now what we have found here, gentlemen, is simply dropsy of the abdomen, with œdema of the legs, and a tumour on the left side of the abdomen. The questions are, first, what is the nature of this enlargement on the left side? What is the cause of the dropsy? and of the tumour here in this region? You would think at once of an enlarged spleen or kidney. When I saw this patient with Dr. Hingston and Dr. Trenholme, the doubt was whether it was renal or splenic. It is so far back in the lumbar region; it is not very moveable; and it was thought that perhaps it might be an enlarged kidney. But, on the other hand, against that are the facts that the border can be felt very distinctly; a notch is evident; and on percussing and palpating towards the left hypochondriac region, it is found that this mass emerges from below the ribs on the left side; the dull line extends nearly to the level of the nipple. From its position, the distinct feel of the edge of the notch, and the way it emerges from the left hypochondrium, there is no doubt about its being an enlarged spleen.

As to the cause of that enlargement, you have, in the first place, to think of chronic malaria; then, in the second place, of simple splenic enlargement not induced by malaria, but, by causes unknown to us, accompanied by anæmia, and sometimes called splenic anæmia; and, thirdly, whether this is the enlarged spleen of leucocythemia. Now, the only possible way in which you can decide between these conditions is by examination of the blood with the microscope. It is impossible for you to make an accurate diagnosis unless you proceed to this. You can say now, so far as we have got, that it is a case of enlargement of the spleen, with dropsy, but that is all until you examine his blood. If you examine this, and find that there is simply a decrease in the number of red-blood corpuscles, you will call it a case of splenic anæmia, whether dependent on malaria or not; but if you examine it, and find the number of white corpuscles greatly increased, so that the ratio is one white corpuscle to twenty, or less, red-blood corpuscles, you will call it a case of leucocythemia. In this instance the blood has been examined, and we find that the ratio is about one white-blood corpuscle to eight red ones. There is very great leukæmia. The examination of the blood decides the question of the nature of the affection, namely, that it is a case of splenic leukæmia. We find also that, in addition to the disproportion of the white and red blood corpuscles, the latter are greatly diminished in number. There is also marked anæmia.

Of the causation or etiology of the disease we have almost everything to learn. It occurs most frequently in individuals of middle period of life, though it is met with not unfrequently in children. The youngest case I have known is that of an infant eight months old, a case of Dr. Howard's. It affects males more frequently than females. Of circumstances which have been stated to influence it, in some respect, malaria is one which by many is thought to have an important influence. I have lately been going over a large number of leukæmia records, particularly of American cases, and I have been surprised to find how few were the cases in which any definite connection with malaria could be ascertained. We know very little, indeed, of the circumstances which induce this affection. Of the morbid anatomy, in the splenic form the spleen is chiefly involved, and it forms a large *cake*, as it is called. The size of the tumour may range from a couple of pounds to 16 or 17 pounds. Some of the largest abdominal tumours are of this splenic variety. This one, from a patient who died under the care of the late

Dr. John Bell, is the largest specimen we have in our museum; it weighed 7 pounds when it was fresh. Here is a second, not so large, and a third, larger in proportion than the others, as it was taken from an infant eight months old. The organ in this affection is large and hard. It is in a condition of what is called chronic hyperplasia. It cuts with difficulty; the section is uniform and the trabeculæ of the gland are unusually distinct. On examination with the microscope, we find that the change is chiefly in the network of adenoid tissue of the gland, which is greatly increased; and between the little meshes are the spleen corpuscles. In a large number of cases the lymphatic glands are also enlarged, more particularly the lymphatic glands in the neck and in the axillia, less frequently in the groins and in the internal glands. The enlargement in the lymphatic glands is simply hyperplasia. They are enlarged and firm, but otherwise look natural. In addition, in a very considerable number of cases of leukæmia, there are definite growths of lymphoid tissues in organs in which we do not usually see such growths. Thus, for instance, in the liver you may have definite tumours, whitish in appearance, varying in size from a walnut to a hen's egg, composed entirely of new growth of lymphoid tissue. These may also occur in the lungs. The glandular elements in the small intestines are sometimes enlarged. The tissue of the bone-marrow has attracted attention in this disease. It is converted into a reddish, soft, pulpy material very much resembling spleen pulp. It is beheved to play a very active part in the production of many of the features of the disease Neuman, Mosler and others speak of a myelogenous form of leukæmia, induced by changes in the bone-marrow. These are the chief changes in the organs and parts of the body. In *post-mortems* the condition of the blood is often found most remarkable, owing to the increase of the white corpuscles. The blood, when clotted, may present a greyish-red appearance, or in clots where the corpuscles have separated from the liquor sanguinis, before coagulation has taken place, you may have the auricle of the heart filled with a substance looking like pure pus. In the first case reported in Canada (by Dr. John Bell), when we opened the right auricle of the heart, Dr. Bell exclaimed in precisely the same terms as are related to have been used by one of Virchow's assistants in a similar case, "Why, we have an abscess of the heart," so puriform did the clots look that filled the right chambers.

With reference to the symptoms of the disease, the first that attracts attention is usually a sense of fullness and uneasiness in the left hypochondriac region, or in the upper zone of the abdomen. Accompanying this there is usually failing health. The patient becomes languid, the appetite is impaired, and they notice that they are paler than usual. Dropsy of the legs soon succeeds. In the patient you have just seen, dropsy of the legs and of the hands appear to have been his first symptom; and throughout the case it has been the chief trouble. The condition of the blood on examination is, of course, one of the essential symptoms of the affection.

The following are the characters by which you may know leukæmic blood: In the first place, when you prick the finger, you find that, instead of the deep purplish-red drop of the normal blood, the colour is changed to a chocolate brown colour, or even, when the leukæmia is very intense, a greyish-red colour. In this patient the colour is not so marked as one might expect from the number of white-blood corpuscles; but the colour, you must bear in mind, does not depend so much on the increase of the white-blood corpuscles as the decrease of the red-blood corpuscles. In a case where the anæmia is very profound, and the number of red corpuscles much decreased, you find the blood almost of a chocolate colour. On examination with the microscope, the colourless corpuscles are greatly increased in number. Instead of seeing two or three white-blood corpuscles in the field of a No. 7 Hartnack, you may find as many as 60 or 70. In fact, one usually supposes, on first examination of leukæmic blood, that the white-blood corpuscles greatly exceed the red in number. It is rather a hazardous thing to estimate, without accurate measuremnt, the proportion of white-blood corpuscles to the red. The red-blood corpuscles are always more numerous than they appear, for the reason that they collect together in clumps. You do not see how many there are owing to formation of rouleaux; whereas the white corpuscles remain isolated, and so they look much more numerous. Secondly, the colourless corpuscles frequently present great variations in size. You will notice this in the slide of blood which I have here for examination. Some are much larger than normal; others are smaller. In cases in which the lymphatic glands are greatly involved—lymphatic leukæmia—there is a much larger proportion of small white corpuscles. Thirdly, the red-blood corpuscles usually present a somewhat paler appearance than usual; occasionally there are great discrepancies in size and irregularity in the outline. Fourthly, you may have, added to the blood, an element not seen in health, namely, nucleated red-blood corpuscles which exist normally in the bone-marrow. These occur not unfrequently in leukæmic patients. In the last case I had they were remarkably abundant. In one instance, in the field of a No. 9, I counted ten nucleated blood corpuscles. I never before saw them so abundant. Lastly, Schultze's granule-masses are, in certain cases, very numerous. These characters you will see in the specimen of blood which I have taken from this patient.

Among other symptoms in connection with leukæmia, *hemorrhages* take a prominent place. In some instances hemorrhages occur very freely, and may be the very first symptoms which a patient complains of. In one of Dr. Howard's series of cases (Montreal General Hospital Reports, Vol. I), vomiting of blood was the first serious symptom that the lad had. In another instance, which I believe to have been a case of leukæmia, the girl died of the most profuse hæmatemesis. She appeared, prior to this attack, to be in fair health. We found at the autopsy a marked increase in the colourless blood corpuscles. The hemorrhage may occur early in the disease, or as a late symptom, and is a grave omen. There is usually vomiting; it may be due simply to the pressure of the large spleen on the stomach. In one case of Dr. Howard's, the vomiting was a persistent symptom throughout. Diarrhœa is occasionally met with. Most of these patients are febrile. There is a slight evening elevation of temperature. This patient has not had much fever. I have taken his temperature several times. The dropsy in this man has been marked. This may, in great part, be anæmic, depending upon the condition of his blood. The marked dropsy of the belly is doubtless due to interference with the portal circulation. Perhaps he has enlarged glands in the gastro-hepatic omentum, which would account for the dropsy in this case. But bear in mind that enlargement of the spleen alone, without any pressure on the portal vein, may account for the dropsy in the belly. This patient has a heart murmur, anæmic in character.

The pathology of the affection is still, unhappily, very obscure, largely depending upon the fact that our knowledge of the growth and development of the corpuscles is still wanting in so many particulars. It is only natural to suppose that the condition of the blood and of the blood-making organs should be intimately associated.

The treatment of this disease is highly unsatisfactory. It is a hopelessly incurable affection. The patient usually goes from bad to worse. Two years sees the termination. There are occasional intermissions of the symptoms, periods during which the patient improves a good deal. It is one of these intermissions that the patient you have just seen is in. It may be, of course, due to the remedies; but these intermissions are known to occur without being influenced by the medicines. Excision of the spleen was the remedy proposed many years ago; it was carried out in some 18 or 20 cases without any success. The patients either died on the table or shortly afterwards. The chief remedies which have been used have been directed either towards reducing the size of the spleen or improving the general condition of the patient's health. Among the remedies used to reduce the size of the spleen have been electricity, which has proved very serviceable in reducing the size of the organ. Quinine, also, and ergot, given internally or injected into the substance of the organ, have been used. Of the medicines used to improve the general condition of the patient and the blood-making powers, iron, arsenic and phosphorus are the ones commonly employed. This patient was on arsenic for some time, and also, I believe, on phosphorus. He is now on iron, and attributes largely his improvement to the large doses of iron he has been obtaining. Tranfusion has been practiced in some cases, in the hope, perhaps, of giving the patient a better blood; but this has proved futile. In a patient—as in this one whom you saw here—with extensive dropsy, you have to relieve the distressing symptoms by tapping. This man has been tapped four or five times.

There is one symptom that I did not refer to, namely, the condition of the retina. This comes in under the symptom of hemorrhage. Many of these cases have a form of retinitis which consists of hemorrhages into the substance of the retina. This man's retinæ are normal. The patient has been sent to one of the wards. We will go in, and some of you will have an opportunity of examining him. These cases rarely occur in the hospital. There has been only one in the past ten years; and I am sure we are much indebted to Dr. Smith for allowing his patient to come up here, and giving us an opportunity of seeing him.

THE TREATMENT OF DIPHTHERIA.

BY JAS. BELL, M.D., Medical Superintendent Montreal General Hospital.

(Read before the Medico-Chirurgical Society of Montreal.)

MR. PRESIDENT AND GENTLEMEN,—I wish to call your attention to the subject of the treatment of diphtheria, not for the purpose of introducing anything new, but with the intention of criticizing some of the established plans of treatment, and eliciting discussion upon them. I only propose to discuss two or three practices which I believe to be not only irrational in theory, but in practice as a rule productive of harm rather than good. I refer, in the first place, to the use of steam in the treatment of diphtheria. Steam, in one form or another, is recommended by most authors for all cases of laryngeal diphtheria (and laryngitis generally), and its use has been extended by many practitioners to ordinary pharyngeal diphtheria, so that there are at the present time probably few of the many plans of treatment more universal than the use of steam, and although, of course, it is only a part of the treatment in any case, it is looked upon by many as a most important part, and has the sanction of many great authorities. Oertel recommends hot steam at a temperature of 113°F. to 122°F. to be inhaled and kept in the mouth as much as possible, and holds that it promotes suppuration, and hastens the separation of the membrane. He has the steam conducted through a tube directly to the mouth—a very important matter in my opinion, because for this reason his theory and the practice based upon it are rational, whatever we may say of the practice, as a desirable or undesirable mode of treatment. English and American authorities recommend, in a general way, that the air of the room be kept warm and moist by the generation of steam, or that a tent be made over the patient's bed and the steam directed into it—in short, some contrivance by which steam may be generated in the neighborhood of the patient, and dissipated into the air about him. Some recommend that the air of the room be kept at a temperature of 60°F. to 80°F. (Roberts), others at a temperature of about 90°F. (Flint.)

Now, it is clear that the explanation given by Oertel cannot be applied to the treatment by steam used in this way, because evaporation is a cooling process, and as the steam issues from the spout of the kettle or from the surface of water boiling in an open vessel, it cools the air instead of warming it and surcharges it with moisture. Every one is familiar with the sensation of cold which is produced by holding the hand in a jet of steam a few inches from its exit into the air. This is due to the fact that in the change of the physical condition of water a certain amount of sensible heat is converted into latent heat, and steam entering the air passages as such is really colder than the air of the room. The advantages claimed for the use of steam diffused in the air are: 1st. That, by surcharging the air with vapor of water, it is rendered more respirable and more agreeable to the inflamed mucous membrane, and that in cases when tracheaotomy has been performed it prevents the unnatural dryness of the trachea which is obviated in health by the air passing through the moist buccal and nasal cavities. 2nd. As a means of conveying volatile medicinal agents to the inflamed part, as carbolic acid, &c.

Now, atmospheric air, as is well known, is a mixture of oxygen and hydrogen, of which oxygen is the important or life-sustaining part, and hydrogen merely an innocuous gas diluting it. It also contains on an average in every 1000 parts 84 parts by volume of aqueous vapor and about 4 parts by volume of carbonic acid, the latter derived chiefly from the respiration of animals; also, at certain times and in certain places, a variable amount of ozone, which is only an allotropic form of oxygen. It is admitted by all physicians that to obtain pure air in the most respirable form and in large quantities is one of the most important indications in the treatment of disease, and more especially in diseases of the respiratory apparatus, when the signs of deficient æration of the blood are looked upon as most ominous; and there is, perhaps, no condition when this indication is more important than in diphtheria of the larynx and air passages. Now, physicists have shown that the moisture of the atmosphere varies greatly in different parts of the world, and in the same places at different times; and from careful observations on animals in different climates, the effect of a dry atmosphere on the animal economy has been determined, and is expressed by Ganot in the following words: "The liquids evaporate more rapidly, by which the circulation and the assimilation are accelerated, and the whole character is more nervous. For evaporation is quicker the drier the air and the more frequently it is renewed; it is, moreover, more rapid the higher the temperature and the less the pressure." Our own normal sensations in health also tell us that the greatest bodily comfort and the greatest mental and physical activity are experienced in a pure and dry atmosphere. A strange inconsistency in the treatment of diphtheria, especially when both are employed at the same time, is the slaking of lime in the neighborhood of the patient—a chemical process which absorbs moisture and dries the air. Of course, a small amount of the freshly slaked lime may be inhaled by the patient, if the process is carried on very close to his bed, and the lime will also consume a small quantity of the carbonic acid of the sick chamber, but the dehydration of the air is probably the chief result of this process. Another inconsistency in medical treatment is the sending of consumptives to the high and dry climate of Colorado, while we surcharge the atmosphere with moisture for patients with diphtheritic laryngitis. In both diseases the ultimate difficulty is the same—the deficient oxygenation of the blood;—in the one case killing slowly by interfering with assimilation and nutrition; in the other, killing rapidly by asphyxia. As a means of conveying medication to the affected parts little need be said, as all the volatile substances which are used for this purpose are quite as volatile by heat alone as with water, and for ordinary local medication by drugs in watery solution a hand spray will answer the purpose much better than a jet of steam. The conclusions, therefore, which I would draw with regard to steam in the treatment of diphtheria are:—

1. That to apply it as recommended by Oertel must be so difficult, so disagreeable, and accompanied by so much risk on account of the high temperature of the steam and the necessary difficulty in accurately determining its temperature, that it is very doubtful if the advantages resulting from its use more than counterbalance their disadvantages.

2. That by the use of steam in the general atmosphere of the room, or under a tent, none of the advantages of moist heat are secured, but, on the contrary, the air is rendered less invigorating, and evaporation and assimilation are retarded, as well as oxygenation of the blood.

3. That in the production of steam a large amount of oxygen is consumed in feeding the flame which boils the water, and deleterious gases are disseminated in the air from the consumed gas or oil used for this purpose.

4. That no local indication can be satisfactorily accomplished by this means.

(I ought to say here that I have never seen steam applied in the manner recommended by Oertel.)

The next point to which I take exception in the treatment of diphtheria is the use of excito-motor agents, such as strychnia and electricity in the early stages of diphtheritic paralysis. It is true that we know almost nothing of the pathology of this affection, and have therefore very little to theorize upon; but there is a strong presumption that the paralysis is due to organic changes in the nerve centres, or at their roots, or in their substance, and that this change is probably of an inflammatory nature. At least no more probable theory has been advanced, and skilled observers claim to have discovered "softening at the roots of the spinal nerves," "capillary hemorrhages into the nerve centres," "exudation and proliferation into the nerve sheaths," &c. Now if these facts were well established, the use of strychnia and electricity (knowing, as we do, that they are powerful excitants of the spinal cord) would be distinctly contra-indicated while the lesion was progressive, and until it had been dormant a sufficient length of time to justify us in assuming that this treatment would not excite fresh inflammatory action. Fortunately, strychnia is one of the very few drugs whose physiological action is capable of experimental demonstration, while the action of electricity is well understood. Taking all the facts into consideration, I think we ought to aim at giving physiological rest to the nervous and muscular apparatus in the progressive stages of diphtheritic paralysis, and reserve excitation and stimulation for a later period, when we can feel satisfied that all inflammatory action has subsided.

Now, Mr. President, I am well aware that in introducing these questions I am dealing with matters of opinion rather than with matters of fact which are capable of demonstration; but as I have been gradually convinced by the observation of a large number of cases that these two special forms of treatment have almost uniformly yielded bad results, I have been led to protest against them, and I now solicit your opinions upon them.

Another question which I wish to raise is: What is the best form of tracheotomy tube or appliance (because it is not necessarily a tube) when tracheotomy is required in children for croup or diphtheria? I do not speak of those cases when tracheotomy is required for chronic destructive disease of the larynx and when the instrument has to be worn for a length of time, because I think a tube is the best form of instrument in these cases, and after the immediate effects of the operation are over it can be adapted to suit the special circumstances of the case. Moreover, the operation in these cases is generally performed in adult life, which very much simplifies the after-treatment. I refer, however, to those cases of croup or diphtheria generally in children, in which the operation is performed to enable the patient to breathe freely and thus tide time over a few days while the inflammation of the mucous membrane is subsiding and the exudation is being separated and thrown off, and when the wound in the trachea can be closed in a week or two at most. The operation itself in these cases is, as a rule, very simple, but the after-treatment for the first few days is extremely difficult, chiefly, I beheve, because no tube ever fits the trachea properly. The depth of the trachea from the surface varies so much, both on account of the natural differences in the amount of adipose tissue, shape of the shoulders, &c., and the amount of swelling of the neck, which is sometimes very great, that the point of the tube hardly ever enters the trachea, so as to form a continuous and uninterrupted channel for the exit of secretion. As a rule, it is either tilted forward against the anterior part of the trachea when the neck is thin, or rests on its posterior part when the neck is fat or swollen and the trachea deeply situated, and often in this way interferes with deglutition. Under any circumstances, it considerably diminishes the already lessened calibre of the trachea, and in a day or two, or perhaps in a few hours, a tough, viscid secretion collects at the point of the tube, caused, I believe, by the irritation which it produces, and obstructs it to such a degree that it is often forcibly expelled by efforts at coughing. This secretion is also deposited on the tracheal walls, just beyond the point of the tube, and causes such obstruction that the patient frequently dies of asphyxia, while the tough, gummy exudation remains just beyond our reach. I believe, therefore, that if we could dispense with the tube altogether and substitute some contrivance which would simply keep the cut segments of the tracheal cartilages separated, so as to allow of the free expulsion of the secretions and keep these secretions carefully swabbed away, tracheotomy would be a far simpler and a far more successful operation than it now is. A wire speculum answers every purpose, but the great difficulty in keeping it *in situ* is a serious objection to its use. I have thought that a clasp to catch the edge of the trachea and conneeted to a few broad metallic links, so as to be applicable to a trachea at any depth, and which would draw its edges apart and the whole trachea slightly forward, would be better than any contrivance I have yet seen.

Reviews and Notices of Books.

Diseases of Women, including their Pathology, Causation, Symptoms, Diagnosis and Treatment: A Manual for Students and Practitioners.—By ARTHUR W. EDIS, M.D., Lond., F.R.C.P., M.R.C.S., Assistant Obstetric Physician to the Middlesex Hospital, Consulting Obstetric Physician to the City Provident Dispensary, &c. With 148 illustrations. Philadelphia: Henry C. Lea's Son & Co. Montreal: Dawson Brothers.

The author claims to have endeavoured to make this a reliable, practical clinical guide to the study of these important affections. From as careful an examination as has been possible of many of the chapters, we think he has good reason to congratulate himself upon the successful manner in which his intention has been carried into effect. All the most recent methods of operating, and the most efficient found useful in these procedures, are very fully explained and illustrated. The diagnosis of abdominal tumors, being generally one of much difficulty to the student, has been given most exhaustively. The author has evidently drawn freely from American sources, as we should expect seeing the high place our neighbours hold in this particular specialty. This fact will no doubt render Dr. Edis' work all the more popular in this country. It is well and clearly written, and well put together. On the whole, we consider it an excellent addition to the text-books of gynæcology, and can highly recommend it.

Nervous Diseases: their Description and Treatment. A Manual for Students and Practitioners and Students of Medicine.—By ALLAN MCLANE HAMILTON, M.D., Fellow of the New York Academy of Medicine; one of the attending physicians of the Hospital for Epileptics and Paralytics, Blackwell's Island, New York. Second edition, revised and enlarged. With 72 illustrations. Philadelphia: Henry C. Lea's Son & Co. Montreal: Dawson Brothers.

It is such a short time since we had the pleasure of giving a commendatory notice of the first edition of Dr. Hamilton's work that it cannot be necessary here to do more than draw attention to the fact of the issue of this second edition. The rapid exhaustion of the original issue of course speaks for itself of the favourable reception it has met with at the hands of the profession. The present edition has been enlarged by nearly 100 pages, and contains many new illustrations. The most important additions are those relative to the localization of diseases of the brain and spinal cord, on which so much work has recently been done. Most of the other chapters have also been revised, and any addition made necessary to bring it up to the level of the most recent published writings.

Elements of Pharmacy, Materia-Medica and Therapeutics.—By WILLIAM WHITLA, M.D., L.R.C.P. & S., Ed., (gold medallist) Queen's University, Ireland; Physician to the Ulster Hospital for Sick Children, &c. With lithograph and woodcuts. London: Henry Renshaw.

The special object of this book is evidently to condense, and this has been accomplished without impairing its accuracy or leading to important omissions. It really consists of three distinct treatises, each one of which is quite separate from the others. The very important branch of practical pharmacy is that contained in the first section. All the various proceedings and manipulations are described, and several suitable woodcuts used to aid the descriptions. The materia-medica portion is very full, and is arranged alphabetically, like a pharmacopœia. The same arrangement is followed in the department of therapeutics, each drug being found in its place, with a short description of the diseases in which it has been beneficially employed. This part is well done, and evidently contains the results of the best therapeutical writers of the present day. The whole is concluded by some very useful chapters upon the administration of medicines and upon prescription-writing. For those commencing practice it would be worth possessing this book, if it were only for their concluding parts, for they are exactly what a beginner requires to know.

It is, on the whole, a nice, compact, handy text-book, which can safely be recommended to all.

Society Proceedings.

MEDICO-CHIRURGICAL SOCIETY OF MONTREAL.

Stated Meeting, June 9th, 1882.

GEORGE ROSS, M.D., PRESIDENT, IN THE CHAIR.

Dr. R. P. Howard said that before the regular business of the meeting was taken up, he thought it was fitting that some notice should be taken of the recent death of the late Dr. George W. Campbell. He therefore moved the following resolution, seconded by Dr. F. W. Campbell :—

" That the Medico-Chirurgical Society of Montreal have heard with deep regret of the unexpected death of the late George W. Campbell, A.M., M.D., LL.D., Emeritus Professor of Surgery, Dean of the Faculty of Medicine of McGill University, and for many years a member of this Society and its first president since its reorganization. A practitioner of medicine for nearly fifty years in this city, he acquired the confidence, the respect, and regard of his professional brethren of the past and the present generations by his eminent qualifications as a physician and surgeon, by his loyalty to, and respect for, the interests of the colleagues whom he met in consultation, and by the consideration and kindness with which he invariably behaved towards all, and especially the younger members of the profession. That it is with profound sorrow that this Society tenders its sincere sympathy to Mrs. Campbell and her family in the severe affliction which the loss of such a husband and father implies, and desires to assure them that the members of the medical profession of this city and country feel it to be an irreparable loss to them."

Further remarks expressive of the esteem and respect in which the late Dr. Campbell was universally held were then made by several members of the Society. On the suggestion of Dr. Trenholme, the resolution was carried by a rising vote.

Dr. R. P. Howard moved that, as a practical expression of their sorrow, the members of the Society should wear some badge of mourning for one month.

Pathological Specimens.—Dr. Bell exhibted: 1st, A case of obstruction in the transverse colon by a cicatricial stricture from ulceration; adhesions had formed between the bowel and the peritoneum, which was ulcerated, resulting in the formation of an abscess between the peritoneum and the abdominal wall. The specimen was obtained from a middle-aged woman, a patient of Dr. Wilkins, who had her admitted into the Hospital some six weeks before with symptoms of obstruction. On her admission a tumour was evident, about the size of a hen's egg, one inch below the umbilicus and half an inch to the right of the median line. A purgative was administered, followed by considerable collapse, but free action of the bowels was produced; there being nothing peculiar noticeable about the stools, the bowels continued to act freely, but there was no diminution in size of tumour, which was hard and painless. Patient was kept exclusively on peptonized milk for about four weeks, when she had violent attacks of vomiting; being unable to retain any nourishment, rectal enemata of peptonized milk and brandy were now used. About this time the swelling became more superficial, and gave evidence of pointing externally. An incision was made a few days after, and a small amount of pus escaped, pus escaping continually in small amounts up to the time of her death, which occurred a week later. There was no enlargement of the glands. 2nd, A case of fractured 11th and 12th dorsal vertebra, from a fall down a hoist: patient died in days. 3rd, Uterus of a patient seven days after confinement; whole interior covered with diphtheritic membrane. 4th, Abnormal distribution of the obtruator artery which would encircle the neck of a hernia. 5th, Secondary cancer of ovaries and retro-peritoneal glands.

Subject of Paper.—Dr. Roddick then read a paper on "Remarks on Hemorrhoids, Fistula in Ano, and Fissure of the Anus." He first called attention to the subject of rectal examination; he considered stooping to be the most favourable position for the male, as the condition of the prostate could also be made out; and the usual obstetric position on the left side for the female. He recommended the use of Reid's Speculum, made with a fenestrated opening running its entire length, and fitted with a glass plate, which can be removed *in situ.* In the treatment of *External Piles*, he invariably incised the tumour and turned out the clot, or injected one or two drops of carbolic acid, and subsequently a sponge, wrung out of hot water, was applied for some hours. He strongly deprecated the use of the ligature for *Internal Piles* on account of the irritation which is produced and the length of time it takes for the mass to come away. He follows Smith's method, viz., the clamp and cautery, employing the thermo-cautère instead of Smith's cautery irons. The pain after the operation is very slight and of short duration, and the patient is seldom confined to bed for more than four days. In old standing piles, with much thickened tissue, he removes the mass by an elliptical incision, radiating from the anus, and brings the edges together by means of catgut sutures, and, if necessary, introduces a catgut drain. *Fistula in Ano*—The treatment of the ordinary single and uncomplicated fistula is easy and satisfactory, but when there has been burrowing of an abscess, and the condition known as horse-shoe fistula produced, caution must be shown. Always divide the sphincter at right angles, never obliquely, and never in more than one place at a time; if it be a long-standing fistula, scrape away the granulating tissue well by means of a Volkman's spoon; would not hesitate to operate on a phthisical patient, if the phthisis happened to be in an early stage. *Fissure of the Rectum*—In treating this disease, he incises through its entire length, passing well into the fibres of the sphincter, and, if necessary, scraping the surface of the ulcer with a spoon. The application of nitric acid or the actual cautery is often of service in obstinate cases. He employs iodoform largely in rectal surgery, both in the form of powder and suppository.

Discussion on Paper.—Dr. Hingston, while agreeing with Dr. Roddick on many points, objected to the actual cautery in treating piles; he recommended the removal of the mass by the ecraseur; he also considered the ligature very objectionable. In fistula, instead of scraping with the spoon, he found that the application of equal parts of caustic potash and water answered well. For fissure of the rectum, he would not use the knife; he favoured forcible tearing of the sphincter by the thumbs.—Dr. Trenholme would not hesitate to operate for fistula in the earlier stages of phthisis. In fissure of the rectum, he recommended the use of suppositories of subnitrate of lead and tannic acid.—Dr. Blackader's experience while in the Brompton Hospital for Consumption was that the operation was considered favourable in the early stages of phthisis.—Dr. Ross thought it often very difficult to decide as to the advisability of operating in phthisical conditions; all the circumstances should be carefully considered before interfering; he related a case of a strong, healthy-looking young man on whom he had operated, not knowing of his being phthisical at the time. Shortly after he developed phthisis, which ran a rapid course; the wound never healed up. Drs. Alloway, Wilkins and Kennedy also took part in the discussion.

Stated Meeting, June 23rd, 1882.

GEORGE ROSS, M.D., PRESIDENT, IN THE CHAIR.

The Secretary read a letter from Dr. Lorne Campbell, thanking the Society for the kind words of sympathy sent to his late father's family.

Treatment of Diphtheria.—Dr. Jas. Bell read a paper on this subject (*see page* 727), and spoke strongly against the use of steam during any stage of the disease. He also condemned, on theoretical grounds, the use of strychnia and electricity in the progressive stages of diphtheritic paralysis. Dr. Bell exhibited a live dog on which he had performed tracheotomy, and applied a new instrument to keep the trachea open without narrowing, as is done with the different tubes in use. His apparatus consists of two clamps which seize the cut edges of the trachea, and are held apart by a flat chain going round the neck.

Dr. Stephen believed that steam in a room would raise the temperature of the air; he also remarked that there was very little danger of McGill graduates using either strychnia or electricity in the progressive stages of diphtheritic paralysis, as they were particularly cautioned by the Professor of Practice of Medicine against this.

Dr. Major said he did not use steam in diphtheria, but that the dry process was used now—gum or resin, with ether,—and desiccation of the membrane encouraged. Steam, he claimed, made the membranes more œdematous.

Dr. Fenwick said that many years ago Marshall Hall lectured in Montreal on epilepsy, holding that it was often caused by asphyxia, and advocated opening the trachea, but objected to the use of tubes; he used a wire and bent clips similar to those used by Dr. Bell.

Dr. Roddick uses steam after tracheotomy only to make the air humid and so prevent the secretions becoming dry. He also spoke of the good results he has always seen follow the use of sulphurous acid in diphtheria. He also burns sulphur in the room. He is a strong advocate of the germ theory of diphtheria, and believes that the vapor of sulphur becomes deposited on the mucous membrane of the larynx and trachea, and in that way anticipates the deposits of micrococci and destroys them when they arrive there. He gives internally Tinct. Ferri Mur. He is not at all satisfied with any of the tubes in use, as sometimes they cause mischief from ulceration, and perhaps perforation of the trachea. Pancoast's speculum, made after the fashion of the eye speculum, is the instrument which comes nearest to perfection in his opinion, but the great objection to it is, that after a few days the granulations crowd in and block up the opening. He would congratulate Dr. Bell on the ingenious instrument displayed by him, but saw one great objection to it, namely, the difficulty in keeping it in position during the violent fits of coughing which so constantly occur in these cases. In the meantime, he knew of no instrument with fewer objections than the ordinary Trousseau's tube, with and without fenestra.

Dr. Hingston said all tubes should have a fenestra on upper surface to test when the patient can do without tube by putting finger on the outer opening. He uses Goodwillie's Nasal Specula, which are of three sizes, each having three prongs, and are easily introduced. He performed tracheotomy after the method of a German surgeon, which is to make a free incision through the skin and fascia, then make a nick down to the crico-thyroid membrane; push a director down along the trachea, under the thyroid; then raise the upper end of the director, and dislocate the thyroid downwards. This exposes three or four rings.

Dr. F. W. Campbell for years has used the treatment advocated by Dr. Bell of Glasgow. He believes it to be almost a specific.

Dr. Kennedy also spoke of the good results following Dr. Bell's (of Glasgow) iron treatment. He believed steam to be worse than useless. Thought Dr. Jas. Bell's clamps must in a short time cause sloughing of that portion of trachea held by them.

Dr. Mills beheved that steam is sometimes useful in diphtheria. If sloughing is threatened, then steam as a poultice or vehicle might be of service.

Dr. Ross suggested caution in making sweeping assertions. He thought that steam was undoubtedly useful in some cases of diphtheria by promoting relaxation and secretion.

Dr. Blackader said the use of steam was very beneficial in the early stages, especially when the larynx is implicated.

Dr. Bell then replied to the different criticisms. He said the production of steam made the air in the room impure by removing the oxygen and adding noxious gases.

Cases in Practice.—Dr. Hingston mentioned having a few days previously removed a naso-pharyngeal fibroid after a method suggested to him by Dr. Frank Hamilton, jun., of New York, who was present at the operation, and which was done by detaching it with the index finger of right hand pushed through the nostril, helped by index finger of left hand in the mouth. The small bones of the nose were crushed; there was very great hemorrhage, but after an hour's hard work he got it away. The patient recovered perfectly, without disfigurement. Dr. H. thought the shock very great, as it could not be done under an anæsthetic.

Dr. Fenwick did not like this operation at all, but much preferred Langenbeck's method as being easier for the patient who is anæsthetized, and also for the surgeon. He has performed the operation once with very little disfigurement to the patient.

Dr. G. T. Ross asked for information regarding the relation between scarlet fever and diphtheria, as he had a case of diphtheritic sore throat in a child having also an erythematous blush over the skin, followed by one or two other cases of undoubted scarlet fever in the same family, and also another member having diphtheritic sore throat, but no rash.

The President said the relation was very close. He believed all the cases were true scarlet fever.

Dr. Kennedy brought forward a recommendation from the Council in reference to entertaining the medical delegates of A. A. S. to Montreal. The matter was referred to the Council.

It was moved by Dr. Kennedy, seconded by Dr. Roddick,—"That whereas the present Customs duties upon medical and other scientific books is found to be burdensome to the medical profession, and tending to retard the progress of scientific research, while at the same time it affords no protection to any industry, as such works are not reproduced in the Dominion. Therefore be it resolved, that this Society, through its Secretary, communicate with the other Medical Societies and Scientific Associations with the object of taking conjoint action in petitioning the Government to abolish these duties ; and that a petition be drawn up for this purpose and forwarded to each Association for signature."—*Carried.*

The meeting then adjourned.

BATHURST AND RIDEAU MEDICAL ASSOCIATION.

The summer gathering of members of the Ontario College of Physicians and Surgeons, residing in the Bathurst and Rideau district, took place at Smith's Falls on Wednesday, the 28th

June. Members were present from Arnprior. Almonte, Carleton Place, Pakenham, Smith's Falls, and Ottawa.

After routine business had been disposed of, the President, Dr. Cranston, delivered an able and appropriate address. He referred to the many changes that had occurred in the district, dwelling upon the death of Dr. Blackwood, who for forty years had practised his profession at Pakenham. As representative in the Medical Council of Ontario, he reviewed the proceedings of the recent session, explaining the changes that had been made, and expressed his satisfaction at the harmonious manner in which that august body had performed its duties. The association was also informed that an inspector for the district had been appointed, who since accepting the office had convicted two illegally practicing "doctors." He concluded his remarks by pointing out the benefit to be derived from such gatherings, and hoped each member would take a personal interest in the success of this association.

The officers for the ensuing year were then elected as follows: *President*, Dr. Cranston, Arnprior. *Vice-Presidents*, Dr. Horsey, Ottawa, and Dr. Burns, Almonte. *Treasurer*, Dr. Hill, Ottawa. *Secretary*, Dr. Small, Ottawa. *Council*, Drs. Baird, Pakenham; Dickson, Pembroke; McCallum, Smith's Falls; Groves, Carp; Lynch, Almonte; Preston, Carleton Place; Sweetland, Grant, and H. P. Wright, Ottawa.

Dr. Powell read an excellent paper on Heart Disease, the significance of murmurs and the prognosis that might be given, received his chief attention. The thanks of the meeting were unanimously voted, and a general discussion took place on many of the points brought forward.

Dr. Wright reported a case of Diabetes Mellitus, also one of Phantom Abdominal Tumor. Dr. Cranston reported a unique case of gravid uterus with cervix unusually elongated. Some microscopical preparations of *Taenia solium* were exhibited by Dr. Small.

Drs. Baird, Burns, Horsey, and Prevost were appointed to prepare papers, and the meeting then adjourned to meet at Ottawa, in January next.

Before separating, the visiting members were entertained by Dr. Atchison of Smith's Falls, who by his hearty manner added greatly to the success of a day already pleasant and profitable.

H. B. SMALL, *Secretary.*

Extracts from British and Foreign Journals.

Unless otherwise stated the translations are made specially for this Journal.

Experimental Discoveries.—The studies of Chauveau and Burdon Saunderson upon pure vaccine lymph, which in its action is so much like the behaviour of syphilis, shows the contagious principle to reside in certain minute rounded bodies, which strongly refract the light, and which seem to be heavier than the lymph. Other workers beheve they have found in the bacterial theory the most conclusive proofs that diphtheria, scarlet fever, erysipelas and other contagious diseases owe their existence to the diffusion of these minute organisms. Syphilis, too, has its advocates for a bacterial origin. "Klebs, (Keyes Venereal Diseases, page 62,) a well-known and thoroughly capable observer, cultivates a spore which he finds in syphilitic blood (apparently a moving bacterium), produces a plant, inoculates it upon an ape, produces consecutive ulcers recalling the ulcers of syphilis clinically and histologically, shows them to Professor Pick, who recognizes their resemblance to syphilitic ulcers, kills the animal, and finds between the dura mater and the skull a material much resembling gumma, and a quantity of organic germs analogous to the forms which had been inoculated upon the animal. Klebs placed a portion of a freshly extirpated syphilitic chancre under the skin of another ape; the wound healed without suppuration, the glands swelled lightly. In six weeks the animal had fever, and shortly afterwards a crop of papules came out upon the neck, head and face. The papules were flat, two or three millimetres in diameter, and of a brownish colour. These lesions scaled off, but did not ulcerate, and the papules, together with the fever, disappeared, leaving no trace." Indisputable evidences of syphilis were found *post-mortem*, and the blood of this ape contained plants looking very fungus which had been inoculated upon the first ape. The conclusions and researches of Klebs, however, must still be held *sub judice*. Beale (Disease, Germs, &c., p. 143), in speaking of the poison of syphilis, says: "It is a molecule of living matter derived by direct descent from the living matter of man's organism—living matter which retains its life after the death of the organism in which it was produced; living matter which has descended from the living matter of health, but which has acquired the property of retaining its life under new conditions; living matter destroyed with difficulty, and possessing such wonderful energy that it will grow and multiply when removed from its seat of development and transferred to another situation, provided only that it be furnished with suitable nutrient pabulum." Professor Otis (Otis on Syphilis), recognizing the pathological teachings of Verson and Beisiadecki, accepts the theory of Beale that the virus is living matter, and accounts for the induration partly by the rapid proliferation of the degraded and diseased cells derived from a syphilitic individual, and finds also an ample explanation for the incubative stage in the absorption and conveyance of the proliferated matters from the point of inoculation to the nearest lymphatic glands through the lymphatic vessels. Whatever the poison may be, whether bacterial, diseased germs, or some undiscovered entity, there can be but little doubt, I think, that the incubative stage marks the period during which only local changes are taking place; or during which the poison is developing, is being taken up by the lymphatics and through them distributed to the system at large. This incubative period is known to be rather irregular in duration, and it has been noticed that the incubative stage is longest when the point of inoculation is near or upon parts feebly supplied by lymph vessels; and is short when located amid these vessels, as near the frenum. It would seem logical to infer from these statements that the syphilitic poison always remained local during the incubative period or developmental stage; that it always infected the system only through the lymphatics, and hence if removed prior to the time the lymphatic glands became involved, should afford complete protection to the constitution. There is no doubt that the glands do play a most important *rôle* in the distribution of the poison, but evidently the blood-vessels too are largely instrumental in the process. Auspitz is perhaps the most enthusiastic admirer of the practice of excision; he reports 23 cases, in 14 of which no secondary symptoms were met with. Kölliker sanctions the practice, and has recorded 8 cases, 3 of which remained free. Unna reports 3 cases. 2 being successful. The treatment by excision in properly selected cases can certainly do no harm; it more rapidly cures the initial lesion than by any other method, and tends thereby to check the further conveyance of the disease to others, and finally it holds out some hope of being actually a curative procedure.—*Maryland Med. Journal.*

Sewer Gas.—At the meeting of the Academy of Medicine on the evening of March 16, Dr. F. H. Hamilton presented a paper on "The Struggle for Life against Civilization and Estheticism: A Supplement to the Discussion on Plumbing, etc." The doctor took a most gloomy view of our chances of life, and presented to the world the alternative either of returning to the simple mode of living of our forefathers or else of winding up its affairs and retiring from existence altogether. He reviewed the paper of Mr. Wingate and the discussion which followed it, and concluded upon the strength of the statements there made that there was nothing but danger in plumbing. We cannot ensure the exclusion of sewer-gas; none of the pipes in use are permanently impervious to gas; gas passes through the water of the traps with the greatest ease; and any means of disinfection we may employ is liable at some time or other to get out of order: consequently we have no safety except in the banishment of plumbers.

Upon the conclusion of Dr. Hamilton's paper, the President of the Academy called upon Dr. J. S. Billings, U.S.A., to favor the members with his views upon the subject under discussion. Dr. Billings thought there was altogether too much of a scare about sewer-gas. In the first place there is no such thing as sewer-gas, as an entity; there are certainly gases in the sewers, but they are ever-changing—one kind now, another an hour hence—some harmless, some injurious if inhaled in large quantities. There are two questions, however, to be considered: first, whether any of these gases are ever inhaled in sufficiently concentrated form by the inmates of our dwellings to be injurious; and secondly, whether, any of the organic diseases are ever caused by gases, in however large quantities they may be inhaled. In regard to the quantity of gas escaping through the traps into the atmosphere of a dwelling, Dr. Billings related the results of some experiments which had been lately undertaken in Glasgow to determine this very question. When the soil-pipe was ventilated, it was found by the experimenter that the gas escaping through the trap was almost inappreciable in amount, and even where there was no ventilation the amount was too small to be injurious. These experiments were conducted in an old house, the soil-pipes of which were ascertained subsequently to be unusually foul. Dr. Billings thought that in all probability, though he would not at the present time assert it positively, the zymotic diseases were caused, *not* by gases resulting from the decomposition of animal or vegetable matter, but by minute organie particles—germs so-called. If such be the case (and there can be but little doubt that it is) it would be interesting to quote further from the Glasgow experimenter as to the possibility of these minute particles—the specific contagia—passing up through the water in the traps of the waste-pipes. In a second series of experiments, conducted in the usual way with a "culture-fluid," it was found that not one single germ passed through the traps—the fluid remaining perfectly clear after weeks of exposure in the open mouth of the soil-pipe above the trap. The speaker did not wish to be understood as asserting that the gases coming from our sewers, if inhaled in concentrated form, were innocuous, but he believed that their injurious effects were seen, when seen at all, not in the production of acute diseases, but in a general lowering of the system, rendering the subject exposed to their influence more liable, perhaps, to take a contagious disease and less able to resist it when once established. He believed, however, that with good plumbing the amount of these gases escaping into a dwelling was too small to be a source of danger to the inmates, and he deprecated the exaggerated view of the evils of sewer gases as expressed by many of the profession as well as by the majority of the laity.

People may cry out against the dangers to which we are exposed on all sides by reason of the advance of civilization, and of the increase in home comforts or luxuries—but what are the facts? Are we worse off now than our fathers were? The rising generation in our cities is not a sickly and puny race, but the reverse—athletic sports are the fashion, not for the young men alone, but also for the women—sallow complexions, hollow chests and weak frames are the exception and not the rule, and one looks in vain in the faces of those he meets in the streets for the evidences of poisoning by the deadly gases, which the alarmists assure us are filling our dwellings and sapping our health and strength. Of course defective plumbing should be guarded against by every means in our power, and we would not recommend sewer-gas as a tonic to our patients, (though, as Dr. A. H. Smith very pertinently asked the Academy, if sewer gas is such a deadly poison, how comes it that plumbers are not carried off by it?) yet it certainly is a pessimistic view to take of the subject to cry that our lives are endangered if we allow a water-closet or a bath-tub or a sink to be placed or to remain in our houses. The whole question of house sanitation and drainage demands a more careful study at the hands of the medical profession than it has hitherto received, and when it receives this attention, it is safe to say there will be less of an outcry against the "modern improvements." When the writer was residing in one of the cities of Connecticut he was invited to attend a meeting of the physicians of the place, called for the purpose of investigating the cause of an epidemic of diphtheria. The city had an abundant supply of pure water, but no system of sewerage, and in the consequent soil pollution undoubtedly lay the solution of the problem. It was proposed by some of the gentlemen present to urge upon the city authorities the introduction of a sewer system—for which the city by reason of its situation was admirably adapted—but the suggestion was not acted upon, the majority of the medical faculty thinking that open cesspools, foul vaults and a filth-soaked earth were far preferable to the horrors of sewer-gas.—*N. Y. Cor. New England Med. Monthly.*

Formation of Hyaline Tube-Casts.—V. Cornil has (*The Practitioner*, Feb., 1882,) studied the morbid kidney changes in albuminous nephritis by aid of pathological specimens from a case occurring spontaneously in man, which also demonstrates the mode of formation of hyaline cylinders. The patient, after exposure to cold, had an attack of acute Bright's disease. Death, preceded by anasarca and uræmic coma, occurred seven weeks later. Examination of the swollen, injected kidneys showed very plainly the *rôle* of the renal cells in the production of intra-tubular exudation. A vacuole filled with liquid first forms in the interior of the epithelial cells, which projects; then the wall of the cell breaks, and a little drop falls into the cavity of the tubule. These clear or granular globules are observed in greater or less quantity, in a greater or less number of tubules, in every case of albuminuria. The chemical nature of these globules has not as yet been perfectly determined. The exudation, besides, is composed of red blood corpuscles, leucocytes and blood-serum, the latter constituents being more manifest in these glomeruli. The farther these different parts of the exudation pass on from the place where they have been poured out, the more they become mixed into a homogenous mass, which coagulates. So originate hyaline casts. The narrow parts of the tubule composing Henle's loop form a kind of wire-drawing apparatus, and as the colloid coagulum passes through these it is drawn out, taking a regular form, which it preserves in the wide intermediate convoluted parts of the tubule and in the straight tubule. Thus constituting veritable hyaline casts.

Experimental Production of Abdominal Pregnancy.—Dr. Leopold of Leipzig, Germany (*Archiv für Gynakologie*), has produced artificially, in rabbits, abdominal pregnancy by transferring to the abdomen of a non-pregnant rabbit the embryo only in some cases, and in others the embryo, its membranes, and placenta. Embryos two and a half, five, six and eight centimetres long were transplanted; those of the latter size being as near maturity as could be obtained. The experiments resulted in two ways. In one, peritonitis followed, from which the animal soon died; in the other case, the animal survived and the fœtus became encapsulated. In the cases where peritonitis was excited, the fœtus underwent rapid disintegration. Of the smallest embryo, no trace was found on the death of the animal on the second day. Where no peritonitis was excited, the animals were killed at periods ranging from three to seventy days after the operation. The fœtus had, as a rule, become encapsulated, but the very early embryos were absorbed, no trace of them being left. In the older embryos there was more or less absorption of the soft parts; the skeleton was left and there was growth of bone or cartilage. Dr. Leopold concludes that cases of extra-uterine gestation ending in rupture of the sac and escape of the fœtus into the abdominal cavity are, perhaps, much commoner than is generally believed, the symptoms being those of pelvic hæmatocele, and the case ending in the absorption of the fœtus.—*Chicago Med. Review.*

Roasted Coffee as a Disinfectant.—Dr. Barbier, in the *Journal de Medecine et Pharmacie de l'Algerie*, relates his first experience with roasted coffee as a disinfectant, and presents it in a manner that leaves little room to doubt its efficacy in this regard. Some 19 or 20 years ago his services were called into requisition as a medical expert, and in the performance of his duty he found himself one day in company with the magistrate of Roaune and his suite, at a country inn, in which a man had been assassinated the evening before. It was excessively hot, so much so as to surpass the highest temperature known to Algeria. The party was introduced into a closed chamber, where the body of the victim lay on the ground, but they were all seized with so alarming a sense of asphyxiation on entrance, that they incontinently beat a retreat, and the physician was the first to lead the inglorious movement. In a moment, however, the magistrate, without being much disconcerted, asked for some ground coffee from the innkeeper, who at once brought a plate full, and the worthy magistrate proceeded to liberally spread it over the cadaver, around the walls and the floor. Instantly the odor disappeared and the physician was enabled to make the autopsy without further inconvenience. The surprise of the medical authority at this unexpected change in the surroundings was only equalled by that of the legal light on learning that such a method of disinfection was unknown. Some time after, Dr. Barbier had occasion to make another autopsy upon the body of an infant which had been fully a week in the water, and he met with the same success in removing the intolerable effluvium. In another instance, in which the remains of an old clergyman were exposed in a *chapelle ardente*, the mephitic exhalations present were completely neutralized by a quantity of Mocha coffee, much to the general astonishment.

Dr. Barbier expresses his regret that it had not occurred to him to use coffee, either in powder or decoction, at an earlier date, in the treatment of foul ulcers, or as an addition to the applications necessary after surgical operations; but he has recently given it a successful trial in a case of ulcer of the sacrum in an old Jew suffering from tabes, and intends hereafter, to replace the usual classical combinations of charcoal, quinine and chloride of lime in poultices by this new agent, wherever these last have been applicable, as in all ulcers of a sluggish nature, anthrax, etc. It is to be further regretted, he feels, that the delicious aromatic principle of coffee should be lost in the process of torrefaction, and an effort should be made to utilize it as much as possible in purifying our households with it. Dr. Barbier notes also the neutralizing effects of coffee in the narcotism produced by tobacco and other noxious *solaneæ*. There is no better antidote. Every one addicted to smoking knows how quickly the narcotic drowsiness frequently experienced is dissipated by half a cupful of that beverage. Whether this useful berry exhibits its virtue as a disinfectant by reason of simple absorbing powers, rather than any chemical action, is not known, but its usefulness as a neutralizing agent cannot be questioned.—(*La France Medicale.*)—*Therapeutic Gazette.*

Therapeutical Action of Ergot.—From its action on the circulation and the nervous system it is evident that ergot possesses a wide therapeutical range. In mentioning a few diseases in which I have found it useful, I would place at the head of the list—*Pertussis*. I am aware that in this disease a vast number of remedies are useful, but after a pretty extensive trial both in hospital and private practice I am inclined to regard ergot as the best and safest. Up to the time when I began to use ergot I regarded the combination of bromide of potassium and tincture of belladonna, or sulphate of zinc and tincture of belladonna, as the best remedies with which I was acquainted, but that sometimes necessitated the belladonna being pushed to its physiological action before the disease would yield. That was sometimes not unattended with danger in young children unless they were carefully watched, which cannot be easily done in hospital or dispensary practice. Ergot seldom fails to cure whooping-cough in from one to three weeks; the cases that are longer in getting better are those complicated with bronchitis, or with troublesome bronchial catarrh. I give from four to fifteen minims of the liquid extract every three or four hours to children of three months and upwards. The benefit of the secale is at once apparent, the fits of coughing occur less frequently, and are not so severe when they do occur. I usually give it alone with a little sugar, but in complicated cases it may be combined with other remedies, and especially with the compound syrup of the phosphates, to complete the cure when there is debility. —*Dr. Dewar in Practitioner.*

On the Treatment of Phthisis by Inhalation.—Dr. S. Dowse read a paper on this subject. He prefaced his paper by referring to the recent very valuable discovery of Dr. Koch, concerning the tubercle-bacillus; and he thought that the inflammatory theory of tubercle, and Dr. Sanderson's recent lectures at the College of Physicians on Inflammation, tended to support rather than to detract from the results of Dr. Koch's original investigations. Dr. Dowse, through the kindness of Dr. Blake, was enabled to show to the members present many forms of respirators, including one of Dr. Blake's invention, which were useful and adapted for the purposes of inhalation. Dr. Dowse said that it was more than ten years ago when he first began to treat pulmonary consumption by inhalation; and he regretted that, until recently, he had not carried out his experiments with that care which so important a subject demanded. During the months of September, October, November and December, 1881, he had treated his patients in the North London Hospital for consumption, by several forms of inhalation, and he almost invariably had good results He thought, however, that the process of inhalation was far from perfect, and he hoped for better results in the future. Short histories and notes of several cases were brought forward as evidence in favor of this mode of treatment. He spoke particularly of the value of acetic ether as an inhalant; in fact, he went so far as to say this drug was, in his opinion, capable of dissolving nascent tubercle. The mixture which he generally used had the following composition: ℞ Thymol, ʒiij; ætheris acetici, ʒiij; ætheris sulph., ʒi; creasoti, ʒiij; acidi carbolici, ♏xv; terebine ad ℥iv. Ten drops to be used at a time for an inhalation. He laid great stress upon continuous inhalation: for instance, two hours in the morning, afternoon and evening, as well as during the whole night. The subject appeared to be of consideraule interest. A lively discussion followed.—*Brit. Med. Journal.*

A Method of Removing Benign Tumors of the Breast without Mutilation.—Prof. T. Gaillard Thomas, surgeon to the New York State Woman's Hospital, contributes to the April number of the *New York Medical Journal and Obstetrical Review* a paper, in which he expresses himself in favor of removing benign tumors of the breast as a rule, because the mere presence of a tumor in the breast usually renders the patient apprehensive, nervous, and often gloomy, while, with our present improved methods of operating, the patient is exposed to slight risks, the danger of growth of the tumor is removed, and with this disappears at the same time that of the subsequent degeneration of a benign into a malignant growth. If, in addition to these advantages, we can add the avoidance of all mutilation to the person, we have strong grounds for departing from the practice of non-interference. The method of operation described, Dr. Thomas has practiced thus far in a dozen cases. He distinctly states that it is entirely inappropriate for tumors of malignant character, and that it is applicable neither to very large nor to very small benign growths, being insufficient for the former and unnecessarily radical in its character for the latter. The growths for the removal of which he has resorted to it have been fibromata, lipomata, cysts, and adenomata, and have varied in size from that of a hen's egg to that of a duck's egg or a little larger. The operation is thus performed: The patient standing erect and the mamma being completely exposed, a semicircular line is drawn with pen and ink exactly in the fold which is created by the fall of the organ upon the thorax. This line encircles the lower half of the breast at its junction with the trunk. As soon as it has dried the patient is anæsthetized, and with the bistoury the skin and areolar tissue are cut through, the knife exactly following the ink-line until the thoracic muscles are reached. From these the mamma is now dissected away until the line of dissection represents the chord of an arc extending from extremity to extremity of the semi-circular incision. The lower half of the mamma which is now dissected off is, after ligation of all bleeding vessels, turned upward by an assistant and laid upon the chest-walls just below the clavicle. An incision is then made upon the tumor from underneath by the bistoury, a pair of short vulsella forceps is firmly fixed into it, and, while traction is made with it, its connections are snipped with scissors, the body of the tumor being closely adhered to in this process, and the growth is removed. All hæmorrhage is then checked, and the breast is put back into its original position. Its outer or cutaneous surface is entirely uninjured, and the only alteration consists in a cavity at the former situation of the tumor. A glass tube with small holes at its upper extremity and along its sides, about 3 inches in length and of about the size of a No. 10 urethral sound, is then passed into this cavity between the lips of the incision, and its lower extremity is fixed to the thoracic walls by India-rubber adhesive plaster, and the line of incision is closed with interrupted sutures. In doing this, to avoid cicatrices as much as possible, very small round sewing-needles are employed: these are inserted as near as possible to the edges of the incision, and carry the finest Chinese silk. After enough of them have been employed to bring the lips of the wound into accurate contact, the line of incision is covered with gutta-percha and collodion, and the ordinary antiseptic dressing is applied. If the glass drainage-tube acts perfectly, there is no offensive odor to the discharge, and the temperature does not rise above 100° ; the tube is in no way interfered with until the ninth day, when the stitches are removed. If, on the other hand, the tube does not appear to perform its function satisfactorily, it is manipulated so as to cause it to drain all parts of the cavity, and warm carbolized water is freely injected through it every eight hours. On the ninth day, when the stitches are removed, the tube is removed likewise.

Muscular Action in the Pathology of Hip Disease.—In the July number of the *New York Medical Journal and Obstetrical Review* Dr. A. B. Judson, Orthopædic Surgeon to the Out-Patient Department of the New York Hospital, discusses some points in the morbid anatomy of hip disease, with special reference to the supposed effect of muscular contraction in promoting the progress of pathological changes in the articular structures. A careful review of the most important observations on record leads him to the inference that the crowding of the articular surfaces together by muscular action has no such effect. What mainly points to this inference is the fact that the primary lesions are not usually to be found in the superficial structures that enter immediately into the formation of the joint, but rather in the cancellous texture of the bones. This conclusion, however, casts no doubt upon the utility of the extension treatment, but simply leads to this interpretation of its beneficial action : Aside from the fact that we are compelled, empirically, by reason of its anodyne quality, to use traction, there is ample rational ground for its use. Traction, however applied, is unavoidably accompanied by fixation. The most efficient apparatus for the application of traction is, at the same time, the most efficient means known to surgery for the solution of that difficult problem, the immobilization of the hip joint ; and, finally, immobilization is indicated by every feature of the pathology as revealed in morbid specimens.

Listerism.—Here antiseptic surgery in its protean forms occupies a prominent position, and in the different hospitals, and often in the same hospital, one hears the most contradictory views and sees the most varied practices. At St. Bartholomew's, Mr. Willet observes the strictest antiseptic precautions in everything; others of the staff use some of the modified forms of dressing in particular cases, while Mr. Savory smilingly claims that he obtains better results without disturbing the comfort of a single bacteria that may chance to float around his operating-table. At the Samaritan, Mr. Thornton practices Listerism at every step of his ovariotomies by the side of Dr. Bantock, who, believing that this method is not only useless but hurtful, simply puts his instruments and sponges in clean water to keep them moist, uses no spray, and dresses the abdominal wound with thymol gauze and plain cotton wool. Much the same condition of things is seen at Soho Square, the London, and other hospitals, exceptions being at King's College, where Mr. Lister and Mr. Wood show germs no quarter, and at the British Lying-in Hospital, where Dr. Fancourt Barnes, warmly encouraged by Dr. Robert Barnes, delivers every woman under the spray, keeps one playing in the wards day and night, and uses a carbolic solution for instruments, hands, and injections from the beginning of labor to the discharge of the patient, in utter disregard of the belief of the majority of the profession that the poison which makes the puerperal state hazardous is autogenetic and not from without. Then, as if to calm the medical Siloam, Mr. Lawson Tait, whose boldness and success seems to act as a chronic irritant to the profession here, which is nothing if not conservative, comes forward, and in an able paper, bristling with facts and statistics, admits the germ-theory on which Listerism is based as applied to dead matter, totally denies it in its application to living tissue and consequently to surgical practice, and, after detailing his own large experience with it, plants himself by the side of Bantock and Keith in the position that Listerism, in abdominal surgery particularly, is not only unnecessary but dangerous, producing death from nephritis in some cases, almost uniformly increasing the temperature, and otherwise retarding the convalescence. It has been currently reported recently that Mr. Lister was giving up the use of the spray, but having seen him operate many times, and having the pleasure a few evenings since of being at his house, where he showed me his latest method of preparing the ligatures and other materials connected with his dressing, supplemented by an interesting history of the evolution of his discovery from its small beginning, it is safe to say that while he fully appreciates some of the disadvantages which are urged against his method, and is experimenting with other substances in the hope of finding something which will possess all the power for good and none for harm of carbolic acid, his faith in antiseptics is unshaken, and he believes that much of the present scepticism in regard to its value has grown out of the imperfect manner in which many surgeons carry it out and to the bad results of modifications of it, which are only antiseptic in name. Hopes were entertained for a time that iodoform would meet the "long-felt want" for a safe dressing, but although it has never been dished into amputation and other large flesh-wounds here with the freedom which Billroth and other continental surgeons use it, but is simply dusted over the surface from a pepper-box or applied on gauze to the outside after the wound has been closed, unpleasant results have been of sufficient frequency to point out that great caution is necessary in its use. For smaller wounds, particularly those made in operations in the mouth, throat, rectum and uterus, to which the carbolic dressing cannot be applied efficiently, the iodoform is much used, particularly by Mr. Heath, and with a success which seems strongly to attest its antiseptic power. What the outcome of this whole question will be, of course no one can foretell, but for the present I think it may be safely said that while many of the best surgeons here believe in and practice strict Listerism most zealously, and a still larger number do so to a greater or less extent to give their patients the benefit of all doubts, there is an unmistakeable drifting into the belief that cleanliness is the great object to be aimed at, and that that method is best which most certainly secures this end.—*London Cor. Amer. Practitioner*.

The Treatment of Typhoid Fever in the past Four Years.—A review of the literature covering the subject of typhoid fever since 1878 is communicated to Schmidt's *Jahrbucher* by Dr. Arthur Geissler. It is interesting to note that a very large proportion of this literature is devoted to the subject of etiology and prophylaxis. Too much, indeed, is said to permit of any adequate criticism of it here. The subject of therapeutics of the disease occupies a much less space. Indeed, considering the extensive prevalence of the disease and the mortality therefrom (four per 100,000 inhabitants in German cities), the question as to how it is best to be dealt with by the physician has received surprisingly little attention. In the articles that have been contributed we find that the measures recommended may be classed under three heads—the antipyretic treatment, the antiseptic treatment, and miscellaneous methods. The antipyretic treatment still excites the most discussion. In Germany it means the use of baths, of quinine, and of salicylic acid. In this country other means of cooling the body than baths are resorted to, the most frequent being probably sponge-bathing. It is noticeable that there is very little literature regarding the efficacy of baths, and Geissler states that in German hospitals the mortality from typhoid fever has considerably increased since eight years ago. In 1877 it was 12.8 per cent. among 10,901 cases; in 1878 it was 13.5 per cent. among 12,406. In the years 1879-81 the figures are still more unfavourable. In Dresden, between the years 1850 and 1870, before the antipyretic treatment was introduced, the mortality was 12.6 per cent. among 3,387.

Those authors who have written recently upon this subject continue for the most part still to recommend it, but not with the exaggerated praise heard eight years ago. A. Vogel had a mortality of one in seventy cases treated with baths; Morf speaks guardedly regarding their employment; Henoch and Asby all caution against frequent cold baths for children; Keulich is enthusiastic over wet-packs combined with systematic high feeding; Steffin was only moderately successful with wet-packs; Zenetti advocates Ziemssen's treatment with calomel, baths, and quinine. One finds little said about the antipyretic value of quinine. There has been a tendency to substitute salicylic acid for it, but the results obtained seem discouraging. Of five authors who report their experience only one advocates its use.

The drug in large doses reduces temperature, but its action is temporary, and is likely to weaken the heart and disturb digestion. Hallopeau and a few others think that by alternating salicylic acid with quinine better results are obtained. A survey of the recent literature collected by Geissler upon the antipyretic treatment of typhoid fever leads to the impression that the roseate views once entertained for it are not being justified. Certainly no American statistics have been collected which show positively that the treatment by baths or by large doses of quinine has any real influence upon the mortality in American typhoid. The measure seems to be helpful in some cases. That is all that can be said.

We referred some time ago to the antiseptic treatment of typhoid fever advocated by Roth. Dr. B. Bell claims good results from a similar method. in which he uses eucalyptus. But the antiseptic treatment, as a special remedial method, has as yet no solid basis. The " water-diet " treatment, strenuously advocated by Dr. Luton, of Rheims, has a curious interest only. He gives his patients only cold water, but this in large quantity, for the first four or eight days. In this way he " washes out " all the disease-germs from the bowels and the blood. Whether he cures his patients may be considered doubtful. The medical profession cannot be said to have yet formulated a treatment for enteric fever which receives any unanimous adoption. This is not to our credit, for it is very largely due to the fact that we do not work as a body, and our individual experiences are not therefore utilized.—*N. Y. Med. Record.*

Dermatolysis : Fibroma Pendulum.—At the University Medical College, March 28th, 1882, Dr. H. G. Piffard, Professor of Dermatology, presented a unique illustration of " dermatolysis " in the person of Herr Haag, the so-called "India Rubber Man," or the man with an elastic skin. In comparison, a man who had a fibroma pendulum of the scalp, was exhibited, the disease consisting of hypertrophy of the white connective tissue of the skin. In this instance the integument has no more than the normal amount of elasticity. This condition has, by some, been called dermatolysis, but when compared with the case of Herr Haag, it was readily seen that the fibroma pendulum is not a true dermatolysis, or loosening of the skin.

Two hundred and twenty-five years ago a case of loosening of the skin, or true dermatolysis, existed, and has been described by Makron (?), who says that "in 1657 a Spaniard, twenty-five years of age, presented himself to our hospital, who could grasp the skin of the right breast, or shoulders, and stretch it out until it covered his mouth, and a like elasticity existed in other parts of the body." The skin of Herr Haag has the normal appearance, except that the small veins show much more distinctly than normal. He has always been aware that his skin was looser than that of other persons, and noticed it when compared with the skin of other boys, When drafted for military service in his native country, the surgeon in examining him noticed, to his surprise, that the skin could be stretched out in broad folds, and on account of his abnormality regarded him as entitled to exemption from doing military duty, and he was discharged. While under the observation of dermatologists in Vienna, a section of skin was removed from the anterior aspect of the right arm, for microscopical examination, and the report was that there was no change in the skin itself, but there was a decided absence of the subcutaneous fat and cellular tissue, which permitted the skin to slide and be stretched over the body. At any part of the body the skin did not stretch to a very great extent longitudinally, but transversely or laterally it could be drawn out to five or six, or more times the normal distance, and as soon as the traction was removed it returned to the normal position and appearance.

By the aid of a calcium light, arranged by Dr. M. N. Miller, and a prism, Prof. Piffard was able to ascertain the spectrum of the blood in the human circulation, and it was demonstrated that it yielded the ordinary *double* absorption bands of oxy-hemoglobin, and not the spectrum of reduced hemoglobin.—*N. Y. Med. Record.*

Baptiste-Jacob, the new Siamese Twins.—The brothers Tocci, born in Turin in 1877, are considered to be even more curious than the famous Siamese twins. They have two well-formed heads, two pairs of arms, and two thoraces, with all the internal organs; but at the level of the sixth rib they coalesce into one body. They have only one body, one umbilicus, one anus, one right and one left leg. Their genital organs consist of a penis and scrotum, and at the back there is a rudimentary male genital organ, from which urine sometimes escapes. It is a curious fact that the right leg moves only under the control of the right twin (Baptiste), whilst the other leg is movable only by the left twin (named Jacob). As a result they are unable to walk. The left foot is deformed, and is an example of talipes equinus. Each infant has a distinct moral personality: one cries while the other is laughing, and one is awake while the other sleeps. When one is sitting up, the other is in a position almost horizontal.—*Presse Médicale Belge.*—*Medical Times.*

American Gynæcology.—Who reads an American book? was once asked by a notorious English satirist and cynic. The question now asked in England and in Europe is, who is there that does not read American books? There are few good books, even in medicine, published in this country, which are not read abroad. More than this, many of them are republished there. Perhaps one of the most interesting facts in this connection is, that Mr. Keith, the celebrated ovariotomist, one not excelled anywhere, has sent his son to take a course in gynæcology in New York! He says that in England, France, and Germany, they "know a thing or two," but that in no city of the world is gynæcology so well taught and illustrated in practice as it is in the city of New York! Who, twenty years ago, could have believed such a fact to be possible? And to whom is all this honor primarily due? To Marion Sims, the founder of this great specialty; *palmam qui meruit ferat.* For a century American medical literature and American medical practice has been ridiculed abroad: now the great change has come; medical Europe looks to America, and offers her praise and gratulation.

> "Let the kettle to the trumpet speak;
> The trumpet to the cannons without;
> The cannons to the Heavens, the Heavens to earth,
> *Now the king drinks to Hamlet.*"

—*American Medical Weekly.*

CANADA

Medical and Surgical Journal.

MONTREAL, JULY, 1882.

PHYSIOLOGICAL KNOWLEDGE.

We have received a circular, and have also seen in some of the daily papers the announcement of the formation of the "Society for the Diffusion of Physiological Knowledge of Canada." From its title it might be supposed that the object of this Association was to encourage the teaching of elementary physiology and biology in schools and colleges—to institute courses of popular lectures on these important subjects in the various towns and cities, &c. Not so, however, for we find that the object, as stated in its prospectus, is to scatter broadcast throughout Canada pamphlets and tracts concerning the ill effects following upon what is known as the secret evil. Any well-directed effort in this direction would have been sure to meet with the cordial co-operation of the medical profession throughout the country, but we think there are the best of reasons why the names of physicians are conspicuous by their absence in the published list of members. It is but a short time since we drew attention to the proceedings of the Quebec Provincial Medical Board, in which the Medical Director of the concern whose title is given above was the subject of very severe remarks on the part of several prominent members. The occasion was a discussion on the propriety of any individual circulating such tracts as are here spoken of. The views then expressed are those of the whole profession. They do not believe that a good end is to be served by this process, but rather that it is constantly open to great abuse. A noticeable feature of the Society is the predominance of the clerical element, a majority of the whole being pastors of congregations. The very best intentions must be credited to these gentlemen, but it will occur to many to observe with what singular want of judgment and discrimination clergymen are apt to think and act when their sympathies are appealed to. Surely it would have been the part of wisdom to have ascertained who were the promoters of this Society, what was their record, and what standing the proposition had with the medical profession, before lending to the scheme the deservedly great influence of their names. We believe that the more this scheme is investigated, the less it will be found worthy of support, and the quicker the true inwardness of it is understood, the more rapidly will its membership decline. We do not wish to say more. The above is simply enough to convey the estimation in which it is held by the profession generally, and to warn benevolent-minded persons from joining in doing that which they might subsequently regret.

—The Bacillus of Tuberculosis described by Koch—the translation of whose article we have been able to give our readers through the kindness of our old friend Dr. Oakley—has been successfully demonstrated by Prof. Osler at the Physiological Laboratory of McGill College before the class of senior students. It was found, as stated by the author, extremely small and quite unlike either the bacillus of putrefaction or that from the blood of splenic fever. The specimen examined was taken from the lung of a man who had died of rapid general tuberculosis.

AMERICAN DRUGS.—Some weeks ago I referred to the fact that the American drug houses, through their agencies in this country, appear to be slowly, yet none the less surely, supplanting our English drug houses. This is being done by persistent and extensive, one might almost say reckless, advertising. In the matter of pushing business, Brother Jonathan is far and away ahead of John Bull; and if John of the drug stores does not mind what he is about, he will wake up one fine morning and find that, whilst he has been sleeping, Jonathan has improved the occasion by securing all his best customers. Some of our old, and at one time famous, druggists never advertise or issue an announcement to let the new race of practitioners know where they are to be found, and would think it a gross breach of business etiquette if they informed the ignorant what they have to sell, or the price of their wares.—*Students' Journal.*

A CORRECTION.

To the Editor of THE CANADA MEDICAL & SURGICAL JOURNAL.

SIR,—Through some unaccountable proceeding on the part of the "devil" who is supposed to haunt printing offices and vex the souls of writers who have not read their own proofs, I am made, in an article in your last number, to say that a *stillborn* child performed various movements and facial contortions. Please state for me that the word I have italicized nowhere appears in my manuscript. The only comfort is, the error is so absurd that my worst enemy could hardly think I really meant it.

J. J. GUERIN.

[Dr. Guerin's correction of an error in our June No. had been received when the following poetical effusion on the same subject also arrived. *N.B.*—Stillborn is not synonymous with dead, as the poet seems to think.—ED.]

DEAD OR ALIVE?

(*Vide* CANADA MEDICAL & SURGICAL JOURNAL—
P. 655, "The child came into the world stillborn."
P. 656, "There was inability to open the left eye, but the child was able to move both arms and legs.")

I reside at Beaver Mountain, and my name is Truthful James,
I am not up to small deceit or any sinful games;
And I'll tell in simple language, or rather I will try,
The story of a stillborn—an abnormality.

But first I would remark, that it's not a proper plan
For a scientific gent to mislead his fellow-man,
By using language hidden, instead of that what's plain,
And thus to lose in sorrow his exempliary name.

It was the month of May, and the lilacs were in bloom,
When there came unto my portal in the evening's dusky gloom,

One calling for a doctor, to come with him along
To Mrs. B— in labor, and whose pains were getting strong.

The painful part soon over, joy ushered in the morn,
But, alas! its stay was fleeting—the infant was *still-born!*
Its puny size I noticed, as it safely crossed the "pons,"
And I thought me of the fable of the mouse and groaning "mons."

Its left face had a mournful look, because I'll tell you why,
Its mother had been frightened by a man with a *sinister* eye;
That it was an abnormality is not difficult to prove,
For though the kiddie was *still-born*, its arms and legs did move!

And this is all I have to say of this abnormality,
That moved its little arms and legs and winked its dexter eye;
For I live at Beaver Mountain, and my name's Veracity Jim,
And I've told in simple language, the story of a whim. H. B.

Obituary.

DR. PEACOCK.—The death of Dr. Peacock removes a London physician widely known throughout Canada, not only by his writings, but personally to the many students who have profited by his teachings at St. Thomas' Hospital, to which school, for years past, the majority of Canadians have resorted. He was an accurate observer and a sound clinical teacher, not brilliant, but to the earnest student always profitable and suggestive. He was specially interested in diseases of the heart and lungs, and his writings deal largely with these subjects. Like so many of the leading London physicians, he was a thorough pathologist, and collected a large number of valuable specimens, chiefly illustrating cardiac pathology, which are now in the College of Surgeons Museum. His death was from apoplexy, the third attack; the first having been in 1877.

DR. HAYES W. LLOYD.—The Class of '79 has lost a favorite member by the death of Dr. Lloyd, which took place in London Ont., on the 18th ult. He began practice in London, and just as success seemed assured, symptoms of phthisis developed, and he went South in search of health, but in vain. The disease made rapid progress, and he returned home and died in a few days. As a student, he distinguished himself by diligent attention to his studies, and he took a prominent part in the establishment of the McGill Medical Society. His genial manner endeared him to his fellow-students, one of whom, in writing to tell of his death, well said "that the profession had lost an honourable member and McGill a worthy son."

Medical Items.

PERSONAL.

APPOINTMENTS MONTREAL GENERAL HOSPITAL.—Dr. J. A. MacMonald has been reappointed for another year, and Drs. T. N. McLean and W. T. Duncan have been appointed Resident Medical Officers.

Dr. Gardner has returned from his wedding-tour.

J. T. Halliday, M.D. (McGill, '65), of Grafton, Ont., is about to remove to Peterboro.

H. C. Burritt, M.D. (McGill, '63), is about to remove to Toronto.

H. V. Ogden, B.A., M.D. (McGill, '82), has joined Dr. Rankine Dawson on a Section of C.P.R., Manitoba.

W. A. Thompson, M.D. (McGill, '82), has been appointed Assistant Surgeon to the Eastern Section of C.P.R.

Herman E. Heyd, M.D. ('81), Reuben Levi, M.D. ('76), and W. D. Oakley, M.D. ('77), are in Vienna.

R. A. Alexander, M.D. ('71), of Granby, has left for a short trip to Europe.

Edward W. Smith, A.B., M.D. ('82), has commenced practice in West Meriden, Conn.

Dr. Henry Howard, Med. Supt. of Longue Pointe Asylum, has a work on Insanity in the press.

Prof. Wm. Osler has been elected an honorary member of the New York Pathological Society.

Dr. A. Henderson has sailed as surgeon to the S.S. *Desirade*, belonging to the new Brazilian line.

H. A. Higginson, M.D. ('81), has returned from Portage La Prairie all the better in health and pocket for his attack of "Manitoba fever."

Dr. J. A. Grant, of Ottawa, was elected, on the 1st June last, a Fellow of the Royal College of Physicians. Dr. Grant has been a member since 1864.

Mrs. O'Reilly, for so many years a nurse at the General Hospital, died at the Winnipeg General Hospital on the 20th June. She had only been there a few months.

The following members of the Class '82 have gone to London to pursue their studies: R. J. B. Howard, B.A.; J. A. Grant, B.A.; H. W. Thornton, B.A.: B. F. W. Hurdman, and W. C. Cousens.

Among the distinguished visitors at the American Association for the Advancement of Science, which meets in Montreal on the 23rd of August, will be Dr. W. B. Carpenter and Dr. Morrell Mackenzie.

We were pleased to have a visit from Dr. Lomer, of Berlin, son of our esteemed fellow-citizen, G. Lomer, Esq. Dr. Lomer has deserted his native country for the "Vaterland," and has before him a distinguished career. He has already been Prof. Credé's assistant in the Gynecological Clinique at Leipzig, and now returns to Berlin, where he has received the important appointment of assistant in Prof. Schroeder's Gynecological Department.

James Robertson, M.D. ('65), and P. A. McIntyre, M.D. ('67), have been returned members of the House of Commons from P. E. Island constituencies. Dr. Robertson was elected a few weeks ago to the Local House, but has resigned this seat for the Dominion one.

DEATH FROM NERVE-STRETCHING.—Socin, Langenbeck, Billroth, Weiss, Berger, and Benedict have each killed his man through nerve-stretching in locomotor ataxia. Violence had been done the spinal cord in these cases, as was evidenced by vomiting, singultus, and paralysis of the bladder. Billroth has abandoned the operation, and Althaus considers it an unsafe measure.—*Gaillard's Journal.*

THE MEDICAL STUDENT'S PRIMER.—What place is this? This is the Pathological Society. How does one know it is the Pathological Society? You know it by the specimens and smells. What does that gentleman say? He says he has made a post-mortem. All the gentlemen make post-mortems. They would rather make a post-mortem than go to a party. What is that on the plate? That is a tumor. It is a very large tumor. It weighs one hundred and twelve pounds. The patient weighed eighty-eight pounds Was the tumor removed from the patient? No, the patient was removed from the tumor. Did they save the patient? No, but they saved the tumor. What is this in the bottle? It is a tapeworm. It is three-quarters of a mile long. Is that much for a tapeworm? It is, indeed, much for a tapeworm, but not much for the Pathological Society.—*Medical Record.*

—The following rather good finish to a speech was made by a student at a social meeting, which was convened to show the regard in which the students held Dr. H. Chiari. "In many here will the unspoken wish arise, that, should fate lead any one of us to the marble table, it may be granted him to have the *post mortem* examination performed by Dr. Chiari's hand." This was not mere flattery: for his rapidity and dexterity in performing necropsies is something remarkable. Out of curiosity I timed several, and found the average for an examination—including brain, larynx, stomach, three or four feet of intestines, and bladder—to be seven minutes.—*Ex.*

—Nothing is worse than a vacillating physician, whom each notion, each wish of the patient, each suggestion of nurse or family affects. Blown hither and thither by every breath, incapable of taking a broad view of the case, his treatment soon becomes as irresolute as himself, and directions and accumulate with bewildering rapidity. The fewer drug are used the better; the greater the decision with which are used the better.—*Da Costa.*

—M. Lecorche, in a communication to the Acadé Médecine, affirms that grave structural changes in th will arrest diabetes. Hepatic congestion is invariable, ar on, secondary structural changes occur. At the same M. Magitot stated that diabetics are extremely liable to affection, which he names alveolar osteo-periostitis, whi begin with the onset of the disease and continue througl This jaw trouble begins by a deviation of the teeth fr perpendicular, they then loosen and fall out. The borders are absorbed, sometimes after gangrene of th which latter symptom usually precedes death.—*America of Neurology.*

—Dumontpallier (Societé de Biologie) asserted that h make certain muscles contract in a patient in his service- hypnotized and prepared for experiment by the applicati silver brass plate on the left side of the forehead--by looking at the muscle. The effect is due, he claims, "ocular influx."

—A brother of Bishop Clark was one of the wittiest me He once went to see one of his parishioners, a lady with digious family, which had recently been increased. As to leave, the lady stopped him with—"But you haven't s last baby." "No," he quickly replied, "and I never to!" Then he fled.—*W. London Observer.*

—Messrs. Wood & Co. and Appleton & Co., of New Presley Blakiston & Co., and L. C. Lea's Son & Co formed a combination to print medical books at the rate cents each. This combination will be a fearful oppos Bermingham & Co., engaged in the same business.

CATHARTIC ELIXIR,

OR

Compound Laxative Elixir.

AGREEABLE TO THE TASTE AND CERTAIN IN ITS EFFECTS.

Physicians will find this Cathartic supply a want long felt by them. It is effective in small doses, acts without griping, does not occasion nausea, and is less apt to create irritation and congestion than any of the usual Cathartics administered. The combination consists of an Extract prepared from Alcoholized Tinnevelly Senna, Butternut (*Juglans Cinerea*), Podophyllin, Rochelle Salt, Bicarb. Soda, with Aromatics; using, in addition, Tamarinds to disguise the disagreeable taste and increase the efficiency. We avoid, by our process of treating the Senna, the danger of rendering it inert, as is so often the case with the Fluid Extract and Decoction. The mild, but certain action of this Cathartic makes it specially valuable as a remedy for habitual constipation, as it will be found in small doses to act promptly, with a tendency to lessen the disposition to costiveness, instead of increasing it, as is so often the case with Drastic purgatives.

DOSE.—As a Cathartic, adults should take a tablespoonful at night on going to bed, or before breakfast in the morning, unless directed otherwise by the physician. For constipation, where a gentle, but regular action is desired, it will be well to take at first one or two teaspoonsful, as it is impossible to lay down any fixed rules for persons suffering from habitual costiveness.

The above directions, naturally, will often be modified by the attending physician, as he alone can judge intelligently of the susceptibilities of the patient.

Children from 4 to 12 years of age should take one or two teaspoonsful, when an efficient cathartic is desired.

MANUFACTURED BY

JOHN WYETH & BROTHER,

PHILADELPHIA.

Chemical Glassware & Apparatus.

The Subscribers have on hand a complete assortment of every description of **CHEMICAL APPARATUS**, comprising

CHEMICAL GLASSWARE FROM BOHEMIA,

PORCELAIN FROM THE ROYAL FACTORY AT BERLIN,

SUPPORTS FOR APPARATUS OF EVERY KIND,

And a full line of

PURE CHEMICALS AND RE-AGENTS.

All at Low Prices.

An Illustrated Catalogue will be sent on application.

LYMAN, SONS & CO.

Wholesale Druggists & Manufacturing Chemists

382, 384 & 386 *ST. PAUL STREET*,

MONTREAL.

DR. MARTIN'S
VACCINE VIRUS

PRICE REDUCED.

TRUE ANIMAL VACCINE VIRUS, (BEAUGENCY STOCK.)

15 Large Ivory "Lancet" points,...... .... $2.00
7 " " " " 1.00

All VIRUS fully warranted. It is hoped that the profession will appreciate the importance of fully supporting PHYSICIANS devoted to this laborious and EXPENSIVE specialty, and responsible for the quality of all virus issued. If the patronage of Physicians is distributed among all who—often without any fitness—offer to supply true animal virus, the simple result will be that no ONE will receive enough to maintain a proper establishment.

Our senior partner has been for over twenty years devoted to the specialty of vaccine supply. He introduced TRUE animal vaccination into America in 1870, and our establishment is by far the most perfect and extensive in the world.

ADDRESS—

DR. HENRY A. MARTIN & SON,

THE MEDICAL HALL

ST. JAMES STREET.

BRANCH: *Phillip's Square.*

MONTREAL.

WINDSOR BRANCH *Windsor Hotel.*

THE NEW MEDICINAL NUTRITIVE

Powdered Extract of Malt.

MORE CONCENTRATED, MORE AGREEABLE & MORE EFFICACIOUS THAN THE LIQUID EXTRACT.

JUST RECEIVED FROM GERMANY.

It may be had also in the following combinations:—

POWDERED MALT EXTRACT, with PEPSINE.
" " " " HYPOPHOSPHITES.
" " FERRATED.

THE GAZETTE.

(MONTREAL),

Has a circulation more than *double* that of any other Morning Newspaper published in the Province.

NO MERCHANT, BANKER, OR OTHER BUSINESS MAN CAN AFFORD TO BE WITHOUT

The Gazette.

DAILY, per annum, ... **$6.00**

WEEKLY EDITION, per annum, ... **1.00**

Address—

RICHARD WHITE, *Managing Director*
GAZETTE PRINTING COMPANY,
MONTREAL.

"Concentration of a y, espec . . . . .
deleterious, is obviously an advance in Pharmacy."

PEPSINA PRORSA:

An Absolute Pepsin, without Sugar of Milk, Starch, or other dilutant.

Our Process—Which is novel and peculiar to our laboratory, yields the full *active* strength of pure Pepsin in the highest degree of perfection, entirely obviating those pharmaceutical and therapeutical objections which attach to even pure Pepsins as usually produced.

PEPSINA PRORSA *is designed exclusively for the use of Physicians and Pharmacists desiring a pure and exact base for fine Pepsinated combinations.*

We find that physicians who have not given the subject especial attention do not, in all cases, realize the difference between *pure* Pepsin and what is commercially known as *saccharated* Pepsin. Standard saccharated Pepsin contains only *one* part of Pepsin to *nine* parts of sugar of milk. Our Absolute Pepsin (Pepsina Prorsa) contains no dilutant whatever, and is not only ten times stronger than saccharated, but has the further advantage, resulting from our method of production, of greater intensity and increased activity of the agent. Concentration is doubtless as valuable to Pepsin as to Cinchona Bark; and the increased power of Quinia, separated from its associated alkaloids, is parallel with the augmented activity of Pepsina Prorsa resulting from the peculiarities of our process.

Relative to Saccharated Pepsin, it would seem sufficient to simply point out the above difference between absolute purity and *ninety per cent.* dilution.

Physicians generally have *greatly enlarged* the dose of Pepsin.

Expert medical opinion authorizes the statement that the therapeutic value of Pepsin is best obtained when *no* dilutant is employed, and experience has determined that *celerity of action* is vastly greater with Pepsina Prorsa than with pure Pepsins that have been isoluted by ordinary processes. The sugar of milk being largely *fermentable*, and quickly affected upon entering the stomach, establishes medicinal incompatibility with the Pepsin. The power of the small percentage of real Pepsin employed is in many cases expended in counteracting the damage done by the milk sugar.

Eminent practitioners have found Pepsina Prorsa to far exceed their expectations in ordinary practice, and especially in cases of young children violently attacked by destructive summer complaints. Well marked cases of cholera infantum, apparently beyond control or hope, have been recently cured by Pepsina Prorsa. Among others, Dr. Stephen H. Roof, New York, had an experience of this kind.

We have the best reasons for knowing that our process of preparation distinguishes Pepsina Prorsa above the brands of pure Pepsin hitherto offered. Its exceptional activity is largely referable to this, without doubt.

That Pepsin has been regarded with disfavor by some is largely due to errors of manufacture. We hazard nothing in saying that five grains of Pepsina Prorsa are of more real medicinal value than 100 grains of standard Saccharated Pepsin, to say nothing of the fact that its bulk is but 1-20th of the latter.

NOTE.—If the natural taste of Pepsina Prorsa be found objectionable to any sensitive stomach, we suggest its administration in a little Glycerole Cherry, made by mixing 1 part Fluid Extract Wild Cherry with 5 parts Glycerine.

BRENT GOOD & CO.,

MANUFACTURERS,

NEW YORK.

N.B.—In ordering please be careful not to confound *Pepsina* PRORSA with "Pepsina *Porci.*"

WHOLESALE AGENTS:

KENNETH CAMPBELL & CO.,

MONTREAL, QUE.

With an Introductory Account

OF THE

FEMALE PELVIS

AND THE

MECHANISM OF LABOR.

By H. G. LANDIS, A.M., M.D.,

Prof. of Obstetrics and Diseases of Women and Children in Starling Medical College, Columbus, O.

The New York Medical Record says: "Prof. LANDIS has given us a very practical comprehensive, and interesting work upon the mechanism of labor and the use of the forceps. It can be read and studied with profit by every general practitioner."

The subject is discussed from an entirely *new standpoint*. A clear and forcible argument is made for the proper use of the forceps. It is endorsed by our best informed obstetricians. Issued in a handy volume convenient to consult, and much more full than the section on this subject in most of the obstetrical works.

12mo volume, with 28 practical illustrations. In extra cloth binding. Price, $1.50 by mail.

E. B. TREAT, Publisher, 757 Broadway, NEW YORK.

FOSSILINE.

(REGISTERED.)

FOSSILINE is a PURE HYDROCARBON JELLY, prepared from Petroleum and purified by special processes, which render it *odourless and tasteless*. It is unsurpassed by any other substance as A SIMPLE DRESSING FOR WOUNDS. It possesses remarkable antiseptic, restorative, and healing properties, which render it infinitely superior to simple ointment and other dressings.

FOSSILINE CANNOT BECOME RANCID, hence Ointments, Pomades, &c., prepared with it will keep indefinitely.

FOSSILINE is CONSIDERABLY CHEAPER than any other HYDROCARBON JELLY yet introduced, and is second to none in purity.

FOSSILINE is put up in 1lb., 2lb., 7lb. tins & upwards. Price 40c. per lb.

SOLE MANUFACTURERS

EVANS, SONS & CO.,
56 Hanover Street,
LONDON, ENG.

EVANS, LESCHER & WEBB,
60 Bartholomew Close,
LONDON, ENG.

H. SUGDEN EVANS & CO.

MONTREAL, CANADA.

Toronto Agency: 19 Front Street West, TORONTO.

(No. 3.)

NESTLÉ'S MILK FOOD

AS A SUBSTITUTE FOR

WOMAN'S MILK OR COW'S MILK.

The Elements entering into the composition of Nestlé's Milk Food, and the scientific principles upon which it is manufactured (see Nos. 1 and 2) render it an unequalled substitute for the

Mother's Milk in all cases where the mother is unable to nurse the child, or the physician prescribes an artificial food. Until quite recently the usual substitute for woman's milk has been

Cow's Milk, more or less diluted with water. The analysis of cow's milk and human milk shows in 1,000 parts of each 106 parts of solid constituents in woman's milk, against 127 parts of solids in cow's milk; but of these solids, cow's milk has 51 parts *casein* (the most indigestible of all the constituents) against only 34 parts *casein* in human milk, or just 50 per cent. more *casein* in cow's milk; and it is for the sole purpose of reducing this *casein* that cow's milk is diluted, usually half and half. In this proportion, in a stomachful, whether of woman's milk or of cow's milk, the *casein* is nearly equal. A moment's thought, though, will show that the other solids—Butter, albumen, Sugar of Milk, &c., in the stomachful of diluted cow's milk—are over 50 per cent *less* than in the same quantity of woman's milk, which readily explains why so many infants fed on diluted cow's milk gradually fade and pine away, actually starved to death. Moreover, in all cities the adulteration of cow's milk is notorious, and to it are traceable many cases of typhoid, diphtheria, and incipient consumption, to say nothing of the almost universal practice of feeding the cows, in the neighborhood of large cities, on brewers' grains, distillery mash, and city garbage. All these dangers are positively removed by the use of **NESTLE'S MILK FOOD.**

We hope to address you shortly with reference to Nestlé's Milk Food as compared with other Infant Foods. For Pamphlet giving fuller information on Nestlé's Milk Food, address,

THOMAS LEEMING & CO., Sole Agents,

MONTREAL, P.Q.

For purity and richness, **NESTLE'S CONDENSED SWISS MILK** is unequalled for all purposes.

Canada Medical and Surgical Journal

MONTREAL.

EDITORS:

GEORGE ROSS, A.M., M.D.,

W. A. MOLSON, M.D., M.R.C.S., Eng.

SUBSCRIPTION, - - - $3.00 PER ANNUM

PAYABLE IN ADVANCE.

ADVERTISING SCALE OF PRICES:

One Page (8vo. Demy)—	12 Months	$60—	6 Months	- - - - - -	$30
Half "	"	"	35	"	- - - - - - - -	25
Quarter Page	"	"	20	"	- - - - - - - -	12
Eight "	"	"	10	"	- - - - - - - -	6

INSERTING INSTITCHES:

12 Months, $75.00; 6 Months, $40.00; 3 Months, $25.00.

☞ Monthly, two monthly or three monthly Advertisements payable in advance; half-yearly and yearly Advertisements payable quarterly in advance. Any omission of insertion during contract to be made up by extra insertion at end of term. Business communications to be addressed to the Publisher,

RICHARD WHITE,

GAZETTE PRINTING CO.,

MONTREAL, CANADA

To the Medical Profession.

LACTOPEPTINE.

We take pleasure in calling the attention of the Profession to LACTOPEPTINE. After a long series of careful experiments, we are able to produce its various components in an absolutely pure state, thus removing all unpleasant odor and taste, (also slightly changing the color). We can confidently claim that its digestive properties are largely increased thereby, and can assert without hesitation that it is as perfect a digestive as can be produced.

LACTOPEPTINE is the most important remedial agent ever presented to the Profession for Indigestion, Dyspepsia, Vomiting in Pregnancy, Cholera Infantum, Constipation, and all diseases arising from imperfect nutrition. It contains the five active agents of digestion, viz: Pepsin, Pancreatine, Diastase, or Veg Ptyalin, Lactic and Hydrochloric Acids, in combination with Sugar of Milk.

FORMULA OF LACTOPEPTINE.

Sugar of Milk	40 ounces	Veg. Ptyalin or Diastase	4 drachms.
Pepsin	8 "	Lactic Acid	5 fl "
Pancreatine	6 "	Hydrochloric Acid	5 fl "

LACTOPEPTINE is sold entirely by Physicians' Prescriptions, and its almost universal adoption by physicians is the strongest guarantee we can give that its therapeutic value has been most thoroughly established.

The undersigned having tested LACTOPEPTINE, recommend it to the profession.

ALFRED L. LOOMIS, M.D.,
Professor of Pathology and Practice of Medicine, University of the City of New York.

SAMUEL R. PERCY, M.D.,
Professor Materia Medica, New York Medical College.

F. LE ROY SATTERLEE, M. D., PH. D.
Prof. Che., Mat. Med. and Therap. in N.Y. Col. of Dent.; Prof. Chem. & Hyg. in Am. Vet. Col. etc.

JAS. AITKEN MEIGS, M.D., PHILADELPHIA, PA.
Prof. of the Institutes of Med. & Med. Juris., Jeff. Medical College; Phy. to Penn. Hos.

W. W. DAWSON, M.D., CINCINNATI, OHIO.
Prof. Prin. & Prac. Surg. Med. Col. of Ohio; Surg. to Good Samaritan Hospital.

ALFRED F. A. KING, M.D., WASHINGTON, D.C.
Prof. of Obstetrics, Univ. of Vermont.

D. W. YANDELL, M.D.,
Prof. of the Science & Art of Surg. and Clinical Surg., University of Louisville, Ky.

L. P. YANDELL, M.D.,
Prof. of Clin. Med., Dis. of Children, and Dermatology, Univ. of Louisville, Ky.

ROBT. BATTEY, M.D., ROME, GA.
Emeritus Prof. of Obstetrics, Atlanta Med. Col., Ex Pres. Med. As'n of Ga.

CLAUDE H. MASTIN, M.D., LL.D., MOBILE, ALA.
PROF. H. C. BARTLETT, PH.D., F.C.S., LONDON, ENGLAND.

THE NEW YORK PHARMACAL ASSOCIATION,

P. O. Box 1574. 10 & 12 COLLEGE PLACE, NEW YORK

Canada Branch—H. P. GISBORNE, 10 Colborne Street, TORONTO.

FORMULÆ AND THERAPEUTICS

—OF—

WM. R. WARNER & CO.'S

PHOSPHORUS PILLS.

(PREPARED FOR PHYSICIANS' PRESCRIPTIONS.)

1.—PIL. PHOSPHORI 1-100 gr., 1-50 gr., or 1-25 gr. [Warner & Co.]

DOSE.—One pill, two or three times a day, at meals.

THERAPEUTICS.—When deemed expedient to prescribe phosphorus alone, these pills will constitute a convenient and safe method of administering it.

2.—PIL. PHOSPHORI CO. [Warner & Co.]

℞ Phosphori, 1-100 gr; Ext. Nucis Vomicæ, ¼ gr.

DOSE.—One or two pills, to be taken three times a day, after meals.

THERAPEUTICS.—As a nerve tonic and stimulant this form of pill is well adapted for such nervous disorders as are associated with impaired nutrition and spinal debility, increasing the appetite and stimulating digestion.

3.—PIL. PHOSPHORI CUM NUC. VOM. [Warner & Co.]

℞ Phosphori, 1-50 gr.; Ext Nucis Vom., ⅛ gr.

DOSE—One or two, three times a day, at meals.

THERAPEUTICS—This pill is especially applicable to *atonic dyspepsia*, depression, and in exhaustion from overwork, or fatigue of the mind. PHOSPHORUS and NUX VOMICA are *sexual stimulants*, but their use requires circumspection as to the dose which should be given. As a general rule, they should not be continued for more than two or three weeks at a time, one or two pills being taken three times a day.

4.—PIL. PHOSPHORI CUM FERRO. [Warner & Co.]

℞ Phosphori, 1-50 gr.; Ferri Redacti, 1 gr.

DOSE.—*For Adults*—Two, twice or three times a day, at meals; *for children between* 8 *and* 12 *years of age*—one, twice or three times daily, with food.

THERAPEUTICS—This combination is particularly indicated in *consumption*, *scrofula* and the scrofulous diseases and debilitated and anæmic condition of children; and in *anæmia*, *chlorosis*, *sciatica*, and other forms of neuralgia; also in carbuncles, boils, etc. It may be administered also to a patient under cod-liver oil treatment.

5.—PIL. PHOSPHORI CUM FERRO ET NUC. VOM. [Warner & C

℞ Phosphori, 1-100 gr.; Ferri Carb., 1 gr.; Ext. Nucis Vom., ¼ gr.

DOSE.—One or two pills may be taken three times a day, at meals.

THERAPEUTICS.—This pill is applicable to conditions referred to in the p vious paragraph as well as to anæmic conditions generally, to sexual weakn neuralgia in dissipated patients, etc.; and Mr. Hogg considers it of great va in atrophy of the optic nerve.

6.—PIL. PHOSPHORI CUM FERRO ET QUINIA. [Warner & C

℞ Phosphori, 1-100 gr.; Ferri Carb., 1 gr.; Quiniæ Sulph., 1 gr.

DOSE.—One pill may be taken three times a day, at meals.

THERAPEUTICS.—PHOSPHORUS increases the tonic action of the iron and q nine, in addition to its specific action on the nervous system. In general debil cerebral anæmia, and spinal irritation, this combination is especially indicate

7.—PIL. PHOSPHORI CUM FERRO ET QUINIA ET NUC. VOM. [Warner & C

℞ Phosphori, 1-100 gr.; Ferri Carb., 1 gr.; Ext Nuc. Vom., ¼ gr.; Quiniæ Sul., 1 gr.

DOSE.—One pill, to be taken three times a day, at meals.

THERAPEUTICS.—The therapeutic action of this combination of tonics, a mented by the specific effect of phosphorus, on the nervous system, may readily appreciated.

8.—PIL. PHOSPHORI CUM QUINIA. [Warner &

℞ Phosphori, 1-50 gr.; Quiniæ Sulph., 1 gr.

DOSE.—*For Adults*—Two pills may be given to an adult twice or three ti a day, with food; and one pill, three times a day, to a child from 8 to 10 year age.

THERAPEUTICS.—This pill improves the tone of the digestive organs, and i general tonic to the whole nervous system.

9.—PIL. PHOSPHORI CUM QUINIA CO. [Warner &

℞ Phosphori, 1-50 gr.; Ferri Redacti, 1 gr.; Quiniæ Sulph., ½ gr.; Strychniæ, 1-60 gr.

DOSE.—One pill, to be taken three times a day, at meals.

THERAPEUTICS.—This excellent combination of tonics is indicated in a la class of nervous disorders accompanied with anæmia, debility, etc., especi when dependent on dissipation, overwork, etc. Each ingredient is capabl making a powerful tonic impression in these cases.

10.—PIL. PHOSPHORI CUM QUINIA ET NUC. VOM. [Warner &

℞ Phosphori, 1-50 gr.; Quiniæ Sulph., 1 gr.; Ext. Nucis Vom., ¼ gr.

DOSE.—One or two pills may be given to an adult twice or three times a d at meals; to children, from 8 to 12 years of age, one pill, two or three times a d

THERAPEUTICS.—The therapeutic virtues of this combination do not need spe mention.

WARNER & CO.'S PHOSPHORUS PILLS.

11.—PIL. PHOSPHORI CUM QUINIA ET DIGITAL. CO. [Warner & Co.]

℞ Phosphori, 1-50 gr.; Quiniæ Sulph., ½ gr.; Pulv. Digitalis, ¼ gr.; Pulv. Opii, ¼ gr.; Pulv. Ipecac., ¼ gr.

DOSE.—One or two pills may be taken three or four times daily, at meals.

THERAPEUTICS.—This combination is especially valuable in cases of consumption, accompanied daily with periodical febrile symptoms, quinine and digitalis exerting a specific action in reducing animal heat. Digitalis should, however, be prescribed only under the advice of a physician.

12.—PIL. PHOSPHORI CUM DIGITAL. CO. [Warner & Co.]

℞ Phosphori, 1-50 gr.; Pulv. Digitalis, 1 gr.; Ext. Hyoscyami, 1 gr.

DOSE.—One pill may be taken three or four times in twenty-four hours.

THERAPEUTICS.—The effect of digitalis as a cardiac tonic renders it particularly applicable, in combination with phosphorus, in cases of overwork, attended with derangement of the heart's action. In excessive irritability of the nervous system, in *palpitation of the heart valvular disease aneurism, etc.*, it may be employed beneficially, while the diuretic action of digitalis renders it applicable to various forms of dropsy. The same caution in regard to the use of digitalis may be repeated here.

13.—PIL. PHOSPHORI CUM DIGITAL. ET FERRO. [Warner & Co.]

℞ Phosphori, 1-50 gr.; Pulv. Digitalis, 1 gr.; Ferri Redacti, 1 gr.

DOSE.—One pill, to be taken three or four times a day, at meals.

THERAPEUTICS.—This combination may be employed in the cases referred to in the previous paragraph, especially when accompanied with anæmia.

14.—PIL. PHOSPHORI CUM CANNABE INDICA. [Warner & Co.]

℞ Phosphori, 1-50 gr.; Ext. Cannibis Ind., ¼ gr.

DOSE.—One or two pills, to be taken twice or three times a day, at meals.

THERAPEUTICS.—The Indian Hemp is added as a calmative and soporific in cases in which morphia is inadmissible from idiosyncrasy or other cause, as well as for its aphrodisiac effect.

15.—PIL. PHOSPHORI CUM MORPHIA ET ZINCI VAL. [Warner & Co.]

℞ Phosphori, 1-50 gr.; Morphiæ Sulph., 1-12 gr.; Zinc. Valer., 1 gr.

DOSE.—One pill may be taken twice or thrice daily, or two, at bedtime.

THERAPEUTICS.—Applicable in consumption attended with nervous irritability and annoying cough; in hysterical cough and neuralgia it may be given at the same time with *cod liver oil.*

16.—PIL. PHOSPHORI CUM ALOE ET NUC. VOM. [Warner & Co.]

℞ Phosphori, 1-50 gr.; Ext. Aloes Aquosæ' ½ gr.; Ext. Nucis Vomicæ, ¼ gr.

DOSE.—One may be given daily at or immediately after dinner.

WAR O.'S

SOLUBLE SUGAR-COATED

PHOSPHORUS PILLS

Observe the following Trade Mark on each label as a guarantee of genuineness.

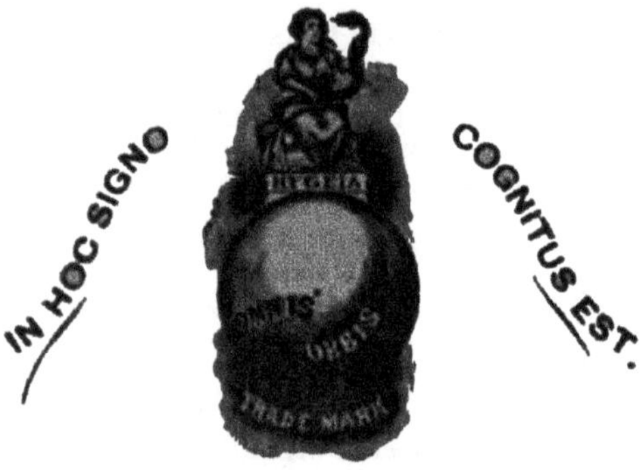
IN HOC SIGNO
COGNITUS EST.
TRADE MARK

The method of preparing Phosphorus in pilular form has been discovered brought to perfection by us, without the necessity of combining it with resi which forms an insoluble compound. The element is in a perfect state of sul division and incorporated with the excipient while in solution. The non-poro coating of sugar protects it thoroughly from oxidation, so that the pill is not im paired by age It is the most pleasant and acceptable form for the administratio of Phosphorus.

Specify WARNER & CO. when prescribing, and order i

substitution of cheaper and inferior brands.

PILLS SENT BY MAIL ON RECEIPT OF LIST PRICE.

WM. R. WARNER & CO., CHEMISTS, PHILADELPHI

Messrs. WM R. WARNER & CO. NEW YORK, November 11, 1877.

GENTLEMEN.—The Phosphorus Pills submitted to me for chemical analysis and microscop examination, afford only traces of Phosphoric Acid, and contain the one-twenty-fifth of a grai (gr. 1-25) of the element in each Pill, as expressed upon the label: they do not exhibit partich of undivided Phosphorus, the mass being perfectly homogeneous in composition, soft in consis ence and thoroughly protected by the non-porous coating of sugar from the oxidising influence of the air. Each pill is an example o what skill, care and elegant Pharmacy can do.—I regar them as a marvel of perfection.

Very respectfully, A. E. McLEAN,
Analytical Chemist and Microscopist.

(Late of Edinburgh, Scotland.) 40 and 42 Broadway, N. Y

CENTENNIAL WORLD'S FAIR AWARD.

"The Sugar-Coated Pills of Wm. R. Warner & Co. are Soluble, Reliable and Unsurpassed in th perfection of Sugar-Coating, thorough composition and accurate subdivision."

"The pills of Phosphorus are worthy of special notice. The element is thoroughly diffused and sub divided, yet perfectly protected from oxidation."

Attest, *A. T. GOSHORN, Director-Genera*

[SEAL] *J. L. CAMPBELL.* *J. R. HAWLEY, President.*

Complete list of W. R. Warner & Co.'s Phosphorus Pills mailed on application.

MALTINE is a concentrated extract of malted Barley, Wheat and Oats. In its preparation t temperature does not exceed 150 deg. Fahr., thereby retaining all the nutritive and digestive agen unimpaired. Extracts of Malt are made from Barley alone, by the German process, which directs th the mash be heated to 212 deg. Fahr., thereby coagulating the Albuminoids and almost wholly destroyi the starch digestive principle, Diastase.

LIST OF MALTINE PREPARATIONS.

MALTINE (Plain).
MALTINE with Hops.
MALTINE with Alteratives.
MALTINE with Beef and Iron.
MALTINE with Cod Liver Oil.
MALTINE with Cod Liver Oil and Pancreatine.
MALTINE with Hypophosphites.
MALTINE with Phosphorus Comp.
MALTINE with Peptones.
MALTINE with Pepsin and Pancreatine.
MALTINE with Phosphates.
MALTINE with Phosphates Iron and Quinia.
MALTINE with Phosphates Iron, Quinia & Stryc
MALTINE Ferrated.
MALTINE WINE.
MALTINE WINE with Pepsin and Pancreatir
MALTO-YERBINE.
MALTO-VIBURNIN.

MEDICAL ENDORSEMENTS.

We append, *by permission*, a few names of the many prominent Members of the Med cal Profession who are prescribing our Maltine Preparations:

J. K. BAUDY, M.D., St. Louis, Mo., Physician to St. Vincent's Insane Asylum, and Prof. Nervous Diseases and Clinical Medicine, Missouri Medical College.

WM. PORTER, A.M., M.D., St. Louis, Mo.

E. S. DUNSTER, M.D., Ann Harbor, Mich., Prof. Obs. and Dis. Women and Children University and in Dartmouth College.

THOS. H. ANDREWS, M.D., Philadelphia, Pa., Demonstrator of Anatomy, Jefferson Medical College.

B. F. HAMMEL, M.D., Philadelphia, Pa., Supt. Hospital of the University of Penn.

F. R. PALMER, M.D., Louisville, Ky., Prof. of Physiology and Personal Diagnosis, University of Louisville.

HUNTER McGUIRE, M.D., Richmond, Va., Prof. of Surgery, Med. Col. of Virginia.

F. A. MARDEN, M.D., Milwaukee, Wis., Supt. and Physic'n, Milwaukee County Hospital.

L. P. YANDELL, M.D., Louisville, Ky., Prof. of Clinical Medicine and Diseases of Children, University, Louisville.

JOHN A. LARRABEE, M.D., Louisville, Ky., Prof. of Materia Medica and Therapeutics, and Clinical Lecturer on Diseases of Children in the Hospital College of Medicine.

R. OGDEN DOREMUS, M.D., L.L.D., New York, Prof. of Chemistry and Toxicology, Bellevue Hospital Medical College; Prof. of Chemistry and Physics, College of the City of New York.

WALTER S. HAINES, M.D., Chicago, Ill., Prof. of Chemistry, and Toxicology, Rush Medical College, Chicago.

E. F. INGALLS, A.M., M.D., Chicago, Ill., Clinical Professor of Diseases of Chest and Throat, Woman's Medical College.

A. A. MEUNIER, M.D., Montreal, Canada, Prof. Victoria University.

H. F. BIGGAR, M.D., Prof. of Surgical and Me cal Diseases of Women, Homœpathic H pital College, Cleveland, Ohio.

DR. DOBELL, London, England, Consulting Ph sician to Royal Hospital for Diseases the Chest.

DR. T. F. GRIMSDALE, Liverpool, Eng., Co sulting Physician, Ladies' Charity a Lying-in-Hospital.

WM. ROBERTS, M.D., F.R.C.P., F.R.S., Ma chester, England, Prof. of Clinical Me cine, Owens' College School of Medicin Physician Manchester Royal Infirmary a Lunatic Hospital.

J. C. THOROWGOOD, M.D., F.R.C.P., Londo England, Physician City of London H pital for Chest Diseases; Physician W London Hospital.

W. C. PLAYFAIR, M.D., F.R.C.P., London, En Prof. of Obstetric Medicine in King's C lege, and Physician for the Diseases Women and Children to King's Colle Hospital.

W. H. WALSHE, M.D., F.R.C.P., Brompton, Er land, Consulting Physician Consumpti Hospital, Brompton, and to the Universi College Hospital.

A. WYNN WILLIAMS, M.D., M.R.C.S., Londo England, Physician Samaritan Free H pital for Diseases of Women and Childre

A. C. MACRAE, M.D., Calcutta, Ind., Dep. In Gen. Hosp. Ind. Service, late Pres. Sur Calcutta.

EDWARD SHOPPEE, M.D., L.R.C.P., M.R.C. London, England.

LENNOX BROWN, F.R.C.S., London, Eng., Se Surgeon, Central Throat and Ear Hospit

J. CARRICK MURRAY, M.D., Newcastle-o Tyne, England, Physician to the N. C. for Diseases of Chest.

J. A. GRANT, M.D., F.R.C.S., Ottawa, Canada.

MALTINE is prescribed by the most eminent members of the Medical Professi in the United States, Great Britain, India, China and the English Colonies, and is large used at the principal Hospitals in preference to any of the Extracts of Malt.

☞ We will forward gratuitously a 1-lb. bottle of any of the above preparations to Physicians, w will pay the express charges. Send for our 28 page Pamphlet on Maltine for further particulars.

Address ***REED & CARNRICK,***

[redacted] 182 Fulton St., New Yo

MALTINE IN PULMONARY PHTHISIS.

HE great value of **MALTINE** *in all wasting diseases, and especially in Pulmonary affections, is becoming more and more apparent to the ical Profession.*

Any Physician who will test **MALTINE,** *Plain, in comparison with Liver Oil, in a case of Pulmonary Phthisis, will find that it will increase ht and build up the system far more rapidly. There are, however, many s where the compounds with Hypophosphites, Phosphates, Peptones, Malto-ine, and Pepsin and Pancreatine are strongly indicated.*

---

fter a full trial of the different Oils and Extract of Malt preparations, in both hospital and private ice, I find MALTINE most applicable to the largest number of patients, and superior to any remedy class. Theoretically, we would expect this preparation, which has become *practically official*, to great value in chronic conditions of waste and mal-nutrition, especially as exemplified in phthisis. rich in Diastase, albumenoids and phosphates, according to careful analysis, it aids in digesting ceous food, while in itself it is a brain, nerve and muscle producer.

WM. PORTER, A.M., M.D., *St. Louis, Mo.*

---

123 *Landsdowne Road, Notting Hill, W., London, October* [illegible]*, 18*[illegible]*.*

have used MALTINE with Cod Liver Oil with the happiest results in a case of tuberculosis attended tubercular peritonitis, in which the temperature of the patient rose to 105 1-5° and persistently ined above 100° for upwards of two months. The only medicine taken was MALTINE with Cod Liver nd an occasional dose of Carbonate of Bismuth, to check diarrhœa. She gradually improved and n perfect recovery. I find MALTINE with Cod Liver Oil is more readily taken and more easily assi-ed than Cod Liver Oil in any other form.

EDMUND NASH, M.D.

Brülge House, Revesby, Boston, Lincolnshire.

he trial of your MALTINE I made in the case of a lady suffering from phthisis pulmonalis has been satisfactory. Her left lung had been in the last stage of disease for some time, and her temperature d for many months between 101° and 104°. After taking the MALTINE for a few days the temperature down to 100°, and to-day it stands below 90°, which makes me feel sanguine that the disease is ed.

THOMAS HUNTER, L.R.C.P.

Kensington Dispensary, London, Nov. [illegible]*, 187*[illegible]*.*

using your MALTINE among our patients, and find *great benefit* from it, especially in cases

DR. CHIPPENDALE, *Resident Medical Officer.*

The Berches, Northwold, July [illegible]*, 1879.*

t my patients can readily digest your MALTINE with Cod Liver Oil without causing any un-r-feeling. I have full confidence in the virtue it possesses to sustain the system during nged diseases of a tubercular or atrophic nature.

FREDERICK JOY, L.R.C.P., M.R.C.S.

ROF. L. P. YANDELL, in *Louisville Medical News, Jan. 3rd*, 1880:—MALTINE is one of the most ble remedies ever introduced to the Medical Profession. Wherever a constructive is indicated, INE will be found excellent. In pulmonary phthisis and other scrofulous diseases, in chronic syphilis, n the various cachectic conditions, it is invaluable.

Adrian, Mich., Feb. [illegible]*, 18*[illegible]*.*

have used your MALTINE preparations in my practice for the past year and consider them su-ior to the Extract of Malt. I have used your Malto-Yerbine in my own case of severe bronchitis as troubled me for the past five years. It has done me more good than anything I have ever taken.

J. TRIPP, M.D.

Received 52 Awards from Exhibitions and Scientific Soci

JOHANN HOFF'

SCHUTZMARKE.

GENUINE

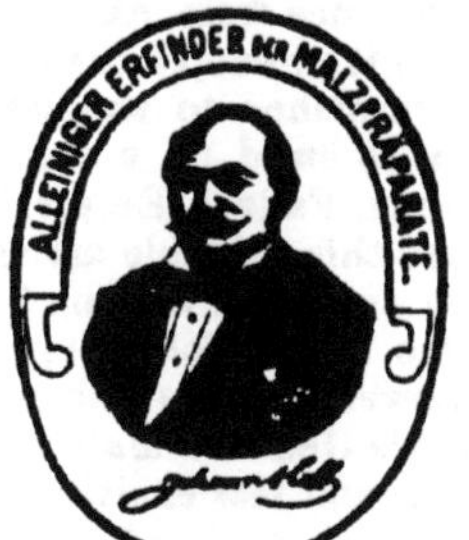

IMPORTE

Deutsches Reichsgesetz vom. 30. 11. 74.

MALT EXTRAC

BEWARE OF IMITATIONS.

ESTABLISHED 1847,

BY

JOHANN HOFF,

Royal Prussian Counsellor, Owner of the Cross of Merit, Pur
to the Emperors of Germany and Austria, to the
Prince of Wales, etc., Berlin, Germany.

MORITZ EISNER,

Sole Agent for the U.S. of A. and Canada,

No. 320 RACE STREET, PHILADELPH

KERRY, WATSON & CO., Montreal,

GENUINE MALT EXTRACT.

Abstract from "The Rational Treatment of Phthisis and Pulmonary Diseases," by Dr. Prosper de Pietra Santa, Paris, (formerly House Physician to the late Emperor Napoleon III). French Edition. 1876.

(*Traitment rationale de la phtisie pulmonaire par le docteur Prosper de Pietra Santa, Paris, Octave Doin, libraire editeur.* 1876.)

Page 147.—"Johann Hoff's Malt Extract is highly esteemed by the medical faculty as an unexcelled Nutritive and Digestive Agent, indicated in certain forms of Dyspepsia, Phthisis, Bronchitis, Asthma, Loss of Appetite, Chronic Diarrhœa, Debility, and in convalescence from exhausting diseases.

In chronic affections it promotes the contraction of the muscles, invigorates the digestive organs, and furnishes to the body those nourishing and strengthening parts, so much essential to build up a weakened constitution. Drs. Blache, Barth, Gueneau de Muffy, Pidoux, Fauvel, Empis, Danet, Robert de Latour, Bouchet, Piorry and Tardieuse, have used this valuable article daily in derangements of the digestive organs, and through my own observations I am induced to adopt the opinion of Dr. Laverau, which I resume in the following: 'As a great many patients experience the want of sufficient power to assimilate and digest food properly, and therefore fail in strength, Johann Hoff's Genuine Malt Extract will be found a valuable remedy, better than all decoctions and less exciting than wine or spirituous liquors.'"

GERMAN HOSPITAL, PHILADELPHIA.

To MR. MORITZ EISNER,

Sole Agent for Johann Hoff's Malt Extract for the U.S.A., 320 Race St., Philadelphia.

DEAR SIR.—Please send one dozen of Johann Hoff's Malt Extract to the above Hospital. I am very much pleased with it, and my patient could not do without it.

E. RAAB, M.D.,

Resident Physician of the German Hospital, Philadelphia.

PHILADELPHIA, May 12, 1881.

To MR. M. EISNER,

Agent for Johann Hoff's Genuine Malt Extract, 320 Race Street, Philadelphia.

DEAR SIR.—Dr. E. Wilson recommended Johann Hoff's Malt Extract AS THE BEST AND ONLY KIND FOR OUR PURPOSE.

With kind regards I am yours truly,

CHAS. S. TURNBULL, M.D.,

Asst. Prof. Jefferson Medical College, Philadelphia.

Suffering from an attack of illness which had not only reduced my strength, but brought on extreme exhaustion from inability to assimilate food, I tried the effect of Hoff's Malt Extract, in the usual dose of a wine-glassful twice or three times a day. Its use was followed by marked effects: (1) Food, which had been found to pass the alimentary canal unchanged, digested properly; (2) there appeared an increased power of evolving animal heat and storing up fat.

PROF. COLEMAN,

Before the Philosophical Society of Glasgow.

GARRISON HOSPITAL, Vienna, Austria, Dec. 21, 1880.

Johann Hoff's Malt Extract has been largely used in the above Hospital, and we cheerfully endorse its use to the medical profession, for general debility and convalescence, for which it has proved to be a most estimable remedy.

(Signed,) DR. LOEFF,

Chief Physician of H. M. the Emperor's Garrison Hospital.

DR. PORIAS, House Physician.

Johann Hoff's Genuine Malt Extract has been chemically investigated in the Laboratory of Professor von Kletzinsky, and has been found to contain only articles which are of great benefit in cases of imperfect digestion and bad nutrition, also affections of the chest, for convalesence and general debility.

PROF. DR. GRANICHSTETTER,
University of Vienna, Austria.

I ordered Johann Hoff's Genuine Extract of Malt for a lady of very weak constitution while NURSING; after using it for about five weeks I found it to be very wholesome to mother and child, and have also recommended it often and with marked good results for individuals suffering from faulty nutrition and digestion, and general debility.

DR. J. E. VON GOTTSCHALL,
St. Gall, Switzerland.

To the "Wiener Medicinische Wochenschrift."

I have found Johann Hoff's Liquid Extract of Malt to be of great value in convalescence as a nutritive, and have used it for years with marked effects.

FELIX PAUL RITTERFELD,
Doctor Med. and Phil., Frankfort-on-the-Main.

Johann Hoff's Liquid Extract of Malt is used in most of the Hospitals throughout the German and Austrian Empires.

DR. GEORGE M. SPORER,
Imperial Austrian Proto-Medicus and Gubernatorial Counsel, writes:

Since the introduction of Johann Hoff's Liquid Extract of Malt into the Hospitals and Lazarettos of the Austrian Empire, I have had occasion in very many instances to test its value as a nutritive for general debility, and its restorative powers, and I most heartily endorse the use of the same.

DIRECTIONS:

Use a small wine-glassful three times a day, before or after meals, according to the advice of Physician. Dose for children—one teaspoonful.

BEWARE OF IMITATIONS.

None genuine without the signature of MORITZ EISNER, Sole agent for the U.S. on the neck of each bottle.

MORITZ EISNER,

SOLE AGENT FOR THE U. S.

No. 320 RACE STREET, PHILADELPHIA.

M. EISNER'S TAMARINDUS CARAMELS.

A Laxative, Refreshing and Chocolate Coated Fruit Lozenge,

FOR THE

RELIEF AND CURE OF CONSTIPATION,

AND ITS ATTENDANT MALADIES, SUCH AS

HEMORRHOIDS, HEADACHE, &c., &c.

PREPARED AFTER PROF. HAGER'S FORMULÆ.

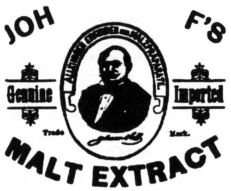

JOH F'S

Genuine Imported

Trade Mark.

MALT EXTRACT

[Registered at the U. S. Patent Office, March 19th, 1879.]

BERLIN, August 31st, 1880.

To whom it may concern:

This is to Certify that I have on the above date appointed MR. MORITZ EISNER, Philadelphia, Pa., No. 320 Race Street, as my sole agent for the United States of America and Canada, for the sale of genuine "Johann Hoff's Extract of Malt." All orders for the above named "Johann Hoff's Extract of Malt," will in future be supplied by him, or through agents appointed by him, as I have bound myself by special contract not to sell hereafter to any individual or firm in the United States of America or Canada any of my gooos.

Every bottle sent by me to the United States of America or Canada, after the above date, will have the signature of my sose agent, Mr. M. Eisner, imprinted on the label, specially certified by my own signature underneath.

In future, therefore, I will only guarantee those bottles bearing the *signature of Mr. Moritz Eisner*, 320 Race Street, Philadelphia, *as well as my own signature*, as being fresh and genuine, and as being obtained direct from my own manufactory in Berlin, Germany. All others I declare to be worthless imitations, and I warn the public and dealers from buying the same.

(Signed,) JOHANN HOFF.

LEGATION OF THE UNITED STATES OF AMERICA.

Berlin, German Empire.

On this fourth day of September, eighteen hundred and eighty, personally appeared before me, Chapman Coleman, second secretary of the above mentioned Legation, Johann Hoff, to me known to be the person who executed the aforegoing instrument, and acknowledged that he executed the same for the purpose therein mentioned.

Witness my hand and official Seal, this 4th day of September, 1880.

CHAPMAN COLEMAN.

KERRY, WATSON & CO., Montreal,

SOLE CONSIGNEES, CANADA.

MEAD'S
ADHESIVE PLASTER

This article is intended to take the place of the ordinary Emp. Adhesive, on account of its superior quality and cheapness. It is pliable, water-proof, non-irritating, very strong and extra adhesive. It is not affected by heat or cold, is spread on honest cotton cloth, and never cracks or peels off; salicylic acid is incorporated with it, which makes it antiseptic. It is indispensable where strength and firm adhesion are required, as in counter-extension, or in the treatment of a broken clavicle. It has been adopted by the New York, Bellevue, and other large hospitals, and by many of our leading surgeons.

Furnished in rolls 5 yards long, by 14 inches wide.
" " 1 " " 7½ "

Price by Mail, per yard roll, 50 cts.; 5 yards, 40 cts. per yard.

BELLADONNA PLASTER

IN RUBBER COMBINATION.

Recent analytical tests conducted by Prof. R. O. Doremus, of Bellevue Hospital Medical College, and J. P. Battershall, Ph. D., analytical chemists, New York, to determine the comparative quantities of atropine in Belladonna Plaster, prepared by the different American manufacturers, disclosed in each case that our article contains a greater proportion of the active principle of Belladonna than any other manufactured. Samples of the various manufactures, including our own, for this test, were procured in open market by the above named chemists themselves. In the preparation of this article, we incorporate the best alcoholic extract of Belladonna only, with the rubber base. It is packed in elegant tin cases (one yard in each case,) which can be forwarded by mail to any part of the country.

Price, by mail, post-paid, $1.00.

BLISTERING PLASTER

IN RUBBER COMBINATION.

We incorporate, by a cold process the whole fly (best selected Russian), with the rubber base, which constitutes, we believe, the most reliable cantharidal plaster known. It is superior to the cerate, and other cantharidal preparations, the value of which is frequently greatly impaired by the excessive heat used in preparing them, which volatilizes or drives off an active principle of the fly. By our peculiar process, no heat is used.

Price, by mail, per yard, $1.00.

MUSTARD PLASTER

IN COTTON CLOTH.

Superior to the best French makes; does not crack or peel off, or tear when wet. Can be removed without soiling the skin. Always reliable.

OFFICE, 21 Platt Street, New York. Samples sent on application.

In October, 1880, I read an advertisement of Hydroleine in some Medical jou The formula being given, I was somewhat favorably impressed, and procured pamphlets: One on "The Digestion and Assimilation of Fats in the Human B and the other on "The Effects of Hydrated Oil in Consumption and Wasting eases." They are ably written, and afforded an interesting study. Their doctrine so reasonable, that I got up faith enough to have my druggist order a sufficient su to thoroughly test the merits of the preparation.

I was ready to catch at anything to take the place of cod-liver oil. In my hands i proved an utter and abominable failure in ninety-five per cent. of all my cases in w I have prescribed it since I have been engaged in country practice, and it never ben ted more than forty per cent. of my city patients.

The inland people, who seldom eat fish, can rarely digest cod-liver oil. Almost e week I am consulted by some victim of the *cod oil mania*, who has swallowed the tents of from one to twenty-five bottles, and who has been growing leaner, paler weaker all the while, until from a state of only slight indisposition, these patients become mere "living skeletons." Nearly all complain of rancid eructations, and bearable fishy taste in their mouth, from one dose to another. They not only f digest the cod oil, but this failure overloads the digestive organs to such an extent digestion and assimilation of all food becomes an impossibility, the patient langu and pines and finally dies of *literal starvation*. In the comparatively small number whom I have found cod-liver oil to agree, it has proved very gratifying in its results. my practice, by far the largest number receiving benefit from it have been chil Those who have, previous to their illness, been accustomed, to some extent, to a ' diet," will be more likely to digest the oil, and more notably so in cold climates. the innumerable efforts that have been made in the shape of "pure cod-liver 'palatable cod-liver oil," "cod-liver oil with pepsin," "cod-liver oil with pancrea "cod-liver oil emulsions," etc., and so on, *ad infinitum*, attest the fact that the *desideratum* after all is to render cod-liver oil capable of retention by the stomach digestible when it is retained.

As Hydroleine is partially digested oil, and this partial digestion is brought abo a combination of factors suggested by actual physiological experiments, these facts mend it to my confidence, and a trial of the preparation in seven typical cases conv me that it possesses a high degree of merit, and I feel that it is a duty incumbent me to call the attention of my medical brethren to the subject.

The first case in which I prescribed it was that of a married lady 28 years of blonde, and the mother of four children, the eldest 9 and the youngest 1 year old. the birth of this last child she dated her illness, for she made a tardy convalesc remaining unable to walk for a month. Soon after she began to grow weaker, and resumed her bed, which she had not left to any extent since, not any time being a sit up longer than fifteen or twenty minutes. During all this time she was under c of a skillful physician. He had tried many remedies to check the rapid emacia among these were several different brands of malt extract, cod-liver oil, and va mixtures of the oil. None of the oils and their mixtures agreed with her. In Ma was called and prescribed Hydroleine, a bottle of which I delivered at the time, d ing her to commence with teaspoonful doses, to be gradually increased to twi amount. It agreed with her finely, and by the time the first bottle was used sh greatly improved. She procured and used two additional bottles, and, at this wi June 15th, is considered well.

The above case was one of general and persisting emaciation, unaccompani any cough or perceptible thoracic trouble. The ensuing case was one of diagnosed

The patient, a married lady, æt. 32, had been married about 14 years, and was the mother of six children, the youngest two years of age, several of her sisters had died of the above mentioned disease. Her medical adviser prescribed cod-liver oil, and she had taken a full dozen bottles with plenty of whiskey. The oil had not been digested, although it had been retained by the stomach. Her cough had grown constantly worse, and she grew rapidly weaker, week by week. I prescribed Hydroleine for her, and she commenced to take it in April, about the 15th. It agreed with her finely. She rapidly gained weight and strength, her cough was relieved and has now nearly ceased. She has used nearly four bottles, and continues to use it, though apparently well.

I have prescribed it in three other cases, in two of which the results have been equally gratifying, but in the other case it produced nausea and greasy eructations.

From these trials I am led to think quite favorably of the hydrated oil, and I am led to believe that although it may not agree with all, it will be found of great and permanent benefit to a very large per cent. of consumption and other "wasting" diseases, and that it is destined, and no distant day, to very largely supplant the undigested oils.

HAZEN MORSE, 57 Front Street East, TORONTO,

SOLE AGENT FOR CANADA.

TUBERCULOSIS RESULTING FROM DEFICIENT NUTRITION.

Various as are the opinions regarding the treatment of consumption, all writers concur in the belief that whatever measure is adopted, the strength of the patient must be husbanded with the greatest care, and the most efficient means employed to supply the system with that element which the symptoms indicate as being required to keep up the vitality while such course of treatment is being pursued as is considered suitable. The most striking indication of the presence of this dreadful disease is rapid loss of weight. The patient himself, prone as he is to disregard premonitory warnings of this insidious malady, cannot but observe an extraordinary difference in the appearance of his form, as first the face, then the trunk, and lastly, the limbs become soft and flabby, and the once well-fitting garments hang loosely about him, his flesh seeming to melt away, so rapid is the change.

EMACIATION.

A natural course of reasoning as to the cause and effect of emaciation under these circumstances has developed the fact that the abnormal consumption of the tissues is the result of nature's efforts to supply the waste, through the blood from the fatty tissues of the body with the requisite amount of material whose oxidation is the source of heat and nerve force, the natural supply, through the assimilation of food, having failed in consequence of an unhealthy condition of the pancreatic secretions causing an insufficient supply of chyle, or a failure on the part of the lacteal tubes, through fever or some cause, to absorb sufficient nutriment.

TUBERCLE.

As the attack upon the tissues of the body progresses, not only fatty tissue is absorbed into the circulation from unnatural sources, causing loss of strength, but particles of albuminoid tissue are carried by the blood and being deposited in channels where the system has no provision for throwing them off, from desquamatious centres of disease which, in their turn, throw off infectious matter to be absorbed into the general system. The immense extent of delicate mucuous surface in the respiratory passages of the lungs exposed to the contents of the minute blood-vessels which permeate their entire texture, offers the greatest and most susceptible field for the reposition of a large amount of this effete albuminoid tissue. This deposit forms the tubercle whose establishment in the lung is the beginning of that train of circumstances which characterizes the progress of that fatal malady—consumption. Thus it is seen that tuberculosis is either due to the defective action of the pancreatic juice on the fatty elements action of the gastric juice, but passes, together with the chyme or digested fibrinous and albuminous matter, to the duodenum, where it comes into contact with the pancreatic juice, and is thereby transformed into chyle, which is a very delicate saponaceous emulsion or suspension of the oleaginous portion of fat. It is when in *this condition only* that fat is capable of absorption by the lacteals, thence passing directly to the venous blood which is supplied to the lungs through the right cavity of the heart, the lungs then absorb from that blood the hydrocarbons or fatty portion, and return the nitrogenous portion to the heart, to form the globulin of arterial blood before passing into the circulation.

This function of partly saponifying and partly emulsifying fats is enjoyed by no other secretion of the alimentary canal but the pancreatic juice, unless we take into consideration the action of the saliva, which is somewhat of that nature; but as the food in most instances is subjected to the action of the saliva in the mouth for so short a time, this feature in the economy is almost inappreciable.

TREATMENT.

The close relations of non-assimilation of the fatty elements of food to wasting diseases, and especially to consumption, is understood, and reason would indicate that if by any artificial means the absorption of fat could be assisted by supplying, as chyle, a proper amount of oleginous or fatty matter, a nutritive progress would be established which would modify the unhealthy action of the pancreas, and not only relieve the body from the depleting effects of the disorder, but afford an opportunity for treatment and recovery. With the assistance of a thorough knowledge of the chemical process which fat undergoes from the time of its introduction into the duodenum to absorption, a preparation has been introduced and extensively used by the profession in England with highly successful results, indicated by the flattering commendations of it from many physicians who, having given the treatment of pulmonary disorders their special attention, are peculiarly qualified to attest its efficacy.

HYDROLEINE.

This preparation, to which the distinctive name of hydroleine (hydrated oil) has been given, is not a simple emulsion of cod-liver oil, but a permanent and perfect saponaceous emulsion of oil, in combination with pancreatin soluble in water, the saponification producing a cream-like preparation, possessing all the necessary qualities of chyle, including extreme delicacy and solubility, whereby a ready and perfect assimilation is afforded.

FORMULA OF HYDROLEINE.

Each dose of two teaspoonfuls, equal to 120 drops, contains:

Pure oil	80 m (drops)
Distilled water	35 "
Soluble pancreatin	5 grains
Soda	$\frac{1}{3}$ "
Boric acid	$\frac{1}{4}$ "
Hyocholic acid	1-20 "

DOSE.—Two teaspoonfuls alone, or mixed with twice the quantity of soft water, wine or whiskey, to be taken thrice daily with meals.

The use of the so-called emulsions of cod-liver oil during the extremely sensitive condition of the digestive organs always accompanying consumption does not usually afford beneficial results. Those of the profession in this country who have under their care cases of consumption, diabetes, chlorosis, Bright's disease, hysteria, and, in short, any disease where a loss of appetite is followed by a rapid breaking down of the tissues of the body in its effort to support the combustion supplying animal heat, are urged to give this preparation a trial. It is supplied by the agent for Canada, Hazen Morse, No. 57 Front Street East, Toronto, who will forward literature relating to the subject upon application.

tion of the life-giving properties of food interferes with recovery from sever
baffling the best directed efforts of the physician, points the necessity for a
combination of agents sufficiently potent to replace the deficient principle and
in renewing the degenerated tissues.

Realizing this need, the science of chemistry produced pepsine. Richard T
C. S., Professor of Chemistry, London, England, in the *Lancet*, Aug. 23, 1879,
this remedy: "Since the introduction of Corvisart and Boudault's powder
into medicine, in the year 1854, Pepsine, obtained from the stomach of the p
sheep, in a state of greater or less impurity has been extensively prescribed in
and certain other affections. According to the testimony of some authoriti
standing, long experience in the use of this agent fully justifies Corvisart's p
relative to its therapeutic value, which were based on physiological reasoning.

There are other authorities who express doubts as to the efficacy of Pepsi
difference of opinion undoubtedly arises from the circumstance that pharm
supply medical men with various preparations, all bearing the specific name of
but differing very considerably in their digestive powers and other qualities.
I find those who speak favorably of its employment in the treatment of disease h
scribed that prepared by the best makers, while those who express a doubtful
have been in the habit of prescribing those varieties or makes, which the experi
myself and others have proved to be practically without any digestive pow
worthless. Under these circumstances it is *absolutely* necessary for the practiti
be certain of the *make* of Pepsine he uses. *Pure* Pepsine, thoroughly tritura
finely powdered sugar of milk (saccharated pepsine) will undoubtedly pro
best results.

Experience in diseases of the stomach, dyspepsia, etc., has demonstrated
cases, the lack of other agents required to promote a healthy digestion besides
namely Pancreatine and Diastase or veg. Ptyalin. Pancreatine the active prin
the sweet bread or pancreas possesses the wonderful power of emulsifying the
oils of food, rendering them easily assimilated by the system not affected by pe
the slightest degree. Diastase or veg. Ptyalin, as obtained from malted barley,
dry extract of malt, represents the saliva, and has the remarkable property of co
the insoluable starchy portions of food into the soluable glucose, thus render
indigestible and innutritious article starch into the nutritive and easily assimila
glucose.

The value of these different ingredients and the difficulty of procuring them of
quality led Hazen Morse, 57 Front Street East, Toronto, to experiment with
combinations during seven years' employment in the manufacture of Pepsine on
scale, and with the assistance of several prominent physicians he was finally ena
present to the profession the following formula.

Sacchar
"
Acid La
Exsiccat

Said formula has been registered at Ottawa under the distinctive name Malto
thus giving the physician a guarantee of always procuring the same standard prep
and preventing their being imposed upon by imitations of inferior quality, and
same time putting it at as low a figure (fifty cents for 1½ ozs.) as possible for
formula to be compounded from the ingredients of the *best* possible manufacture.

Maltopepsyn has digestive power ten times greater than the best Pepsine in th
ket, as it digests Fibrin and Caseine, emulsifies the fat of food taken into the st
thus rendering it assimilable, converts starch into glucose, in fact it combines
agents that act upon food, from mastication to its conversion into chyle, digest
ailment used by mankind while Pepsine acts only upon plastic food. Maltopeps
combines with the above the nutritive qualities of Extract of Malt, and the bra
nerve strengthening powers of the Acid Phosphates.

It has been found that a free acid, like Hydrochloric, does not combine well
Saccharated Mixture, and renders it liable to decomposition. I, therefore, do not
in my formula. It can be easily prescribed in solution, (say 20 drops of acid to 4
of water) one half-ounce with each dose, in cases where its use is indicated.

For infants, however, Maltopepsyn will be found to yield the most satisfactory
and the acid should be dispensed with. The necessity for the absence of acid
would tend to produce harmful results, will be recognised, when it is consider
even the slight acidity of most cows' milk, when used as food for infants, is suffic
disagree with them.

With regard to the proper time for its administration, as before or after taking
opinions vary, but reason would suggest that about half an hour before eating wil
the ferment a sufficient time to combine with the existing condition of the stomac
... the most natural effect upon the food

The rapidly increasing demand for our IMPROVED EXTRACT OF MALT, during the four years that it has been manufactured and offered to the medical profession in America, justifies the belief that in its production here we are meeting a generally felt want.

Long experience in manufacturing Malt Extract has enabled us to completely overcome the many difficulties attending its manufacture in large quantity: and we positively assure the profession that our Extract of Malt is not only perfectly pure and reliable, but that it will keep for years, in any climate, without fermenting or molding, and that its flavor actually improves by age. Our Extract is guaranteed to equal, in every respect, the best German make, while, by avoiding the expenses of importation, it is afforded at less than half the price of the foreign article.

The Malt from which it is made is obtained by carefully malting the very best quality of selected Toronto (Canada) Barley. The extract is prepared by an *improved process*, which prevents injury to its properties or flavor by excess of heat. **It represents the soluble constituents of Malt and Hops,** viz., MALT SUGAR, DEXTRINE, DIASTASE, RESIN and BITTER OF HOPS, PHOSPHATES OF LIME and MAGNESIA, and ALKALINE SALTS.

Attention is invited to the following analysis of this Extract, as given by S. H. Douglas, Professor of Chemistry, University of Michigan, Ann Arbor:—

TROMMER EXTRACT OF MALT CO.—I enclose herewith my analysis of your Extract of Malt:

Malt Sugar, 45·1; Dextrine, Hop-bitter, Extractive Matter, 23·6; Albuminous Matter (Diastase), 2·469. Ash—Phosphates, 1·712; Alkalies, ·377. Water, 25·7. Total, 99·958.

In comparing the above analysis with that of the Extract of Malt of the German Pharmacopœa, as given by Hager, that has been generally received by the profession, I find it to substantially agree with this article.

Yours truly, SILAS H. DOUGLAS,

Prof. of Analytical and Applied Chemistry.

This invaluable preparation is highly recommended by the medical profession, as a most effective therapeutic agent, for the restoration of delicate and exhausted constitutions. It is very nutritious, being rich in both muscle and fat-producing materials.

The very large proportion of *Diastase* renders it most effective in those forms of disease originating in *imperfect digestion of the starchy elements* of food.

A single dose of the Improved Trommer's Extract of Malt contains a larger quantity of the active properties of Malt than a pint of the best ale or porter; and not having undergone fermentation, is absolutely free from alcohol and carbonic acid.

The dose for adults is from a dessert to a tablespoonful three times daily. It is best taken after meals, pure, or mixed with a glass of milk, or in water, wine or any kind of spirituous liquor. Each bottle contains 1½ lbs. of the Extract.

Our preparations of Malt are for sale by druggists generally throughout the United States and Canadas, at the following prices:—

EXTRACT OF MALT,	*With Hops (Plain),*	$1 00
" " "	*Pyrophosphate of Iron (Ferrated),*	1 00
" " "	*Cod Liver Oil,*	1 00
" " "	*Cod Liver Oil and Iodide of Iron,*	1 00
" " "	*Cod Liver Oil and Phosphorus,*	1 00
" " "	*Hypophosphites,*	1 50
" " "	*Iodides,*	1 50
" " "	*Alteratives,*	1 50
" " "	*Citrate of Iron and Quinia,*	1 50
" "	*Pepsin,*	1 50

Manufactured by

TROMMER EXTRACT OF MALT CO

FREMONT, OHIO.

In corresponding with advertisers please mention Canada M. & S. Journal.

Europe, and adopted by the United States Government. More of them sold than any other Battery in the World.

McINTOSH

COMBINED GALVANIC AND FARADIC BATTERY.

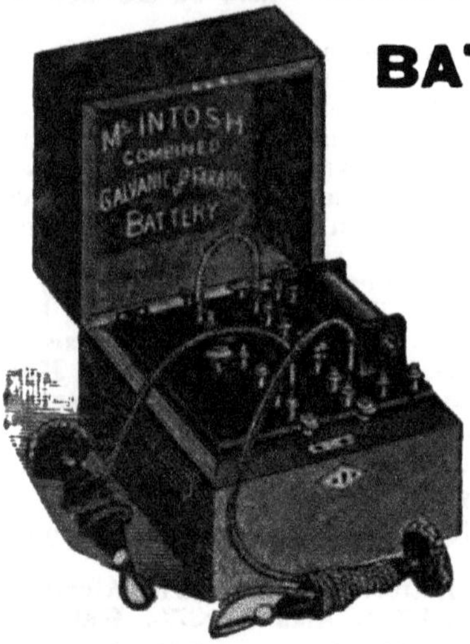

☛ The First and only **PORTABLE BATTERY** ever invented which gives both the Galvanic and Faradic Current, thus combining two distinct Batteries in one case.

NO PHYSICIAN CAN AFFORD TO BE WITHOUT ONE.

This celebrated Battery is constructed on an improved plan. The zincs and carbons are fastened to hard rubber plates in sections of six each; this manner of connecting brings the plates nearer together than in any other battery, thus giving less internal resistance. The rubber plate or cover will not warp or break, and is not affected by the fluid.

The cells are composed of one piece of hard rubber, and are made in sections of six each with a drip-cup, thus one section can be handled, emptied and cleaned as easily and quickly as one cell.

The fluid cannot spill or run between the cells, and there is no danger of breaking as with glass cells. The drip-cup is to receive the elements when the battery is not in use. The Faradic coil is fastened to the hard rubber plate or cover.

The rubber plate to which the zincs and carbons are attached is securely fastened over the cells when not in use, making it impossible for any of the fluid to be spilled in carrying.

An extra large cell (with a zinc and carbon element) is added to the combined batteries for the purpose of producing the Faradic current. This cell gives as much power as is ever needed, and avoids exhausting the current from the Galvanic cells.

Our Batteries weigh less, occupy less space, give a current of greater intensity and quantity than any other Battery manufactured. For simplicity of construction they cannot be surpassed, and any person reading our directions will have no trouble in operating them.

This is the only Battery in which the zinc and carbon plates can be kept clean and always in order by simply rinsing them.

All the metal work is finely nickel-plated and highly polished, and every part is put together so that it can be easily replaced by the operator.

We have the most complete line of electrodes yet offered to the profession. We also manufacture various styles of Table and Office Batteries, Bath Apparatus, &c., &c. Our manufacturing facilities are the largest of the kind in America, and we employ none but skilled mechanics, and men of scientific experience.

Our Illustrated Catalogue, a handsome book giving full description of all our goods, and other valuable information, sent free on application.

McIntosh Galvanic & Faradic Battery Co.,

192 & 194 JACKSON ST., CHICAGO, ILL.

Or, **ELLIOTT & CO., Chemists, 3 Front St., TORONTO,**

And **F. GROSS, 682 to 690 Craig Street, MONTREAL,**

WHOLESALE AGENTS FOR CANADA.

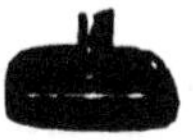

DR. McINTOSH'S

NATURAL UTERINE SUPPORTER

No Instrument has ever been placed before the Medical Profession which has given such Universal Satisfaction.

Every Indication of Uterine Displacements is met by this combination: Prolapsus, Anteversion, Retroversion and Flexions are overcome by this instrument when others fail. This is proven by the fact that since its introduction to the profession it has come into more general use than all other instruments combined.

Union of External and Internal Support.—The abdomen is held up by the broad morocco leather belt with concave front and elastic straps to buckle around the hips. The Uterine Support is a cup and stem made of highly polished hard rubber, very light and durable, shaped to fit the neck of the womb, with openings for the secretions to pass out, as shown by the cuts. Cups are made with extended lips to correct flexions and versions of the womb.

Adaptability to Varying Positions of the Body.—The cup and stem are suspended from the belt by two soft elastic Rubber Tubes, which are fastened to the front of the belt by simple loops, pass down and through the stem of the cup and up to the back of the belt. These soft rubber tubes being elastic, adapt themselves to all the varying positions of the body, and perform the service of the ligaments of the womb.

Self-Adjusting.—One of the many reasons which recommend this Supporter to the physician is that it is self-adjusting. The physician, after applying it, need have no fear that he will be called in haste to remove or readjust it, (as is often the case with rings and various pessaries held in position by pressure against the vaginal wall), as the patient can remove it at will, and replace it without assistance.

It can be worn at all times, will not interfere with nature's necessities, will not corrode, and is lighter than metal. It will answer for all cases of Anteversion, Retroversion, or any Flexion of the womb, and is used by the leading physicians with unfailing success, even in the most difficult cases.

Our Reduced Prices are, to Physicians, $7.00; to Patients, $10.00.

Instruments sent by mail at our risk, on receipt of price, with 35 cents added for Canadian postage; or we can send by express, C. O. D.

Physicians in the Dominion can obtain these instruments at above prices from

F. GROSS, 682 & 690 Craig Street, MONTREAL,

Or **ELLIOTT & CO., Chemists, 3 Front Street, TORONTO.**

CAUTION.—We call particular attention of Physicians to the fact, that unscrupulous parties are manufacturing a worthless imitation of this Supporter, and some dishonest dealers, for the sake of gain, are trying to sell them, knowing they are deceiving both Physician and patient.

Persons receiving a Supporter will find, if it is genuine, the directions pasted in the cover of the box, with the head-line, "DR. L. D. McINTOSH'S NATURAL UTERINE SUPPORTER;" a cut on the right, showing the Supporter and on the left its application, also the *fac-simile* Signature of DR. L. D. McINTOSH. Each pad of the abdominal belt is stamped in gilt letters, DR. McINTOSH'S NATURAL UTERINE SUPPORTER CO., CHICAGO, ILL. Each box also contains our pamphlet on "DISPLACEMENTS OF THE WOMB," and an extra pair of RUBBER TUBES.

DR. McINTOSH NATURAL UTERINE SUPPORTER CO.,

192 & 194 JACKSON ST., CHICAGO, ILL.

Our valuable pamphlet, "Some Practical Facts about Displacements of the Womb," will be sent you free on application.

COLONIAL HOUSE.

HENRY MORGAN & CO

Importers of

FANCY & STAPLE DRY GOODS

Carpets, Oilcloths, Drapery,

UPHOLSTERING MATERIALS, &c.

AGENTS *for* **MARKS'**

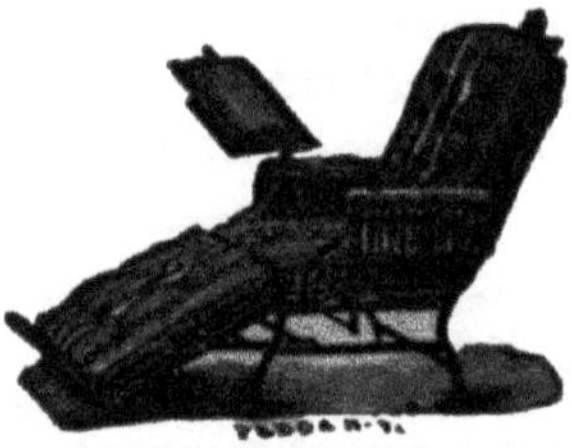

ADJUSTABLI FOLDING CHAIR.

Combining in one an elegant Parlor, Library, Smoking, Invalid or Reclinin Chair, Lounge and Full Length Bed, and the Physician's Operating Chair, a thoroughly effective article.

☞ A Full Line in Stock of Rattan and Wicker-work Chairs, Beds Couches, Children's Cots, Cradles, Work-Baskets and other Article from the celebrated Factories of the Wakefield Rattan Co., Boston Heywood Bros. & Co., Gardner, Mass., and the Delaware Chair Co. Delaware, Ohio.

TO PHYSICIANS & SURGEONS.

JUST RECEIVED FULL SUPPLIES OF

BEST ENGLISH & GERMAN CHEMICAL

—AND—

French, English and American Pharmaceutical Preparations and Specialties.

New remedies and rare Chemicals added to stock as soon as reports i Medical Journals warrant it.

Nitrate of Pilocarpine; Tannate of Pelletierine; Tannate of Bismuth Resorcin; Glonoin & Glonoin Pills; Benger's Natural Digestive Ferments an Peptonized Beef Jelly; Pepsina Prorsa; Wyeth's Saccharated Pepsine; Dess cated Blood; Powell's Cod Liver Oil Beef and Pepsine Elixir; Squibb Anæsthetic Æther; Squibb's Hydrobromic Acid; Squibb's Nitrite of Amyl.

—ALSO—

ROBERT GARDNER'S SYRUP OF HYDRIODIC ACII

Containing all the Therapeutic Effects of Iodine without its irritating properties.

HENRY R. GRAY, Chemist,

144 St. Lawrence Main Street.

[ESTABLISHED 1859.]

BELLEVUE HOSPITAL MEDICAL COLLEGE.

CITY OF NEW YORK.

SESSIONS OF 1882-'83.

The COLLEGIATE YEAR in this institution embraces the Regular Winter Session and a Spring Session. The REGULAR SESSION will begin on Wednesday, September 20, 1882, and end about the middle of March, 1883. During this Session, in addition to four didactic Lectures on every week-day except Saturday, two or three hours are daily allotted to clinical instruction. Attendance upon two regular courses of lectures is required for graduation. The SPRING SESSION consists chiefly of recitations from Text-Books. This Session begins about the middle of March and continues until the middle of June. During this Session, daily recitations in all the departments are held by a corps of examiners appointed by the Faculty. Short courses of lectures are given on special subjects, and regular clinics are held in the Hospital and in the College building.

Faculty.

ISAAC E. TAYLOR, M. D.,
Emeritus Professor of Obstetrics and Diseases of Women and Children, and President of the Faculty.

FORDYCE BARKER, M.D., LL.D.,
Professor of Clinical Midwifery and Diseases of Women.

BENJAMIN W. McCREADY, M.D.,
Emeritus Professor of Materia Medica and Therapeutics, and Professor of Clinical Medicine.

AUSTIN FLINT, M.D., LL.D.,
Professor of the Principles and Practice of Medicine and Clinical Medicine.

W. H. VAN BUREN, M.D., LL.D.,
Prof. of Principles and Practice of Surgery and Clinical Surgery.

LEWIS A. SAYRE, M.D.,
Professor of Orthopedic Surgery, and Clinical Surgery.

ALEXANDER B. MOTT, M.D.,
Professor of Clinical and Operative Surgery.

WILLIAM T. LUSK, M.D.,
Professor of Obstetrics & Diseases of Women and Children and Clinical Midwifery.

A. A. SMITH, M.D.,
Prof. of Materia Medica and Therapeutics, and Clinical Medicine.

AUSTIN FLINT, Jr., M.D.
Professor of Physiology and Physiological Anatomy, and Secretary of the Faculty.

JOSEPH . BRYANT, M.D.,
Professor of General, Descriptive & Surgical Anatomy.

R. OGDEN DOREMUS, M.D., LL.D.,
Professor of Chemistry and Toxicology.

EDWARD G. JANEWAY, M.D.,
Prof. of Diseases of the Nervous System and Clinical Medicine, and Associate Professor of Principles and Practice of Medicine.

PROFESSORS OF SPECIAL DEPARTMENTS, Etc.

HENRY D. NOYES, M.D.,
Professor of Opthalmology and Otology.

EDWARD L. KEYES, M.D.,
Professor of Cutaneous and Genito-Urinary Diseases.

JOHN P. GRAY, M.D., LL.D.,
Professor of Psychological Medicine and Medical Jurisprudence.

FREDERICK S. DENNIS, M.D., M.R.C.S.,
Professor Adjunct to the Chair of Principles and Practice of Surgery.

WILLIAM H. WELCH, M.D.,
Professor of Pathological Anatomy and General Pathology.

J. LEWIS SMITH, M.D.,
Clinical Professor of Diseases of Children.

JOSEPH W. HOWE, M.D.,
Clinical Professor of Surgery.

LEROY MILTON YALE, M.D.,
Lecturer Adjunct on Orthopedic Surgery.

BEVERLY ROBINSON, M.D.,
Professor of Clinical Medicine.

FRANCKE H. BOSWORTH, M.D.,
Professor of Diseases of the Throat.

CHARLES A. DOREMUS, M D., Ph D.,
Professor Adjunct to the Chair of Chemistry and Toxicology.

FREDERIC S. DENNIS, M.D., M.R.C S.,
WILLIAM H. WELCH, M.D.,
Demonstrators of Anatomy.

FACULTY FOR THE SPRING SESSION.

FREDERICK A. CASTLE, M.D.,
Lecturer on Pharmacology.

WILLIAM H. WELCH, M.D.,
Lecturer on Pathological Histology.

T. HERRING BURCHARD, M.D.,
Lecturer on Surgical Emergencies.

CHARLES S. BULL, M.D.,
Lecturer on Ophthalmology and Otology.

CHARLES A. DOREMUS, M.D., Ph.D., Lecturer on Animal Chemistry.

FEES FOR THE REGULAR SESSION.

Fees for Tickets to all the Lectures, Clinical and Didactic	$140 00
Fees for Students who have attended two full courses at other Medical Colleges, and for Graduates of less than three years' standing of other Medical Colleges	70 00
Matriculation Fee	5 00
Dissection Fee (including material for dissection)	10 00
Graduation Fee	30 00

No Fees for Lectures are required of Graduates of three years' standing, or of third-course Students who have attended their second course at the Bellevue Hospital Medical College.

FEES FOR THE SPRING SESSION.

Matriculation (Ticket valid for the following Winter)	$ 5 00
Recitations, Clinics and Lectures	40 00
Dissection (Ticket valid for the following Winter)	10 00

☞ For the Annual Circular and Catalogue giving Regulation [illegible]

McGILL UNIVERSITY, MONTREA

FACULTY OF MEDICINE.

FIFTIETH SESSION, 1882–83.

The Collegiate Courses of this School are a Winter Session, extending from the 1 October to the end of March, and a Summer Session from the end of the first week in A to end of the first week in July.

Founded in 1824, and organised as a Faculty of McGill University in 1828, this School enjoyed, in an unusual degree, the confidence of the Profession throughout Canada and neighboring States. One of the distinctive features in the teaching of this School, and one to which its prosperity is largely due, is the prominence given to Clinical Instruc Based on the Edinburgh model, it is chiefly bed-side, and the Student personally investig the cases under the supervision of special Professors of Clinical Medicine and Surgery.

Among important changes in the past few years may be mentioned: The provision systematic practical instruction in Gynæcology; the thorough re-modelling of the Dep ment of Practical Anatomy on the plan of the best European schools; the establishmen an extensive Physiological Laboratory, with well arranged courses, and the establishmen a Demonstration-course in Morbid Anatomy.

FACULTY:

WM. E. SCOTT, M.D., Prof. of Anatomy.

WM. WRIGHT, M.D., L.R.C.S., Edin., Prof. of Materia Medica and Therapeutics.

ROBT. P. HOWARD, M.D., L.R.C.S., Edin., Professor of the Theory and Practice of Medicine, and Acting Dean.

DUNCAN C. McCALLUM, M.D., M.R.C.S., Eng., Professor of Midwifery and the Diseases of Women and Children.

J. W. DAWSON, LL.D., F.R.S., Professor of Botany and Zoology.

ROBT. CRAIK, M.D., Emeritus Professor.

G. E. FENWICK, M.D., Prof. of Surgery.

JOSEPH M. DRAKE, M.D., Emeritus Professor.

O. P. GIRDWOOD, M.D., M.R.C.S., Eng., Professor of Chemistry.

GEORGE ROSS, A.M., M.D., Professor of Clinical Medicine.

WM. OSLER, M.D., M.R.C.P., Lond., fessor of the Institutes of Medicine.

THOS. G. RODDICK, M.D., Professo Clinical Surgery.

WM. GARDNER, M.D., Professor of M cal Jurisprudence and Hygiene.

F. BULLER, M.D., M.R.C.S., Eng., turer on Ophthalmology.

F. J. SHEPHERD, M.D., M.R.C.S., E Demonstrator of Anatomy.

RICHARD L. MACDONNELL, B.A., M M.R.C.S., Eng., Assistant Demonstrato

WM. SUTHERLAND, M.D., L.R.C Lond., Curator of the Museum.

ARTHUR A. BROWNE, B.A., M.D., structor in Obstetrics.

GEO. W. MAJOR, B.A., M.D., Instru in Laryngology.

A. D. BLACKADER, B.A., M.D., M.R. Eng., Instructor in Diseases of Childre

MATRICULATION.—Students from Ontario and Quebec are advised to pass Matriculation Examination of the Medical Councils of their respective Provinces be entering upon their studies. Students from the United States and Maritime Provinces present themselves for the Matriculation Examination of the University, on the first Fr of October, or the last Friday of March.

HOSPITALS.—The Montreal General Hospital has an average number of 150 pati in the wards, the majority of whom are affected with diseases of an acute character. shipping and large manufactories contribute a great many examples of accidents and su cal cases. In the Out-Door Department there is a daily attendance of between 75 and patients, which affords excellent instruction in minor surgery, routine medical prac venereal diseases, and the diseases of children. Clinical clerkships and dresserships ca obtained on application to the members of the Hospital staff.

UNIVERSITY DISPENSARY.—This was established four years ago for the purpo affording to senior students practical instruction in Diseases of Women, and has proved successful. Two other special departments have been added, viz., Diseases of Children Diseases of the Skin.

CLINICS.—The clinical teaching is conducted in the wards and theatre of the Gen Hospital, daily, throughout the Session. Ample opportunities are afforded to the Stu to investigate the cases, medical and surgical.

The *DISSECTING ROOM* is large, well ventilated, and abundantly provided material. The Demonstrators are skilled teachers, trained in the best anatomical sch of Europe, and are in attendance daily from 10 to 12 a.m., and from 8 to 10 p.m.

REQUIREMENTS FOR DEGREE.—Every candidate must be 21 years of age, studied Medicine *four years*, one Session being at this School, and must pass the neces examinations. Graduates in Arts of recognised Universities, and Students who pro evidence of having *studied a year* with a physician subsequent to passing the Matricula examination, can qualify for examination after attendance on three Sessions.

FEES, arranged according to years, are as follows:—

First Year, $76; Second Year, $89; Third Year, $74; Fourth Year, $64; Hosp Ticket (6 months), $8; Lying-in Hospital (6 months), $8; Graduation, $2

All Fees are payable strictly in advance.

For further information, or Annual Announcement, apply to

WILLIAM OSLER, M.D., *Registrar*,
1351 St. Catherine Street, MONTRE

VASELINE!

A pure and highly concentrated essence of Petroleum refined without distillation or Chemicals.

PREPARED EXPRESSLY FOR

Medicinal, Phamaceutical and Toilet

PURPOSES.

An INVALUABLE REMEDY and the BEST EMOLIENT yet discovered.

☞IT IS NOT A PATENT MEDICINE.☜

The Chesebrough Manufacturing Comp'y,

CONSOLIDATED.

No. 110 Front Street, - - NEW YORK.
" 41 Holborn Viaduct, - - LONDON, E.C.
" 246 Notre Dame Street, - MONTREAL.

☞ The attention of Physicians is called to this new and valuable product. Vaseline is a dense oleaginous substance, of the consistency of butter or Jelly; it melts at 94° Farenheit, evaporates at about 500° Farenheit, does not crytalize or oxydize, and will never become *rancid*. It contains no admixture, is chemically pure, perfectly neutral, has neither odor or taste, and is in color of a light translucent opal.

Its therapeutic qualities are so thoroughly established that it is largely prescribed by physicians of the highest standing in their private practice, as well as in the leading Hospitals of the American and European Continents, where VASELINE, in its various forms, is regarded as the most important recent addition to the *materia medica*.

A pamphlet containing extracts from English, American and French Medical Journals, together with the expressed opinion of eminent physicians, will be forwarded (with a sample bottle of VASELINE) *free* to the profession on application.

CHEMISTS keep *VASELINE* in its many forms in stock

The high character and wide reputation **Scott's Emulsion** has attained through th
agency of the Medical Profession, and the hearty support they have given it since its fir
introduction, is a sufficient guarantee of its superior virtues. The claims we have made a
to its permanency—perfection and palatableness—we believe have been fully sustained, an
we can positively assure the profession that its high standard of excellence will be full
maintained. We believe the profession will bear us out in the statement that no combina
tion has produced as good results in the wasting disorders incident to childhood; in th
latter, as well as in the incipient stages of Phthisis, and in Scrofula, Anæmia and Gener
Debility. We would respectfully ask the profession for a continuance of their patronag
and those who have not prescribed it to give it a trial. Samples will be furnished free upo
application.

FORMULA.—Fifty per cent. of pure Cod Liver Oil, six grains of the Hypophosphite o
Lime, and three grains of the Hypophosphite of Soda to a fluid ounce.

AMHERST, N. S., November, 1890.

MESSRS. SCOTT & BOWNE:

For nearly two years I have been acquainted with "Scott's Emulsion of Cod Liver O
with Hypophosphites," and consider it one of the finest preparations now before the publi
Its permanency as an emulsion, with its pleasant flavor, makes it the great favorite for chi
dren, and I do highly recommend it for all wasting diseases of the system.

Yours truly,

C. A. BLACK, M. I

HALIFAX, N. S., November 19, 1890.

MESSRS SCOTT & BOWNE:

I have prescribed your "Emulsion of Cod Liver Oil with Hypophosphites" for the pa
two years, and found it more agreeable to the stomach, and have better results from its us
than from any other preparation of the kind I have tried.

WM. CAMERON, M. D.

SCOTT & BOWNE, Manufacturing Chemists,
NEW YORK.

A LARGE STOCK OF

TRUSSES, OF ALL SIZES

With Hard Rubber, Metal, Leather or Ivory Pads,

BY THE BEST ENGLISH AND AMERICAN MAKERS.

ALSO,

**Shoulder Braces, Abdominal Supporters, Body Belts, Umbilica
Bands, &c.**

J. GOULDEN, { 175 ST. LAWRENCE STREET.
595 ST. CATHERINE STREET.

THIS JOURNAL may be found on file at GEO. P. ROWELL & CO.'S News
paper Advertising Bureau (10 Spruce Street), where Advertising Contract
may be made for it in NEW YORK.

---

410 East Twenty-Sixth Street, opposite Bellevue Hospital, New York City.

FORTY-SECOND SESSION, 1882–83.

FACULTY OF MEDICINE.

REV. JOHN HALL, D.D., LL.D., *Chancellor of the University, pro tem.*

ALFRED C. POST, M.D., LL.D., Professor Emeritus of Clinical Surgery, President of the Faculty.

CHARLES INSLEE PARDEE, M.D., Dean of the Faculty; Professor of Otology; Surgeon to the Manhattan Eye & Ear Hospital.

JOHN C. DRAPER, M.D., LL. D., Professor of Chemistry.

ALFRED L. LOOMIS, M.D., Professor of Pathology and Practice of Medicine; Visiting Physician to Bellevue Hospital.

WM. DARLING, M.D., LL.D., F.R.C.S., Professor of General & Descriptive Anatomy.

WILLIAM H. THOMSON, M.D., professor of Materia Medica; Therapeutics, and Diseases of the Nervous System; Visiting Physician to Bellevue Hospital.

J. W. S. ARNOLD, M.D., Professor of Physiology and Histology.

J. WILLISTON WRIGHT, M.D., Professor of Surgery; Visiting Surgeon to Bellevue Hospital.

WM. M. POLK, M.D., Professor of Obstetrics and Diseases of Women and Children; Gynæcologist to Bellevue Hospital.

LEWIS A. STIMSON, M.D., Professor of Surgical Pathology; Surgeon to Bellevue Hospital; Curator to Bellevue Hospital.

FANEUIL D. WEISSE, M.D., Professor of Practical and Surgical Anatomy; Surgeon to Workhouse Hospital, B.I.

STEPHEN SMITH, M.D., Professor of Clinical Surgery; Surgeon to Bellevue Hospital.

A. E. MACDONALD, LL.B., M.D., Professor of Medical Jurisprudence and Diseases of the Mind; Medical Superintendent of the New York City Asylum for the Insane.

R. A. WITTHAUS, M.D., Professor of Physiological Chemistry.

HERMAN KNAPP, M.D., Professor of Ophthalmology; Surgeon to the Ophthalmic Institute.

AMBROSE L. RANNEY, M.D., Adjunct Professor of Anatomy.

JOSEPH E. WINTERS, M.D., Demonstrator of Anatomy.

THE PRELIMINARY SESSION will begin on Wednesday, September 20, 1882, and end October 4, 1882. It will be conducted on the same plan as the Regular Winter Session.

THE REGULAR WINTER SESSION will begin October 4, 1882, and end about the middle of March, 1883. The Plan of Instruction consists of Didactic and Clinical Lectures, recitations and laboratory work in all subjects in which it is practicable. To put the laboratories on a proper footing a new building has been erected at an expense of thirty thousand dollars. It will contain laboratories fitted for instruction in Chemistry, Histology, Pathology, Materia Medica, Operative Surgery, and Gynæcology.

Two to five Didactic lectures and two or more Clinical lectures will be given each day by members of the Faculty. In addition to the ordinary clinics, *special clinical instruction*, WITHOUT ADDITIONAL EXPENSE, will be given to the candidates for graduation during the latter part of the Regular Session. For this purpose the candidates will be divided into sections of twenty-five members each. All who desire to avail themselves of this valuable privilege must give in their names and pay their examination fee of $30 to the Dean during the first week in November. At these special clinics students will have excellent opportunities to make and verify diagnoses, and watch the effects of treatment. They will be held in the Wards of the Hospitals and at the Public and College Dispensaries.

Each of the seven professors of the Regular Faculty will conduct a recitation on his subject one evening each week. Students are thus enabled to make up for lost lectures and prepare themselves properly for their final examinations without additional expense.

THE SPRING SESSION will begin about the middle of March and end the last week in May. The daily Clinics and Special Practical Courses will be the same as in the Winter Session, and there will be Lectures on Special Subjects by the Members of the Faculty. It is supplementary to the Regular Winter Session. Nine months of continued instruction are thus secured to all students of the University who desire a thorough course.

FEES.

For Course of Lectures	$140.00
Matriculation	5.00
Demonstrator's Fee (including material for dissection)	10.00
Final Examination Fee	30.00

For further particulars and circulars address the Dean,

Prof. CHARLES INSLEE PARDEE, M.D.,

University Medical College, 410 East Twenty-Sixth Street, New York City.

ANGLO-SWISS MILK FOOD.

Decided superiority is claimed for the Anglo-Swiss Milk Food i comparison with any other farinaceous Food for infants. No so called Milk Food consists entirely of milk; all are partly compose of cereal products, involving, when not properly prepared, the pres ence of an injurious amount of starch. The highest authorities agre in condemning starchy food for young children. The Anglo-Swis Condensed Milk Company overcomes this objectionable feature o Milk Food as usually supplied, by meeting an essential requiremen in the method of preparing it. The Anglo-Swiss Milk Food is s prepared that when gradually heated with water, according to th directions for use, the starch contained in the materials used is con verted, in a satisfactory degree, into soluble and easily digestibl dextrine and sugar.

For a simple test, mix one part of the Food with three parts of cold water—taking a smalle proportion of water than usual—occupy from five to eight minutes in bringing it slowly t the boiling point, stirring constantly, and continue the boiling one minute; the result wi not be a pulp or pap, but a liquid resembling milk. Submit other Foods to the same tes and if you obtain a mucilaginous paste, a heavy pasty appearance should not be accepte as evidence or measure of nutriment; it only betrays the raw or unconverted starch containe

That nature does not give to young children the ability t properly digest food containing a large proportion of starch is uni versally conceded, and when we remember that nature designs mil as food for the young, and that milk contains no starch, the con sistency of nature is strikingly apparent.

We should not offend nature's ways by presuming to improv upon them. Obviously there is but one logical conclusion respect ing the use of starchy materials in compounding a proper food fo infants, namely, that starch must be relieved of its individua character by being, in a great degree, converted into soluble an more easily digestible dextrine and sugar. By so doing we effect through our mode of preparation, certain changes in the food itsel which would otherwise be left for the digestive organs to accomplis before healthful assimilation could take place.

The Anglo-Swiss Milk Food will be found to meet these essentia conditions to the satisfaction of anyone who will take the pains t examine it, and we invite critical examination of it in compariso with any other Food.

We do not claim that the starch in this Food is wholly converted but that its transformation has been carried to the greatest practica degree, and it will be found that the comparatively small portion o starch remaining, which chemical analysis will detect, has been s far deprived of its individual type as to render it impossible to forn a paste from the Food by heating it with water. Every chemist i aware that starch in wheaten flour cannot be converted to thi extent by the mere application of ordinary heat in boiling or baking under the usual methods of preparing flour for easy digestion.

Directions for using the Anglo-Swiss Milk Food will be foun upon the labels.

Prepared by the Anglo-Swiss Condensed Milk Co.

CHAM, SWITZERLAND.

Agents for Canada—H. HASWELL & CO.,

Wholesale Druggists. MONTREAL

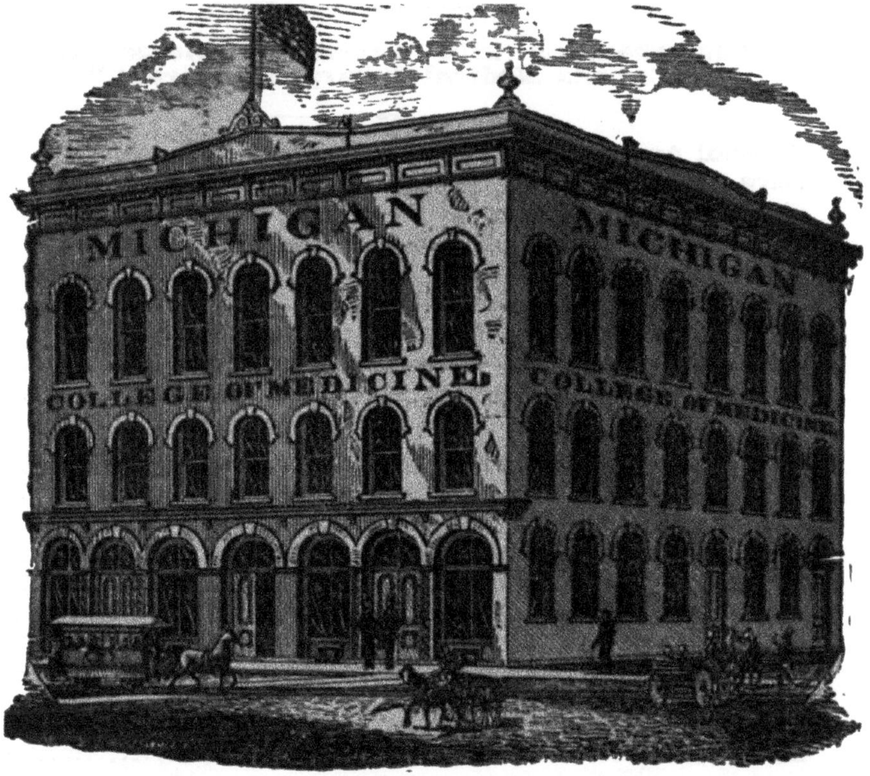

COR. ANTOINE ST. & GRATIOT AVENUE, DETROIT, MICHIGAN.

THE REGULAR SESSION

OF THE

MICHIGAN COLLEGE OF MEDICINE

WILL OPEN

On the First Tuesday in September.

TERMS:

Matriculation Fee (paid but once)	$ 5.0J
Annual Fee	50.00
Graduation Fee	20.00

Chemicals in Laboratory and Anatomical Material at Reasonable Rates.

For Annual Announcement and Catalogue, address—

J. J. MULHERON, *Registrar.*

In Corresponding with Advertisers please mention "Canada Medical & Surgical Journal."

…ponding with advertisers please mention Canada M. & S. Journal.

READ THE LIST OF STANDARD PUBLICATIONS

which we offer to supply with the

Canada Medical & Surgical Journal

at the following greatly reduced rates:

CANADA MEDICAL & SURGICAL JOURNAL

— AND —

Atlantic Monthly	$ 6 00
Appleton's Journal	4 75
" " with Dickens Plate	5 50
Any Visiting List, 25 patients	3 50
" " 50 "	3 75
" " 75 "	4 00
Braithwaite's Retrospect	4 50
Boston Journal Chemistry	3 25
Canadian Illustrated News	5 50
Canadian Journal of Medical Science	4 75
Detroit Lancet	4 50
Frank Leslie's Monthly	5 50
" Ladies' Magazine	5 25
" Weekly	5 50
Graphic (London)	11 50
Gazette Daily	7 00
Gazette Weekly	3 50
Harper's Magazine	5 50
" Weekly	5 75
" Bazar	5 75
London (Eng.) Lancet	10 00
American Edition	5 25
London (Eng.) Practitioner	7 25
London (Eng.) Medical Record	7 00
Lippincott's Magazine	4 75
Michigan Medical News	3 25
Medical and Surgical Reporter	7 00
North American Review	6 25
New York Medical Journal	5 50
Popular Science Monthly	6 50
Philadelphia Medical Times	5 50
Scientific American	5 00
Scientific Supplement	6 50
Scientific American and Supplement (both to one address)	8 00
Scribner's Monthly	5 50
St. Nicholas	4 75
St. Louis Med. & Surg. Journal	5 50
Therapeutic Gazette	3 25
The Living Age	9 00
The Archives of Dermatology	5 50

THESE RATES INCLUDE POSTAGE.

☞ The Magazines in all cases will be sent direct to subscribers from the offices of publication.

Send Orders Early. *Cash must accompany Orders.*

Address, ***GAZETTE PRINTING COMPANY,***

RICHARD WHITE, *Managing Director.* MONTREAL.

In corresponding with advertisers please mention Canada M. & S. Journal.

CONTAINS

The **Essential Elements** to the Animal Organization—P and Lime;

The **Oxidising Agents**—Iron and Manganese;

The **Tonics**—Quinine and Strychnine;

AND

The **Vitalising Constituent**—Phosphorus,

Combined in the form of Syrup, with SLIGHT ALKALINE REACTION.

LETTER FROM ROBERT W. PARKER, M.R.C.S. ENG., F.R. Chir. and Obs. S.; Assist.-Surg. E. Lond. Children's Hos Author of "Tracheotomy in Laryngeal Diphtheria."

8, OLD CAVENDISH STREET,
CAVENDISH SQUARE, LONDO

DEAR SIR,

I have used your Syrup of Hypophosphites in the Children's pital. I find that it is well taken, and consider it an important ad to our Pharmacopœial remedies. Combined either with Glyceri Cod Liver Oil, it has proved itself an efficacious remedy in Scrof diseases affecting bones or joints.

In the debility which often follows on the exanthemata, and cially in that which follows diphtheria, I have found it a very tonic.

I must thank you for the present of the Syrup to the Hospit

Yours faithfully,

MR. FELLOWS. ROBERT WM. PA

Each Bottle of FELLOWS' HYPOPHOSPHITES contains 100 doses.

Prepared by JAMES I. FELLOWS, Chem

PRINCIPAL OFFICES:

ST. ANTOINE STREET,
MONTREAL, CANADA.

48 VESEY STREE
NEW YORK,

8, SNOW HILL, Holborn Viaduct, LONDON.

Pamphlet sent to Physicians on application.

Lightning Source UK Ltd.
Milton Keynes UK
UKHW011141271218
334507UK00011B/560/P

9 781330 303078